Atlas of
GLAUCOMA

Atlas of GLAUCOMA

Edited by

Neil T Choplin MD
Chairman
Department of Ophthalmology
Naval Medical Center
San Diego
California USA

Diane C Lundy MD
Director of Glaucoma Services
Department of Ophthalmology
Naval Medical Center
San Diego
California
USA

MARTIN DUNITZ

First published in the United Kingdom in 1998 by
Martin Dunitz Ltd
The Livery House
7–9 Pratt Street
London NW1 0AE

A CIP catalogue record for this book is available from the British Library

ISBN 1–85317–375–4

Distributed in the United States by:
Blackwell Science Inc.
Commerce Place, 350 Main Street
Malden, MA 02148, USA
Tel: 1-800-215-1000

Distributed in Canada by:
Login Brothers Book Company
324 Salteaux Crescent
Winnipeg, Manitoba, R3J 3T2
Canada
Tel: 204-224-4068

Distributed in Brazil by:
Ernesto Reichmann Distribuidora de Livros, Ltda
Rua Coronel Marques 335, Tatuape 03440-000
Sao Paulo,
Brazil

Composition by Scribe Design, Gillingham, Kent, United Kingdom
Printed and bound in Hong Kong by Imago

Dedication

This book is warmly dedicated to Dr George L Spaeth, Director of the Glaucoma Service of the Wills Eye Hospital in Philadelphia, Pennsylvania and Professor of Ophthalmology at Thomas Jefferson University, and to Dr Donald S Minkler, Director of the Glaucoma Service of the Doheny Eye Institute of the University of Southern California and Professor of Ophthalmology at the University of Southern California, and their associates, who taught us what there is to know and what there is to learn about glaucoma.

Contents

List of Contributors

J Brent Bond MD
Leigh Valley Ophthalmic Associates, 400 N 17th Street, Suite 101, Allentown, PA 18104–5099, USA

Louis B Cantor MD
Department of Ophthalmology, Indiana University Medical Center, 702 Rotary Circle, Room 141, Indianapolis, IN 46202–5175, USA

Neil T Choplin MD
Department of Ophthalmology, Naval Medical Center, 34800 Bob Wilson Drive, San Diego, CA 92134–5000, USA

Anne L Coleman MD
Jules Stein Eye Institute, 100 Stein Plaza, Los Angeles, CA 90095, USA

James William Doyle MD
Department of Ophthalmology, University of Florida, Box J284, Gainesville, FL 32610, USA

Maher M Fanous MD
Department of Ophthalmology, University of Florida, Box J284, Gainesville, FL 32610, USA

Robert D Fechtner MD
Kentucky Lions Eye Research Institute, 301 East Muhammad Ali Boulevard, Louisville, KY 40202, USA

Ronald L Fellman MD
7150 Greenville Avenue, Suite 300, Dallas, TX 75231, USA

Gustavo E Gamero MD
Kentucky Lions Eye Research Institute, 301 East Muhammad Ali Boulevard, Louisville, KY 40202, USA

David S Greenfield MD
Glaucoma Associates of New York, The New York Eye and Ear Infirmary, 310 East 14th Street, New York, NY 10003, USA

Alon Harris PhD
Department of Ophthalmology, Indiana University Medical Center, 702 Rotary Circle, Room 141, Indianapolis, IN 46202–5175, USA

Richard A Hill MD
Department of Ophthalmology, University of California at Irvine, 101 City Drive, Orange, CA 92668, USA

L Jay Katz MD
Wills Eye Hospital, 9th and Walnut, Philadelphia, PA 19107, USA

Paul P Lee MD
Estelle Doheny Eye Institute, 1450 San Pablo Street, Los Angeles, CA 90033–4666, USA

Jeffrey M Liebmann MD
Glaucoma Associates of New York, The New York Eye and Ear Infirmary, 310 East 14th Street, New York, NY 10003, USA

Diane C Lundy MD
Department of Ophthalmology, Naval Medical Center, 34800 Bob Wilson Drive, San Diego, CA 92134–5000, USA

Jonathan Myers MD
Wills Eye Hospital, 9th and Walnut, Philadelphia, PA 19107, USA

Gary D Novack PhD
Pharma Logic Development Inc, 17 Bridgegate Drive, San Rafael, CA 94903–1093, USA

Robert Ritch MD
Glaucoma Associates of New York, The New York Eye and Ear Infirmary, 310 East 14th Street, New York, NY 10003, USA

Alan L Robin MD
3rd Floor, 6115 Falls Road, Baltimore, MD 21209–2226, USA

Mark B Sherwood MD
Department of Ophthalmology, University of Florida, Box J284, Gainesville, FL 32610, USA

Mary Fran Smith MD
Department of Ophthalmology, University of Florida, Box J284, Gainesville, FL 32610, USA

Richard Tamesis MD
University of Nebraska Medical Center, 600 South 42nd Street, Omaha, NB 68198–5540, USA

Carol B Toris MD
University of Nebraska Medical Center, 600 South 42nd Street, Omaha, NB 68198–5540, USA

Carlo E Traverso MD
Clinica Oculista, PAD 9 Ospedale San Martino, 16132 Genova, Italy

Richard P Wilson MD
Wills Eye Hospital, 9th and Walnut, Philadelphia, PA 19107, USA

Darrell WuDunn MD
Department of Ophthalmology, Indiana University Medical Center, 702 Rotary Circle, Room 141, Indianapolis, IN 46202–5175, USA

Michael E Yablonski MD
University of Nebraska Medical Center, 600 South 42nd Street, Omaha, NB 68198–5540, USA

Foreword

Since 'glaucoma' encompasses a wide variety of clinical findings, diagnostic techniques, and treatment options, we thought it best to assemble a book like this one from many parts, each manufactured by someone who is an expert in that particular subject matter. Although at times it felt like we were trying to herd mercury, this project has come together in a way that has exceeded our expectations.

Editing a project like this can be trying; the big benefit comes from having the material to teach us as part of the editorial process. We learned a lot about glaucoma as we went through the individual chapters, and trust that the readers will likewise benefit. The chapters were written by authors recognized for their clinical and research expertise, particularly in their subject areas: Drs Toris and Yablonski (two of the world's experts on fluorophotometry) from the University of Nebraska on aqueous humor dynamics, Ron Fellman on gonioscopy, Rob Fechtner from the University of Louisville on the optic nerve (Rob was one of the first people in the world to work with scanning laser polarimetry), Paul Lee from the Doheny Eye Institute of the University of Southern California (an expert in epidemiology as well as glaucoma) on primary open-angle glaucoma, Jonathan Myers and L Jay Katz from the Wills Eye Hospital in Philadelphia, PA, on secondary glaucoma, Jeff Liebmann and the group from the New York Eye and Ear Infirmary on the angle-closure glaucomas (pioneering experts on ultrasound biomicroscopy), Lou Cantor and the group from the University of Indiana on normal-tension glaucoma (experts in ocular blood flow), Carlo Traverso from the University of Genoa, Italy, on developmental glaucoma and its treatment (Carlo's experience with the subject while in Saudi Arabia is staggering, where he saw something like 300 cases of congenital and developmental glaucoma in a three-year period!), Al Robin from the Wilmer Eye Institute of the Johns Hopkins University, and Gary Novack, on medical treatment, Rick Hill from the University of California, Irvine (who has done outstanding work in laser sclerostomy and ciliodestruction), on laser therapy, J Brent Bond and Rick Wilson on filtering surgery (Rick was one of Dr Choplin's mentors on the art of trabeculectomy), Anne Coleman from the University of California, Los Angeles, on aqueous shunts (Anne was one of the original investigators for the Ahmed Glaucoma Valve, and was the senior author on the first published paper dealing with the device), and Mark Sherwood and co-workers from the University of Florida, Gainesville (superb clinicians and experienced glaucoma researchers), on the co-management of cataract and glaucoma.

Having a diversity of authors makes for a diversity of styles. Although the editors wielded a broad editorial pen, attempting to maintain a consistent style throughout the book, the reader will note that each chapter has its own unique character. Some chapters have much text and a few illustrations, while others are almost exclusively graphical, with extensive legends written to bring out the teaching point of the picture. The material, it is hoped, no matter how it is presented, will add to the reader's knowledge of glaucoma, as it has to ours.

Disclaimer

The editors are both active duty medical officers in the United States Navy. This book was not written as part of our official duties. Neither of us has any financial or proprietary interest in any company, product, drug, machine, or device mentioned in the book, nor is any commercial endorsement of any product by the United States Navy intended. The views and opinions expressed in this work are ours or those of the individual authors, and are not intended to be construed as official opinions of the Department of the Navy, the Department of Defense, nor of the United States Government.

Neil T Choplin
Diane C Lundy

Preface

What is glaucoma? It is becoming clear to us that glaucoma is a spectrum of clinical entities that encompasses many ocular and systemic conditions. It may be regarded as a primary eye disease, or a manifestation of some other ocular or systemic disease. Most ophthalmologists have come to recognize that glaucoma is an optic nerve disease, with 'characteristic' progressive structural changes leading to loss of visual function in a 'characteristic' way. The use of intraocular pressure levels to define the disease has pretty much gone away, and now pressure is used to gauge the risk of having, or developing, glaucoma. Does that mean that the 65-year-old patient with 'cupped out' optic nerves, central and temporal islands in the visual fields, and an untreated intraocular pressure of 12 mmHg has glaucoma, while the 45-year-old myopic male with pigment dispersion syndrome and an initial intraocular pressure of 52 mmHg in each eye, with normal optic nerves and visual fields doesn't? The former patient may be in the 'burned out' stage of glaucoma or may have suffered visual loss from anterior ischemic optic neuropathy, while the latter may be in the early stages of glaucoma or may have simply had a transient rise in pressure following a brisk walk. To try to describe multiple disease, conditions, and scenarios in a widely disparate group of patients with a single term 'glaucoma' is subject to frustration. 'Glaucomologists' do not deal with a single disease.

While the definition of glaucoma remains in a state of flux, so does comprehension of its pathophysiology and its treatment. We are at the dawn of a new era in glaucoma research, focusing on the cellular mechanisms responsible for the death of optic nerve axons. The research is proceeding on many different fronts: genetic, biochemical, and cellular biological, to name but a few. New ideas are emerging. Perhaps intraocular pressure (in some people) is the initiating event that damages a handful of neurons, with the bulk of the damage then done by the propagation of environmental toxin released when those cells die. Perhaps glaucoma is the genetically predetermined self-destruction of the optic nerve, with similar genetically determined mechanisms in the trabecular meshwork responsible for the observed increase in intraocular pressure, with no causal relationship between intraocular pressure and optic nerve damage. Perhaps glaucoma is a condition in which the blood flow to the optic nerve is insufficient for its nutritional requirements, leading to its ultimate demise. How different these ideas are from the concept that 'glaucoma is a disease in which the intraocular pressure rises and this causes optic nerve damage'.

This book illustrates what we know about 'glaucoma' today. It encompasses a wide variety of subjects, as one would expect for a disease that encompasses a wide variety of clinical conditions, syndromes, and findings.

Neil T Choplin

Acknowledgements

Thank you to our residents, co-workers, spouses, and families for your patience as this project evolved. We would also like to acknowledge the hard work and effort employed by the contributors and their co-workers, without whom this book would not have been possible. Lastly, we are extremely grateful to Alan Burgess, our commissioning editor at Martin Dunitz Ltd, for his help, advice, and constant encouragement; and to Tanya Wheatley for her invaluable editorial assistance.

1 Introduction to glaucoma

Diane C Lundy and Neil T Choplin

Introduction

Glaucoma is a diagnosis that may be readily and perhaps too frequently made, based upon a variety of clinical findings by different eye-care providers. It is not a single disease, but rather a group of diseases with some common characteristics. The hallmarks of glaucoma are typical, often progressive, optic nerve head changes and visual field loss (Fig. 1.1) or the potential for them. Optic nerve damage (discussed in Chapter 6), and its corresponding visual field loss (discussed in Chapter 7), is often, but not always, reached in the setting of intraocular pressure deemed to be too high for the affected eye (Chapters 3, 4 and 8). All glaucomatous disease may have a common end point, that being irreversible loss of visual function and even blindness. Since 'glaucoma' is not a single disease, there is no typical 'glaucoma patient' or single best 'glaucoma treatment'.

The spectrum of glaucoma

The manifestations of glaucoma are protean regardless of which parameter is considered. At one end of the clinical spectrum is the white, quiet, painless eye of a patient with primary open-angle glaucoma (POAG) who may, in fact, be unaware of the presence of the disease (Chapter 8). At the other extreme is the patient with acute angle closure glaucoma who is distraught with eye pain, decreased vision, and possibly even systemic symptoms such as nausea and vomiting (Chapter 10). The age of the glaucoma patient at the time of clinical presentations is likewise variable. Congenital glaucoma (Chapter 13) presents in the newborn, while typical patients with glaucoma due to the exfoliation syndrome (Chapter 9) are usually in their seventh or eighth decade of life. Although the glaucomas share a common end point, their proximal etiologies range from acute macroscopic

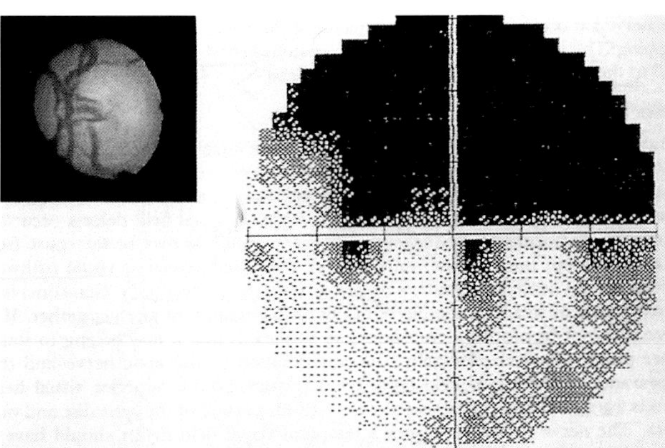

Figure 1.1 Optic disc and corresponding visual field from a patient with glaucoma
Note the thinning of the temporal rim of this left optic disc with extension of the cup to the inferior rim. The visual field shows a superior altitudinal hemianopia, corresponding to the loss of the inferior rim.

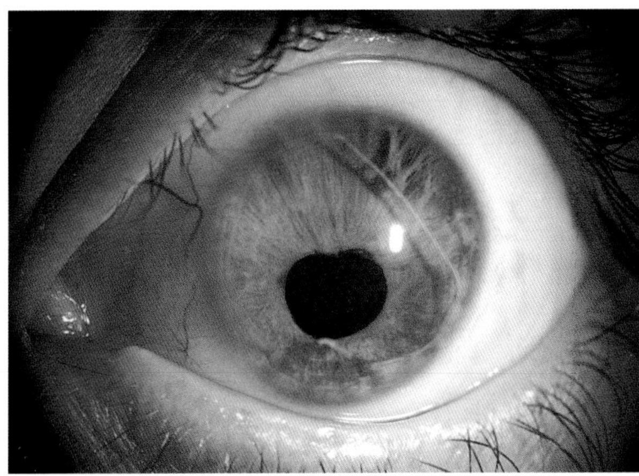

Figure 1.2 Rieger's syndrome
This eye shows many of the structural abnormalities of anterior segment dysgenesis affecting the iris, cornea, anterior chamber angle, and pupil. See Chapter 13 for a complete discussion of this syndrome and other developmental glaucomas.

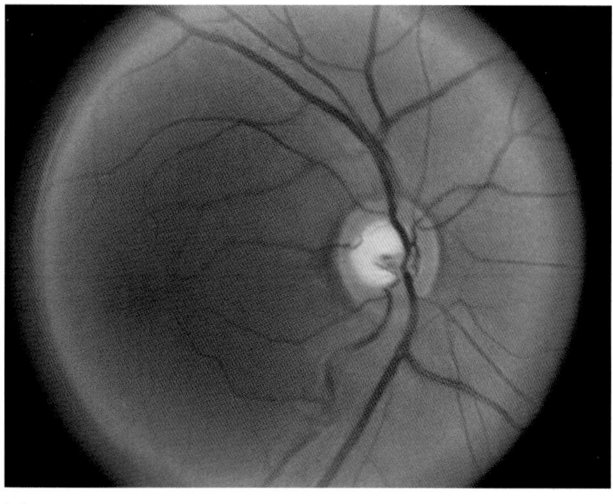

(a)

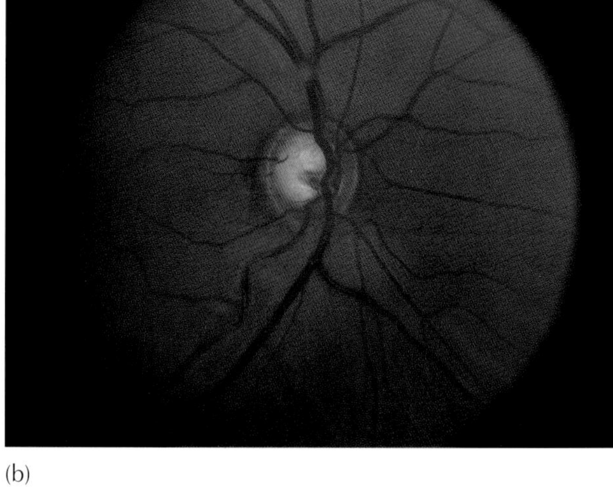

(b)

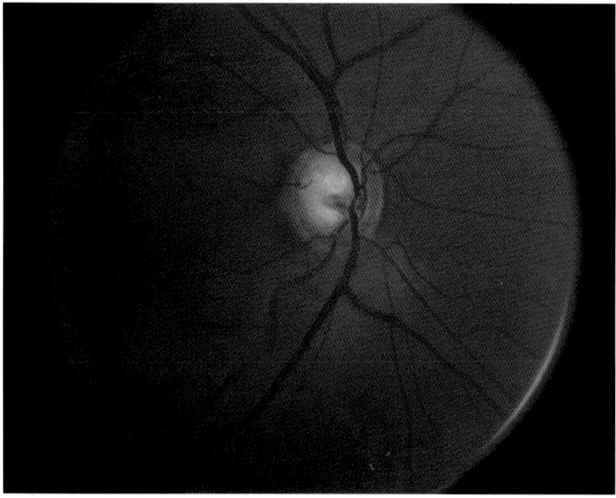

(c)

Figure 1.3 ((a), (b), and (c)) Progressive glaucoma This series of disc photographs demonstrates concentric enlargement of the cup in a patient initially thought to have ocular hypertension. The baseline photograph is (a), with follow-up photographs taken 7 (b) and 9 (c) years later.

mechanical closure of the outflow structures as in acute angle closure, to a macroscopically open angle with increased resistance to outflow at the microscopic and cellular level as in POAG. Newer evidence points towards the possible role of neurotoxins as a distal part of the route to glaucomatous optic neuropathy and field loss.

The differing manifestations of glaucoma are reflected in the clinical examination findings. The examination findings of a 'glaucoma patient' can range from the normal-appearing anterior segment of the POAG patient to the markedly abnormal examination of the patient with uveitic glaucoma or iridocorneal endothelial syndrome (ICE). (Consider the appearance of the eye of a patient with Rieger's syndrome shown in Figure 1.2). Intraocular pressure may be quite elevated, as in the case of acute angle closure, or well within the 'average' range (Chapter 11). The visual field examination of the glaucoma patient may likewise represent a spectrum of findings (Chapter 7). At one extreme is the mild diffuse loss of early POAG while the patient with advanced normal tension glaucoma (NTG) may demonstrate focal defects which are deep and close to fixation (Chapter 11).

Befitting such a diverse group of diseases, treatment of the glaucomas ranges from careful observation in the patient with ocular hypertension (Chapter 8) to cyclodestructive surgery and tube shunts (Chapter 16) for neovascular glaucoma. Medical therapy (Chapter 14), the mainstay of treatment for most types of glaucoma at this time, ranges from topical beta blockers in POAG to oral calcium channel blockers in normal tension glaucoma to intravenous carbonic anhydrase inhibitors in acute angle closure. Laser surgery (Chapter 15) may be offered to the

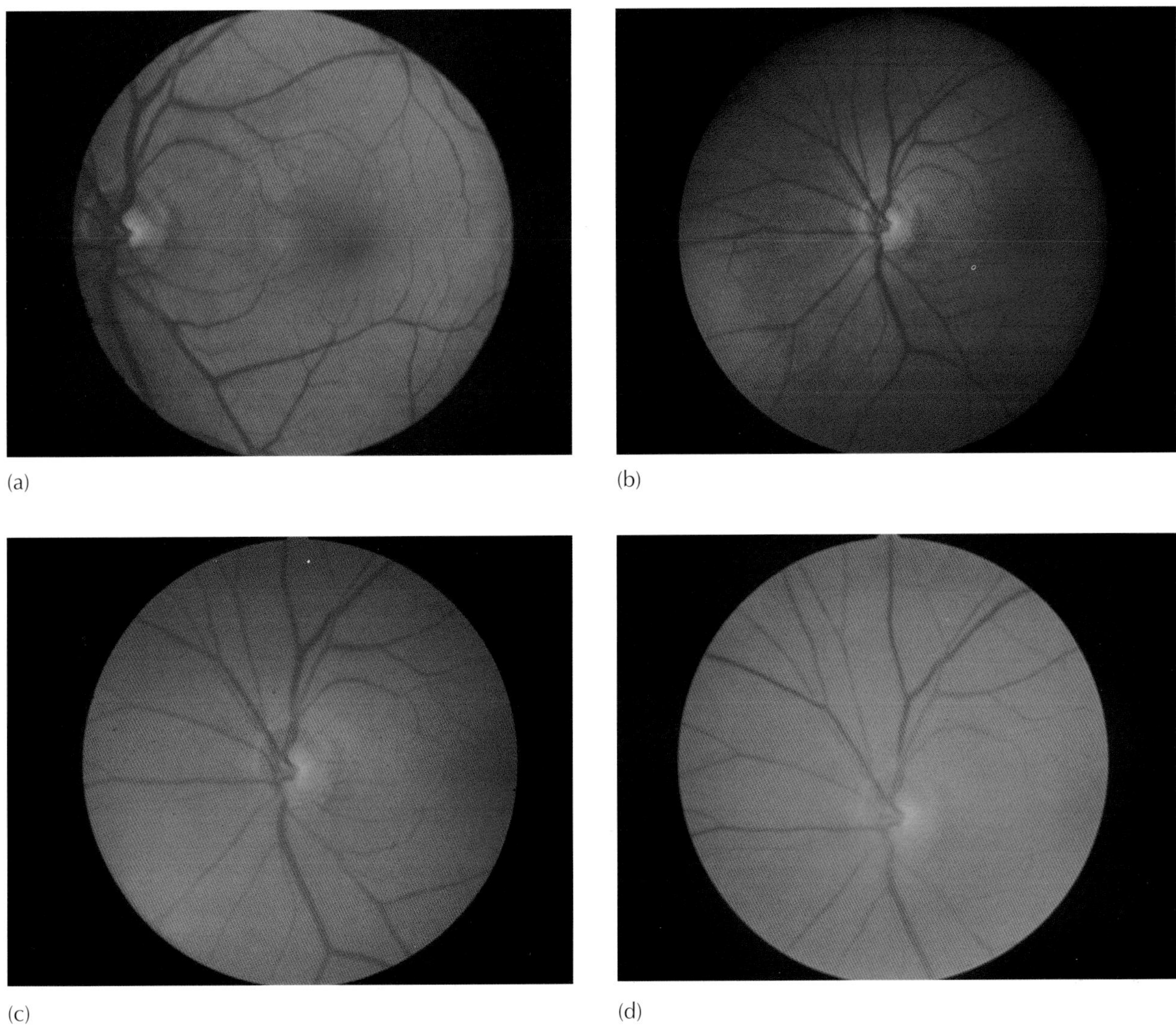

Figure 1.4 ((a), (b), (c), and (d)) Progressive glaucoma This series of disc photographs demonstrates progressive extension of the cup inferiorly and temporally, with eventual loss of rim. The baseline photograph (a) was taken because of a congenital optic nerve pit in the fellow eye. Follow-up photographs were obtained 6 (b), 7 (c), and 8 (d) years following the baseline after the patient developed giant cell arteritis.

glaucoma patient—laser peripheral iridotomy (LPI) for primary angle closure glaucoma, argon laser iridoplasty (ALT) for exfoliation glaucoma, iridoplasty for plateau iris, or ciliary body destruction as an end-stage procedure in all types of glaucoma. Surgery may be the primary treatment modality as in goniotomy for congenital glaucoma (Chapter 19) or an end-stage procedure as in enucleation for the patient with a blind painful eye as the result of a central retinal vein occlusion and recalcitrant neovascular glaucoma. More often, surgery such as a trabeculectomy or a tube shunt is offered after medical and laser treatment fail adequately to control progression of optic nerve damage (Chapters 16–18).

In spite of the broad range of treatment modalities available, the prognosis of the glaucomas is variable and reflects the broad scope of underlying etiologies. The typical myopic male patient with onset of pigment dispersion glaucoma in his forties has a much better prognosis than the patient with absolute glaucoma as the result of an ischemic central retinal vein occlusion and complete angle closure from iris neovascularization. POAG is the most common type of glaucoma and has a fairly good prognosis in most cases once the diagnosis is made. However, delay in diagnosis can lead to blindness or significant visual disability.

The diagnosis of glaucoma may be difficult to make, particularly on a single examination. Considering

Table 1.1 Risk factors for glaucoma (other than POAG).

Risk factor	Associated glaucoma
Race	
Caucasian	Exfoliation syndrome
Asian	Primary angle closure, normal tension glaucoma
Refractive error	
Hyperopia	Primary angle closure
Myopia	Pigmentary glaucoma
Family history	
	Anterior segment dysgenesis syndromes (Axenfeld's, Rieger's)
Vasospastic conditions	
Migraine	Normal tension glaucoma
Raynaud's phenomenon	Normal tension glaucoma

the progressive nature of the disease, observation of its progression may be necessary to confirm the diagnosis. Consider the patient whose photograph of the right optic disc is shown in Figure 1.3a. This patient is an African-American male in his mid-fifties with elevated intraocular pressure (mid-20s) in both eyes. His visual field examination is entirely within normal limits, and the other eye is identical, i.e. symmetrical. He was started on medical therapy to lower his pressure, and followed at regular intervals. Figures 1.3b and c are disc photographs of the same eye were taken 7 and 9 years later, respectively. Each time the visual field remained normal, although there was a very subtle but steady decrease in mean sensitivity. The optic discs remained symmetrical. Taken as a series, these photographs demonstrate concentric enlargement of the cup over time corresponding to the diffuse loss of sensitivity in the visual field. Each individual time period, viewed independently of the rest, is consistent with 'ocular hypertension' and might be treated by periodic follow-up visits, as with this patient. Viewed as a series, however, this patient clearly has progressive open-angle glaucoma. Glaucoma, therefore, may be like a movie depicting the destruction of the optic nerve, with each examination but one frame from the movie.

Further difficulty in making a diagnosis arises when the patient's examination is seemingly normal. The photograph in Figure 1.4a was obtained because the fellow eye had a congenital optic nerve pit. Additional photographs were obtained when the patient developed giant cell arteritis (biopsy proven), but without any evidence of acute anterior ischemic optic neuropathy. Figures 1.4b–d were obtained 6, 7 and 8 years after Figure 1.4a respectively. There is a steady concentric enlargement of the cup, with extension inferiorly, eventually reaching the inferior disc rim. Intraocular pressure in this eye was never greater than 18 mmHg. This would most likely be termed 'normal tension glaucoma', and in this case may be due to chronic ischemia. Again, it is the observed progression over time that leads to the diagnosis, not the individual examinations.

Risk factors for glaucomatous disease

POAG is the most common of the glaucomas and affects an estimated two million Americans, half of whom are unaware they have the disease. Since it is often asymptomatic in the early to moderately advanced stages, patients may suffer substantial irreversible vision loss prior to diagnosis and treatment. Therefore, considerable effort has been made to identify at-risk populations and develop accurate screening tests to make the diagnosis in order that sight-preserving treatment can begin early in the disease process. Several population-based studies have been carried out to determine the prevalence of POAG as well as identify risk factors for the disease (Chapter 8). Some of the information from these studies is conflicting but race and intraocular pressure consistently appear as risk factors. In one

US urban population, the age-adjusted prevalence of POAG was four times greater for African-Americans as opposed to Caucasians. Elevated intraocular pressure (>22 mmHg) was also associated with a greater incidence of glaucoma. However, in this same group, 16% of persons with glaucomatous nerve changes and field loss never had an intraocular pressure greater than 20 mmHg on multiple examinations. Unfortunately, intraocular pressure, while easy to measure in a mass-screening setting, is a much poorer predictor of disease than visual field or optic nerve examination. Visual fields and dilated optic nerve examinations, while more sensitive and specific, are time and labor intensive, and therefore not conducive to screening large numbers of people. Newer methods of optic nerve examination, which can be performed rapidly through the nondilated pupil, may offer better means of screening for POAG (Chapter 6). Myopia, systemic hypertension, diabetes mellitus, or a family history of glaucoma have long been associated with an increased risk for POAG, although results of recent studies have questioned the strength of these associations. Many still consider these as risk factors, although to a lesser degree than race and elevated intraocular pressure. There may also be an association between angle-recession (post-traumatic) glaucoma and POAG in the nonrecession eye as well as central vein occlusion (CRVO) and POAG in the non-CRVO eye. In addition, there is good evidence that patients who demonstrate steroid responsiveness (elevated intraocular pressure with chronic steroid use) have a higher incidence of POAG than nonresponders.

Identifying pertinent risk factors and accurate screening criteria for glaucoma are complex issues complicated by the fact that we are dealing with a heterogeneous collection of diseases rather than a single entity. However, the asymptomatic nature of the majority of glaucomas and the irreversible nature of the resulting vision loss demand effective screening strategies if we are to make early vision-preserving interventions.

In summary, the glaucomas are a group of diseases encompassing a broad spectrum of clinical presentation, etiology, and treatment modality. Pathophysiology of the glaucomas remains uncertain and research efforts are hindered by the fact that we are dealing with a heterogeneous group of diseases rather than a single entity but one that results in a common end point. However, as we learn more about the differing routes to their common end point, we hope to be better able to classify and treat this group of vision-threatening diseases.

FURTHER READING

Hollows FC, Graham PA, Intraocular pressure, glaucoma, and glaucoma suspects in a defined population, *Br J Ophthalmol* (1966) **50**:570–86.

Kahn HA, Milton RC, Alternative definitions of open angle glaucoma; effect on prevalence and associations in the Framingham Eye Study, *Arch Ophthalmol* (1980) **98**:2172–7.

Klein BEK, Klein R, Sponsel WE, et al., Prevalence of glaucoma: the Beaver Dam Eye Study, *Ophthalmology* (1992) **99**:1499–504.

Mason RP, Kosoko O, Wilson R, et al., National survey of the prevalence and risk factors of glaucoma in St Lucia, West Indies, *Ophthalmology* (1989) **96**:1363–8.

Quigley HA, Enger C, Katz J, et al., Risk factors for the development of glaucomatous visual field loss in ocular hypertension, *Arch Ophthalmol* (1994) **112**:644–9.

Sheffield VC, Stone EM, Alward WLM, et al., Genetic linkage of familial open single glaucoma to chromosome 1q21–q31, *Nat Genet* (19??) **4**:47–50.

Singh SS, Zimmerman MB, Podhajsky P, et al., Nocturnal arterial hypotension and its role in optic nerve head and ocular ischemic disorders, *Am J Ophthal* (1994) **177**:603–24.

Sommer A, Tielsch JM, Katz J, et al., Relationship between intraocular pressure and primary open angle glaucoma among white and black Americans: the Baltimore Eye Survey, *Arch Ophthalmol* (1991) **109**:1090–5.

Tielsch JM, Katz J, Singh K, et al., A population-based evaluation of glaucoma screening: the Baltimore Eye Survey, *Am J Epidemiol* (1991) **134**:1102–10.

Tielsch JM, Sommer A, Katz J, et al., Racial variations in the prevalence of primary open angle glaucoma: the Baltimore Eye Study, *JAMA* (1991) **266**:369–74.

2 Classification of glaucoma

Neil T Choplin

Introduction

As discussed in Chapter 1, the term 'glaucoma' encompasses a wide variety of diseases and conditions. In order to arrive at a working diagnosis and institute appropriate therapy, the patient's history must be obtained and an examination performed. Classification of diseases such as glaucoma into various categories, each distinguished from the other by some essential characteristic or set of characteristics, allows us to deal with a patient's disease appropriately. For example, the initial treatment of a patient with a pressure of 48 mmHg due to angle-closure glaucoma is very different from that of a patient with the same pressure presenting for the first time with open-angle glaucoma. Similarly, the therapeutic goal set for a patient with extensive visual field loss and optic nerve cupping may be very different if the presenting intraocular pressure was 40 as opposed to 21. Thus, the approach to diagnosis often looks along some sort of classification scheme in which the subcategories have common diagnostic or therapeutic characteristics. Various classification schemes exist, and almost all glaucomatous disease falls somewhere in all of them. Most of the entities will be discussed in other chapters of this atlas.

Classification of glaucoma by mechanism

The mechanistic classification is probably the most common scheme for sorting out the various glaucomatous diseases (Fig. 2.1). The main division of this classification is between open-angle and angle-closure glaucoma. This type of division emphasizes the importance of gonioscopy (Chapter 5) for arriving at the correct diagnosis. It would be impossible to differentiate between primary open-angle glaucoma and primary chronic angle-closure glaucoma (where the patient never had an acute attack) without gonioscopy. The other important differentiation in this classification scheme is between primary (primary disease of the eye with no associated conditions or diseases) and secondary glaucomas (where the glaucoma is attributed to some underlying condition or disorder). This differentiation may be important for therapeutic considerations. For example, primary open-angle glaucoma may

Table 2.1 **Classification of glaucoma by age of onset.**

Age of onset	Distinguishing characteristics
Congenital	Present at birth, related to developmental abnormalities, almost always requires surgical treatment
Infantile	Glaucoma not present at birth but developing before 2 years of age
Juvenile	Onset after age 2, often having identifiable angle abnormalities (such as absence of ciliary body band) that distinguish the condition from adult open-angle glaucoma
Adult	Typical open-angle glaucoma, onset usually in mid-to-late adulthood (after age 35), no identifiable structural abnormalities in the angle

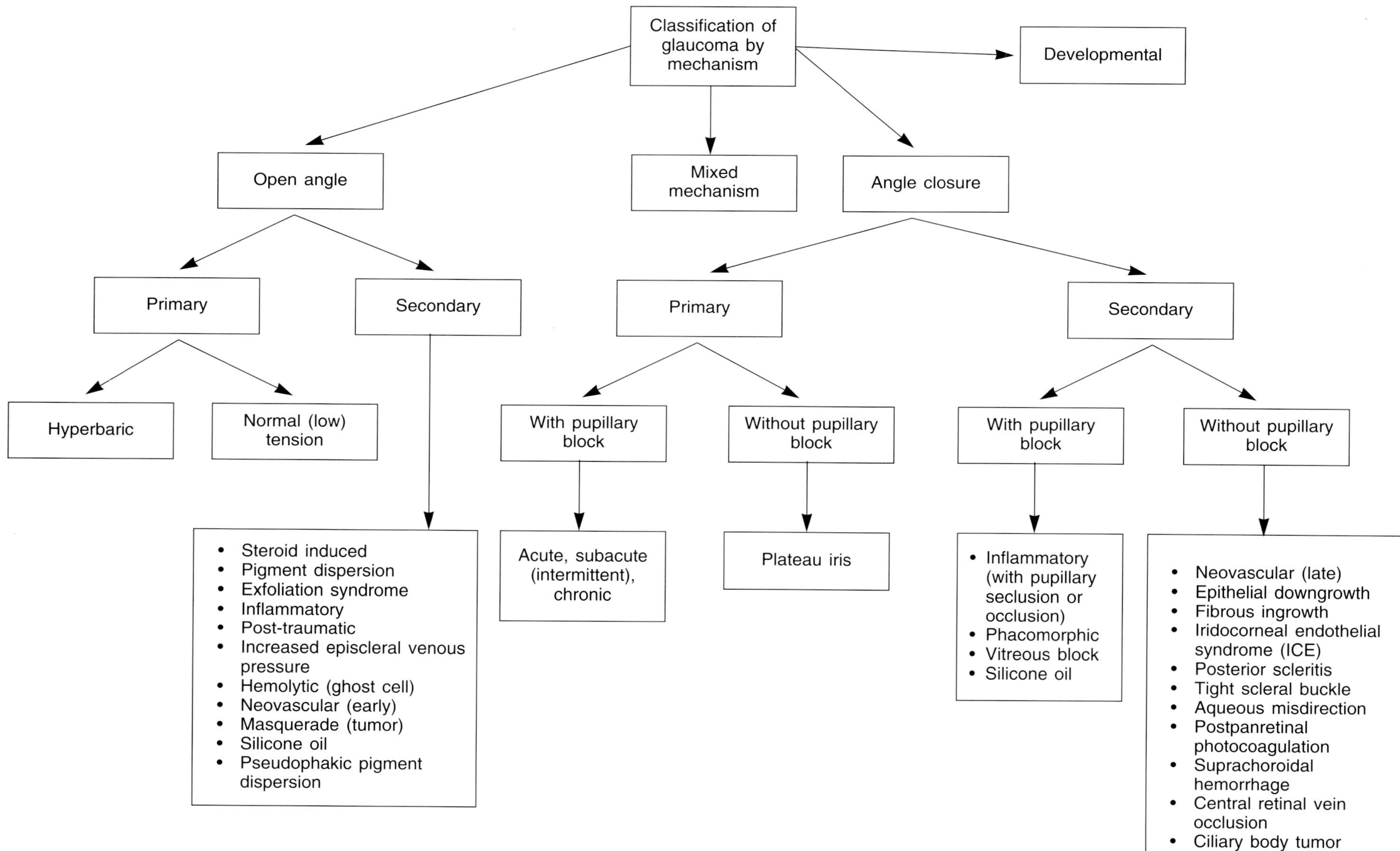

Figure 2.1 Classification of glaucoma by mechanism
Note the main subdivisions are open angle and angle closure.

respond well to miotics such as pilocarpine while inflammatory glaucoma may be worsened by treatment with miotics. Iridotomy is appropriate for treating pupillary block angle closures, but not nonpupillary block angle closure. Note that the classification scheme as presented here does not mention 'narrow angle' glaucoma. The term 'angle closure' is preferred, since 'narrowing' of the anterior chamber angle is really of no significance until the angle becomes closed (partially or completely).

Classification by age of onset

Table 2.1 illustrates a classification of glaucoma by age of onset. The developmental glaucomas are discussed in Chapter 13.

Classification by intraocular pressure

The main subdivisions in this classification are 'hyperbaric' and 'normal or low tension' glaucoma. Table 2.2 lists some distinguishing characteristics. The term 'hyperbaric' is not often used except to distinguish 'garden variety' open-angle glaucoma from normal-tension glaucoma. Open-angle glaucoma is discussed in Chapter 8, while normal-tension glaucoma is discussed in Chapter 11.

Classification by stage of disease

Classification by stage may be important for setting therapeutic goals, for prognosis, or for disability determinations. Table 2.3 illustrates stages of glaucoma.

Classification based upon the International Classification of Diseases (ICD-9)

The International Classification of Diseases, Ninth Revision, Clinical Modification (ICD-9-CM) is derived from a classifications of diseases from the World Health Organization. It uses codes to classify all diseases and disorders, originally intended for indexing of hospital records by disease and operations for the purpose of data storage and retrieval. Coding is used for such things as billing and database management. Codes 360–379 cover the eye and adnexa, and the 365 codes include the glaucomas. Table 2.4 lists the ICD-9 codes for glaucoma.

Table 2.2 **Classification of glaucoma by level of intraocular pressure. Hyperbaric glaucoma is usually synonymous with open-angle glaucoma as the term is usually used. The division between normal-tension and low-tension glaucoma is somewhat arbitrary.**

Level of intraocular pressure (IOP)	Name of condition	Distinguishing characteristics
Low	Low-tension glaucoma	IOP less than 21 mmHg, focal loss of optic disc rim, dense nerve-fiber bundle defects with loss close to fixation, may require very low IOP for stabilization
Normal	Normal-tension glaucoma	Similar to low-tension glaucoma with slightly higher IOP levels
High	Hyperbaric glaucoma (but usually just referred to as 'open-angle glaucoma')	Elevated IOP consistently greater than 22 mmHg and frequently much higher, concentric enlargement of the cup over time, diffuse loss of sensitivity may precede focal loss of visual field, treatment directed at 'normalizing' IOP

Table 2.3 **Classification of glaucoma by stage of disease.**

Stage	Potential characteristics	Possible optic nerve findings	Possible visual field findings
Glaucoma suspect with borderline findings	Borderline intraocular pressure	Borderline cupping	Normal
Ocular hypertension	Intraocular pressure >21 mmHg	Normal	Normal
Mild	Early changes of glaucomatous disease	Mild cup-to-disc asymmetry, vertical cupping with intact rims, concentric enlargement of the cup, mild nerve-fiber layer loss	Normal or mild diffuse loss of sensitivity, defects generally <10 dB in depth, early nasal step or paracentral depressions, increasing short-term fluctuation
Moderate	Definite disease with minimal functional impairment	Extension of cup to rim, disc hemorrhage, bared vessels, diffuse thinning of neuroretinal rim	Loss of sensitivity 10–20 dB diffusely or at isolated points or small clusters, well defined nasal steps, focal defects from loss of nerve fiber bundles
Advanced	Significant disease	Cup to disc >0.8, segmental loss of rim	Loss on both sides of the horizontal, large nerve-fiber bundle defects or altitudinal loss, areas of absolute loss
Far advanced	May be symptomatic with reduced visual acuity, may be aware of visual field loss	Cup to disc >0.9, pallor, undermining of the rim	Requires change to larger stimulus size to measure, temporal and central islands remaining
End stage	Legally or totally blind	Total cup, 4+ pallor	Unmeasurable

Table 2.4 Classification of glaucoma in the International Classification of Diseases, Ninth Revision, Clinical Modification.

365.0 Borderline glaucoma (glaucoma suspect)
- 365.00 Preglaucoma, unspecified
- 365.01 Open angle with borderline findings
  Open angle with: borderline intraocular pressure, cupping of optic discs
- 365.02 Anatomical narrow angle
- 365.03 Steroid responders
- 365.04 Ocular hypertension

365.1 Open-angle glaucoma
- 365.10 Open-angle glaucoma, unspecified
- 365.11 Primary open-angle glaucoma
- 365.12 Low-tension glaucoma
- 365.13 Pigmentary glaucoma
- 365.14 Glaucoma of childhood, infantile or juvenile glaucoma
- 365.15 Residual stage of open-angle glaucoma

365.2 Primary angle-closure glaucoma
- 365.20 Primary angle-closure glaucoma, unspecific
- 365.21 Intermittent angle-closure glaucoma
- 365.22 Acute angle-closure glaucoma
- 365.23 Chronic angle-closure glaucoma
- 365.24 Residual stage of angle-closure glaucoma

365.3 Corticosteroid-induced glaucoma
- 365.31 Glaucomatous stage
- 365.32 Residual stage

365.4 Glaucoma associated with congenital anomalies, dystrophies, and systemic syndromes
- 365.41 Glaucoma associated with chamber-angle anomalies, Axenfeld's anomaly (743.44), Reiger's anomaly or syndrome (743.44)
- 365.42 Glaucoma associated with anomalies of iris aniridia (743.45), essential iris atrophy (364.51)
- 365.43 Glaucoma associated with other anterior segment anomalies, microcornea (743.41)
- 365.45 Glaucoma associated with systemic syndromes, neurofibromatosis (237.7), Sturge–Weber syndrome (759.6)

365.5 Glaucoma associated with disorders of the lens
- 365.51 Phacolytic glaucoma
- 365.52 Pseudoexfoliation glaucoma
- 365.59 Glaucoma associated with other lens disorders

365.6 Glaucoma associated with other ocular disorders
- 365.60 Glaucoma associated with unspecified ocular disorder
- 365.61 Glaucoma associated with pupillary block
- 365.62 Glaucoma associated with ocular inflammation
- 365.63 Glaucoma associated with vascular disorders
- 365.64 Glaucoma associated with tumors or cysts
- 365.65 Glaucoma associated with ocular trauma

365.8 Other specified forms of glaucoma
- 365.81 Hypersecretion glaucoma
- 365.82 Glaucoma associated with increased episcleral venous pressure
- 365.83 Other specific glaucoma

365.9 Unspecified glaucoma

Note:
The codes for some of the associated disorders have not been included in the table.

FURTHER READING

Hoskins HD, Jr, Kass M. *Becker–Shaffer's diagnosis and therapy of the glaucomas*, sixth edition (CV Mosby: St Louis, MO, 1989).

Jones MK, Castillo LA, Hopkins CA, Aaron WS, eds. *ICD-9-CM code book for physician payment* (St Anthony Publishing: Reston, VA, 1995).

3 Aqueous humor dynamics

Carol B Toris, Michael E Yablonski and Richard Tamesis

Introduction

Normal visual function requires the shape of the globe to remain fixed and the optical pathway from the cornea to the retina to remain clear. This requires that the nutrition of the intraocular tissues in the optical pathway must occur with a minimum number of blood vessels. All this is accomplished very efficiently by the production of the clear aqueous humor, its circulation into the anterior chamber, and its drainage through tissues with high resistance. The intraocular pressure thus is maintained, the shape of the eye is preserved, the refracting surfaces are kept in place, and the avascular cornea and lens are provided with nourishment and waste removal.

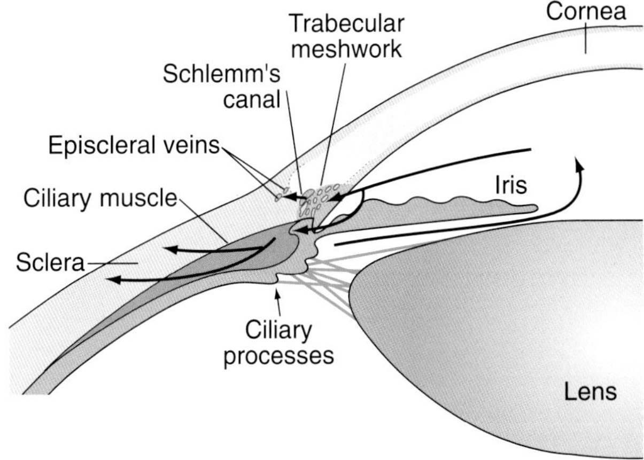

Figure 3.1 Circulation and drainage of aqueous humor Ocular aqueous humor is secreted by the ciliary processes of the ciliary body into the posterior chamber. It circulates between the lens and the iris through the pupil into the anterior chamber (large green arrow). It drains from the anterior chamber by passive bulk flow via two pathways, trabecular outflow and uveoscleral outflow. Trabecular outflow is the drainage of aqueous humor sequentially through the trabecular meshwork, Schlemm's canal, collector channels, episcleral veins, anterior ciliary veins, and into the systemic circulation (small green arrow). Uveoscleral outflow is the drainage of aqueous humor from the chamber angle into the tissue spaces of the ciliary muscle and on into the suprachoroidal space. From there some fluid percolates through the scleral substance or emissarial canals and some fluid is reabsorbed by uveal blood vessels (blue arrows).

Flow of aqueous humor

Aqueous humor is produced by the ciliary body and is secreted into the posterior chamber. Most of this fluid then flows into the anterior chamber and drains out of the chamber angle via the trabecular outflow pathway or the uveoscleral outflow pathway (Fig. 3.1).

Aqueous production mechanisms

The primary function of the ciliary processes is to produce ocular aqueous humor. These processes constitute the internal aspect of the pars plicata of the ciliary body. The anterior portions of the larger processes have increased numbers of capillary fenestrations and epithelial mitochondria, indicating specialization for aqueous humor production. Ciliary processes have a highly vascularized core (Figs 3.2 and 3.3); their perfusion directly regulates the volume of capillary ultrafiltration and indirectly influences active secretion by controlling the supply of blood-borne nutrients to the ciliary epithelium.

The first step in the formation of aqueous humor is the development of a stromal pool of plasma filtrate by ultrafiltration through the ciliary process capillary wall (Fig. 3.3). Next, an active transport of ions out of the cell establishes an osmostic gradient in the intercellular spaces of the ciliary epithelium (Fig. 3.4). Finally, water moves into the posterior chamber along the osmotic gradient (Figs 3.4 and

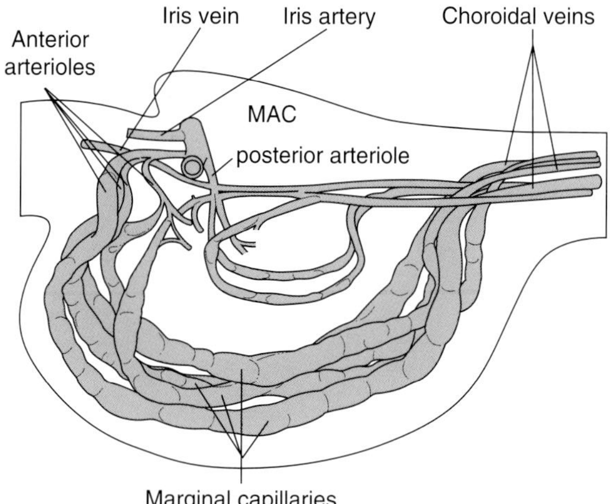

Figure 3.2 Ciliary process vasculature
One ciliary process of a monkey is shown in lateral view. The vasculature consists of a complex anastomotic system supplied by anterior and posterior arterioles radiating from the major arterial circle (MAC). The anterior arterioles supply the anterior aspect of the process and drain posteriorly into the choroidal veins. The posterior arterioles provide posteriorly draining capillaries generally confined to the base of the process. The choroidal veins drain blood from the iris veins, ciliary processes, and the ciliary muscles. (Redrawn from Morrison JC, Van Buskirk EM, Ciliary process microvasculature of the primate eye, *Am J Ophthalmol* (1984) **97**:372–83.)

3.5). The posterior chamber aqueous humor is modified by diffusion of molecules into or out of the surrounding tissue. A small percentage of the modified aqueous humor flows posteriorly through the vitreous and across the retina and retinal pigment epithelium (Fig. 3.6) but most flows through the pupil into the anterior chamber (Figs 3.1 and 3.6). Under steady-state conditions, the net inflow of fluid into the posterior chamber closely estimates the outflow via the pupil, therefore measuring aqueous flow into the chamber gives a good estimation of the aqueous production rate.

The rate at which aqueous enters the anterior chamber in the normal human eye averages about 2.5 μl/min. There is a circadian fluctuation in aqueous flow such that the rate is lowest during sleep at night and highest around noon to 1300 hrs (Fig. 3.7). The circadian rhythm is not affected by eyelid closure, supine posture, sleep deprivation, sleep in a lighted room, or short naps. The factors mediating the reduction in aqueous flow are unclear, but corticosteroids and catecholamines may play a role.

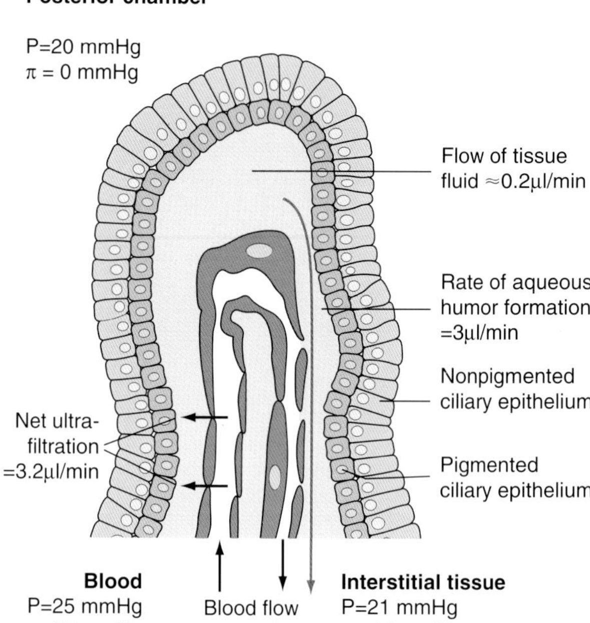

Figure 3.3 Production of aqueous humor
The ciliary process consists of a core containing capillaries and interstitial tissue surrounded by two epithelial layers oriented apex to apex. The outer layer consists of nonpigmented ciliary epithelial cells which are connected to each other by tight junctions and desmosomes. The inner layer consists of pigmented ciliary epithelial cells connected to each other by gap junctions. The production of aqueous humor by the ciliary processes involves both ultrafiltration and active secretion. Plasma filtrate enters the interstitial space through capillary fenestrations (ultrafiltration). The net filtration of fluid from the capillaries (3.2 μl/min) has to correspond to the formation of the aqueous humor (3 μl/min) plus any loss of tissue fluid from the processes (0.2 μl/min). The net filtration of filtrate from the capillaries corresponds to about 4% of plasma flow. The capillary wall is a major barrier for the plasma proteins but the most significant barrier is in the nonpigmented ciliary epithelium where tight junctions occlude the apical region of the intercellular spaces. The outcome of this design is a high protein concentration in the tissue fluid which causes a high oncotic pressure in the tissue fluid and thereby reduces the transcapillary difference in the oncotic pressure. The hydrostatic pressure (P) and colloid osmotic pressure (π) of the blood, interstitial tissue, and posterior chamber are listed for the rabbit. The effect of hydrostatic and oncotic pressure differences across the ciliary epithelium is a pressure of about 13 mmHg tending to move water into the processes from the posterior chamber. Therefore, under normal conditions the movement of fluid into the posterior chamber requires secretion. Because the π is zero in the posterior chamber, the only way to secrete fluid into this chamber is via active transport across the ciliary epithelial layers. (Modified from Bill A, Blood circulation and fluid dynamics in the eye, *Physiol Rev* (1975) **55**:383–417.)

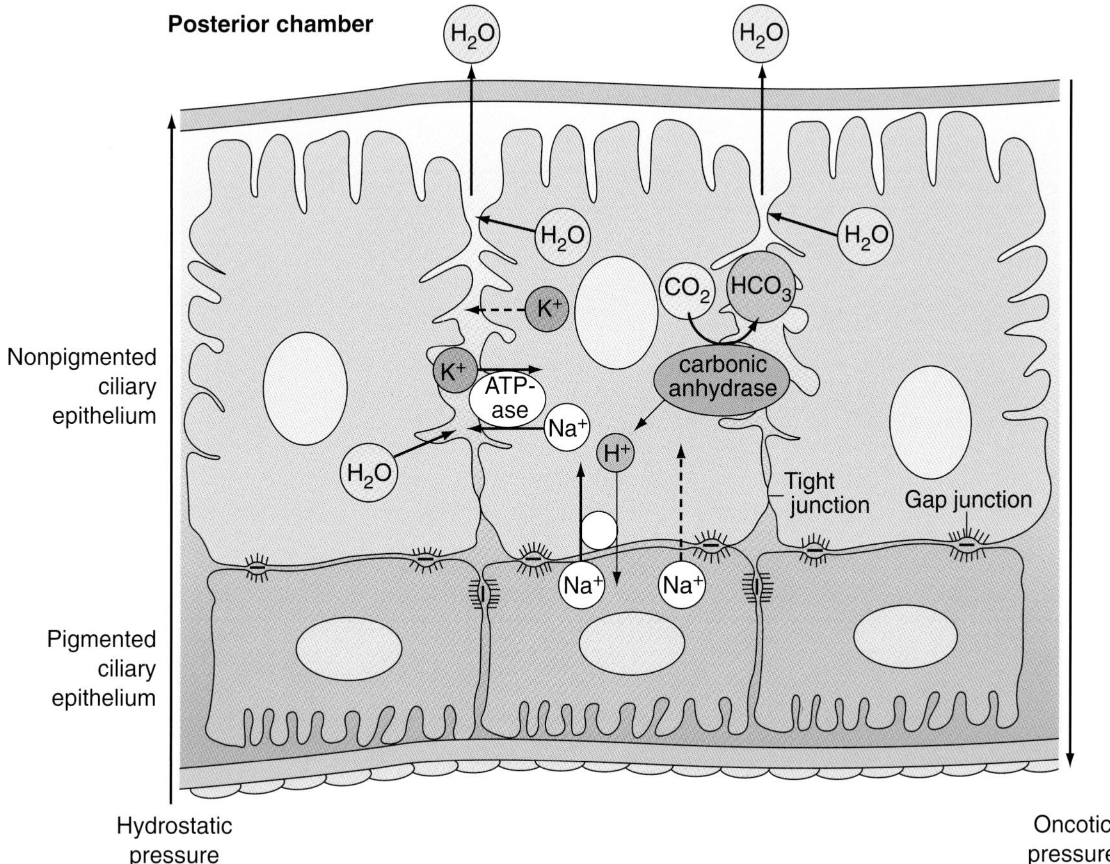

Figure 3.4 Active transport of aqueous humor
Active transport is the work required for the continuous formation of a fluid that is not in thermodynamic equilibrium with the blood plasma. This secretion is accomplished by the active transport of ions from the nonpigmented ciliary epithelium cells into the intercellular clefts. There are indications that the active transport of Na^+ across the NPE is the key process in aqueous humor formation. The active transport of HCO_3^- and Cl^- may also play a role. Enzymatic inhibitors of these transport processes can significantly reduce aqueous flow. Examples include the carbonic anhydrase inhibitor, acetazolamide, and the inhibitor of Na^+–K^+ ATPase, ouabain. The osmotic pressure in the clefts increases as ions are pumped in. The presence of apical tight junctions connecting adjacent nonpigmented ciliary epithelial cells necessitates the movement of water and its solutes out into the posterior chamber.

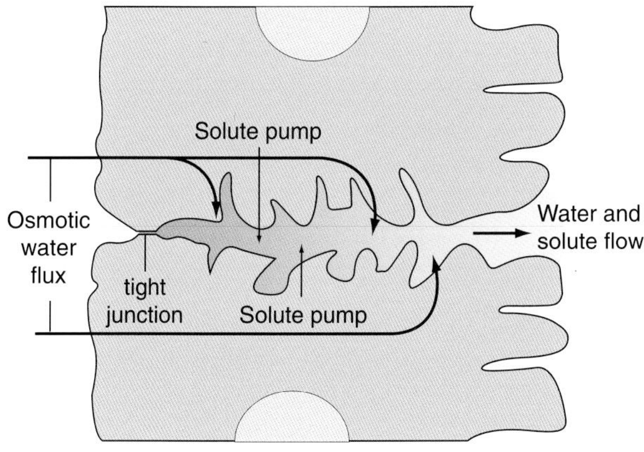

Figure 3.5 Cole's hypothesis of fluid production
A standing gradient osmotic flow system is represented by this diagram. The system consists of a long, narrow channel with a restriction at the apical end (tight junction). Solute pumps line the walls of the channel and solute is continuously and actively transported from the cells into the intercellular channel (blue arrows). This makes the channel fluid hyperosmotic. As water flows along the path of least resistance towards the open end of the channel (black arrow), more water enters across the walls because of the osmotic differential (red arrows). In the steady state a standing gradient is maintained. The relative osmolarity is depicted by the blue color. Volume flow is directed towards the open end of the channel. (Modified from Cole DF, Secretion of the aqueous humour, *Exp Eye Res* (1977) **25 (suppl)**:161–76.)

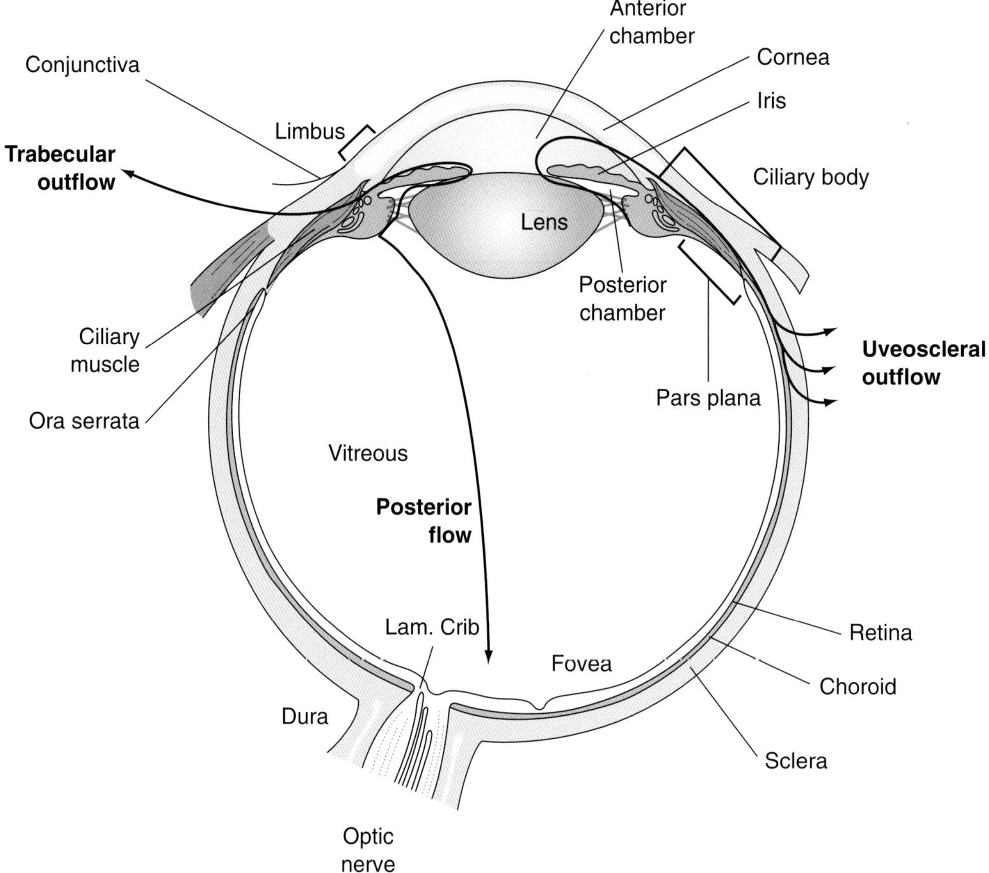

Figure 3.6 Aqueous humor circulation in the eye
Although the bulk of the posterior chamber aqueous humor exits the eye through the pupil, some drains across the vitreous into the retina and retinal pigment epithelium. The active transport of fluid out of the eye by the retinal pigment epithelium utilizes a mechanism similar to that of the nonpigmented epithelium.

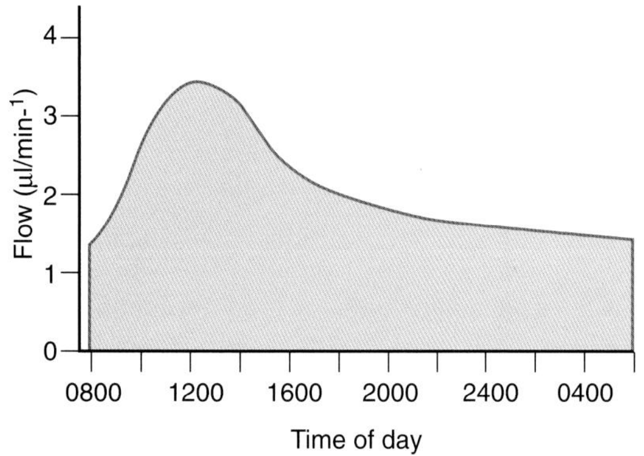

Figure 3.7 Aqueous flow versus time of day
In humans, aqueous humor flow into the anterior chamber is highest between 1200 and 1300 hours peaking at a rate of about 3.1 µl/min. It decreases through the afternoon and into the night to a rate of about 1.6 µl/min at 0400 hours. This represents a 45% reduction in aqueous flow. The magnitude of reduction is greater than that produced by pharmacological aqueous humor suppressants. (Data from Reiss GR, Lee DA, Topper JE, Brubaker RF, Aqueous humor flow during sleep, *Invest Ophthalmol Vis Sci* (1984) **25**:776–8.)

Aqueous outflow pathways

In the anterior chamber, some of the aqueous humor may be lost via the cornea and iris or gained from iris blood vessels, but these gains and losses are very small so that in a steady state, the rate of drainage of aqueous humor through the chamber angle is nearly equal to the rate of inflow of aqueous humor through the pupil. Thus, aqueous flow (F_a) can be defined as the sum of aqueous drainage through two outflow pathways, the trabecular meshwork (F_{trab}) and the uveoscleral tissues (F_u):

$$F_a = F_{trab} + F_u \tag{1}$$

Trabecular outflow

In the primate trabecular outflow pathway, the aqueous humor drains sequentially through the trabecular meshwork, Schlemm's canal, collector channels, episcleral veins, anterior ciliary veins, and into the systemic circulation (Fig. 3.1). It is generally agreed that the tissues between the anterior

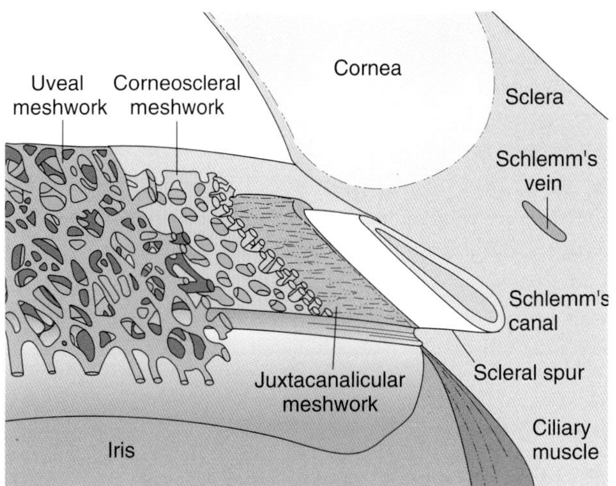

Figure 3.8 Three layers of the trabecular meshwork
Aqueous humor first passes through the inner layer or the uveal meshwork. This layer is a forward extension of the ciliary muscle. It consists of flattened sheets which branch and interconnect in multiple planes. The uveal meshwork does not offer any significant resistance to aqueous drainage because of the presence of large overlapping holes in these sheets. The middle layer, or the corneoscleral meshwork, includes several perforated sheets of connective tissue extending between the scleral spur and Schwalbe's line. Relative to the openings in the uveal meshwork the openings in these sheets are small and do not overlap. The sheets are connected to each other by tissue strands and endothelial cells. The result of this architectural design is a circuitous path of high resistance to the flow of aqueous. The outer layer, or the juxtacanalicular meshwork, lies adjacent to the inner wall of Schlemm's canal. It contains collagen, a ground substance of glycosaminoglycans and glycoproteins, fibroblasts, and endothelial-like juxtacanalicular cells. It also contains elastic fibers that may provide support for the inner wall of Schlemm's canal. This meshwork contains very narrow, irregular openings providing high resistance to fluid drainage.

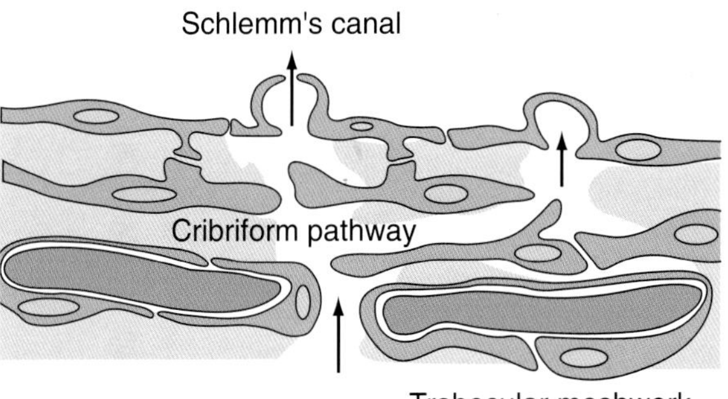

Figure 3.9 Inner wall of Schlemm's canal and the juxtacanalicular meshwork (also called cribriform meshwork)
The inner wall of Schlemm's canal contains a monolayer of spindle-shaped endothelial cells interconnected by tight junctions. One theory is that fluid may move through this area in transcellular channels. These channels may form and recede in a cyclic fashion, beginning as invaginations on the meshwork side of the endothelial cell and progressing to a transcellular channel into Schlemm's canal. Only a few channels appear to open at a time providing the major resistance to trabecular outflow. One channel is drawn as a vacuole and one is shown opened to Schlemm's canal. The arrows indicate the direction of fluid flow. (Modified from Rohen JW, Why is intraocular pressure elevated in chronic simple glaucoma? Anatomical considerations, *Ophthalmology* (1983) **90**:758–65.)

chamber and Schlemm's canal provide the major portion of normal resistance to aqueous drainage. Which tissue constitutes the greatest resistance is somewhat controversial. To exit the eye via Schlemm's canal, aqueous must traverse three layers of trabecular meshwork and the inner wall of Schlemm's canal. The resistance to fluid flow increases along the pathway.

The three layers of meshwork are described in Figure 3.8. The outer layer of the meshwork contains a delicate meshwork of elastic-like fibers which are connected at one end with the endothelium of Schlemm's canal, and at the other end with tendons of the ciliary muscle. Contraction of the ciliary muscle may increase spaces between the plates of the meshwork and reduce resistance to flow. Pilocarpine may reduce trabecular outflow resistance (or increase trabecular outflow facility) by this mechanism.

In humans, trabecular outflow accounts for 65–95% of aqueous drainage, while in monkeys the rate is about 50%. This flow is pressure dependent, meaning that the flow is proportional to the difference between intraocular pressure and the hydrostatic pressure in the canal.

Uveoscleral outflow

Anterior chamber aqueous humor that does not drain through the trabecular meshwork flows from the chamber angle into the supraciliary space, ciliary muscle, and through the scleral substance and emissarial canals or into uveal blood vessels (Fig. 3.1). This aqueous outflow is called 'uveoscleral outflow'. Other names for this drainage include

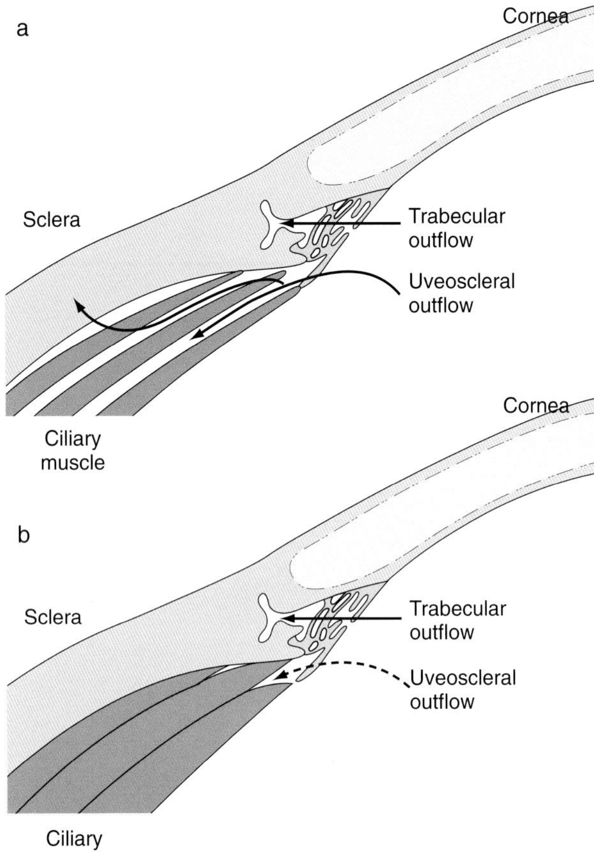

Figure 3.10 Ciliary muscle effects on uveoscleral outflow

(a) The ciliary muscle in the relaxed state. The spaces between muscle bundles are substantial and aqueous can easily pass through the tissue. Drugs that relax the ciliary muscle can increase uveoscleral outflow. Examples include the cholinergic agonist, atropine, and the prostaglandin $F_{2\alpha}$ analog, latanoprost. (b) The ciliary muscle in the contracted state. The spaces between muscle bundles are obliterated and uveoscleral outflow is greatly reduced. Drugs that contract the ciliary muscle reduce uveoscleral outflow. An example is the cholinergic antagonist, pilocarpine. (From Bill A, Blood circulation and fluid dynamics in the eye, *Physiol Rev* (1975) **55**:383–417.)

'unconventional outflow' and 'uveovortex outflow'. These names arose from attempts to describe a relatively undefined seepage route. It would be more accurate to refer to this drainage as simple 'uveal' outflow to include all anterior chamber aqueous humor egress from the uvea. The term appearing most often in the literature is 'uveoscleral outflow'—hence its use in this chapter.

In contrast to trabecular outflow, uveoscleral outflow is effectively pressure independent. At intraocular pressures greater than about 5 mmHg this outflow remains relatively constant and the facility of uveoscleral outflow is very low (approximately 0.02 µl/min/mmHg). Uveoscleral outflow reportedly accounts for anywhere from 4% to 35% of total aqueous drainage in humans. It can be increased by drugs that relax the ciliary muscle and reduced by drugs that contract it (Fig. 3.10). Prostaglandin analogues, such as latamaprost, also increase uveoscleral outflow, possibly by inducing enzymatic breakdown of extracellular matrix material.

Techniques for measuring aqueous flow

Aqueous flow was first measured by injecting a tracer such as para-aminohippuric acid or fluorescein into the blood stream, allowing it to enter the anterior chamber, and then sampling the aqueous humor to determine the rate of its disappearance. The relationship between aqueous humor tracer concentration and plasma tracer concentration was monitored to determine aqueous flow. Subsequently, oral administration of fluorescein was used for the same purpose. Injecting a large molecular weight tracer such as albumin or fluorescein isothiocyanate dextran directly into the anterior chamber and collecting aqueous samples over time provided a more direct measure of aqueous flow. The rate of disappearance of the tracer from the aqueous is a function of aqueous flow.

Another method used to determine aqueous flow in humans was a noninvasive photogrammetric technique. With the anterior chamber filled with fluorescein, freshly secreted aqueous humor appeared as a clear bubble in the pupil. The increase in volume of this bubble was determined by geometric optics and was an indication of the rate of aqueous flow.

Currently the method of choice to assess aqueous flow is fluorophotometry. Fluorescein is administered to the eye either topically (Fig. 3.11) or by corneal iontophoresis. Fluorescein traverses the cornea, enters the anterior chamber, and drains through the chamber angle (Fig. 3.12). When an equilibrium has been established, the concentrations of fluorescein in the cornea (C_c) and the anterior chamber (C_a) decrease over time. A fluorophotometer (Fig. 3.13) is used to monitor these changes. The instrument can focus separately on the cornea (Fig. 3.14a) and then on the anterior chamber (Fig. 13.4b), thus allowing a discrete measurement of each region.

The rate of aqueous flow determines the cornea and anterior chamber fluorescein decay curves. The

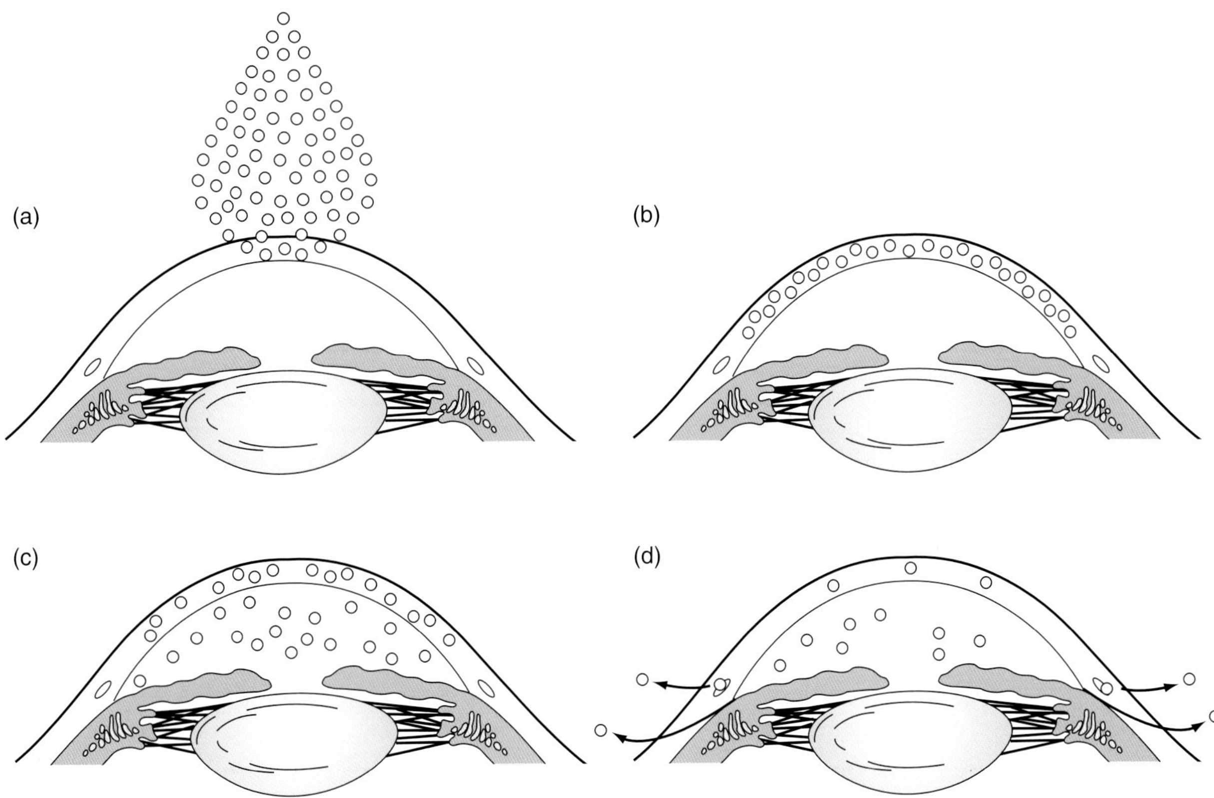

Figure 3.11 Ocular distribution of topically administered fluorescein
Fluorescein (yellow dots) applied to the surface of the cornea (a), penetrates the epithelium and fills the corneal stroma (b). The epithelium is approximately 1000-fold less permeable than the endothelium, hence, once in the stroma, effectively all the fluorescein diffuses into the anterior chamber (c). Diffusional loss into limbal or iridial vessels is very small; hence once in the anterior chamber, approximately 95% of the fluorescein leaves with the bulk of aqueous humor through the two anterior chamber drainage routes (arrows) (d). The rate of disappearance of the fluorescein is a measure of aqueous flow.

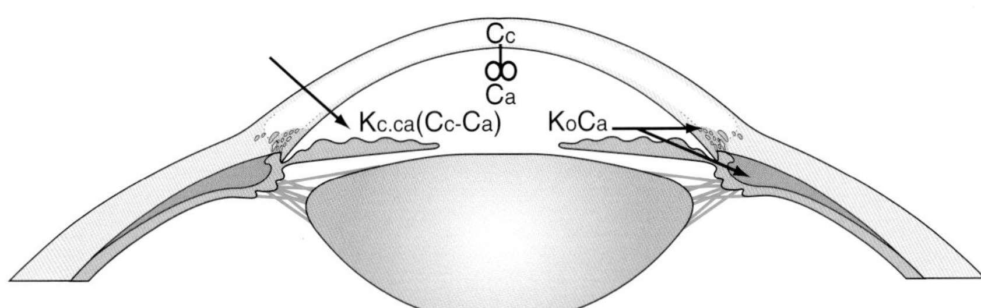

Figure 3.12 The dynamics of topically administered fluorescein
This figure demonstrates some of the important assumptions which are the basis for the fluorophotometric determination of the anterior chamber aqueous humor flow, F_a. The anterior chamber, by virtue of normal thermoconvective streams, is a well mixed (signified by the 'mixer') compartment of uniform fluorescein concentration. The net flux of fluorescein into the anterior chamber is given by $K_{c.ca}$ $(C_c - C_a)$ multiplied by the volume of the anterior chamber. $K_{c.ca}$ is the transfer coefficient for fluorescein between the cornea and anterior chamber per unit volume of the anterior chamber. C_c and C_a are the fluorescein concentrations of the corneal stroma and anterior chamber respectively. The net flux of fluorescein out of the anterior chamber is given by K_oC_a multiplied by the volume of the anterior chamber. K_o is the fraction per minute of anterior chamber volume turned over by aqueous flow.

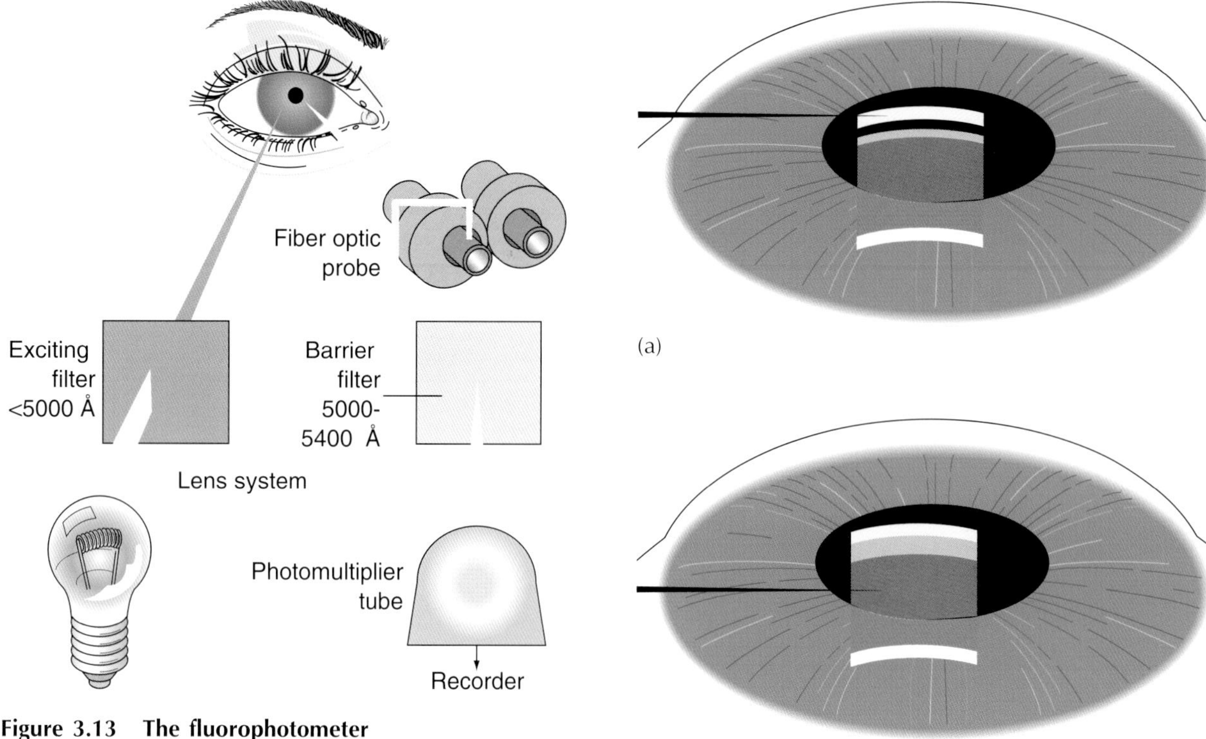

Figure 3.13 The fluorophotometer
Several hours after fluorescein is applied to the eye, cornea measurements are made by focusing a fiber-optic eyepiece probe on the corneal stroma. Anterior chamber measurements are made by focusing the eyepiece probe on the center of the anterior chamber. The eye is intermittently exposed to a blue light to excite the fluorescein. The blue light is produced by placing an excitation filter in the light path. The fluorescence signal is detected by the fluorophotometer and is transformed to an electrical impulse by a photomultiplier tube. The signal is sent to a recorder and converted into units of ng/ml by referencing a standard curve.

Figure 3.14 View of an eye through a slit-lamp fluorophotometer
(a) The slit-lamp beam is focused on the corneal stroma as indicated by the black pointer. A discrete reading of corneal fluorescein concentration is taken. (b) The slit beam is focused in the middle of the anterior chamber as indicated by the black pointer and a discrete reading of anterior chamber fluorescein concentration is taken.

typical time course of the tracer in the corneal stroma and anterior chamber is illustrated in Figure 3.15. The magnitude of the anterior chamber aqueous humor flow (F_a) is a function of the anterior chamber volume (V_a), the absolute value of the slope of the decay curve (A), and the ratio of the mass of fluorescein in the cornea to that in the anterior chamber (M_c/M_a) (Equation 2):

$$F_a = V_a A[1 + M_c/M_a] \qquad (2)$$

M_c can be rewritten as V_c/C_c where V_c is the corneal stroma volume and C_c is the corneal stroma fluorescein concentration. Similarly, M_a can be rewritten as V_a/C_a where C_a is the anterior chamber concentration of fluorescein. Equation 2 then becomes

$$F_a = V_a A[1 + V_c C_c/V_a C_a] \qquad (3)$$

Assuming that V_c and V_a remain constant in the steady state, then F_a is a function of the slope of the decay curve (A) and C_c/C_a. The logarithm of C_c/C_a is represented by the distance between the parallel decay curves (Fig. 3.15). Equation 3 shows that the more rapid the rate of aqueous humor flow (Fa) the steeper will be the decay curves and the larger the magnitude of the distance between the two decay curves. At the other extreme, if F_a becomes zero, the fluorescein concentrations in the anterior chamber

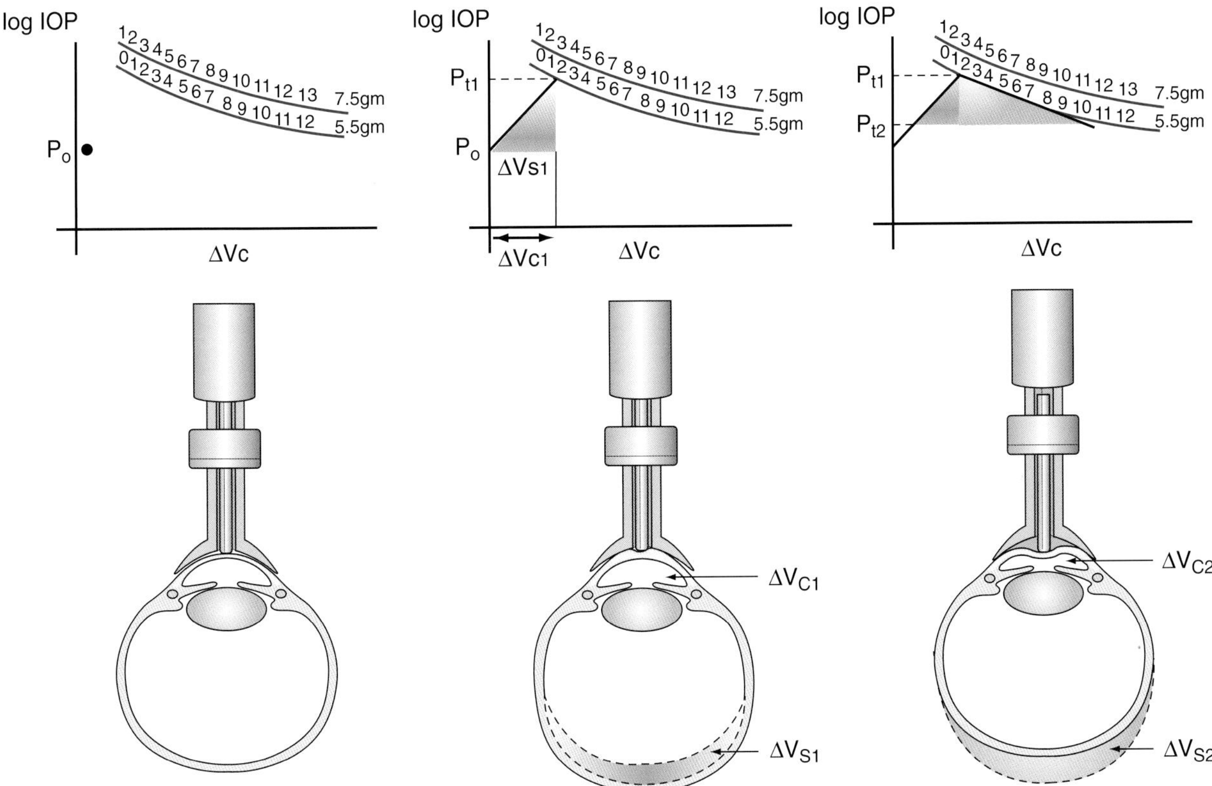

Figure 3.17 Tonography

Tonography exploits the fact that the 16.5 gm weight of the Schiotz tonometer raises IOP while it is being applied to the cornea. This increase in IOP causes an increase in the rate of flow of aqueous humor across the trabecular meshwork. The ratio of the increase in IOP to the increase in flow across the trabecular meshwork is the trabecular outflow facility.

$C_{trab} = \Delta F_{trab}/\Delta \text{IOP}$

The figure on the left shows the eye just before the weight of the tonometer is applied. The baseline intraocular pressure, P_o, before application of the tonometer, is shown on the left graph by the dot indicating that, when measured by the applanation tonometer, the cornea was only slightly indented (about 0.5 µl). Therefore, the applanation tonometer does not change the intraocular pressure during its measurement. In contrast, as shown in the middle figure and graph, the Schiotz tonometer when applied to the eye indents the cornea to decrease appreciably the anterior chamber volume by ΔV_{C1} which pushes fluid posteriorly to expand the sclera by ΔV_{S1}. ΔV_{C1} equals $-\Delta V_{S1}$. The intraocular pressure correspondingly rises, with the above changes in intraocular volumes, to ΔP_{t1} along the line shown in the graph whose slope equals the scleral rigidity, defined as $\Delta \log \text{IOP}/\Delta V_{S1}$. This line connects the point representing the applanation intraocular pressure, P_o, to the number on the appropriate nomogram curve for the Schiotz plunger weight used, which gives the reading of corneal indentation on the Schiotz scales. The figure and graph on the right show the situation after t minutes of tonography. The cornea has further indented to decrease anterior chamber volume by ΔV_{C2} and to show an increased reading on the tonometer scale and on the nomogram curve. ΔV_{C2} is caused by fluid exiting through the trabecular meshwork, in excess of normal trabecular flow, during the period of the tonography. In addition, because intraocular pressure has decreased from P_{t1} to P_{t2}, during the period t of tonography, scleral volume contracts along the same scleral rigidity slope as shown in the middle graph, yielding ΔV_{S2}. This contraction of scleral volume also represents fluid loss from the eye during the tonography period. Total fluid forced out across the trabecular meshwork, above that which normally flows across the trabecular meshwork, is therefore equal to $\Delta V_{C2} + \Delta V_{S2}$. This value is given by the length of the horizontal line connecting the final reading on the nomogram to the scleral rigidity line, as shown in the graph. Dividing this volume by t gives the rate of this excess outflow during tonography. The average IOP during the period of tonography is assumed to equal $(P_{t1} + P_{t2})/2$ and the increase in IOP causing the increase in trabecular flow, above normal flow, is equal to $(P_{t1} + P_{t2})/2 - P_o$. Inserting these values into the above equation yields:

$C_{trab} = \Delta F_{trab}/\Delta \text{IOP} = (\Delta V_{C2} + \Delta V_{S2})/((P_{t1} + P_{t2})/2 - P_o)t$

Pseudofacility is an inherent part of tonography. Some of the assumptions that go into the calculation of outflow facility from tonography are that the rate of aqueous humor production during tonography remains at the normal rate and that the change from P_{t1} to P_{t2} is due to fluid begin forced out of the eye only across the trabecular meshwork. Any decrease in the rate of aqueous humor formation or if fluid is forced out of the eye by nontrabecular routes, for example, decrease in blood volume or extracellular fluid volume would be measured as increased outflow facility and are therefore included in pseudofacility. Therefore the outflow facility measured by tonography equals trabecular outflow facility plus pseudofacility.

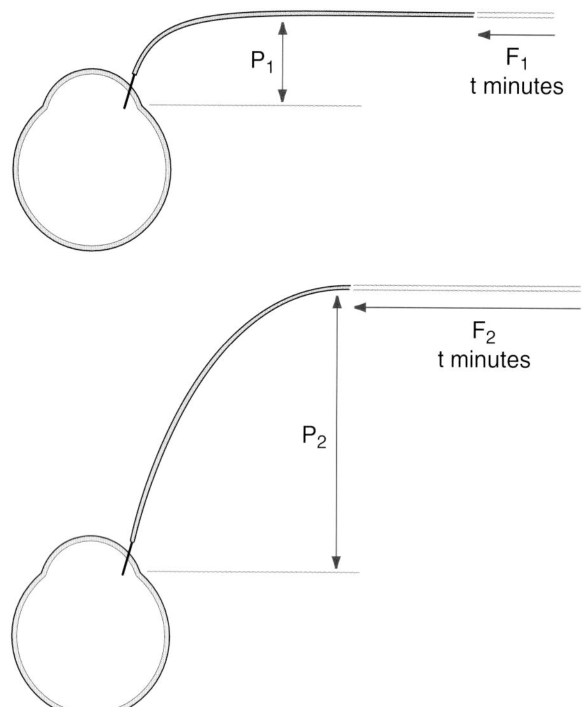

Figure 3.18 Measurement of outflow facility by the two-level constant pressure perfusion method (C_{tot})
In step 1, a cannula filled with mock aqueous humor is inserted into the anterior chamber. The end of the cannula is placed at an exact height above the eye to establish a specific pressure (P_1) above the spontaneous intraocular pressure. The amount of fluid flowing into the eye during time t to maintain P_1 is F_1. In step 2 the cannula end is raised to a new height to establish a new pressure (P_2) and during the next time interval, t, the flow of fluid into the eye to main P_2 is F_2. From these measurements C_{tot} is calculated as $(F_2 - F_1)/(P_2 - P_1)$.

Formula 6 is used again. This is the constant-flow perfusion method.

Two major problems exist with the perfusion method. One is the need to insert needles in the eye which can cause trauma and breakdown of the blood–aqueous barrier in some animals. Also this precludes its use in humans. The other is the 'washout' phenomenon. When an eye is perfused experimentally, the flow resistance of the eye decreases progressively probably from the depletion of proteins in the trabecular meshwork. The consequence of this is an artifactual increase over time in the experimentally measured outflow facility.

Circumventing the problems of the perfusion method is a noninvasive fluorophotometric method to assess C (Fig. 3.19). This method has been used

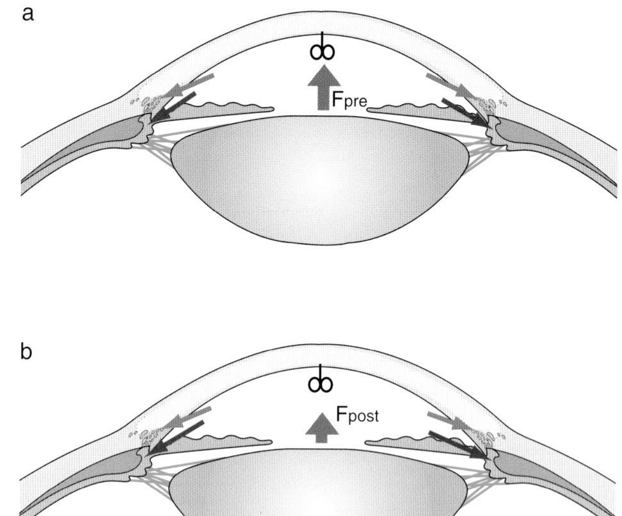

Figure 3.19 Measurement of outflow facility by fluorophotometry
The measurement of outflow facility by fluorophotometry is like that of tonography and of the two-level constant pressure method in that it also attempts to measure a change in flow across the trabecular meshwork caused by a known change in intraocular pressure. After measuring the baseline flow of aqueous humor, F_{pre}, (purple arrow in a), from the equilibrium data, the eye is treated with a topical beta blocker and/or systemic carbonic anhydrase inhibitor causing a decrease in aqueous humor flow to F_{post} (purple arrow in b). It is assumed that the entire difference between F_{pre} and F_{post} causes an equal decrease in trabecular outflow, F_{trab} (green arrow into canal of Schlemm). In other words, it is assumed that the magnitude of uveoscleral flow F_u (red arrows) is unchanged by the administration of topical beta blocker and/or systemic carbonic anhydrase inhibitor. Therefore, unlike tonography or the two-level constant pressure perfusion method, pseudofacility does not contaminate the measurement since the change in flow across the trabecular meshwork is measured more directly. Dividing this change in flow, ΔF_{trab}, by the corresponding change in intraocular pressure yields the fluorophotometrically determined outflow facility:

$C_{trab} = \Delta F_{trab}/\Delta IOP$

It can be assumed that the outflow facility measured by this technique equals the true outflow facility since pseudofacility is bypassed by this method. To determine the magnitude of uveoscleral flow, F_{trab} is calculated by multiplying C_{trab} by outflow pressure ($IOP - P_{ev}$), using the baseline IOP and the episcleral venous pressure (P_{ev}) measured by venomanometry:

$F_{trab} = C_{trab}(IOP - P_{ev})$

Subtracting F_{trab} from baseline F_{pre} yields baseline uveoscleral flow, F_u:

$F_u = F_{pre} - F_{trab}$

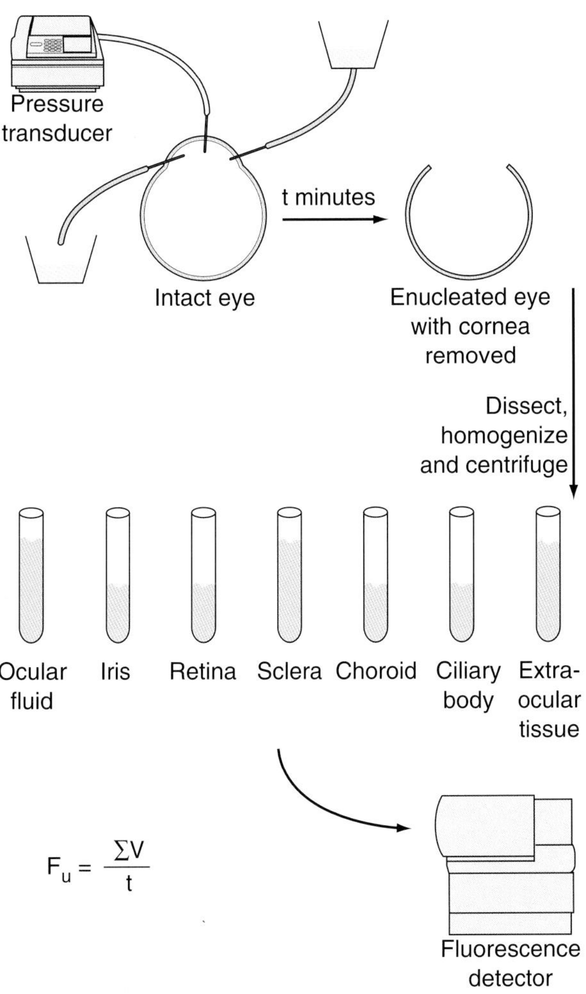

Figure 3.20 Measurement of uveoscleral outflow with infusion of intracameral tracer

A large molecular weight tracer such as fluorescein isothiocyanate dextran is infused into the anterior chamber of an anesthetized animal at a pressure of around spontaneous intraocular pressure (IOP). IOP is monitored with a pressure transducer. After a 30–60 minute time interval (*t*), infusion is stopped, the eye is enucleated, the cornea is removed, and the surface of the iris and lens are rinsed to removal all intracameral tracer. The eye is dissected into the tissues as shown. The supernatant from each homogenized and centrifuged sample is measured with a fluorescence detector. Uveoscleral outflow (F_u) is calculated by dividing the sum of all the tissue tracer values, expressed as equivalent volumes of aqueous (ΣV), by the infusion time (*t*).

productively in humans. After measuring the intraocular pressure (*P*) with tonometry and aqueous flow (*F*) with fluorophotometry, the patient is given either acetazolamide or a beta blocker to reduce *F* and hence reduce *P*. These drugs are known to reduce intraocular pressure solely by reducing aqueous flow, so they are the pharmacological equivalent of lowering the reservoir and slowing the infusion pump. One to three hours after administering the aqueous flow suppressants, intraocular pressure is remeasured and Formula 6 is used to calculate *C*. This method avoids the problems of pseudofacility and scleral rigidity and it can detect changes in trabecular outflow facility that are missed by tonography.

Uveoscleral outflow

One technique for measuring uveoscleral outflow (F_u) involves infusing a large molecular weight tracer, in which the flux can be assumed to be entirely by solvent drag, into the anterior chamber at a predetermined pressure. Usually radioactive-labeled protein or fluorescein-labeled dextran are used as tracers. At a specified time, usually 30–60 minutes, the eye is enucleated and dissected. All tracer collected from the ocular tissues and ocular fluids (minus the anterior chamber fluid) within the given time period is considered to be uveoscleral outflow (Fig. 3.20). If the time of tracer infusion exceeds the time needed to saturate the tissues then there is a risk of loss of tracer from the globe. Some laboratories handle this problem by collecting periocular and periorbital tissues as well but they run the risk of collecting tracer exiting the eye via the trabecular meshwork and thus overestimating F_u. Without collecting these extraocular tissues, however, one runs the risk of underestimating F_u.

The second technique to determine uveoscleral outflow is an indirect assessment. By measuring all other components of aqueous humor dynamics, one can calculate F_u with the formula:

$$F_u = F_a - (C(\mathrm{IOP} - P_{ev})) \quad (7)$$

This provides a means of evaluating F_u without sacrifice of the animal and it can be used safely and repeatedly in animals and humans. The drawback is that mean F_u measured this way has a large standard deviation. This is because of the variability of each of the components defining F_u (Equation 7). This can be overcome by the use of a large number of subjects to minimize the standard error of the mean.

Acknowledgment

Some of the figures were drawn by Allen Toris. His help is greatly appreciated.

FURTHER READING

Araie M, Sawa M, Takase M, Physiological study of the eye as studied by oral fluorescein. I. Oral administration of fluorescein and its pharmacokinetics, *Acta Soc Ophthalmol Jpn* (1980) **84**:1003–11.

Bárány EH, Simultaneous measurement of changing the intraocular pressure and outflow facility in the vervet monkey by constant pressure infusion, *Invest Ophthalmol* (1964) **3**:135–43.

Bárány EH, Kinsey VE, The rate of flow of aqueous humor. I. The rate of disappearance of para-aminohippuric acid, radioactive Rayopake, and radioactive Diodrast from the aqueous humor of rabbits, *Am J Ophthalmol* (1949) **32**:177–88.

Bill A, The aqueous humor drainage mechanism in the cynomolgus monkey (*Macaca irus*) with evidence for unconventional routes, *Invest Ophthalmol* (1965) **4**:911–19.

Bill A, Conventional and uveo-scleral drainage of aqueous humor in the cynomolgus monkey (*Macaca irus*) at normal and high intraocular pressures, *Exp Eye Res* (1966) **5**:45–54.

Bill A, Further studies on the influence of the intraocular pressure on aqueous humor dynamics in cynomolgus monkeys, *Invest Ophthalmol* (1967) **6**:364–72.

Bill A, Aqueous humor dynamics in monkeys (*Macaca irus* and *Cercopithecus ethiops*), *Exp Eye Res* (1971) **11**:195–206.

Bill A, Blood circulation and fluid dynamics in the eye, *Physiol Rev* (1975) **55**:383–417.

Bill A, Basic physiology of the drainage of aqueous humor, *Exp Eye Res* (1977) **25**:291–304.

Bill A, Bárány EH, Gross facility, facility of conventional routes, and pseudofacility of aqueous humor outflow in the cynomolgus monkey, *Arch Ophthalmol* (1966) **75**:665–73.

Bill A, Phillips CI, Uveoscleral drainage of aqueous humor in human eyes, *Exp Eye Res* (1971) **12**:275–81.

Brubaker RF, Flow of aqueous humor in humans, *Invest Ophthalmol Vis Sci* (1991) **32**:3145–66.

Cole DF, Secretion of the aqueous humor, *Exp Eye Res* (1977) **25**:161–76.

Diamond JM, Bossert WH, Standing-gradient osmotic flow. A mechanism for coupling of water and solute transport in epithelia, *J Gen Physiol* (1967) **50**:2061–83.

Friedenwald JS, Some problems with the calibration of tonometers. *Am J Ophthalmol* (1948) **31**:935–44.

Goldmann H, Abflussdruck, minutenvolumen und widerstand der kammerwasser-strömung des menschen, *Doc Ophthalmol* (1951) **5–6**:278–356.

Grant WM, Tonographic method for measuring the facility and rate of aqueous flow in human eyes, *Arch Ophthalmol* (1950) **44**:204–14.

Grant WM, Clinical measurements of aqueous outflow, *Arch Ophthalmol* (1951) **46**:113–31.

Hayashi M, Yablonski ME, Mindel JS, Methods for assessing the effects of pharmacologic agents on aqueous humor dynamics. In Duane TD, ed, *Foundations of Clinical Ophthalmology* (JB Lippincott, 1993).

Hayashi M, Yablonski ME, Novack GD, Trabecular outflow facility determined by fluorophotometry in human subjects, *Exp Eye Res* (1989) **48**:621–5.

Holm O, A photogrammetric method for estimation of the pupillary aqueous flow in the living eye, *Acta Ophthalmol (Copenh)* (1968) **46**:254–83.

Jacob E, FitzSimon JS, Brubaker RF, Combined corticosteroid and catecholamine stimulation of aqueous humor flow, *Ophthalmology* (1996) **103**:1303–8.

Johnson M, Gong H, Freddo TF, et al., Serum proteins and aqueous outflow resistance in bovine eyes, *Invest Ophthalmol Vis Sci* (1993) **34**:3549–57.

Jones RF, Maurice DM, New methods of measuring the rate of aqueous flow in man with fluorescein, *Exp Eye Res* (1966) **5**:208–20.

Kaufman PL, Aqueous humor dynamics. In: Duane TD, ed. *Clinical Ophthalmology* (Philadelphia, PA: Harper & Row, 1985), 1–24.

Langham ME, Taylor CB. The influence of superior cervical ganglionectomy on intraocular dynamics, *J Physiol (Lond)* (1960) **152**:447–58.

Linner E, Friedenwald JS, The appearance time of fluorescein as an index of aqueous flow, *Am J Ophthalmol* (1957) **44**:225–29.

Mäepea O, Bill A, The pressures in the episcleral veins, Schlemm's canal and the trabecular meshwork in monkeys. Effects of changes in intraocular pressure, *Exp Eye Res* (1989) **49**:645–63.

Nagataki S, Effects of adrenergic drugs on aqueous humor dynamics in man, *Acta Soc Ophthalmol Jpn* (1977) **81**:1795–800.

O'Rourke J, Macri FJ, Studies in uveal physiology. II. Clinical studies of the anterior chamber clearance of isotopic tracers. *Arch Ophthalmol* (1970) **84**:415–20.

Reiss GR, Lee DA, Topper JE, et al., Aqueous humor flow during sleep, *Invest Ophthalmol Vis Sci* (1984) **25**:776–8.

Sperber GO, Bill A, A method for near-continuous determination of aqueous humor flow; effects of anaesthetics, temperature and indomethacin, *Exp Eye Res* (1984) **39**:435–53.

Toris CB, Camras CB, Yablonski ME, Effects of PhXA41, a new prostaglandin $F_{2\alpha}$ analog, an aqueous humor dynamics in human eyes, *Ophthalmology* (1993) **100**:1297–304.

Toris CB, Gleason ML, Camras CB, et al. Effects of brimonidine on aqueous humor dynamics in human eyes, *Arch Ophthalmol* (1995) **113**:1514–17.

Toris CB, Pederson JE, Effect of intraocular pressure on uveoscleral outflow following cyclodialysis in the monkey eye, *Invest Ophthalmol Vis Sci* (1985) **26**:1745–9.

Toris CB, Tafoya ME, Camras CB, et al., Effects of apraclonidine on aqueous humor dynamics in human eyes, *Ophthalmology* (1995) **102**:456–61.

Toris CB, Wang Y, Chacko DM, Acetazolamide and the posterior flow of aqueous humor, *Invest Ophthalmol Vis Sci* (1995) **36**:S724 (abst).

Toris CB, Yablonski ME, Wang Y, et al., Prostaglandin A_2 increases uveoscleral outflow and trabecular outflow facility in the cat, *Exp Eye Res* (1995) **61**:649–57.

Townsend DJ, Brubaker RF, Immediate effect of epinephrine on aqueous formation in the normal human eye as measured by fluorophotometry, *Invest Ophthalmol Vis Sci* (1980) **19**:256–66.

Wang Y, Zhan G, Toris CB, et al., Effects of topical epinephrine on aqueous humor dynamics in feline eyes, *Invest Ophthalmol Vis Sci* (1993) **(Suppl) 34**:934 (abst).

Yablonski ME, Zimmerman TJ, Waltman SR, et al., A fluorophotometric study of the effect of topical timolol on aqueous humor dynamics, *Exp Eye Res* (1978) **27**:135–42.

4 Intraocular pressure and its measurement

Neil T Choplin

Introduction

Intraocular pressure is determined by the relative balance between the production and drainage of aqueous humor, discussed in Chapter 3. The range of intraocular pressures in the normal population is fairly wide, showing a quasi-normal distribution with a skew to the right (Fig. 4.1). In the nonglaucomatous population (defined as having normal-appearing optic nerves and without detectable visual field loss) the average intraocular pressure is approximately 16 mmHg with a standard deviation of 2.5. The 'statistical' normal range, defined as the mean ± two standard deviations, would therefore be approximately 11–21 mmHg. Two to three percent of the normal population would be expected to have pressures above the statistical upper limit, and it is this segment of the population that is said to have 'ocular hypertension'.

Intraocular pressure in a given eye is subject to a certain degree of variability from day to day and hour to hour. This 'diurnal variation' in pressure is usually no more than 4 mmHg in normal eyes. However, eyes with glaucoma may show much greater variability in measurement during the course of a day, sometimes spiking very high pressures while measuring within the normal range at other times (Fig. 4.2). Some of this variability has been attributed to, among other things, serum cortisol levels which are also subject

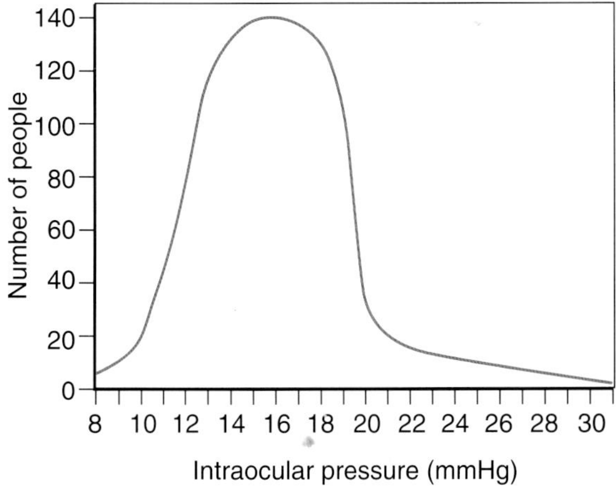

Figure 4.1 Distribution of intraocular pressure in the normal population
The pressure approximates normal distribution around a mean of 16 ± 2.5 mmHg. The tail to the right (above 21 mmHg) represents the segment of the population with 'ocular hypertension'.

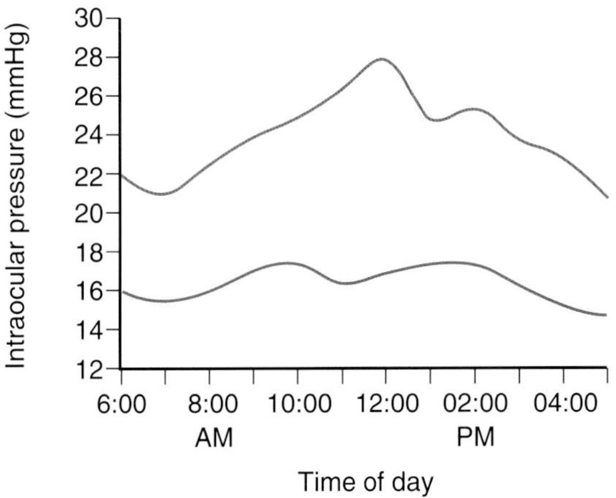

Figure 4.2 Diurnal variation in intraocular pressure
Normal pressure shows limited variation during the course of a day (bottom curve), while eyes with glaucoma may show considerably more variation (top curve).

Table 4.1 **Factors affecting intraocular pressure.**

Site of action	Increased inflow (raising pressure)	Decreased inflow (lowering pressure)	Decreased outflow (raising pressure)	Increased outflow (lowering pressure)
Ciliary body	Increased fluid load Increased blood flow Beta agonists	Decreased body fluid (dehydration) Reduced blood flow Beta blockers Digitalis Cyclitis Age Carbonic anhydrase inhibitors Alpha-two agonists Choroidal detachment, uveal effusion Surgical destructions		
Conventional outflow pathways			Age Prostaglandin E_1 Pigment, debris Anticholinergics, e.g. atropine Corticosteroids	Cholinergics, e.g. pilocarpine Laser trabeculoplasty
Non-conventional outflow pathways			Cholinergics, e.g. pilocarpine	Anticholinergics, e.g. atropine Alpha-two agonists Prostaglandin analogs, e.g. latanoprost
Blood–aqueous barrier	Breakdown of blood–aqueous barrier, e.g. uveitis Osmotic gradients, e.g. protein Cholinergics, e.g. phospholine iodine		Stabilization of blood–aqueous barrier, e.g. anti-inflammatories Anticholinergics, e.g. atropine	
Other			Angle closure Increased episcleral venous pressure	Sclerostomy Rhegmatogenous retinal detachment cyclodialysis cleft

to diurnal variation. Diurnal variation is one of the factors that makes intraocular pressure measurement a poor screening tool for glaucoma, since a pressure reading within the normal range does not rule out glaucoma. The measurement of the 'diurnal curve', with particular attention to uncovering pressure spikes, should be considered in any patient with apparent glaucomatous optic neuropathy in whom the pressure has been measured within the normal range, or in any glaucoma patient who appears to be progressing despite normal pressure readings.

Since intraocular pressure is determined by the relative balance between aqueous humor inflow and outflow, any factors which increase inflow and/or decrease outflow will raise intraocular pressure, while factors decreasing aqueous formation and/or increasing outflow will lower pressure. Some of these factors are listed in Table 4.1.

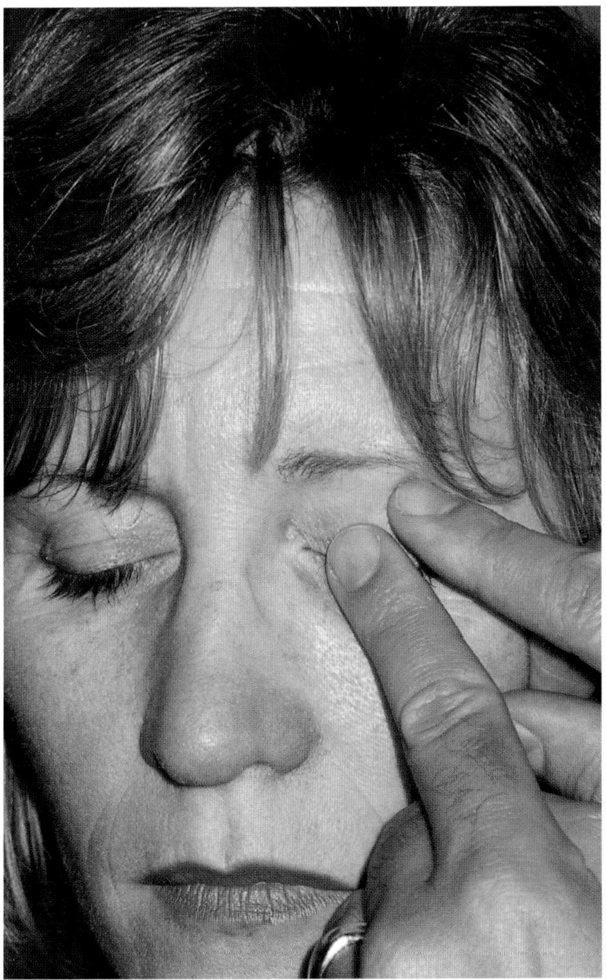

Figure 4.3 Estimation of intraocular pressure by palpation
The patient is instructed to close the eye and look down. The examiner uses the index fingers of both hands, alternately applying slight pressure to estimate the force necessary to indent the globe. The resistance to indentation is provided by the intraocular pressure. By correlating 'finger tension' with applanation readings obtained just prior to palpation, the examiner can learn how much force correlates with varying levels of intraocular pressure, and may be able to estimate intraocular pressure to within 2–3 mmHg.

Measurement of intraocular pressure

The measurement of intraocular pressure should be part of any eye examination. Direct measurement of pressure by cannulation of the anterior chamber using manometric techniques is obviously impractical, and so indirect measurements have been devised. These techniques rely upon the determination of the eye's response to an externally applied force. Tonometers developed for the purpose of measuring intraocular pressure fall into two categories: indentation, in which the amount of corneal or globe deformation in response to an externally applied weight is determined, and applanation, in which the force necessary to flatten a known surface area of cornea is determined. In both cases it is the intraocular pressure that resists the externally applied force.

Estimation of intraocular pressure by palpation

In the absence of an instrument to measure eye pressure, an estimation can be made by palpation. Although not highly accurate, it is usually easy to differentiate between very low and very high pressure. Obviously, this technique should not be employed in cases of suspected globe rupture. It is useful in emergency-room settings when faced with a patient with a red painful eye, and acute glaucoma is in the differential diagnosis.

To estimate intraocular pressure by palpation, the patient should close the eye and look down. The examiner uses the index finger of both hands, alternating pressure to the superior part of the eye through the closed lids, to gently determine the force necessary to indent the eye wall (Fig. 4.3). It is usually obvious whether the eye is rock hard or very soft. If palpation is applied after determining pressure by another technique, the examiner may become quite capable of estimating intraocular pressure to within 2–3 mmHg.

Schiotz tonometry

The Schiotz tonometer is an indentation instrument which measures intraocular pressure by registering the depth of indentation of the cornea produced when the instrument, carrying a known weight, is applied to the anesthetized eye. The instrument is illustrated schematically in Figure 4.4. The weight is carried on a plunger which should move freely within the holder. When the weight is applied to the eye, the intraocular pressure provides a counterbalancing force which pushes back up on the plunger. This causes a deflection of the pointer along the inclined scale transmitted through the convex hammer. Each unit on the scale, which ranges from 1 to 20, corresponds to an indentation of 1/20 of a millimeter in the cornea. High intraocular pressure resists indentation, resulting in low scale readings, while low intraocular pressure allows for easy indentation, manifested by high scale readings. In cases with elevated intraocular pressure (scale readings of less than 4 with any weight), the next higher weight should be placed on top of the standard 5.5 g weight until a scale reading greater

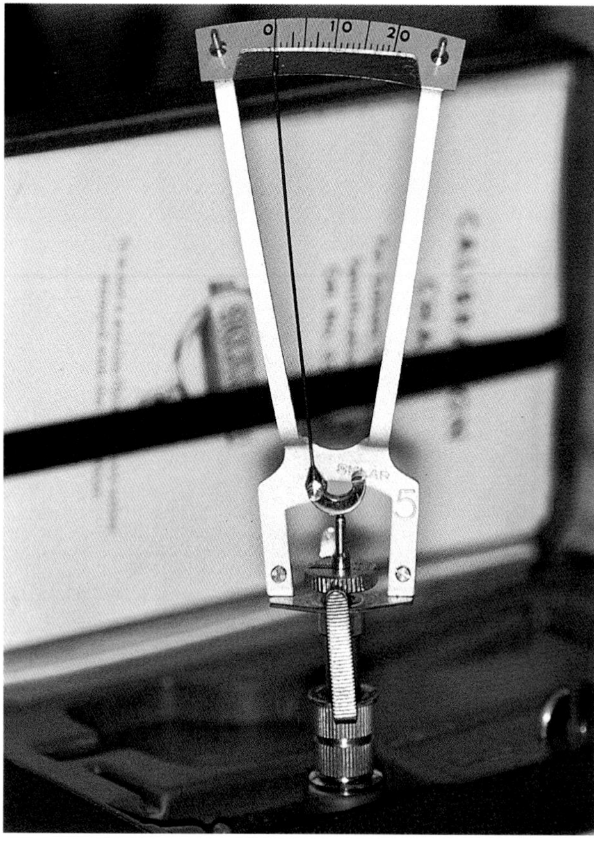

(a)

Mirror
Inclined scale
Lever ratio 1:20
Frame
Pointer
Convex hammer
Fulcrum
Jewel mounted plunger
Load 5.5 gram
Cylinder
Set screw
Handle
Sleeve
Holder
Plunger
Foot plate

(b)

Figure 4.4 The Schiotz tonometer
(a) A Schiotz tonometer resting on the calibration block. Since the block resists indentation, the scale should read zero. (b) Schematic diagram of a Schiotz tonometer. The various parts of the tonometer are labeled.

than 4 is obtained. The intraocular pressure is determined by referring to the calibration chart (Fig. 4.5) and reading the pressure that corresponds to the scale reading for the plunger load applied.

In order to perform a measurement, the patient must be supine (Fig. 4.6). Topical anesthetic is applied. Calibration of the instrument is tested by placing the plunger on the test block provided in the case; a scale reading of zero should be obtained (a set screw is provided on the handle for any necessary adjustments). The examiner then gently holds the patient's lids open (without exerting pressure on the globe), instructs the patient to look straight ahead, and places the instrument on the cornea. The handle is then lowered to a position midway between the top and bottom of the cylinder. The scale reading is determined by lining up the pointer with its mirror image on the inclined scale, thus providing a reading free of parallax. The intraocular pressure is then determined by reading from the chart as above.

Although the Schiotz tonometer is generally accurate, it has largely been replaced by other forms of tonometry. First, the positioning of the patient that is required makes the instrument somewhat awkward to use. More importantly, measurements may be subject to fairly large errors induced by scleral rigidity. For example, myopic eyes are more elastic than other eyes. When an external weight is applied (such as a Schiotz tonometer), some of the weight may be dissipated through the sclera (which lacks resistance to distention), resulting in less resistance to corneal indentation and underestimation of intraocular pressure. The opposite is true of hyperopic (and more rigid) eyes.

Applanation tonometry

Applanation tonometry is the procedure of choice in most clinical situations, and tonometers have been developed for use both at the slit lamp and hand-held for use outside the examining lane. Included in this category are the Goldmann tonometer, the Perkins tonometer, the Mackay–Marg tonometer, the pneumatic tonometer, and the Tonopen. The underlying principle is similar for each instrument. Intraocular pressure is determined by measuring the force necessary to applanate, or flatten, a known surface area of the cornea.

Scale reading	Plunger load (In grams)			
	5.5	7.5	10.0	15.0
0	41	59	82	127
.5	38	54	75	118
1.0	35	50	70	109
1.5	32	46	64	101
2.0	29	42	59	94
2.5	27	39	55	88
3.0	24	36	51	82
3.5	22	33	47	76
4.0	21	30	43	71
4.5	19	28	40	66
5.0	17	26	37	62
5.5	16	24	34	58
6.0	15	22	32	54
6.5	13	20	29	50
7.0	12	19	27	46
7.5	11	17	25	43
8.0	10	16	23	40
8.5	9	14	21	38
9.0	9	13	20	35
9.5	8	12	18	32
10.0	7	11	16	30
10.5	6	10	15	27
11.0	6	9	14	25
11.5	5	8	13	23
12.0		8	11	21
12.5		7	10	20
13.0		6	10	18
13.5		6	9	17
14.0		5	8	15
14.5			7	14
15.0			6	13
15.5			6	11
16.0			5	10
16.5				9
17.0				8
17.5				8
18.0				7

Figure 4.5 Calibration chart for Schiotz tonometers
The amount of corneal indentation is read from the column on the left (corresponding to the scale reading). The intraocular pressure is listed under the load weight used to take the measurement.

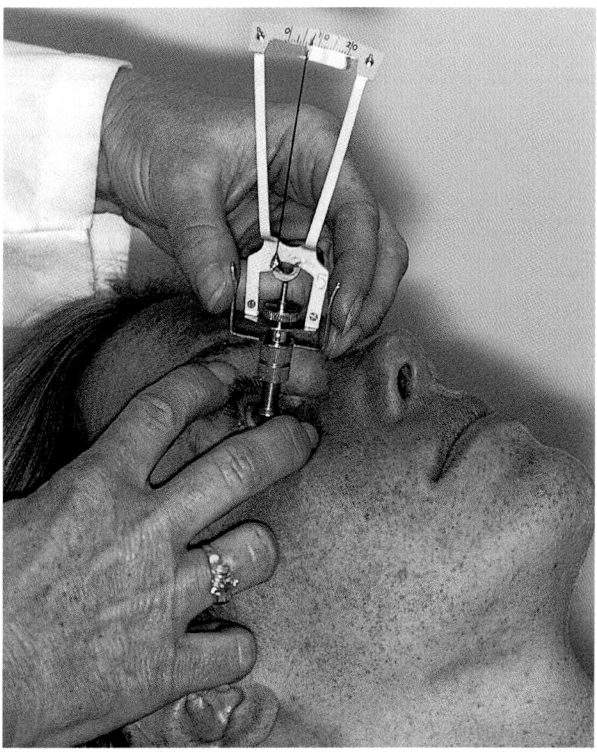

Figure 4.6 Measurement of intraocular pressure with a Schiotz tonometer
The patient is placed in the supine position and topical anesthetic applied. The examiner holds the lids open with the free hand, being careful not to apply any pressure to the globe. The patient is instructed to look straight ahead or fixate on a point on the ceiling with the fellow eye. Holding the instrument by the handles with the other hand, it is gently applied perpendicularly to the cornea until the foot plate rests on the cornea. Usually, when the instrument is properly positioned, there will be a gentle pulsation of the pointer, corresponding to the ocular pulse. The plunger, with the attached load weight, pushes down on the cornea and indents it to the amount allowed by the resistance of the intraocular pressure. This causes the jewel-mounted plunger to push back on the convex hammer, causing the pointer to deflect off zero on the inclined scale. Since the lever ratio is 1:20, the reading corresponds to the amount of corneal indentation × 0.05 mm. Once the scale reading has been determined, the intraocular pressure is read from the calibration chart.

Complete descriptions and instructions for use of each of the following instruments should be found in the manufacturer's documentation provided with the instrument.

Goldmann tonometer

The Goldmann tonometer (Fig. 4.7) is probably the most widely used tonometer and is the international standard for measuring intraocular pressure. The flattening force to the cornea is supplied by a coiled spring contained in the housing of the instrument, controlled by a rotating knob at the base, and is applied to the anesthetized eye by the tip of a split prism device through which the cornea may be viewed with the slit lamp. The area of cornea

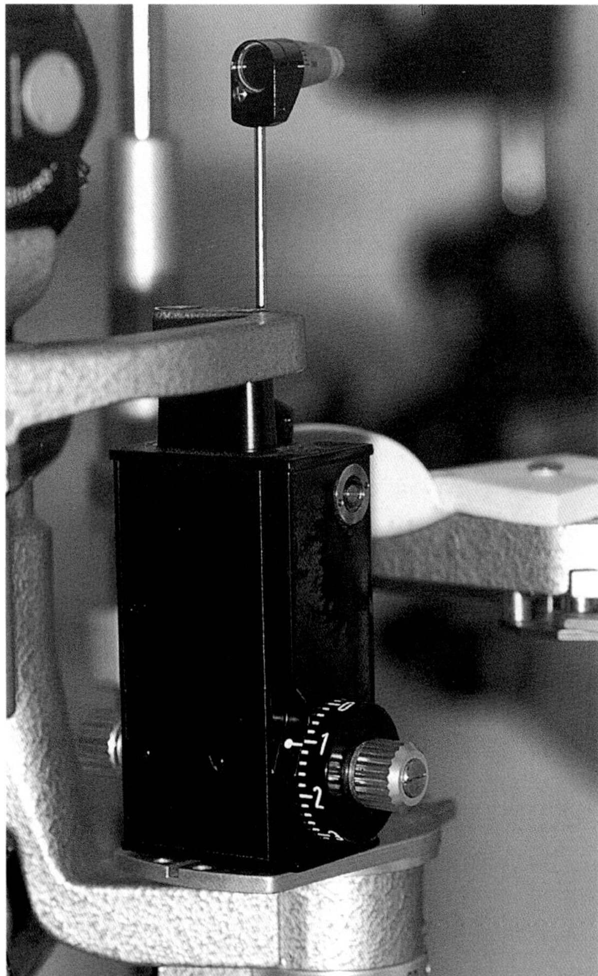

Figure 4.7 The Goldmann tonometer
Mounted on a slit lamp, the Goldmann tonometer consists of a tip attached by a rod to a coiled spring contained within the instrument housing. The tension on the spring, determined by the position of the calibrated knob, supplies the force used to flatten 3.06 mm of the central cornea. The tip contains a prism which splits the circular image of the flattened corneal surface into two semicircles, one above the other.

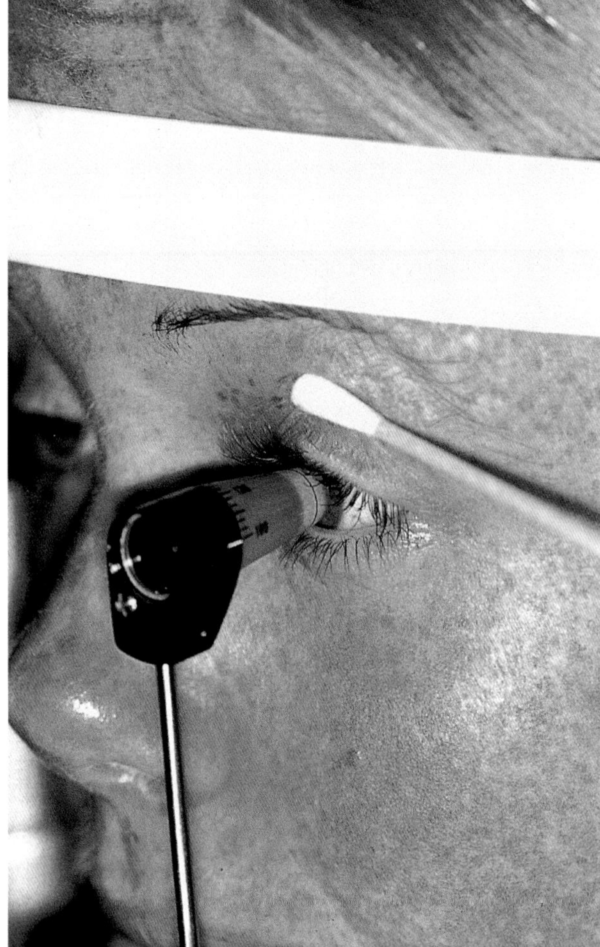

Figure 4.8 Measuring intraocular pressure with the Goldmann tonometer
The eye is anesthetized and the tear film stained with fluorescein. The instrument is then brought into the appropriate position on the slit lamp and the cobalt blue filter placed in the light path. The slit aperture should be opened widely. The tip of the instrument is gently placed against the cornea, and the image of the tear film is viewed through the biomicroscope. The knob is turned until the inner edges of the semicircles are just touching, indicating that 3.06 mm of corneal flattening has been attained, corresponding to the intraocular pressure. The reading on the knob is multiplied by ten to obtain the pressure reading.

flattened is 3.06 mm in diameter. Topical anesthetic and fluorescein are applied to the eye, and the tear film illuminated using the cobalt blue filter of the slit lamp. As the instrument is applied to the eye (Fig. 4.8), the applanating head creates a circular tear film meniscus which may be viewed through the slit lamp. The prism in the applanating head splits the circular image into two semicircles, and the end point of the measurement is determined by adjusting the knob until the inside edges of the semicircles are just touching (Fig. 4.9). The intraocular pressure is then determined by multiplying the reading on the scale on the knob by ten.

Hand-held tonometers

The Perkins tonometer

The Perkins tonometer (Fig. 4.10) is a battery-powered hand-held applanation tonometer which

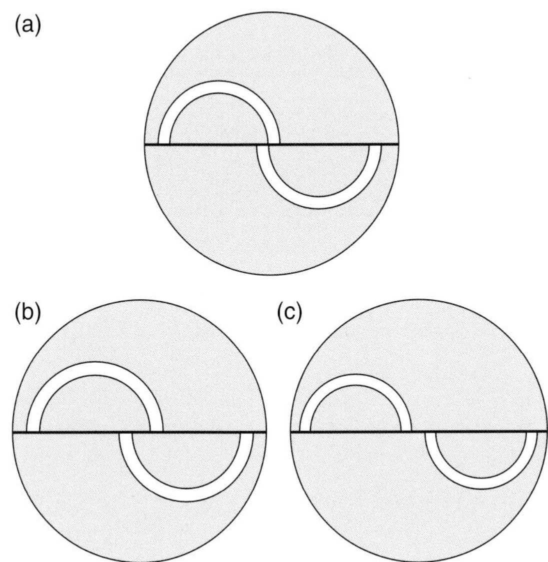

Figure 4.9 Tear film meniscus
Appearance of tear film meniscus as viewed through the Goldmann tonometer during applanation tonometry. (a) Correct appearance of the mires when the applied force to the cornea is equal to the intraocular pressure. (b) Appearance of the mires when the applied force is greater than the intraocular pressure or the instrument is pushed too far into the eye, indicating that the cornea has been overflattened. (c) Appearance of the mires when the applied force is less than the intraocular pressure, indicating that the cornea has been underflattened.

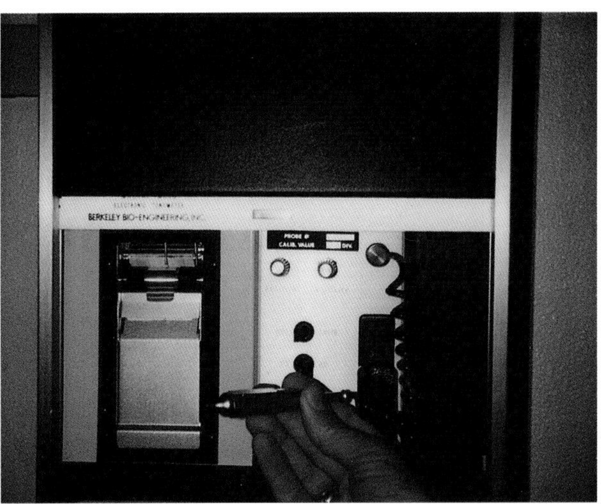

Figure 4.11 The Mackay–Marg tonometer
This is another applanation-type device in which the movement of the tip is sensed by a transducer contained in the hand piece. The bending pressure of the cornea, opposed by the intraocular pressure, is determined. The instrument is useful for measuring the intraocular pressure in scarred, irregular, and/or edematous corneas.

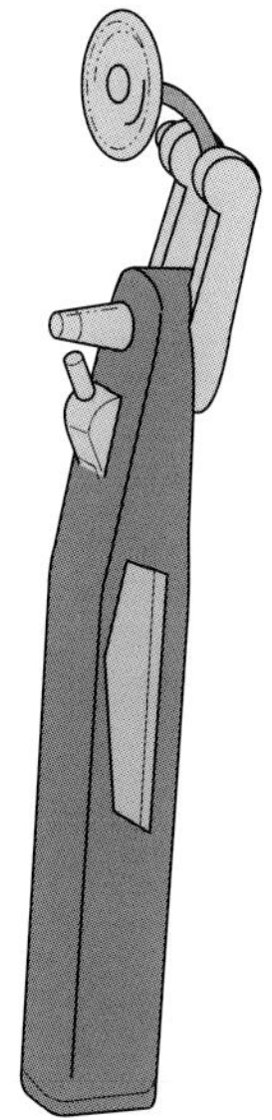

Figure 4.10 The Perkins tonometer
This tonometer employs the same principles as the Goldmann tonometer. The prism is mounted on a counterbalanced arm and the change in force obtained by rotation of a spiral spring. The disc at the top of the instrument is placed against the patient's forehead as a brace. The instrument can be used in any position and does not need to be held vertically.

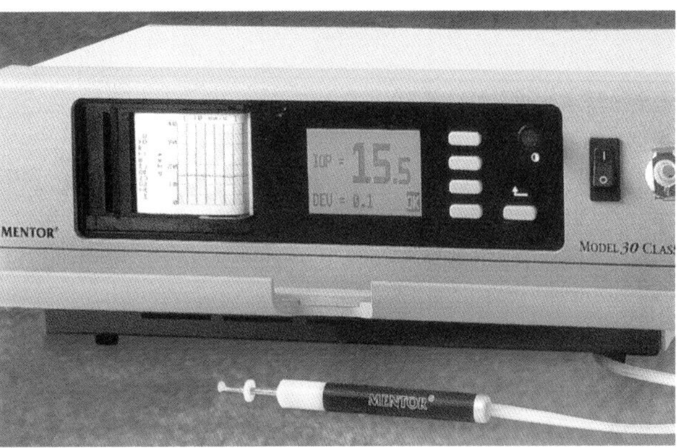

Figure 4.12 The pneumatic tonometer
The measuring device consists of a gas-filled chamber with a transducer capable of sensing the pressure in the chamber. As the device is applied to the eye, the counterpressure in the eye pushes back on the tip, raising the pressure on the gas until the end point is reached and recorded, either on a moving paper strip or displayed on a digital readout. This device may also be used for tonography.

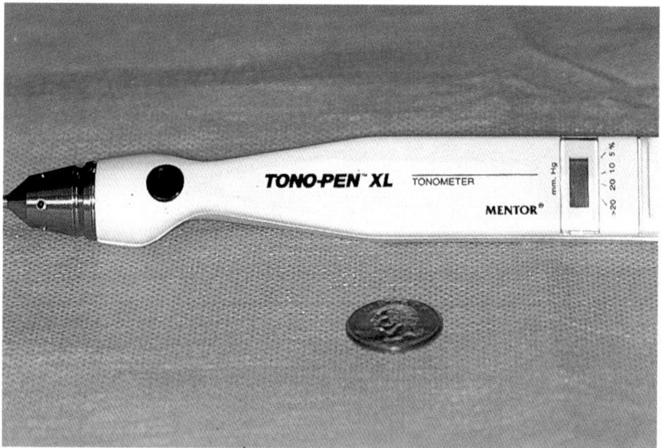

Figure 4.13 The Tonopen™
This miniaturized electronic applanation tonometer is battery powered and can be used in any position. It is very useful for measuring intraocular pressure in patients who cannot sit at a slit lamp. It is also useful for measuring pressures in patients with irregular corneas, since the applanation area is much smaller than that of the Goldmann instrument.

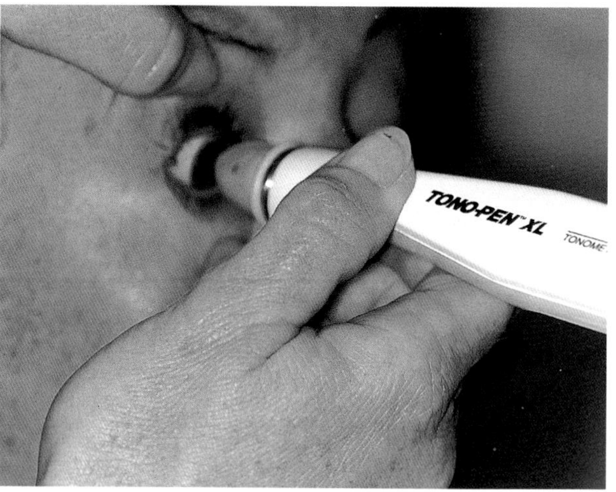

Figure 4.14 Measurement of intraocular pressure with the Tonopen™
The eye is anesthetized and the instrument tip covered with a latex sleeve. The examiner holds the upper lid open, rests the hand holding the instrument on the patient's cheek, and gently and quickly touches the central cornea with the tip, moving the instrument rapidly on to and off the eye. A short beep will be emitted by the instrument when a measurement has been recorded, and the reading displayed when five successful measurements are obtained.

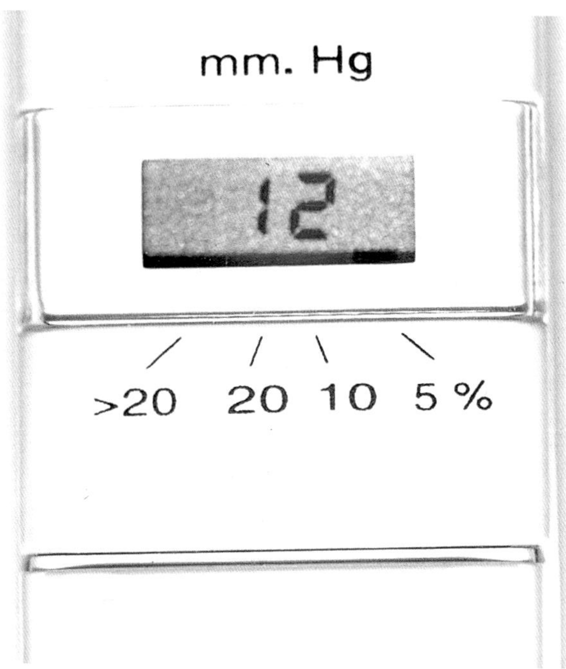

Figure 4.15 Intraocular pressure reading displayed on the Tonopen
The number indicates the average of the five readings in mmHg. A solid line will appear at the bottom of the printout corresponding to the percentage spread of the five readings (5%, 10%, 20%, or >20%).

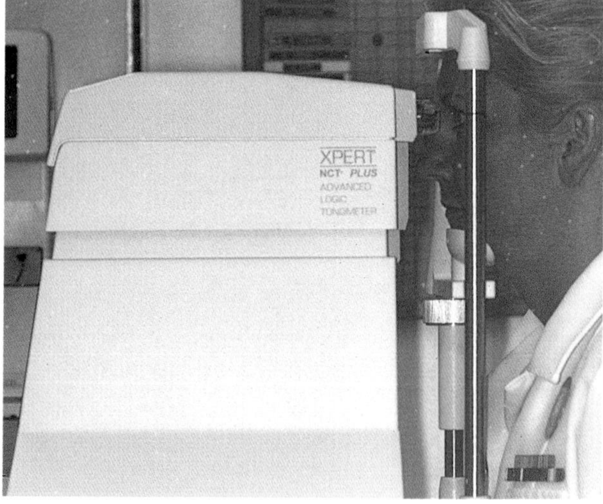

Figure 4.16 The noncontact tonometer
A patient is properly positioned for measurement of intraocular pressure with this instrument. The operator is seated to the left. No anesthetic is used. The eye to be measured is viewed on a CRT monitor, and, when the eye is properly aligned, the operator pushes a button which releases the air jet. Light sensors positioned on either side of the jet determine the degree of corneal flattening and when the end point has been reached. The patients usually react to the air jet with a slight startled response, but the measurement is not uncomfortable.

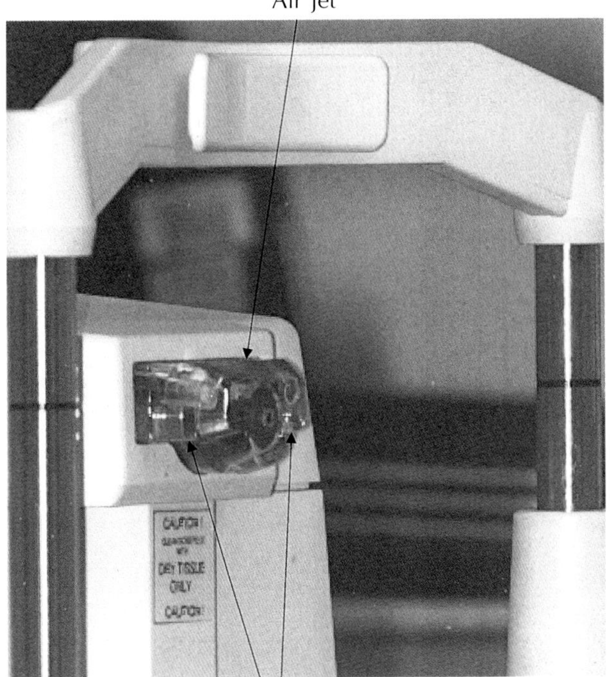

Figure 4.17 The 'business' end of a noncontact tonometer
The air jet is in the middle, with the two sensors on either side. As the air jet increases in force, the sensors determine when the end point of corneal flattening has been reached. The time required to reach this end point is directly related to the force opposing the flattening, i.e. the intraocular pressure.

functions identically to the Goldmann tonometer. The mires are viewed directly through the instrument so a slit lamp is not necessary. It may be used in situations where the patient cannot sit at the slit lamp. The instrument is counterbalanced to allow it to be used in a variety of positions.

The Mackay–Marg tonometer
The Mackay–Marg tonometer (Fig. 4.11) was designed to measure intraocular pressure in eyes with scarred, irregular, or edematous corneas using a tip that is approximately half the diameter of that of the Goldmann tonometer. The movable tip protrudes from a surrounding foot plate and is supported by a spring connected to a transducer. The transducer senses the tension on the spring and translates that tension into a pressure reading. Basically, by advancing the tip on to the cornea, the bending pressure of the cornea (opposed by the intraocular pressure) is measured. Pressure readings are recorded on a moving paper strip.

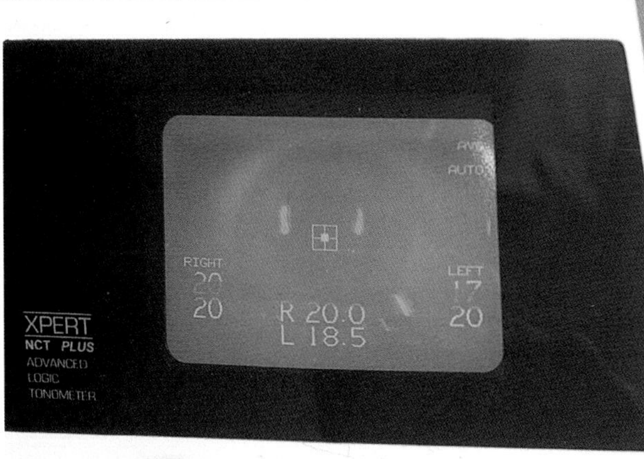

Figure 4.18 The display of a noncontact tonometer
The eye can be seen faintly in the center of the CRT. The pressure readings obtained for each eye are displayed, with the average in the middle.

The pneumatic tonometer
Another device useful for measuring pressure in eyes with scarred, irregular, and/or edematous corneas is the pneumatic tonometer (Fig. 4.12). Measurements can also be made over bandage contact lenses.

The Tonopen™
Advances in electronics and miniaturization have led to the development of a self-contained, compact, hand-held applanation tonometer that works on the same principle as the Mackay–Marg tonometer. This has been marketed as the Tonopen (Fig. 4.13). The device is gently applied to the anesthetized cornea (Fig. 4.14) and intraocular pressure is displayed on a digital readout after five readings have been obtained. The spread of the measurements is also displayed as a percentage (Fig. 4.15).

Noncontact tonometry

The noncontact (or air-puff) tonometer (Fig. 4.16) was originally developed to allow the measurement of intraocular pressure by nonmedical personnel since measurements may be obtained without the use of topical anesthetics. No part of the device touches the eye. The device uses a jet of air to applanate the cornea. Figure 4.17 shows the air jet and the sensors detect corneal flattening by means of reflected light. When activated, an air jet is blown at the cornea with increasing force over time. The cornea is illuminated with a collimated light beam which is reflected back to a detector, which determines when the reflected light reaches a maximum, corresponding to flattening of a corneal area 3.06 mm in diameter. The time required to reach this maximum reflection is directly related to the force of the air jet, counterbalanced by the intraocular pressure, and is translated into the intraocular pressure reading (Fig. 4.18).

FURTHER READING

Brubaker RF, Tonometry. In: *Duane's clinical ophthalmology. Volume 3* (Philadelphia, PA: JB Lippincott, 1994), Chap. 47.

Hitchings RA, Primary glaucoma. In *Slide atlas of ophthalmology. Volume 7* (London: Gower Medical, 1984).

Hoskins HD, Jr, Kass M, eds. *Becker–Shaffer's diagnosis and therapy of the glaucomas* sixth edition (St Louis, MO: Mosby, 1989), 67–88.

5 Gonioscopy

Ronald L Fellman

The classification of glaucoma relies heavily upon knowledge of the anterior segment anatomy, particularly that of the anterior chamber angle. Gonioscopy refers to the techniques used for viewing the anterior chamber angle of the eye for evaluation, management and classification of normal and abnormal angle structures. The *anterior chamber* is commonly evaluated during slit lamp biomicroscopy, but the chamber *angle* is hidden from ordinary view because of total internal reflection of light rays emanating from the angle structures (Fig. 5.1). It requires additional effort, skill and patient co-operation to view the normally concealed chamber angle by either indirect (angle structures (Fig. 5.2) viewed through a mirror) or direct (angle structures (Fig. 5.3) viewed directly) gonioscopic techniques. Without gonioscopy, it is impossible to classify the glaucomas properly.

On a busy patient day, the Zeiss or equivalent gonioprism (Posner, Sussman) is the most convenient contact lens for rapidly evaluating any chamber angle, and the Goldmann or equivalent gonioprism

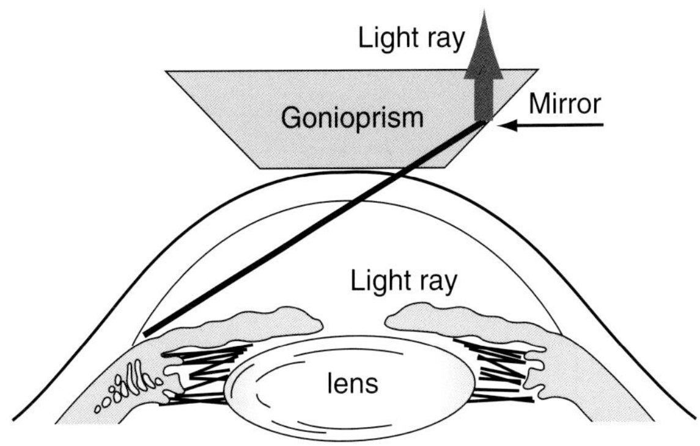

Figure 5.2 Indirect gonioscopy
A special contact lens overcomes the problem of total internal reflection of light rays from the chamber angle. The bending of light rays back into the chamber angle at the cornea–air interface is eliminated when a contact lens (gonioprism) is placed on the cornea. With this method of indirect gonioscopy, the light rays are reflected by a mirror in the gonioprism to the observer and focused with the slit lamp biomicroscope. The Goldmann and Zeiss lenses are examples of indirect goniolenses.

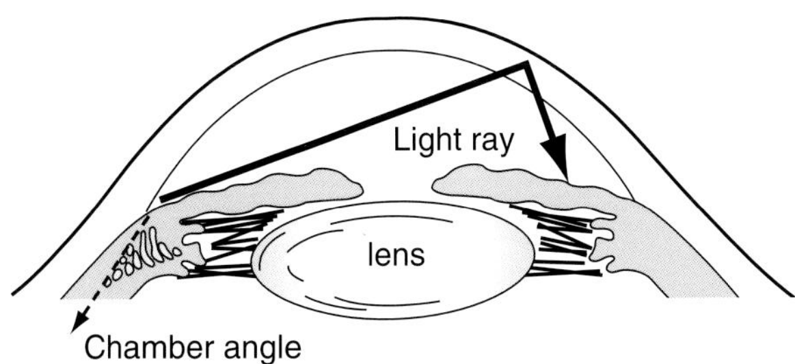

Figure 5.1 The normally hidden anterior chamber angle
The anterior chamber angle is not routinely seen during slit lamp biomicroscopy because light rays emanating from the chamber angle are refracted back into the eye (total internal reflection of light rays). During slit lamp examination, the anterior chamber may be described as 4+ deep, but without gonioscopy, the additional diagnostic clues of disease are forever hidden from ordinary view.

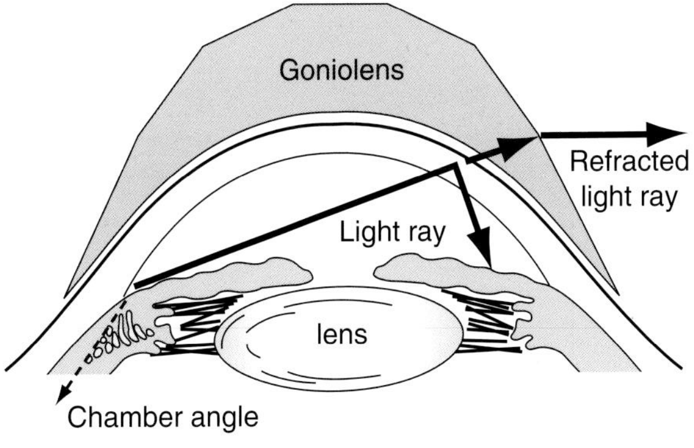

Figure 5.3 Direct gonioscopy
With direct gonioscopy, the goniolens allows chamber-angle light rays to be refracted directly through the cornea–contact lens interface and a hand-held gonioscope is required for magnification and illumination. The Koeppe lens is an example of a direct goniolens.

with antireflective coating is best for laser therapy (Fig. 5.4 and Table 5.1).

Gonioscopic appearance of the normal anterior chamber angle

The variability of the normal chamber angle is as immense as the variability of the normal optic nerve. Without a full appreciation of the diversity of the normal angle, early recognition of angle pathology is impossible. There are several key landmarks that guide the gonioscopist through the anterior chamber angle in a systematic way, otherwise the panoramic view causes confusion. Initially, it is best to envision the angle from a diagram, then master gonioscopy and look for the expected structures. To avoid confusion, try to observe the following six angle structures in order from the iris to the cornea (Fig. 5.5).

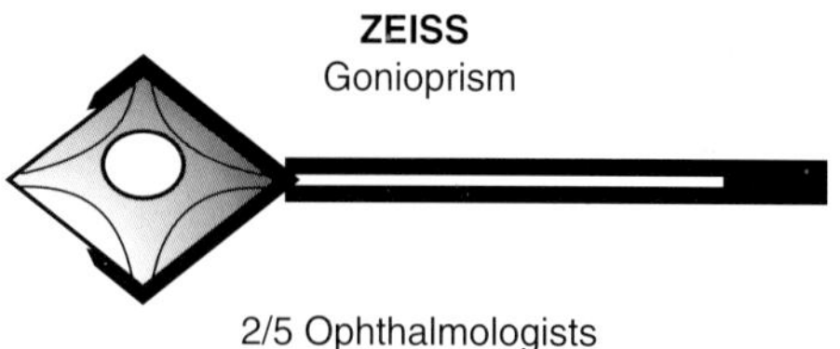

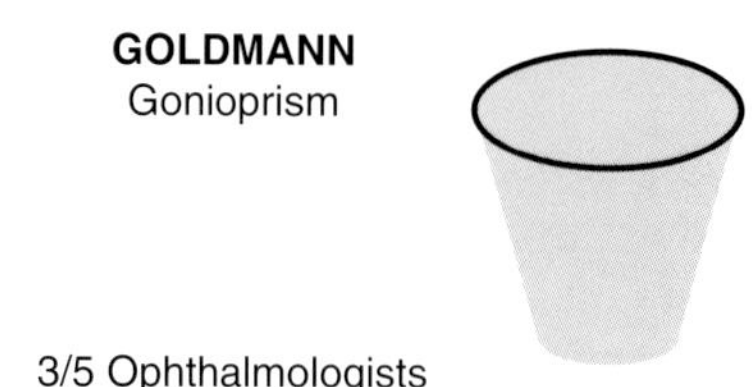

Figure 5.4 The two most common contact lenses for gonioscopy
The Goldmann prism (Table 5.1) has a contact surface of 12 mm, a mirror tilt of approximately 60 degrees and requires a goniogel bridge for optimal viewing. The Zeiss gonioprism uses the patient's tear film as a bridge and is convenient for indentation gonioscopy. On a day-to-day basis, the majority of ophthalmologists still use the Goldmann lens. The additional time and patient inconvenience with this lens inhibit rapid convenient viewing of the angle, and thus many angles go unseen. The Zeiss or equivalent gonioprism allows rapid, easy, convenient viewing but requires additional skill and training. Table 5.1 reviews the advantages and disadvantages of the most common contact lenses used for gonioscopy. On a busy patient day the Zeiss or equivalent gonioprism (Posner, Sussman) is the most convenient contact lens for rapidly evaluating any chamber angle, narrow or open, and the Goldmann or equivalent gonioprism with antireflective coating is best for laser therapy.

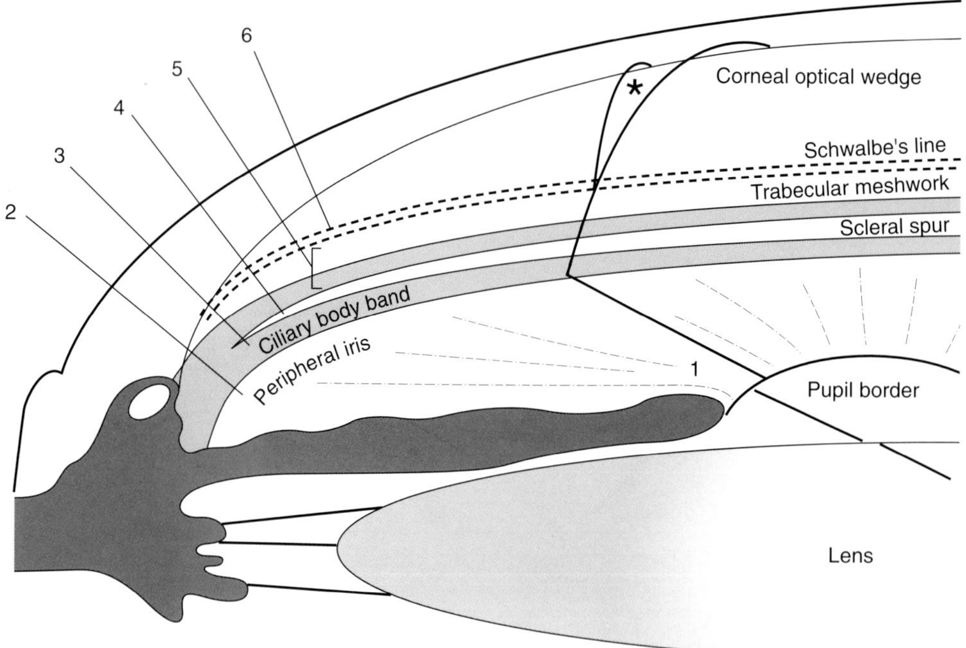

Figure 5.5 Six key landmarks of the anterior chamber angle
If you can identify the six key structures, then all components of the outflow system have been described. The three most important landmarks from a diagnostic and therapeutic viewpoint are the point of insertion of the iris on to the inner wall of the eye, the scleral spur and the trabecular meshwork. The same key for the six landmarks is used for all diagrams. 1 = pupil border; 2 = peripheral iris; 3 = ciliary body band; 4 = scleral spur; 5 = trabecular meshwork; 6 = Schwalbe's line; * = corneal optical wedge.

Table 5.1 **Contact lenses used for gonioscopy**

Contact lens	Type	Advantage	Disadvantage
Koeppe	Direct	Convenient for examination under anesthesia (EUA), no angle distortion, able to view fundus, easiest for angle photography, excellent anatomic view, panoramic view	Patient must be in supine position, laborious examination, patient dislikes, examiner must change position, gonioscope or operating microscope required
Barkan	Direct	Surgical goniolens with blunted side allows access for goniotomy, variable sizes	Same as Koeppe
Goldmann 3-mirror	Indirect	Excellent gonioprism for neophyte to learn angle anatomy, viscous bridge creates suction effect stabilizing eye for examination and laser therapy	Goniogel required for best view which obscures patient's vision and may compromise further same-day diagnostic tests, corneal abrasion in compromised cornea, part of angle hidden in narrow-angled eyes, time consuming when necessary to evaluate both eyes, artifactual narrowing of the angle
Zeiss 4-mirror	Indirect	Rapid evaluation without goniogel, no corneal compromise with goniogel, further same-day diagnostic tests not compromised, indentation or compression gonioscopy allows expert evaluation of narrow-angled eyes with hidden anatomy, patient friendly, slit lamp friendly with minimal movement to see 360°, option for compression to perform indentation gonioscopy	Must first master Goldmann gonioprism, more hand–eye co-ordination necessary than for Goldmann gonioprism, Unger handle required, easy to apply excessive force causing corneal folds with poor view of angle

Six-point gonioscopy checklist

1) *Pupil border* A scan of the iridocorneal angle starts with the pupillary border, looking for blood vessels, iris cysts and dandruff-like particles. At this point, also view the posterior chamber for diagnostic clues of misdirection, tumors or cyclitic membranes. You may also view the fundus through the contact lens.
2) *Peripheral iris* Identify where the iris inserts onto the inner wall of the eye, describe the peripheral configuration of the iris and characterize the angular approach of the iris to the cornea. The peripheral iris may be flat, steep or bow posteriorly; insert anywhere from ciliary body to cornea; and have an angular approach of 0–40 degrees.
3) *Ciliary body band* The ciliary body band is that portion of the ciliary body muscle seen on gonioscopy. The band is usually tan, gray or dark brown, and typically narrow in hyperopes and wide in myopes. The root of the iris usually inserts onto the ciliary body band directly posterior to the scleral spur. If the iris inserts directly on to the scleral spur, the ciliary body band is not seen.
4) *Scleral spur* The scleral spur is the most notable landmark in the chamber angle. This white band represents the attachment of the ciliary body to the sclera and, if found, the trabecular meshwork is directly anterior to it. The scleral spur separates the conventional trabecular outflow pathway from the uveoscleral outflow pathway. Cyclodialysis clefts appear posterior to the spur and laser trabeculoplasty is carried out anterior

Table 5.2 **Classification systems for gonioscopy**

System	System basis	Angle structures	Classification
Scheie (1957)	Extent of angle structures visualized	All structures seen	Wide open
		iris root not seen	Grade I narrow
		ciliary body band not seen	Grade II narrow
		posterior trabeculum obscured	Grade III narrow
		only Schwalbe's line visible	Grade IV narrow
Shaffer (1960)	Angular width of the recess	Wide open (30°–45°)	Grade 3–4, closure improbable
		moderately narrow (20°)	Grade 2 closure possible
		extremely narrow (10°)	Grade 1 closure probable
		partly or totally closed	Grade 0 closure present
Spaeth (1971)	Angular approach to the recess, configuration of peripheral iris, insertion of iris root	Level of iris insertion	
		Anterior to Schwalbe's line	A.
		Behind (posterior) to Schwalbe's	B.
		s**C**leral spur	C.
		Deep into ciliary body band	D.
		Extremely deep	E.
		angular approach to recess	0°–40°
		peripheral iris configuration	
		regular approach	r
		quirk (posterior bowing)	q
		steep, where iris arises	s

to the spur. This is a critical structure in the delineation of iridocorneal anatomy.

5) *Trabecular meshwork* The trabecular meshwork extends from the scleral spur to Schwalbe's line and typically has a ground-glass appearance best seen with sclerotic scatter. Pigment in the meshwork usually accumulates in the posterior division and facilitates identification. However, any angle structure may accumulate pigment. The junction of the mid and posterior meshwork is the favored location for laser trabeculoplasty. When there is no pigment in the meshwork, the characteristic ground-glass appearance can be best seen with sclerotic scatter.

6) *Schwalbe's line* Schwalbe's line is the termination of Descemet's membrane and is the most anterior angle structure identifiable. Schwalbe's line marks the forward limit of the trabecular meshwork and is easily identified where the anterior and posterior reflections of the corneal optical wedge meet: best seen with the Goldmann lens.

Gonioscopic classification systems

A reliable system is crucial to document and follow the chamber angle. Chart documentation should accurately reflect angle findings. The chamber angle is a very complex structure. For example, during a new-patient examination it is not enough to say the angle is 'open', 'narrow' or slit lamp 4+open. This is tantamount to saying the optic nerve is 'normal'. Even if the nerve looks normal, its appearance is documented with a picture, drawing or description in order to establish a baseline for future reference. The chamber angle is no different—it can change yearly or daily, especially if pharmacologically provoked! The standard of care is to document your findings according to one of the angle classification systems or to annotate your descriptive findings completely. Future reference may indicate the angle has not changed and is 'open', but initially a full angle description is required. For example, a more

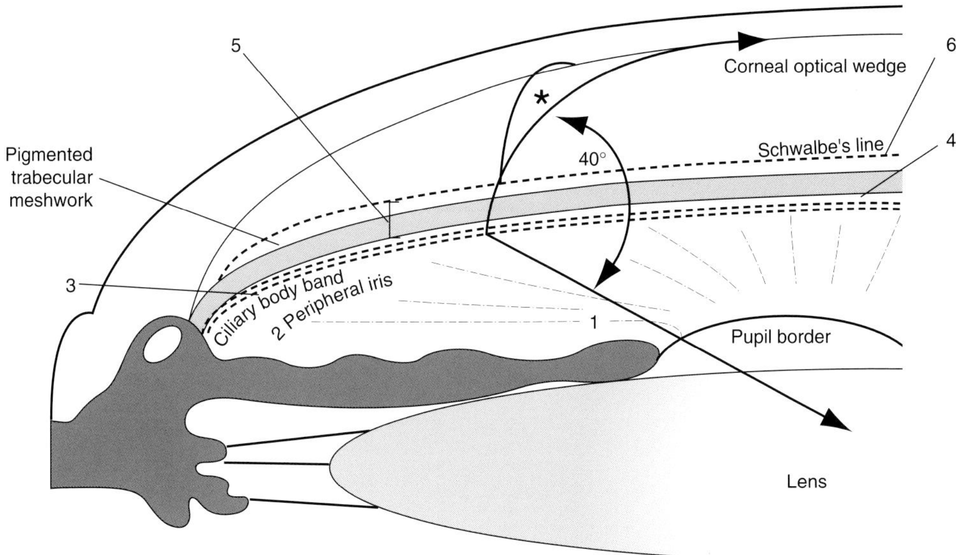

(a)

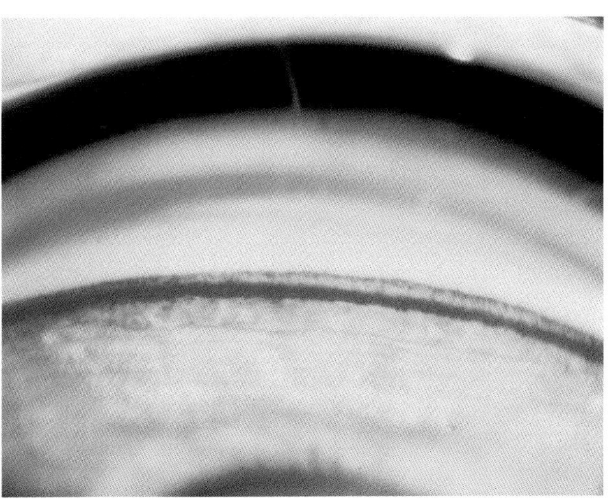

(b)

Figure 5.6 Excessive angle pigmentation
(a) Goniodiagram. (b) Goniophotograph. Grade the angle (refer to Table 5.2). Scheie, wide open; Shaffer Grade 4, wide open, closure improbable; Spaeth, C40r (iris inserts into scleral spur (ciliary body not easily seen)), angular approach 40 degrees, regular (flat) approach of peripheral iris to recess, pigmented meshwork 4+, no synechiae. In normal eyes, trabecular pigmentation is most marked inferiorly. Excessive pigmentation should prompt a search for exfoliation syndrome, pigmentary glaucoma, uveitis, trauma and tumor. 1 = pupil border; 2 = peripheral iris; 3 = ciliary body band; 4 = scleral spur; 5 = trabecular meshwork; 6 = Schwalbe's line; * = corneal optical wedge.

appropriate angle description is 'wide open for 360 degrees, ciliary body band easily seen and moderate trabecular pigmentation'. This angle can be dilated safely and a picture of the angle comes to mind. In addition to classification systems, additional findings such as pigmentation, synechiae, iris processes, clefts, recession, vessels, precipitates, cysts, etc., are noted with their clock-hour location.

Grading the anterior chamber angle

Figures 5.6, 5.7 and 5.8 are all 'open' angles, but their iridocorneal structures vary considerably. Compare the diagram ('a') with the clinical goniophotograph ('b'), and grade the angle.

The challenge of the narrow angle

Additional skills and corneal indentation techniques are necessary to view the crowded or narrow angle. Even with 'routine' gonioscopy there are still unseen vital angle structures. To diagnose and treat the narrow angle adequately, the gonioscopist must understand the relationship between the anterior chamber angle and the viewing mirror and master indentation gonioscopy. A technique for viewing the structures in a crowded anterior chamber angle is illustrated in Figure 5.9.

(a)

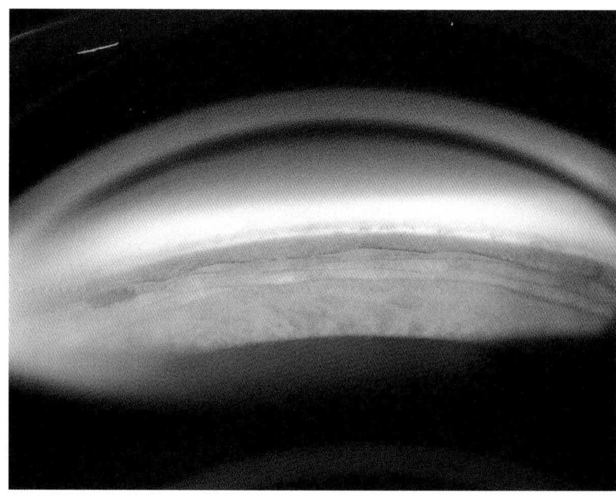

(b)

Figure 5.7 Normal angle
(a) Goniodiagram. (b) Goniophotograph. Grade the angle (see Table 5.2). Scheie, wide open; Shaffer, Grade 4, wide open; Spaeth, D40r. There is minimal pigmentation of the trabecular meshwork, a wide ciliary body band and no synechiae. The ciliary body band is typically wide in myopia, narrow banded in hyperopia and tan in color. The iris inserts deep into the ciliary body band. The trabecular meshwork is difficult to see because it is lightly pigmented. The corneal optical wedge (*) facilitates identification of Schwalbe's line, the anterior extent of the meshwork. In addition, sclerotic scatter (off axis illumination) will help identify the ground-glass appearance of the trabecular meshwork. Without these visual clues, argon laser trabeculoplasty may become argon laser cilioplasty. 1 = pupil border; 2 = peripheral iris; 3 = ciliary body band; 4 = scleral spur; 5 = trabecular meshwork; 6 = Schwalbe's line; * = corneal optical wedge.

Indentation gonioscopy

(Figs 5.10a and b)

Indentation gonioscopy is a technique in which a temporary deepening of the chamber angle due to posterior displacement of aqueous humor by corneal indentation with the Zeiss or equivalent lens is induced. The goal of the technique is to differentiate appositional closure from synechial angle closure in angles which appear to be closed optically. With the gonioprism in the normal position, apply enough force to indent the cornea gently. The amount and force of corneal indentation will vary depending on the level of IOP, shallowness of the chamber and lens thickness. As the iris bows backwards, identify landmarks and remember this is a dynamic process and can be repeated several times. If the iris falls back for 360 degrees and there are no synechiae noted, then optical angle closure exists. If synechiae are identified as the iris bows backwards, then the diagnosis of angle closure disease has been made. Figure 5.11 illustrates many aspects of the narrow angle.

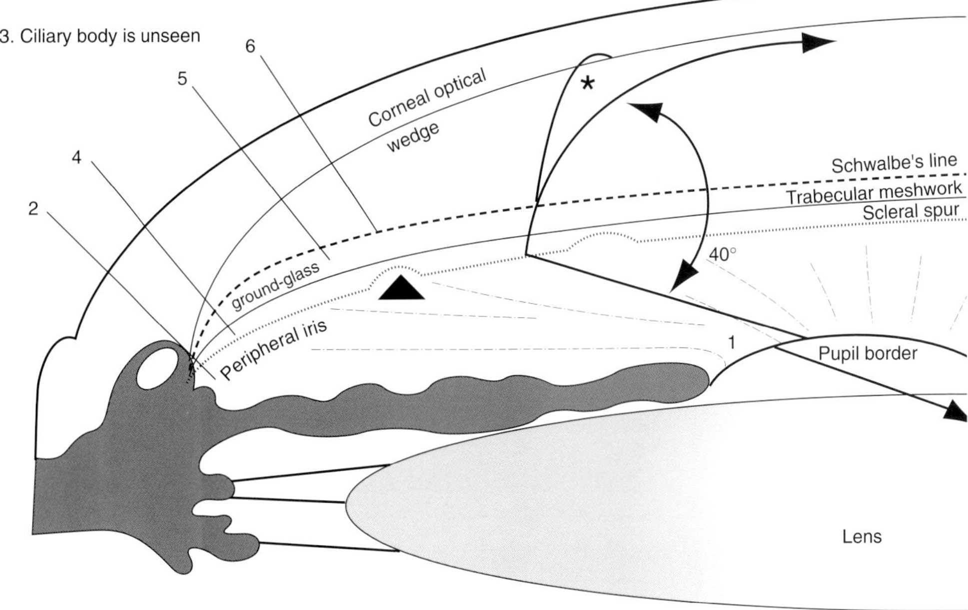

(a)

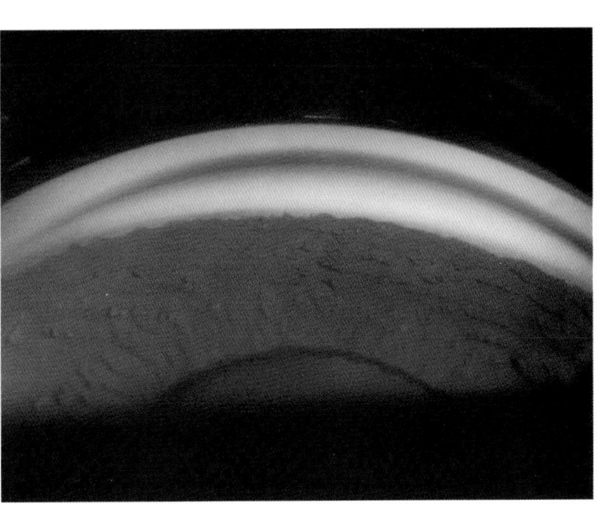

(b)

Figure 5.8 Normal angle
(a) Goniodiagram. (b) Goniophotograph. Grade the angle (refer to Table 5.2). Scheie, wide open; Shaffer, Grade 4, wide open; Spaeth, C40r. This is a difficult angle to evaluate because there are no obvious landmarks. There is no pigmentation to the trabecular meshwork and the ciliary body band is absent (compare to prior goniophotograph). The corneal optical wedge (*) identifies the anterior extent of the meshwork and scleral spur the posterior extent (both require additional gonioscopic skills to see). The iris inserts anteriorly onto the scleral spur in an irregular fashion (▲), creating a high insertion. This increases the likelihood of chronic angle-closure disease, even though the angle is classified as open with the Scheie and Shaffer systems. The Spaeth system identifies the iris as high insertion (C40r), clarifying the exact relationship of iris to chamber recess, adding a warning of some crowding in an 'open angle'. 1 = pupil border; 2 = peripheral iris; 3 = ciliary body band; 4 = scleral spur; 5 = trabecular meshwork; 6 = Schwalbe's line; * = corneal optical wedge.

Normal angle variability

The variability of the normal chamber angle is rarely appreciated because gonioscopy is not routinely performed. Unfortunately, gonioscopy is performed when pathology already exists. Routine gonioscopy reveals wide variation in chamber depth (Figs 5.6b, 5.7b, 5.8b, 5.11a–d); ciliary body band size and color (Figs 5.7b, 5.8b); size, shape and color of iris processes (Fig. 5.12b); angle vessels (Fig. 5.13b); and trabecular pigmentation (Figs 5.6b, 5.7b, 5.8b).

Angle pathology

Gonioscopy significantly added to the diagnosis and management of abnormal and surgical angle findings. Several examples are presented in Figures 5.14–5.19. The use of gonioscopy in laser trabeculoplasty is illustrated in Figure 5.20.

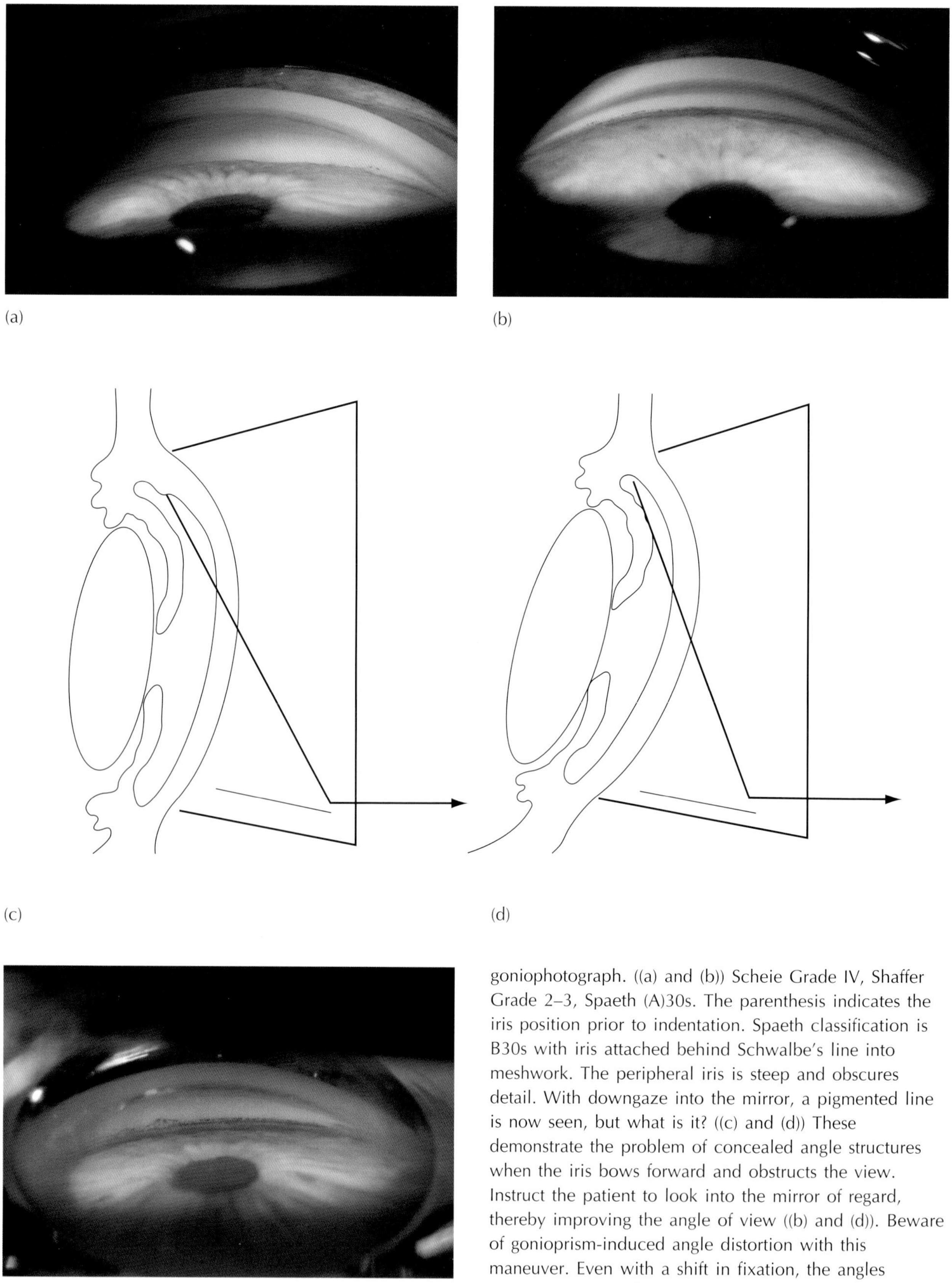

(a)

(b)

(c)

(d)

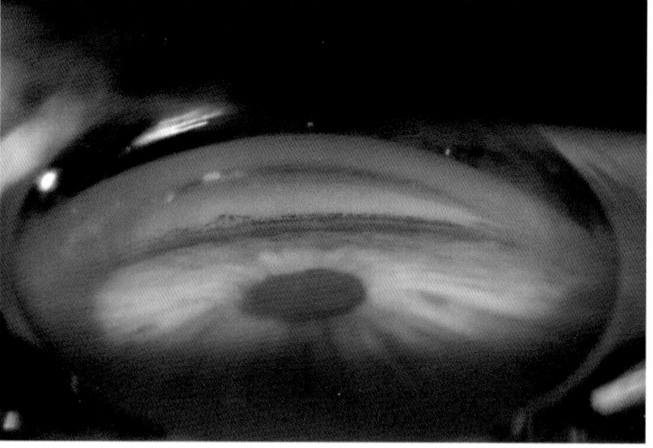

(e)

Figure 5.9 Viewing the crowded angle
(a) Crowded angle Goldmann goniophotograph. (b) Downgaze into mirror. ((c) and (d)) Diagram—eye movement and mirror relationship. (e) Indentation goniophotograph. ((a) and (b)) Scheie Grade IV, Shaffer Grade 2–3, Spaeth (A)30s. The parenthesis indicates the iris position prior to indentation. Spaeth classification is B30s with iris attached behind Schwalbe's line into meshwork. The peripheral iris is steep and obscures detail. With downgaze into the mirror, a pigmented line is now seen, but what is it? ((c) and (d)) These demonstrate the problem of concealed angle structures when the iris bows forward and obstructs the view. Instruct the patient to look into the mirror of regard, thereby improving the angle of view ((b) and (d)). Beware of gonioprism-induced angle distortion with this maneuver. Even with a shift in fixation, the angles structures are poorly seen. However with indentation gonioscopy (e), the pigmented line is actually anterior to Schwalbe's line, and the pigmented posterior meshwork can finally be seen loaded with synechiae. Correct diagnosis and counseling can now begin.

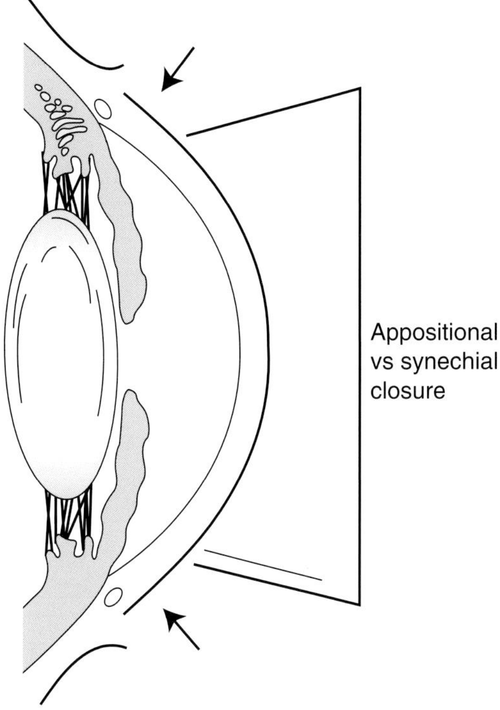

(a)

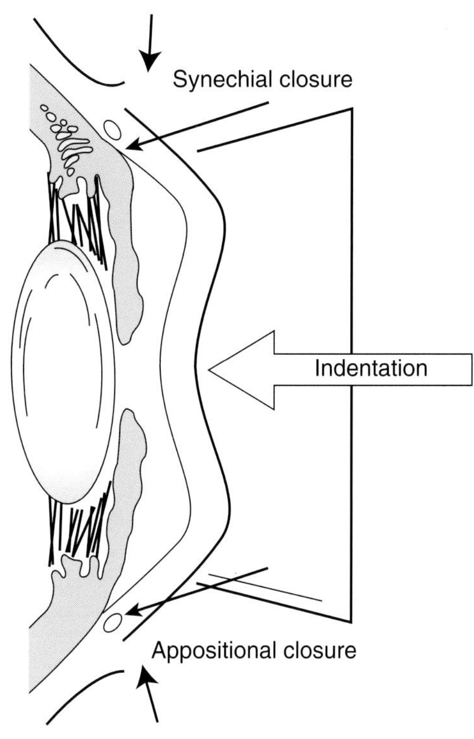

(b)

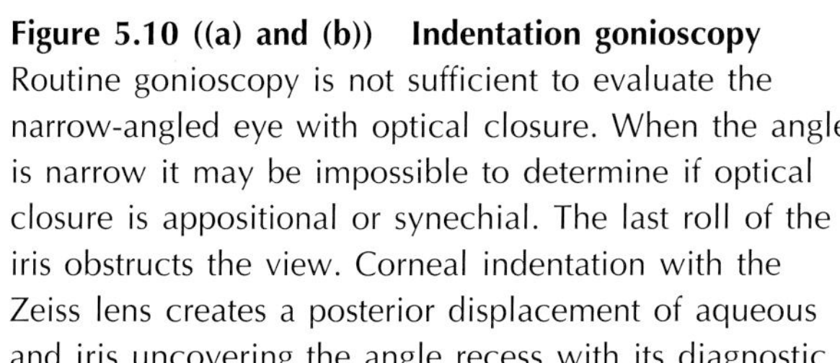

Figure 5.10 ((a) and (b)) Indentation gonioscopy Routine gonioscopy is not sufficient to evaluate the narrow-angled eye with optical closure. When the angle is narrow it may be impossible to determine if optical closure is appositional or synechial. The last roll of the iris obstructs the view. Corneal indentation with the Zeiss lens creates a posterior displacement of aqueous and iris uncovering the angle recess with its diagnostic footprints of disease. Indentation with the Goldmann lens causes distortion of the chamber angle because it has a contact surface of 12 mm and covers the limbus. The Zeiss lens has a contact surface of 9 mm which prevents distortion of the chamber angle. The superior angle in (b) demonstrates synechial closure and the inferior angle appositional closure.

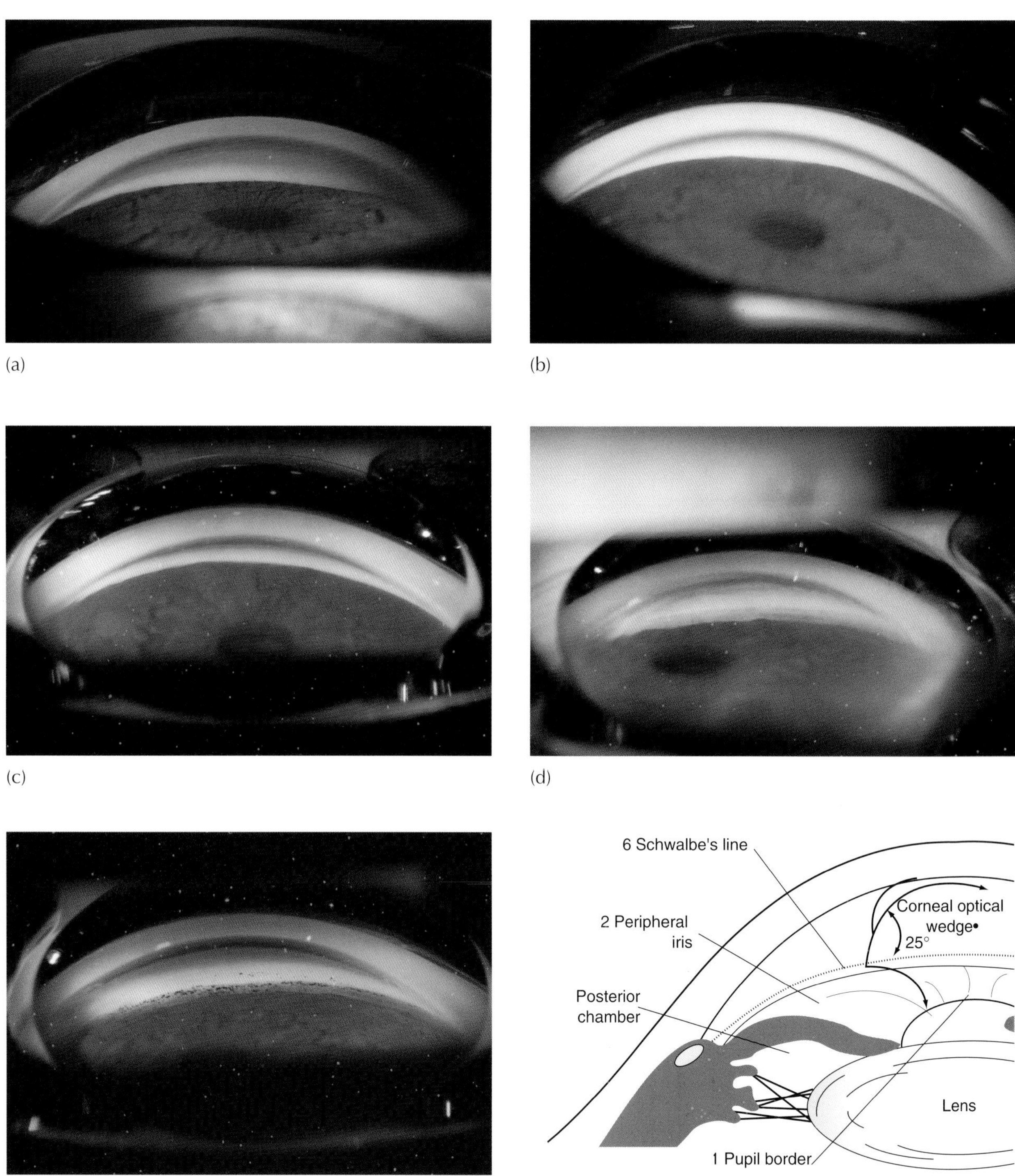

Figure 5.11 The narrow-angled eye as seen with the Goldmann and Zeiss lenses

(a) Narrow angle as seen with the Goldmann lens. (b) Same lens with patient downgaze into the mirror of regard. (c) View of same angle with Zeiss 4-mirror gonioprism. (d) Same lens with indentation view. (e) View of angle post laser iridectomy. (f) Goniodiagram. Views ((a)–(c)) do not differentiate appositional from synechial closure. However with indentation techniques (d), the recess can be seen all the way into scleral spur with minimal pigmentation to the posterior meshwork. The iris is easily displaced posteriorly demonstrating appositional closure. The patient's prognosis can now be explained in meaningful terms. The angle has deepened considerably following laser iridectomy (e). Diagram of angle reveals ciliary body band, scleral spur and trabecular meshwork are all hidden by the iris – Spaeth (A)C25s. (A) in parenthesis implies appearance of iris insertion before indentation and C indicates iris truly inserts into scleral spur.

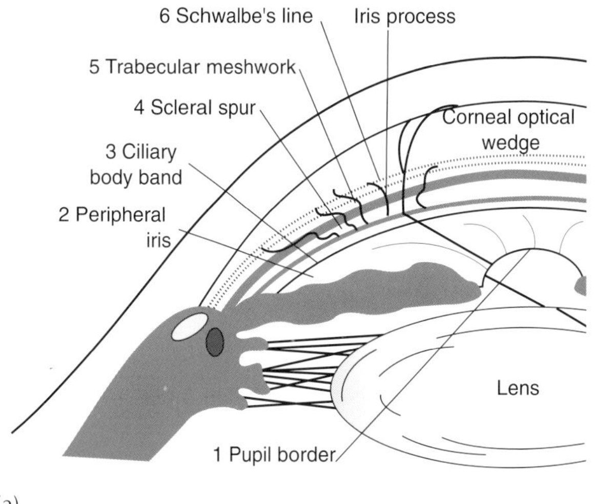

(a)

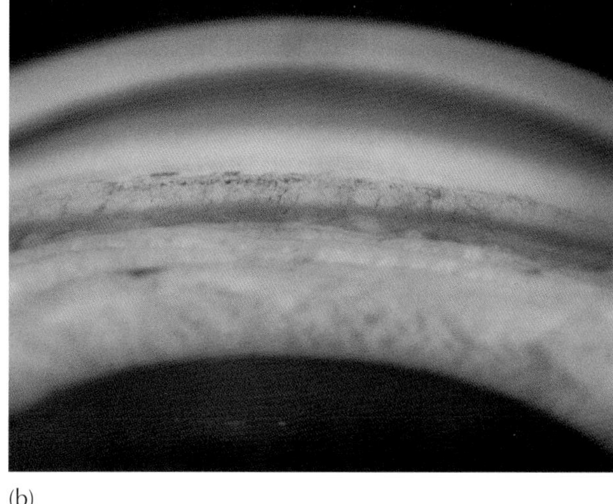

(b)

(c)

Figure 5.12 Iris processes vs peripheral anterior synechiae (PAS)

(a) Goniodiagram of iris processes. (b) Goniophotograph of iris processes. (c) Goniophotograph of PAS. ((a) and (b)) Iris processes are most common nasally, then inferiorly and are present in up to 35% of normals. Iris processes are part of the uveal meshwork, are more common in brown eyes, are filmy and gray in blue eyes and bridge the chamber angle recess. To the neophyte, these normal processes may be confused with peripheral anterior synechiae (PAS). Typically, PAS are most common in the superior angle (c), are broader, denser and obstruct the gonioscopist's view of the scleral spur and trabecular meshwork, even with indentation.

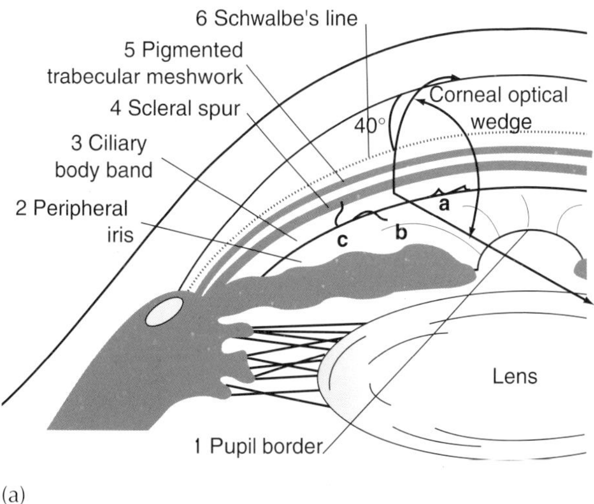

(a)

(b)

Figure 5.13 Normal angle vessels

(a) Goniodiagram. (b) Goniophotograph. Normal angle vessels are most common in blue-eyed individuals and must be differentiated from new vessel formation. Normal angle vessels are gonioscopically visible in 62% of individuals with blue eyes and in 9% with brown eyes. Normal vessels are more common in eyes with deep angles and may take on three different configurations: (a) circular ciliary band vessels (most common); (b) radial iris vessels; and (c) radial ciliary body or rarely trabecular vessels. Normal vessels may bridge the angle recess up to scleral spur but should be considered abnormal if they cross the spur. Abnormal vessels typically arborize and branch out from a feeder vessel and lace the angle structures while crossing the scleral spur. In addition, PAS are frequently associated with abnormal vessels.

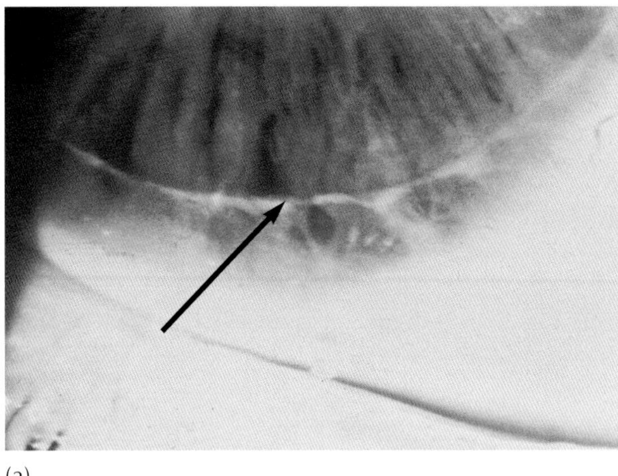
(a)

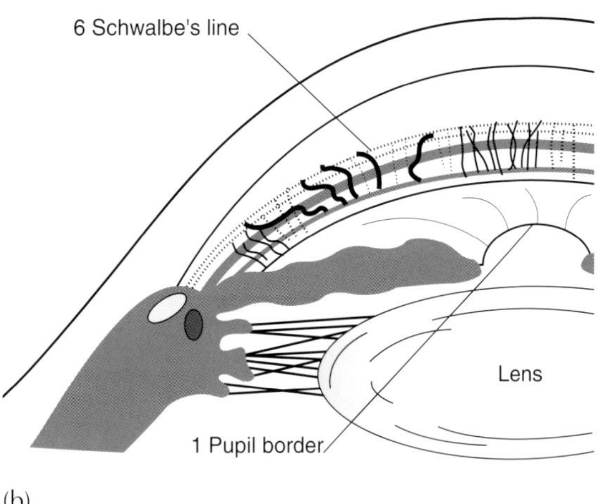

(b)

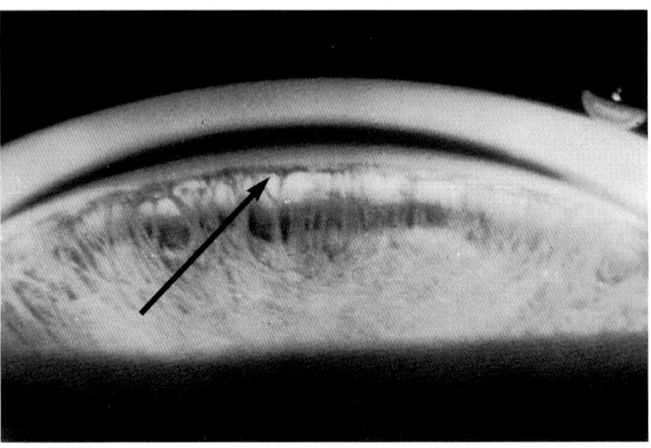
(c)

Figure 5.14 Axenfeld's anomaly
(a) Slit lamp photograph. (b) Goniodiagram. (c) Goniophotograph. Axenfeld's anomaly is a bilateral developmental abnormality of the peripheral cornea, anterior chamber angle and iris stemming from maldevelopment of neural crest cells. The characteristic abnormality of a prominent anteriorly displaced Schwalbe's line (posterior embryotoxon) (arrow) (a) along with bridging prominent iris strands creates the typical picture of this anomaly. These strands may be extremely thick mimicking PAS, (c) arrow. Unless this anomaly is properly recognized, erroneous therapeutic intervention may occur. In addition, this anomaly includes a wide spectrum of developmental abnormalities and may be associated with glaucoma and various systemic abnormalities.

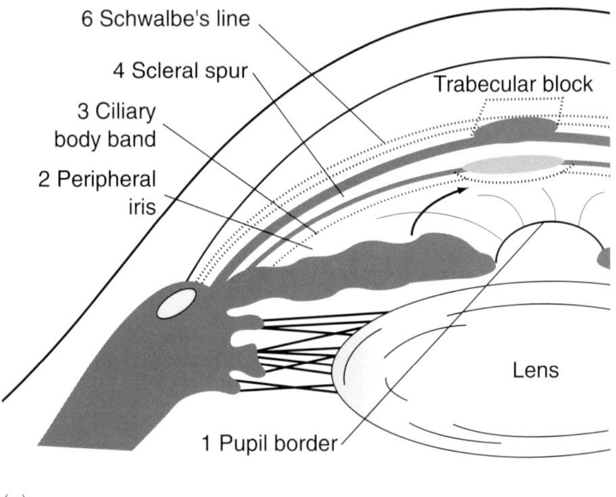

(a)

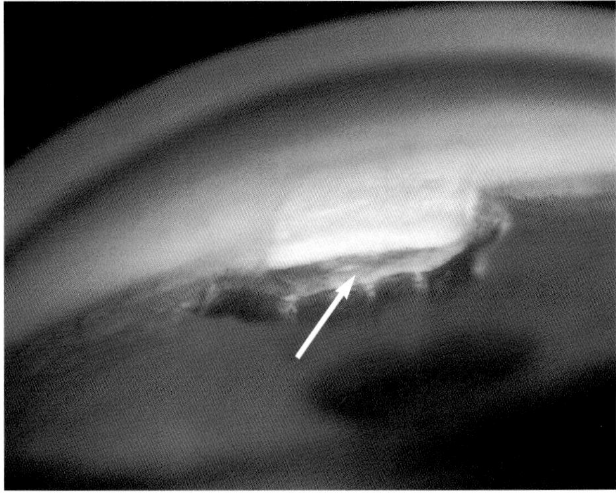
(b)

Figure 5.15 Trabeculectomy block with cyclodialysis cleft
(a) Goniodiagram. (b) Goniophotograph. Gonioscopy following trabeculectomy reveals several alterations to normal anatomy. During trabeculectomy, a block of trabecular tissue including trabecular meshwork and Schwalbe's is removed and can be seen as a rectangular defect. If the scleral spur is excised with the trabecular block, a cyclodialysis cleft may result (arrow). A cyclodialysis cleft is a separation of the ciliary body from its attachment to the scleral spur. These clefts may cause undesirable hypotony and may be traumatic or surgical in origin. In contrast to a cyclodialysis, a separation of the iris root from the scleral spur is an iridodialysis.

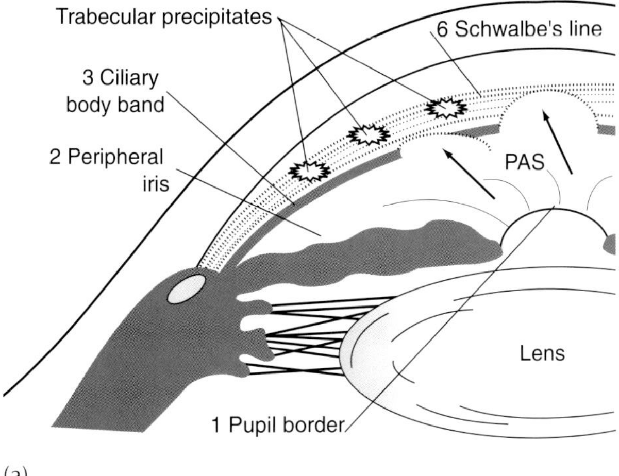

(a)

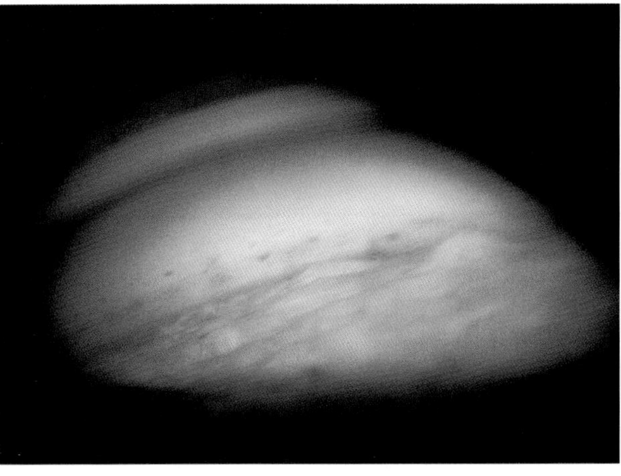

(b)

Figure 5.16 Trabeculitis
(a) Goniodiagram. (b) Goniophotograph. Inflammatory glaucoma due to trabeculitis is impossible to diagnose without gonioscopy. Fresh trabecular precipitates are white and best seen with indirect light and sclerotic scatter. These precipitates are extremely difficult to see, typically bilateral and develop in the lower angle but may be at any clock hour, and may be present without any other signs of anterior segment inflammation. As the precipitates age, they darken, become easier to see and when peripheral iris comes in contact with these inflammatory foci, PAS develop. PAS may start at the ciliary body band and then extend into the trabecular meshwork. Miotic drugs break down the blood–aqueous barrier and worsen this type of glaucoma while topical corticosteroids, or nonsteroidal anti inflammatory agents, decrease trabecular inflammation and prevent further synechial angle closure.

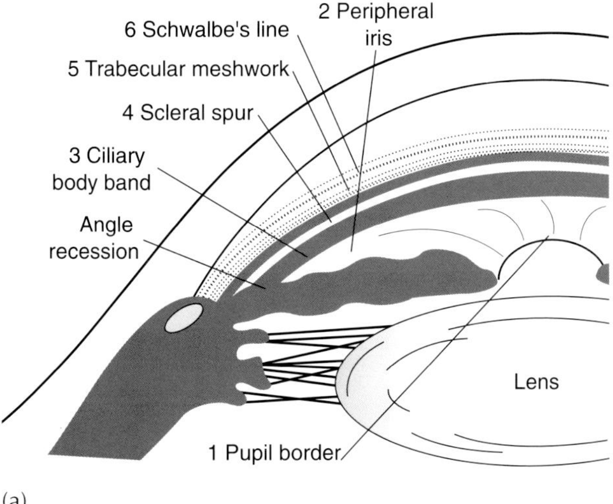

(a)

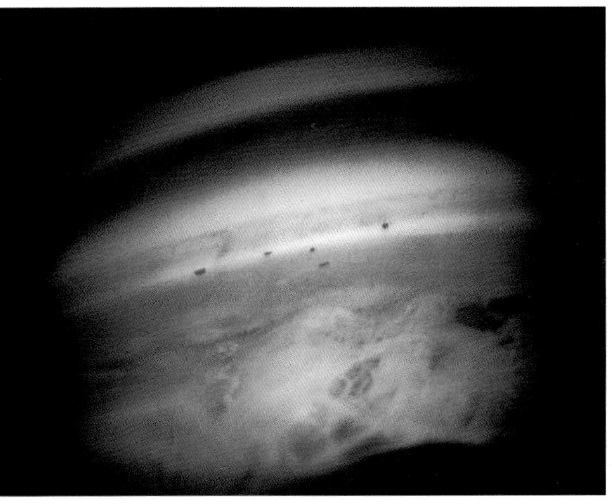

(b)

Figure 5.17 Angle recession
(a) Goniodiagram. (b) Goniophotograph. Gonioscopy is the only method of diagnosing angle recession, a common sequela of blunt ocular trauma. A very wide irregular ciliary body band should raise the question of ocular trauma. Bilateral gonioscopy is the key to make this diagnosis for the ciliary body band will appear normal in one eye and extremely wide in the other. A diagnosis of angle recession requires a lifetime of vigilance for glaucoma. Blunt trauma shears the root of the iris posteriorly past its normal insertion site. Commonly, only part of the angle is recessed, revealing a variable insertion of the iris onto the wall of the eye. Angle recession is a footprint of past trauma that probably altered trabecular anatomy as well.

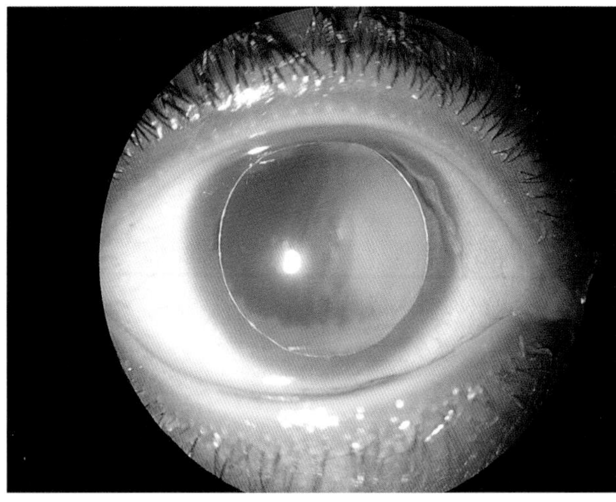

(a)

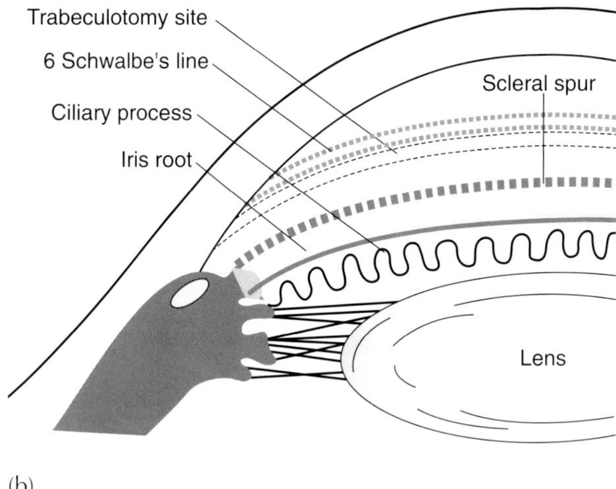

(b)

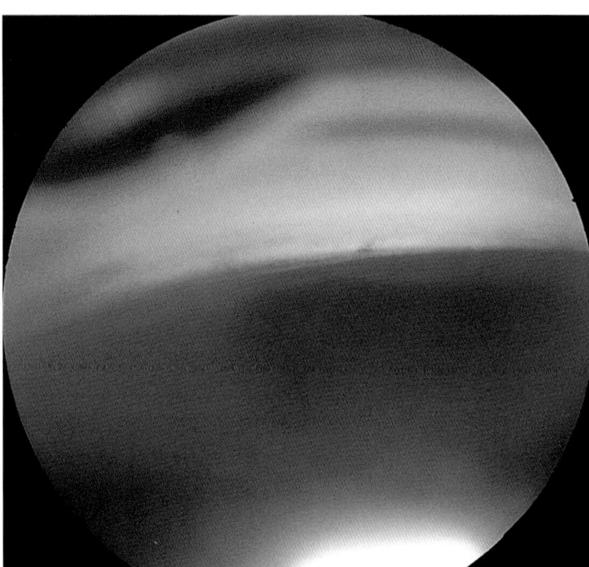

(c)

Figure 5.18 Aniridia

(a) Slit lamp photograph. (b) Goniodiagram. (c) Goniophotograph of trabeculotomy site. Aniridia is a bilateral disorder characterized by congenital absence of the iris, foveal hypoplasia, polar cataract, corneal pannus and refractory glaucoma. The association with Wilm's tumor of the kidney should always be evaluated. (a) This clearly shows the absence of iris with the shimmering edge of the lens. Gonioscopy reveals the root of the iris usually persists and may lead to PAS following angle surgery. Trabeculotomy consists of a mechanical opening of the poorly developed Schlemm's canal and outflow area with either a metal trabeculotome or suture technique (filamentary trabeculotomy). Careful observation of the goniophotograph reveals an area where Schlemm's canal is still open, post trabeculotomy.

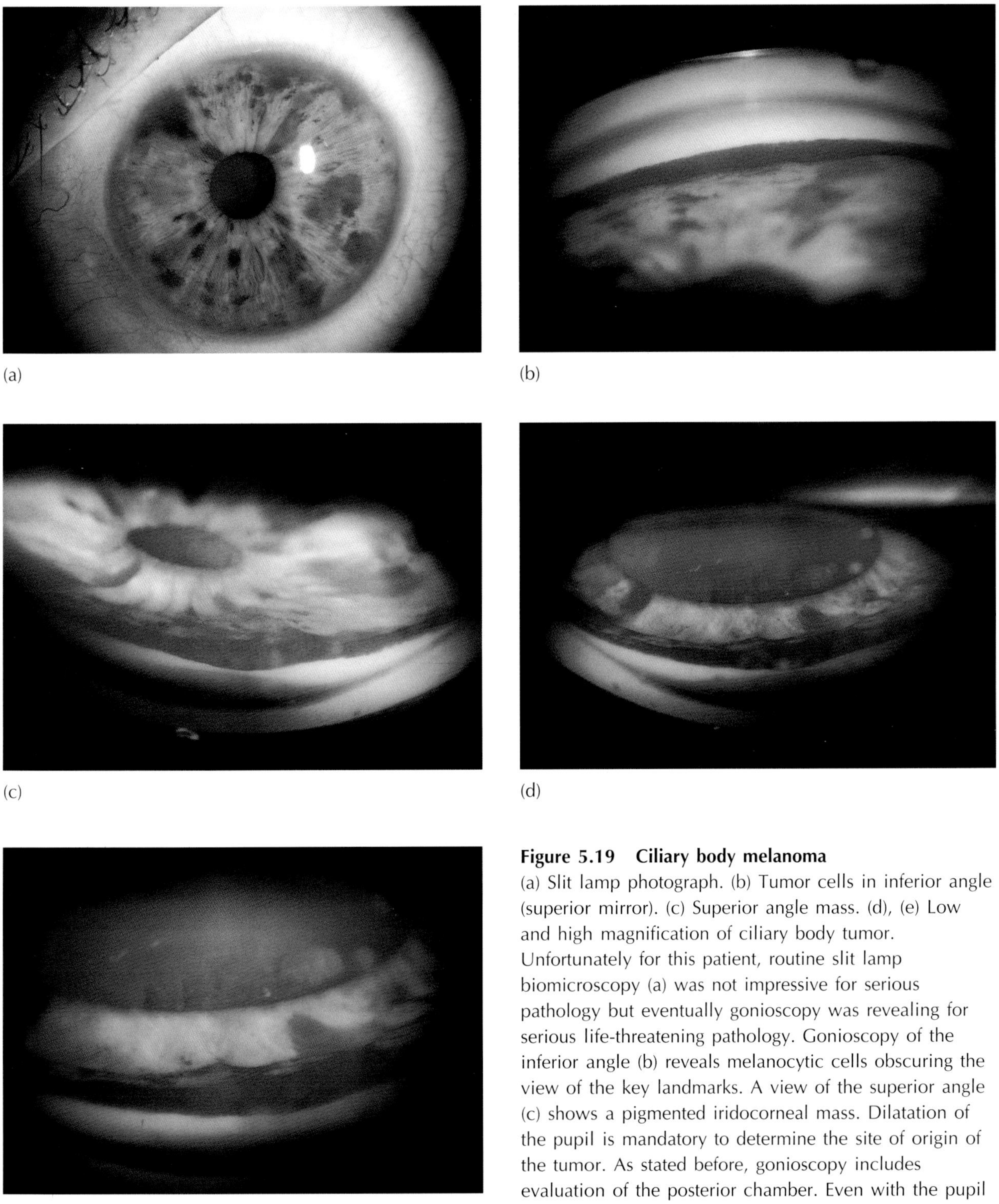

(a)

(b)

(c)

(d)

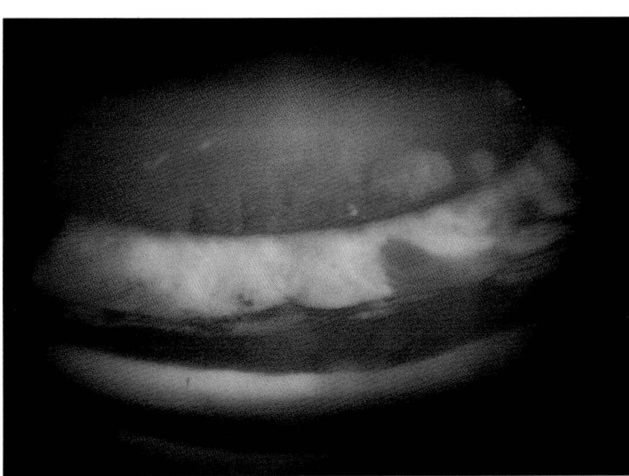

(e)

Figure 5.19 Ciliary body melanoma

(a) Slit lamp photograph. (b) Tumor cells in inferior angle (superior mirror). (c) Superior angle mass. (d), (e) Low and high magnification of ciliary body tumor. Unfortunately for this patient, routine slit lamp biomicroscopy (a) was not impressive for serious pathology but eventually gonioscopy was revealing for serious life-threatening pathology. Gonioscopy of the inferior angle (b) reveals melanocytic cells obscuring the view of the key landmarks. A view of the superior angle (c) shows a pigmented iridocorneal mass. Dilatation of the pupil is mandatory to determine the site of origin of the tumor. As stated before, gonioscopy includes evaluation of the posterior chamber. Even with the pupil dilated, the extent of the tumor cannot be seen without gonioscopy. However, with gonioscopy through a dilated pupil, the tumor-laden ciliary body is easily seen under low (d) and high (e) magnification. This was a highly aggressive ciliary body tumor that seeded the chamber angle. Even with enucleation, the tumor spread to the liver claiming the life of this patient.

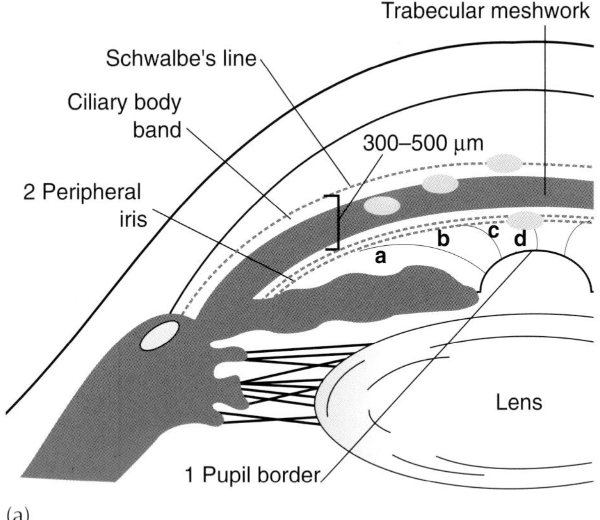

(a)

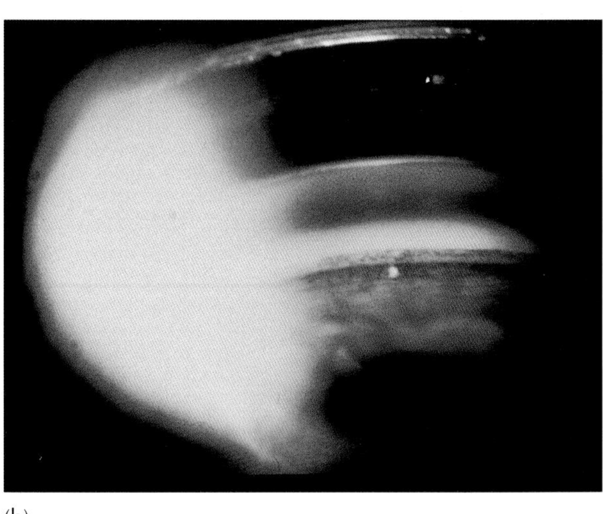

(b)

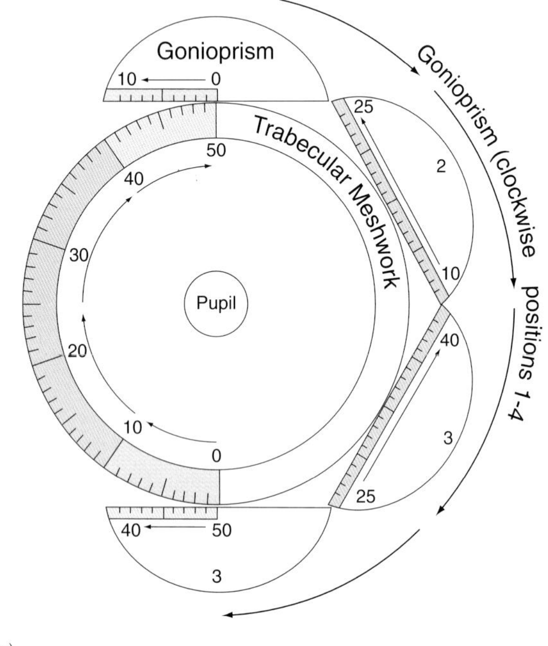

(c)

Figure 5.20 Variable trabeculoplasty location and goniolens rotation

(a) Goniodiagram of variable laser trabeculoplasty sites. (b) Goniophotograph of argon laser trabeculoplasty. (c) Rotation of goniolens during trabeculoplasty. Laser treatment of the chamber angle should be the culmination of understanding normal variability, classifying glaucomas and treating the appropriate structures. A wide-open iridocorneal angle covers 300–500 μm from scleral spur to Schwalbe's line and the laser beam is only 50 μm. Therefore, there may be room to treat the posterior (a), mid (b) or anterior (c) trabecular meshwork. Typically the mid to posterior meshwork is most often treated (b). Avoid treating the scleral spur and ciliary body band (d) which leads to inflammation and PAS formation. The color-coded correlation of gonioprism mirror and angle structures treated is seen in (c). Clockwise treatment of the *patient's* right half of the angle is achieved by rotating the goniolens in a clockwise manner (curved arrows, position 1–4). When treating the right half of the patient's angle, the actual movement of the laser beam in the mirror of the goniolens is in a counterclockwise manner, as illustrated by the straight arrows.

FURTHER READING

Campbell DG, A comparison of diagnostic techniques in angle-closure glaucoma. *Am J Ophthalmol* (1979) **88**:197–204.

Chandler PA, Grant WM, *Lectures on glaucoma* (Philadelphia, PA: Lea & Febiger, 1954).

Fellman RL, Spaeth GL, Starita RJ, Gonioscopy: key to successful management of glaucoma. In: *Focal points 1984: clinical modules for ophthalmologists* (San Francisco, CA: American Academy of Ophthalmology,

Fellman RL, Starita RJ, Spaeth GL, Reopening cyclodialysis cleft with Nd:YAG laser following trabeculectomy, *Ophthalmic Surg* (1984) **15**:285–8.

Forbes M, Gonioscopy with corneal indentation. A method for distinguishing between appositional closure and synechial closure, *Arch Ophthalmol* (1966) **76**:488–92.

Henkind P, Angle vessels in normal eyes. A gonioscopic evaluation and anatomic correlation. *Br J Ophthalmol* (1964) **48**:551–7.

Lichter PR, Iris processes in 340 eyes, *Am J Ophthalmol* (1969) **68**:872–8.

Lynn JR, Fellman RL, Starita RJ, Full circumference trabeculotomy: an improved procedure for primary congenital glaucoma, *Ophthalmology* (1988) 95(suppl):168.

Palmberg P, Gonioscopy. In: Ritch R, Shields MB, Krupin T, eds. *The glaucomas*, 2nd edn. (St Louis, MO: Mosby, 1996), 457.

Scheie H, Width and pigmentation of the angle of the anterior chamber. A system of grading by gonioscopy, *Arch Ophthalmol* (1957) **58**:510–12.

Shaffer RN, Gonioscopy, ophthalmoscopy and perimetry, *Trans Am Acad Ophthalmol Otolaryngol* (1960) **64**:112–25.

Shields MB, Axenfeld–Rieger syndrome. A theory of mechanism and distinctions from the iridocorneal endothelial syndrome, *Trans Am Ophthal Soc* (1983) **81**:736.

Shields MB, Aqueous humor dynamics. II. Techniques for evaluating. In: *Textbook of glaucoma*, 3rd edn. (Baltimore, MD: Williams & Wilkins, 1992), 38–40.

Spaeth GL, The normal development of the human anterior chamber angle: a new system of descriptive grading, *Trans Ophthalmol Soc UK* (1971) **91**:709–39.

Starita RJ, Rodrigues MM, Fellman RL, Spaeth GL, Histopathologic verification of position of laser burns in argon laser trabeculopathy, *Ophthalmic Surg* (1984) **15**:854–8.

Sugar HS, Concerning the chamber angle, *Am J Ophthalmol* (1940) **23**:853–66.

6 The optic nerve in glaucoma

Gustavo E Gamero and Robert D Fechtner

Introduction

The glaucomas are characterized by optic nerve (ON) damage and corresponding changes in visual function as may be seen with visual field testing. An appreciation of the anatomy of the normal ON and the pathologic changes that occur in glaucomatous optic neuropathy (GON) is essential for the detection and monitoring of these diseases.

Anatomy of the optic nerve

Normal nerve

Structure

The optic nerve (cranial nerve II) originates in the ganglion cells of the retina. Their axons (also known as nerve fibers) converge in the posterior pole of the eye and exit through the scleral canal constituting most of the ON tissue. In a healthy middle-aged adult the ON is composed of approximately 0.8–1.2 million axons. This number is higher in the newborn and diminishes gradually throughout life as a result of an estimated loss of 5000 nerve fibers per year, although these figures have been challenged. From its origin in the eye until it reaches the optic chiasm in the anterior cerebral fossa the ON can be divided in four segments as illustrated in Figure 6.1: intraocular (1 mm), which consists of the nerve fiber layer (NFL), prelaminar, laminar and retrolaminar portions; intraorbital (20–25 mm); intracanalicular (4–10 mm); and intracranial (10 mm).

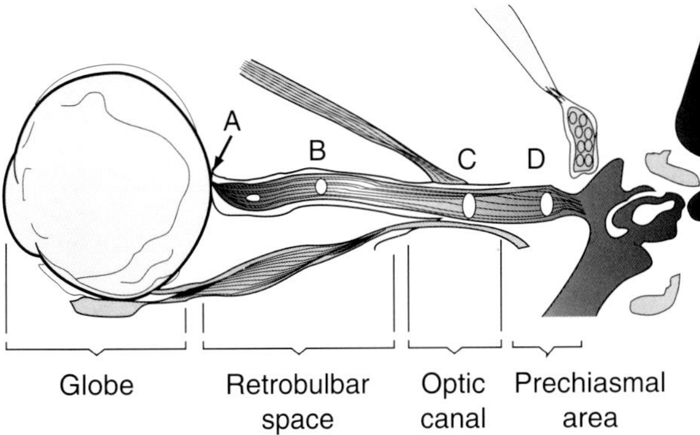

Figure 6.1 Division of the optic nerve
Topographic division of the optic nerve from its origin in the globe to the optic chiasm. A Intraocular. B Intraorbital. C Intracanalicular. D Intracranial. (Adapted from: Hogan MJ, Zimmerman LE, *Ophthalmic pathology. An atlas and textbook.* (Philadelphia, PA: Saunders, 1962), 57.)

The intraocular portion of the ON is also referred to as the optic nerve head (ONH). The visible most anterior part of the ONH is known as the optic disc. The average optic disc is slightly more elongated vertically (1.9 mm) than horizontally (1.7 mm). There is significant variation in the area of normal optic discs. Histologically its most anterior portion, the nerve fiber layer, is composed mainly of unmyelinated axons with some astroglial tissue in between. After traveling on the surface of the retina, these axons turn 90 degrees away from the retinal surface at the scleral canal to exit the eye arranged in approximately 1000 bundles or fascicles. The more peripheral nerve fibers turn into the ON closer to the scleral rim therefore occupying the periphery of the ON. The more central fibers exit the eye closer to the axis of the scleral canal and thus travel more centrally within the ON substance (Fig. 6.2).

As they pass through the prelaminar portion (at the level of the retina and peripapillary choroid), the nerve fibers are still surrounded by astroglia and will exit the eye through a modified region of the eye wall known as the lamina cribrosa. Despite being totally surrounded by scleral tissue the lamina cribrosa has a distinctive histologic structure and collagen configuration. It is composed of 8–12 roughly parallel layers of connective and elastic tissue with 500 to 600 orifices or pores of variable diameter which convey the nerve fascicles. This

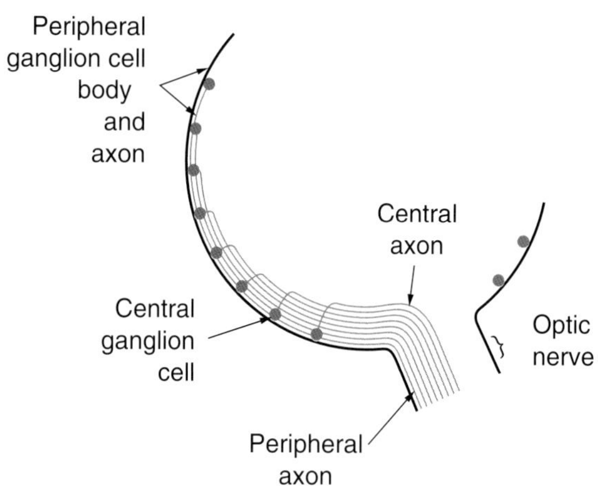

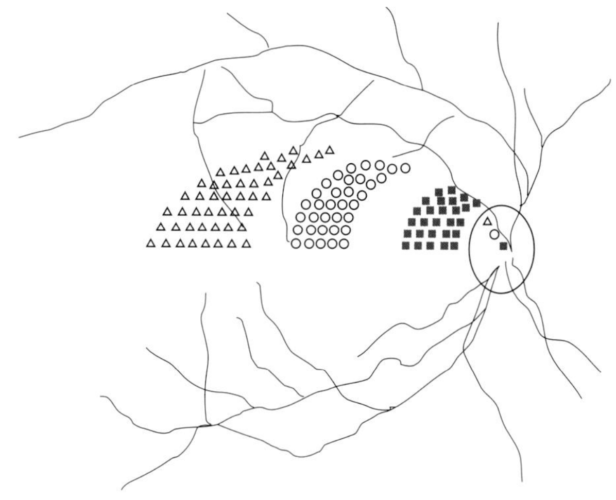

Figure 6.2 Retinotopic organization of the ganglion cell axons
(a) The retinotopic organization of the ganglion cell axons as they enter the optic nerve. Note that axons from peripheral retinal ganglion cells occupy a more peripheral position in the optic nerve. Axons from retinal areas closer to the disc are located more centrally in the nerve. (b) A frontal view of the distribution pattern of axons as shown in (a). The same retina–optic nerve correspondence of fibers is represented. (From Minckler DS, *Arch Ophthalmol* (1980) **98**:1630.)

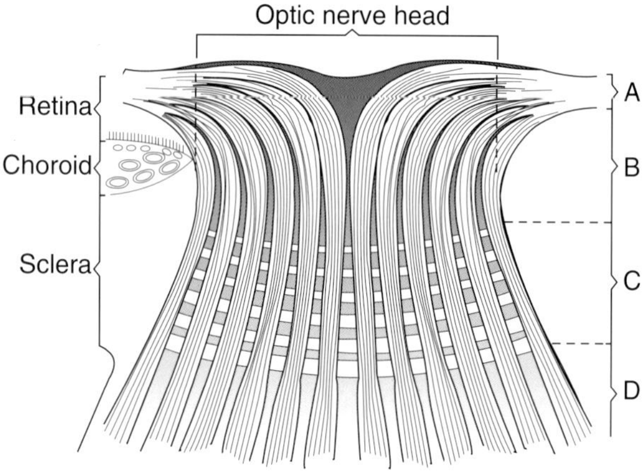

Figure 6.3 Schematic subdivision of the optic nerve head in four portions
A, Nerve fiber layer. B, Prelaminar. C, Laminar. D, Retrolaminar. (Reproduced with permission from Shields MB, *A study guide for glaucoma* (Baltimore, MD: Williams & Wilkins, 1982), 79.)

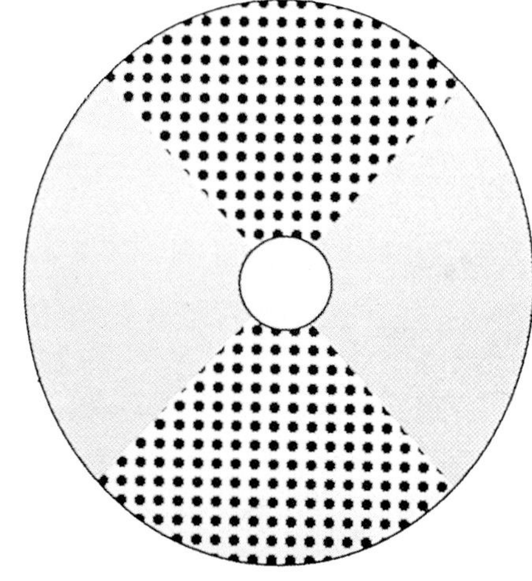

Figure 6.4 Lamina cribrosa
Diagram of the lamina cribrosa showing its laminar orifices and their regional variation. Note the hour-glass distribution of the larger orifices (superiorly and inferiorly) which correspond with the more susceptible areas of ONH damage in glaucoma.

specialized tissue provides mechanical and nutritional support to the axons. The lamina cribrosa along with the nerve bundles, capillaries and astroglia constitute the laminar portion of the ONH (Fig. 6.3). The pores of the lamina cribrosa are larger superiorly and inferiorly than nasally and temporally. These larger pores accommodate thicker nerve fascicles and fibers. This apparently results in less mechanical support as fewer connective and elastic tissues exist between them. This histological feature may have clinical implications in the pattern of development of glaucomatous optic nerve damage (Fig. 6.4). Glaucomatous arcuate visual field defects involve fibers passing through these regions.

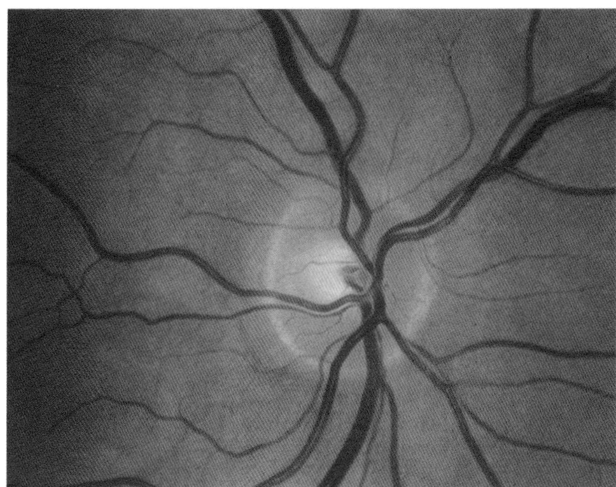

Figure 6.5 Appearance of an average normal optic disc

Note its sharp margins and a pink rim area composed by the ganglion cell axons. The retinal vessels exit from the center of an average-size 0.3 cup.

The optic disc topography is generally described as consisting of the neural rim (the nerve axons) and the optic cup (the central area of the disc surrounded by the neural rim). The optic cup is relatively devoid of nerve fascicles and appears as a round to oval depression of variable size, usually of a lighter color, where the laminar orifices are more noticeable (Fig. 6.5). The diameter of the optic cup divided by the diameter of the optic disc is known as the cup/disc ratio (C/D ratio) and is expressed in decimal notation (0.1, 0.2, etc.). Usually vertical and horizontal C/D ratios are measured and documented. Ninety percent of normal individuals have an average C/D ratio of less than 0.5 measured by direct ophthalmoscopy. However, data obtained by stereoscopic examination and topographic analysis have revealed slightly larger C/D ratios. The size of the optic cup tends to be proportional to the size of the optic disc. Assuming discs of the same size, both cups are quite symmetric in normal individuals, with only 1–2% having more than a 0.2 difference between the eyes. The area occupied by the neural rim is normally pink and ranges from 1.4 to 2.0 mm^2 in normal subjects. It probably diminishes somewhat with age but does not correlate well with the size of the optic disc or the cup. The neural rim is thickest inferiorly, then superiorly, nasally, and is thinnest temporally. The central retinal artery and vein emerge from the nerve near the center of the optic cup in most eyes.

The retrolaminar portion of the optic nerve is short and corresponds to the area where myelin produced by oligodendroglia begins to 'wrap' the nerve nearly doubling its diameter to 3–4 mm. The intraorbital, intracanalicular and intracranial portions of the ON, like the brain, are surrounded by pia mater, arachnoid and dura mater.

Vasculature

Glaucomatous optic neuropathy was once believed primarily to represent a mechanical injury of the ganglion cell axons at the level of the lamina cribrosa induced by elevated intraocular pressure (IOP). In recent years it has been appreciated that GON is probably a multifactorial entity. There has been great interest in the role of microvasculature in the etiology of GON. Emerging technologies are providing new information about blood-flow characteristics in glaucoma. While this information has not yet had an impact on the office management of glaucoma, it may in the future. A thorough knowledge of the blood supply to the ON and its regulatory mechanisms in health and disease may better allow us to understand and treat the causes of glaucoma.

The blood supply of the ONH derives entirely from the ophthalmic artery, mainly through the short posterior ciliary arteries (SPCAs) (Figs 6.6 and 6.7). Some reports have drawn conflicting conclusions regarding the blood supply to the various portions of the ONH. Current evidence shows that the NFL is supplied mainly by branches of the central retinal artery. The prelaminar portion of the ONH is supplied by direct branches of the SPCAs and the circle of Zinn-Haller (an intrascleral vascular structure around the ONH, not always continuous, and originating from branches of the SPCAs). Direct choroidal contribution to the blood supply of the prelaminar region is minimal. The laminar portion is mainly supplied by the SPCAs, with lesser contribution of the circle of Zinn-Haller and occasionally of the peripapillary choroid. The contribution of the choroid to the ONH circulation may have clinical significance. The choroid is a relatively high-flow, low-pressure system with less capacity for autoregulation than the retinal circulation. Consequently, choroidal circulation may be more susceptible to local or systemic factors. The retrolaminar region is supplied by the SPCAs, some intraneural branches of the central retinal artery and perforating pial branches.

Despite regional differences in the architecture of the various capillary plexuses of the ONH they remain interconnected. The endothelial cells of these nonfenestrated capillaries exhibit tight junctions constituting the blood–nerve barrier. The venous drainage of the ONH occurs mainly via the central retinal vein.

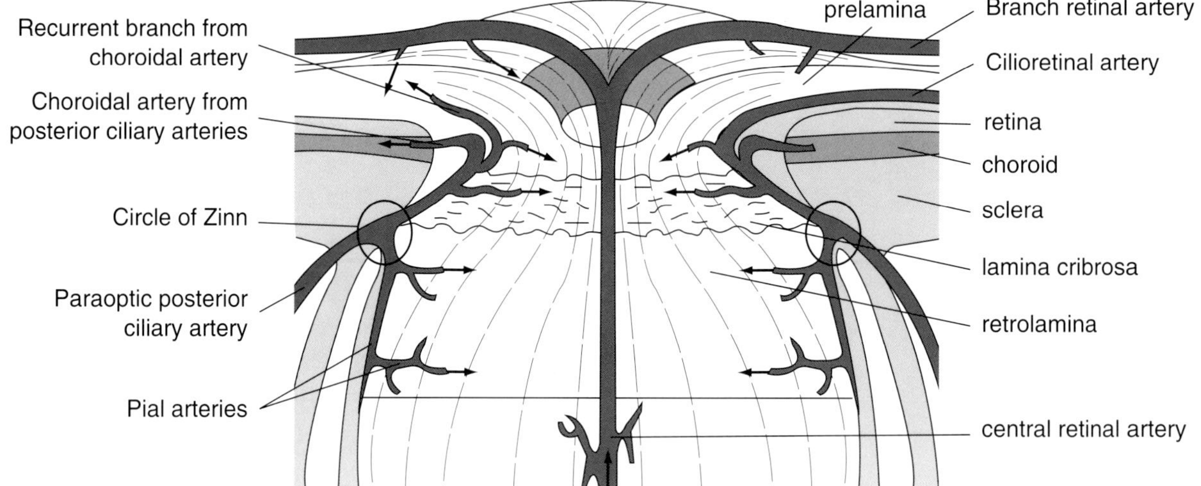

Figure 6.6 The arterial vasculature of the ONH Note the extensive contribution of the short posterior ciliary arteries as well as the intraneural branches from the central retinal artery in the retrolaminar region. (Reproduced with permission from Varma R, Minckler DS, Anatomy and pathophysiology of the retina and optic nerve. In: Ritch R, Shields MB, Krupin T, eds. *The Glaucomas*. 2nd edn. (St Louis, MO: Mosby-Year Book, 1996), 153.)

Variations

The appearance of the ONH depends on the size and shape of the scleral canal, the angle at which the nerve exits the globe, and the number and configuration of axons and vessels passing through this canal. Despite the large variability in the relative sizes of optic discs and cups in normal subjects, the nerve rim area tends to remain fairly constant.

There are a number of factors that affect the appearance of a normal optic nerve head:

- *Age:* optic cups tend to enlarge with age as the number of axons diminishes, although some evidence to the contrary exists.
- *Race:* blacks and Asians have larger discs, cups and C/D ratios than whites, with Hispanics having intermediate sizes. Nonetheless the neural rim area appears to be similar.
- *Gender:* males have slightly larger optic nerves and cups than females, a finding without clinical significance.
- *Refractive error:* hyperopic individuals have smaller globes, discs and cups than emmetropes. High myopes have larger globes, discs and cups even though no direct relationship between disc size and axial length (or refractive error) has been found in lower degrees of myopia. These cups are more difficult to assess due to their shallowness and indistinct margins. Furthermore, these discs tend to be tilted due to an oblique insertion of the ON into the globe (Fig. 6.8).

Glaucomatous optic neuropathy (GON)

The changes in the morphology of the ONH in glaucoma have been characterized extensively in several reviews. The inferior and superior poles of the ONH tend to be affected earlier, causing characteristic arcuate visual field defects. The inferotemporal rim is the most commonly damaged early in the course of the disease. Decreased laminar support in these areas may render nerve fibers more susceptible to damage from elevated IOP.

Even though different patterns of GON have been described, many of the following signs are common to most types of glaucomas and should guide the clinician in the early diagnosis as well as detection of progressive ON damage.

Specific signs

A number of findings are highly suggestive of GON and are important in the diagnosis and follow-up of glaucoma patients:

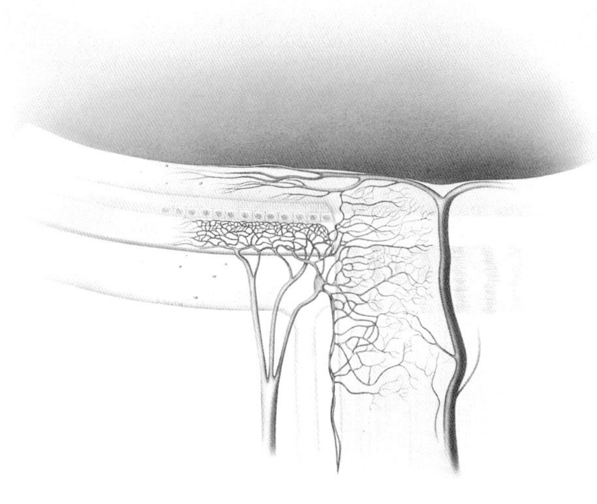

(a)

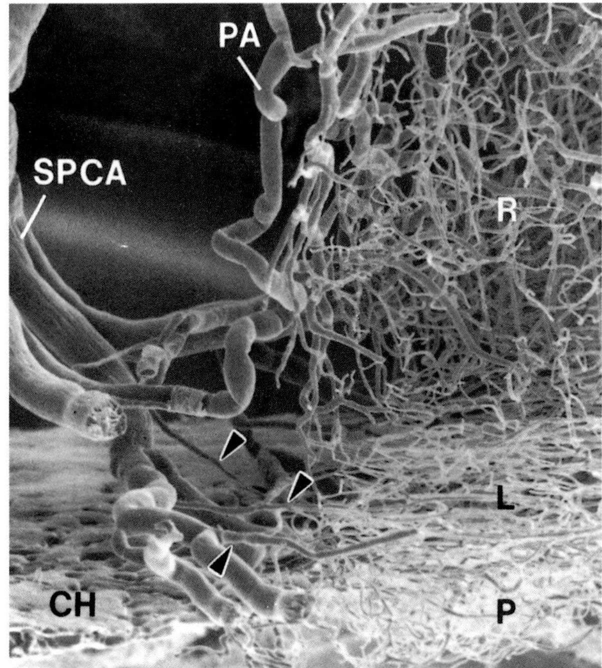

(b)

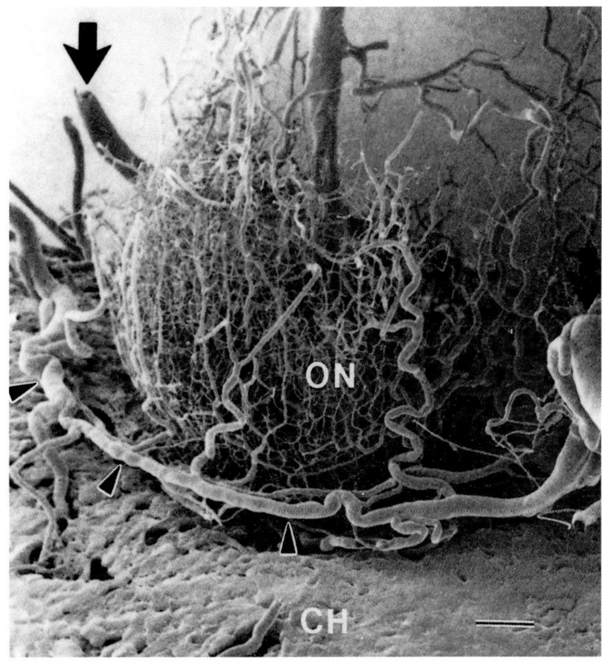

(c)

Figure 6.7 The arterial circulation of the ONH
(a) Note major direct contributions from the short posterior ciliary arteries (SPCA) and from the circle of Zinn-Haller (Z-H), which originates from the SPCA. Additional blood supply derives from pial arteries (PA) and the central retinal artery (CRA). A few choroidal branches contribute to the arterial supply of the ONH (RPE, retinal pigment epithelium; NFL, nerve fiber layer; PL, prelaminar region; L, lamina cribrosa; RL, retrolaminar region; D, dura mater). (b) Microvascular corrosion casting of the human anterior optic nerve. Short posterior ciliary arteries (SPCA) are the main contributors. Some connections (arrowheads) to the pial system (PA) can be seen (CH, choroid; P, prelaminar region; L, lamina cribrosa; R, retrolaminar region). (c) Microvascular corrosion casting of the human anterior optic nerve head (ON). The circle of Zinn-Haller (arrowheads) can be seen originating from the posterior ciliary arteries (black arrows). In this specimen choroidal contributory branches (asterisks) can be seen (CH, choroid). (Reproduced with permission from Cioffi, GA, Van Buskirk, EM, Vasculature of the anterior optic nerve and peripapillary choroid. In: Ritch R, Shields MB, Krupin T, eds. *The Glaucomas.* 2nd edn. (St Louis, MO: Mosby-Year Book, 1996), 179.)

- Progressive enlargement and/or deepening of the cup, when documented, is the hallmark of GON (Fig. 6.9). This appearance is the direct result of axonal loss and backwards bowing of the lamina cribrosa. Some enlarged cups can remain shallow despite extensive axonal loss, but usually advanced cupping produces undermining of the rim, creating what has been called a ‘bean pot’ appearance (Fig. 6.10).
- Vertical elongation of the cup (Fig. 6.9). This change results from preferential loss of the superior and inferior nerve fibers, perhaps due to histological laminar features previously discussed. When present, it represents a highly specific sign of progression.
- Localized nerve rim thinning (‘notching’, Fig. 6.11). A notch of variable magnitude results from focal ON rim damage and usually corresponds to

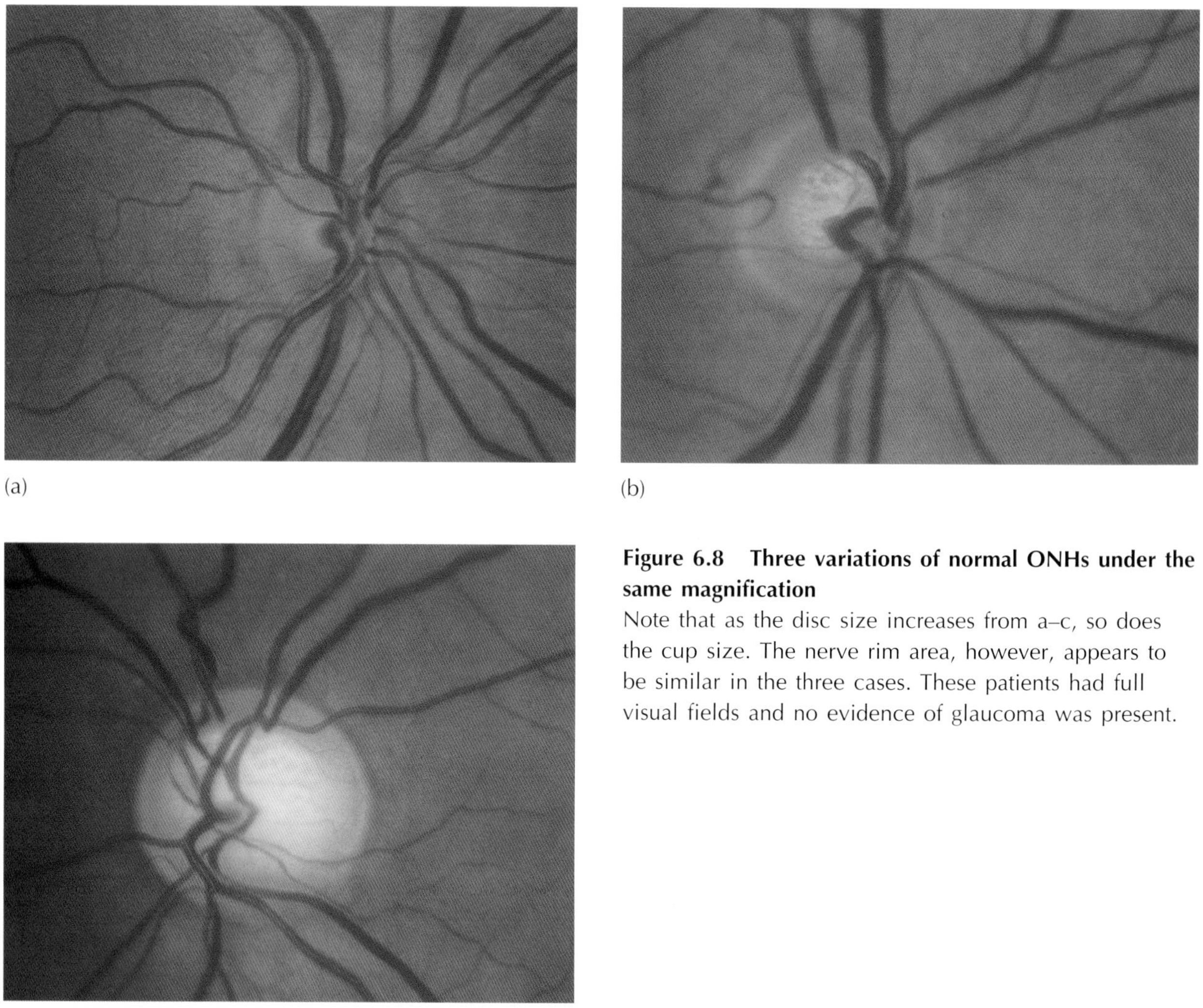

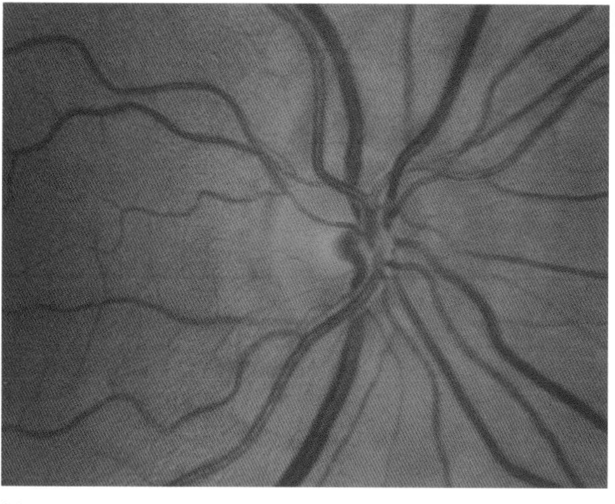
(a)

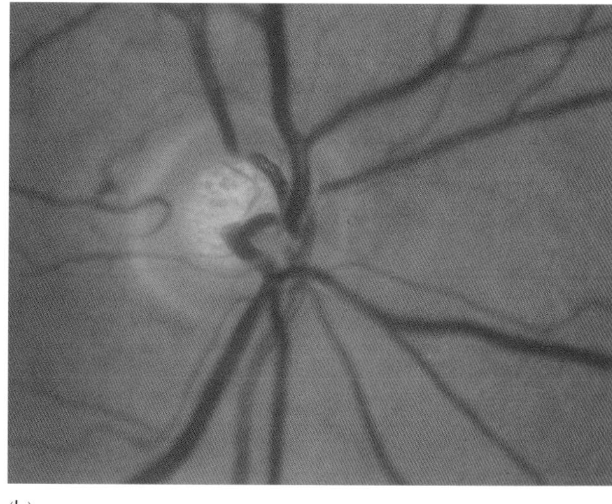
(b)

(c)

Figure 6.8 Three variations of normal ONHs under the same magnification
Note that as the disc size increases from a–c, so does the cup size. The nerve rim area, however, appears to be similar in the three cases. These patients had full visual fields and no evidence of glaucoma was present.

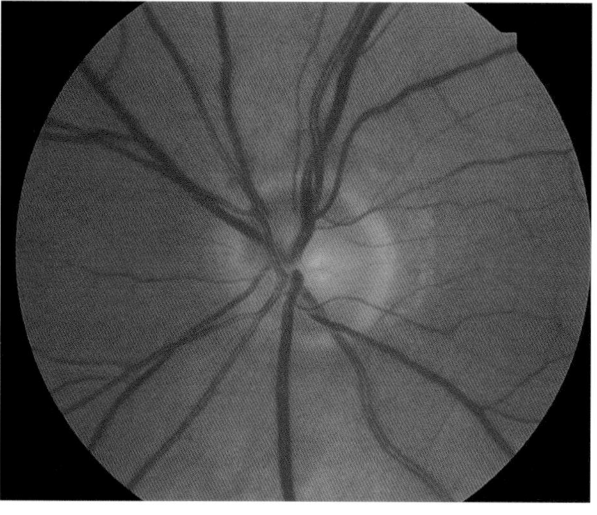
(a)

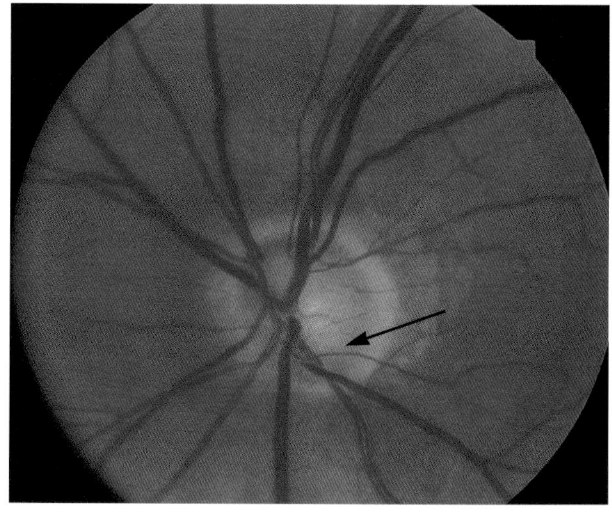
(b)

Figure 6.9 Enlargement of the optic nerve excavation
Sequential photographs showing subtle but definite enlargement of the size of the optic nerve excavation with vertical extension of the cup and a change in the position of a vessel (see arrow). This patient showed a corresponding new visual field defect as a result of this progressive change.

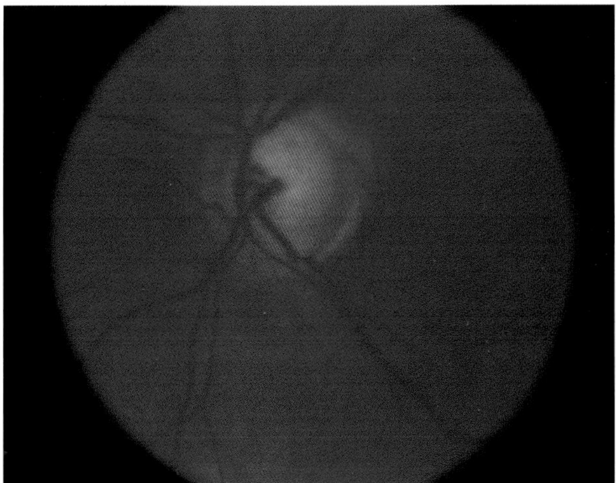

Figure 6.10 'Bean-pot' appearance
Extensive cupping as a result of advanced axonal loss, giving the ONH a 'bean-pot' appearance.

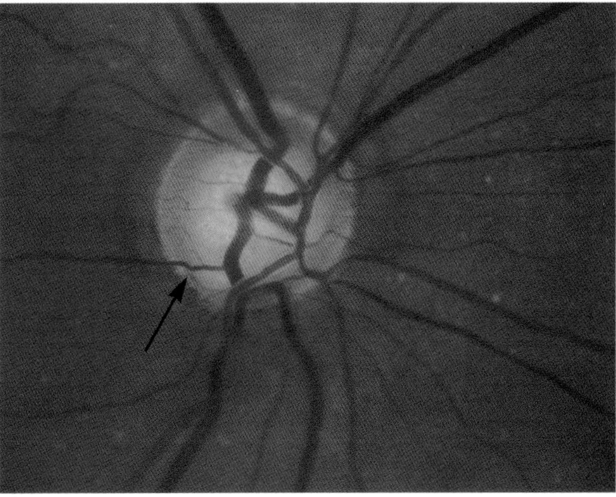

Figure 6.11 Moderately advanced cupping and 'notch'
Moderately advanced cupping in addition to a localized nerve rim loss ('notch') in the inferotemporal region of the ONH (arrow).

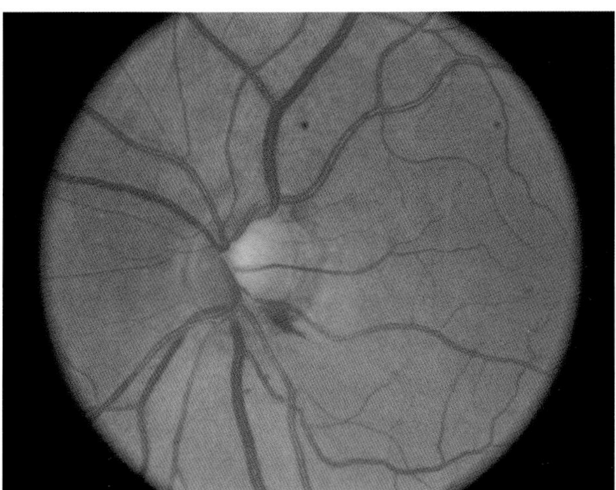

Figure 6.12 Flame-shaped hemorrhage
Characteristic appearance and location of a flame-shaped hemorrhage in the inferotemporal portion of the nerve tim.

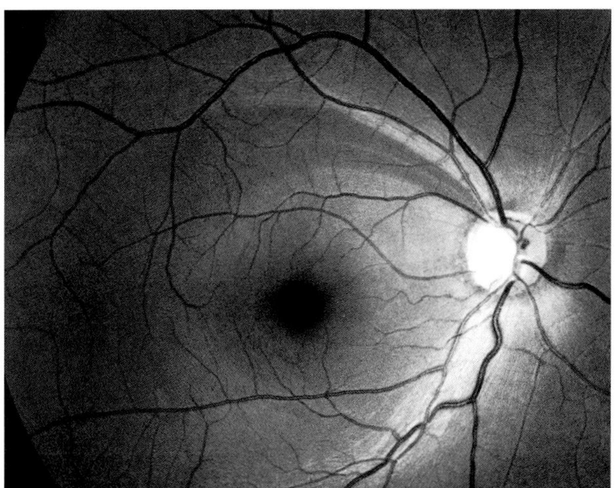

Figure 6.13 Nerve fiber layer defects
Black-and-white nerve fiber layer photograph showing a typical defect in the superior bundle compatible with glaucomatous optic nerve damage. (Courtesy of Frederick Mikelberg, MD.)

visual field changes and NFL loss. Whether this is caused by pressure, focal ischemia or other factors is still controversial.

- Neural rim hemorrhages (Fig. 6.12) are usually small and splinter or flame-shaped and occur at the level of the NFL. They tend to be located on the temporal rim, where they are more common inferiorly than superiorly. Rarely they can occur nasally. They resolve, often leaving a focal NFL loss and, depending on the severity, a corresponding visual field defect. These hemorrhages are more common in eyes with normal-tension glaucoma and have a prognostic significance, usually indicating progression of disease. Since they often precede the occurrence of a focal notch on the ONH, it is possible that both findings originate through the same mechanism.
- Nerve fiber layer defects (Fig. 6.13) can be highly specific for the diagnosis of glaucoma. They occur as a result of axonal loss at the ONH

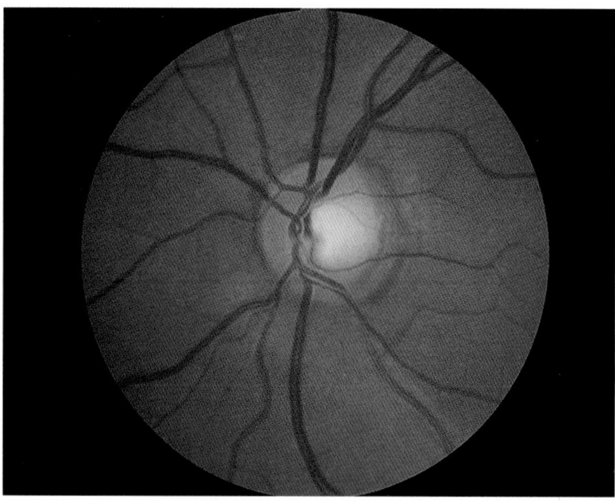
(a)

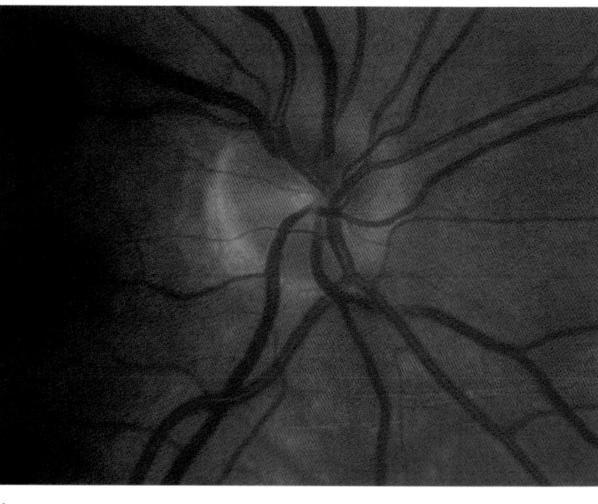
(b)

Figure 6.14 Asymmetric cups in nearly equal-size discs The right cup measures 0.1 and the left cup measures 0.3. Both eyes had normal IOPs, full visual fields and no evidence of glaucoma. Close follow-up of this patient is indicated.

and can precede the appearance of ONH changes or visual field defects. The morphology of these defects follows the normal architectural pattern of the NFL in the retina and will be discussed later.

- Asymmetric cups (Fig. 6.14) are sometimes the first objective sign of glaucoma. As mentioned earlier, it is highly unusual (1–2%) for normal individuals to have a cup asymmetry equal to or greater than 0.2. Comparing two stereo color disc photos is the most effective way of detecting subtle differences between cups.

Nonspecific signs

Less specific but still significant signs in patients suspected of having glaucoma are as follows:

- A large cup/disc ratio (greater than 0.5) in Caucasian individuals is a suspicious finding. Keeping in mind age- and race-related differences in cup size a given C/D ratio bears no clinical significance unless additional signs of ONH damage described here are present.
- Nasal displacement of central vessels can occur in glaucoma. This change is not early, can also occur in large physiological or myopic cups in the absence of glaucoma and is seen in many eyes with advanced disease.
- Segmental ('sloping') or generalized ('saucerization') depression of the ONH surface results from partial nerve tissue loss. These topographic changes can best be recognized by stereoscopic examination under appropriate magnification and illumination.
- An increased space between a vessel and the underlying nerve surface ('overpass sign') can result from localized loss of supporting nerve tissue, although an increased transparency without actual surface change has been suggested.
- Peripapillary atrophy of the choroid and retinal pigment epithelium (Fig. 6.15) has been frequently associated with glaucoma. When atrophy involves the choroid alone it appears as a whitish discoloration of the peripapillary tissue known as zone beta. It often corresponds to areas with greater nerve tissue loss and visual field defects. A retinal pigment epithelium crescent surrounding zone beta may also be present (zone alpha) which is less specific.
- Baring of the lamina cribrosa can result from significant loss of nerve fibers but can also be seen in large nerves with deep, large cups in the absence of glaucoma.
- Optic disc pallor can occur in GON. Typically the degree of cupping will exceed the degree of pallor. When pallor exceeds cupping other ON diseases must be suspected and ruled out. In glaucomatous nerves, pallor can sometimes affect the neural rim in a localized manner. This change is believed to result from thinning of the nerve tissue and capillary dropout. In addition, mild to moderate diffuse disc pallor can result after an attack of acute angle-closure glaucoma.

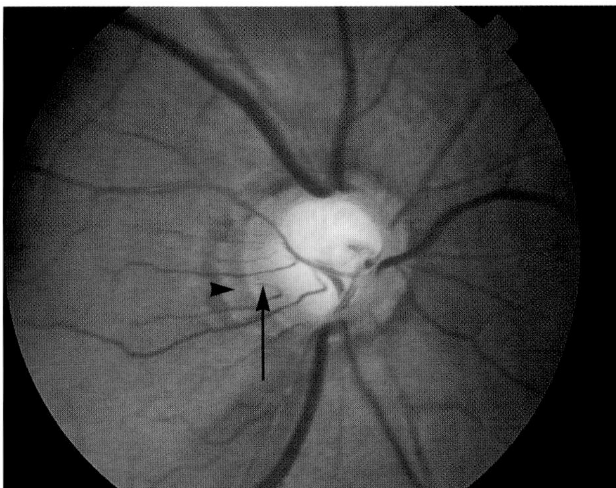

Figure 6.15 Peripapillary changes in glaucoma
Note the whitish area of choroidal sclerosis surrounding the nerve (zone beta, arrow). A pigment epithelium crescent is also present (zone alpha, arrowhead).

- Baring of a circumlinear vessel was once thought to be a specific sign. Such a vessel characteristically follows the margin of the cup and is present in half of normal nerves. A recession of the cup margin as a result of tissue loss will create a space between the vessel and the cup margin known as baring of a circumlinear vessel. This finding can also occur in other conditions.

Differential diagnosis

Careful evaluation of the ONH characteristics and other clinical findings will in most cases allow us to differentiate GON from nonglaucomatous optic neuropathy. Nonetheless, a number of clinical conditions may mimic GON and must be considered and excluded. These include the following:

- A physiological or congenitally large optic cup (Fig. 6.8c). Examination of close relatives may reveal a similar configuration and will help in the differential diagnosis.
- Congenital anomalies of the optic nerve, like congenital pits, colobomas (Fig. 6.16a), the morning glory syndrome and the tilted-disc syndrome, can occasionally mimic the appearance of a glaucomatous nerve.
- Pale, cupped nerves can sometimes result from diseases such as ischemic optic neuropathy (arteritic or nonarteritic), central retinal artery occlusion, toxic optic neuropathy, traumatic optic atrophy and compressive lesions. A detailed history and physical examination will often guide the clinician in the appropriate direction and reveal the underlying condition.
- Tilted nerves in myopic patients (Fig. 6.16b) can simulate glaucomatous cupping and require careful differentiation.

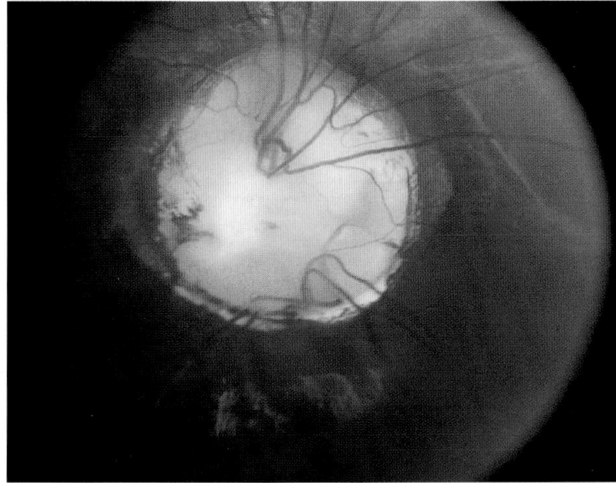

(a)

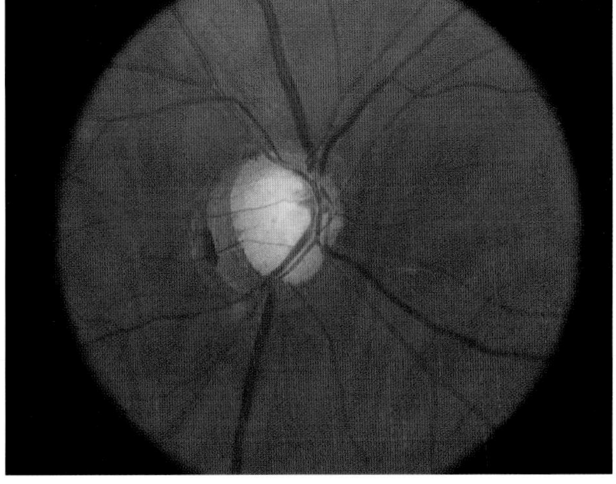

(b)

Figure 6.16 Pseudo-glaucomatous cupping
(a) A congenital anomaly of the optic nerve simulating glaucomatous cupping. The abnormal vascular pattern and colobomatous changes suggest a nonglaucomatous etiology. (b) A tilted disc in a myopic patient can mimic glaucomatous cupping and make the assessment of the cup difficult in true glaucoma cases.

Theories of etiology of glaucomatous optic neuropathy

Glaucomatous optic neuropathy probably represents the final common pathway for various mechanisms of injury. It is generally appreciated that IOP alone cannot explain the occurrence of GON in every patient. As understanding of the pathophysiology of GON expands, so too will diagnostic and therapeutic approaches to these diseases. Outlined briefly below are several of the current theories regarding the mechanisms of damage in GON.

Mechanical

This theory supports that elevated IOP is the primary mechanism responsible for the damage to neural cells through biomechanical or structural factors. It is commonly recognized that IOP is probably the single most important identifiable risk factor in the development of GON and the only one currently treatable. Levels of IOP appear to correlate with degrees of ONH damage in many patients. Disturbances in one or more components of axoplasmic flow at the level of the lamina cribrosa can result in axonal injury and subsequent cell death as a result of increased IOP. The precise mechanisms by which this occurs are not known, but it is thought that backwards bowing of the lamina from elevated IOP causes 'kinking' of the axons within the pores, resulting in a disruption of axoplasmic flow. Left untreated, the nerve fiber eventually dies.

Vascular

This theory proposes that the basic pathogenic mechanism responsible for the death of ganglion cells in glaucoma is an insufficient blood supply to the optic nerve head. Despite extensive investigation, the precise level at which this abnormality occurs is at this time unknown. It is therefore not clear at what location an ischemic injury must occur to produce the characteristic findings of GON. This mechanism has been postulated as responsible for the optic neuropathy seen in many patients with GON and normal IOPs (normal-tension glaucoma). Several noninvasive methods to measure the circulation of the posterior pole of the eye and the orbit have recently been developed. For example, color Doppler ultrasonographic analysis has allowed estimates of blood supply through the ophthalmic artery, nasal and temporal short posterior ciliary arteries and central retinal artery. Posterior ciliary, retinal and choroidal circulation differences between normals and glaucoma patients have been reported, but the precise significance of these findings is at this time of uncertain clinical significance. It is difficult to estimate the degree to which these or other mechanisms play a role in a particular patient since these theories are not exclusive. Decreased circulation and a tendency to an elevated IOP are two known occurrences in elderly individuals in the western world. There is evidence that significant nocturnal systemic arterial hypotension can occur in some individuals, theoretically compromising the blood supply to the optic nerves. It is therefore difficult to separate the mechanical and vascular mechanisms as isolated causes of GON in a given patient.

Neurochemical

It is well known that typical glaucomatous ONH changes occur in eyes without documented elevated IOP or demonstrable circulatory ('vascular') insufficiency. A third proposed mechanism of neuronal injury is of a chemical nature; a number of substances have been shown to have a damaging effect on neural cells and deserve mention.

The excitotoxins (excitatory neurotransmitters) are found in normal neural tissue and in high concentrations have been shown to be toxic to neurons. One of these compounds, glutamate, has been recently found in higher amounts in glaucomatous eyes.

An uncontrolled accumulation of intracellular calcium can cause neuronal damage and subsequent cell death. Calcium channel blockers not only have shown a vasodilating action in cases of normal-tension glaucoma attributed to vasospasm but also decrease the intracellular concentration of calcium.

Vascular endothelial cells produce a number of compounds that exert a variety of vascular and chemical effects. One of them is nitric oxide which, besides acting as a neurotransmitter, has vasodilating effects. It has also shown toxic effects (probably glutamate-mediated) on neurons. A group of substances produced by the vascular endothelium called endothelins have shown a marked vasoconstrictive effect on the ONH and their role in the pathogenesis of GON is being investigated. An increase in oxygen free radicals has been found in certain neurologic diseases, and a role in ganglion cell damage appears possible.

The future importance of these alternative mechanisms in the pathogenesis of glaucoma lies in the possibility of pharmacologic intervention. This may allow us to 'protect' the cells and in some cases halt or even reverse the alleged chemically mediated neuronal damage.

Apoptosis

It has been shown that ganglion cell loss occurs in the optic nerves of normal individuals throughout life at a fairly steady rate. Much attention has been given recently to a specific and distinct process of cellular death called apoptosis that occurs in many cells, including neurons. Each cell carries a predetermined ('programmed') intrinsic self-destruction mechanism that ultimately results in its death. There is evidence that apoptosis occurs in eyes with experimental glaucoma. Glaucoma could theoretically result from accelerated or premature apoptosis due to defective control mechanisms, possibly genetic in origin. Further research will define the possible role of this mechanism in the pathogenesis of glaucoma.

Clinical examination techniques

Glaucomatous optic neuropathy is at this time considered mostly an irreversible process. Its detection at the earliest stages becomes of the utmost importance in order to intervene and halt the pathologic process before functional loss occurs. A number of subjective, qualitative methods of examination have traditionally been used to evaluate glaucomatous damage. Several newer objective methods have been developed to evaluate both the ONH and the NFL. Comparisons between these methods have been conducted, showing that at present no single method is clearly the best in detecting early glaucomatous damage. Like the diagnostic process in most areas of medicine, these techniques appear to complement each other. Evidence has suggested that up to 40% of the nerve fibers may have been destroyed before a diagnostic visual field defect develops. Accordingly, some clinical techniques have detected the presence of ONH and NFL abnormalities prior to the occurrence of typical glaucomatous visual field defects. Still, careful examination by an experienced observer remains one of the best tools to detect glaucomatous damage.

Although a careful observer can obtain excellent reproducibility, the variability between observers using subjective techniques and the lack of standardized terminology to describe various clinical observations have created the need for more objective techniques to record the appearance of the ONH. The following are the examination techniques currently in use by clinicians in the assessment of the ONH.

Direct ophthalmoscopy

Direct ophthalmoscopy has been used for many years to examine the posterior pole of the eye. A direct ophthalmoscope yields a virtual, upright image with a 15× magnification, good illumination but a limited field of view. The major drawback of this monocular technique is the lack of stereopsis. Subtle yet important topographic changes in the ONH may be overlooked. A rough idea of the status of the optic nerve can be obtained by direct ophthalmoscopy, but it remains a suboptimal method to evaluate glaucoma patients. It is nonetheless a useful tool for non-ophthalmologist physicians, for screening purposes and whenever a small pupil precludes other types of ophthalmoscopy.

Standard binocular indirect ophthalmoscopy

In this technique peripheral light rays from the patient's retina are 'captured' by aspheric condensing lenses and projected onto the examiner's retina allowing a much wider field of view. A real and inverted image is formed between the lens and the examiner. The power of the lenses used for indirect ophthalmoscopy vary from 15 to 30 diopters, yielding a lateral magnification that ranges from 2× to 4×. Although a stereoscopic view is obtained, these levels of magnification are inadequate for the evaluation of fine details. Under these conditions the assessment of subtle variations in ONH color and surface is difficult to make. An increase in axial magnification adds to this inconvenience. It is not recommended that one rely on standard indirect ophthalmoscopy when examining glaucoma patients.

Slit lamp biomicroscopy

The excellent illumination, high magnification and stereoscopic view obtainable through a slit lamp biomicroscope makes this type of examination highly desirable for the clinical evaluation of the ONH. The visualization of the fundus requires a supplemental lens.

The Hruby lens (adapted to the slit lamp) is a plano-concave lens of −55 D of power. It provides an upright virtual image with good magnification. Unfortunately, the small field of view makes this technique challenging and may preclude good stereopsis. It is a noncontact technique that has largely been replaced.

The Goldmann fundus contact lens, like the Hruby lens, creates an upright virtual image. Its use requires a coupling material between the lens and the cornea. This allows some control of the globe during the examination. Adequate magnification can be obtained from the optical system of the slit lamp (up to 16× and higher), since the lens itself provides little magnification. With a fully dilated pupil and good illumination, this technique provides the best view available for the clinical assessment of the ONH. Unfortunately the use of a coupling material can affect the view during subsequent examination or fundus photography.

Condensing biconvex aspheric lenses of high power allow the use of the slit lamp for binocular indirect ophthalmoscopy. The availability of high magnification makes this an effective technique ('biomicroscope indirect ophthalmoscopy'). A real, inverted image is created between the examiner and the lens. Lenses of 60D, 78 D and 90 D of power are commonly used today. As a noncontact technique, it is comfortable for the patient and does not interfere with further eye examination since no coupling material is needed. Good illumination and magnification can be obtained from the slit lamp. The 78 D lens gives better magnification while the 90 D lens allows examination through smaller pupils. A reduced depth perception results from the inherent optics of these lenses, which can result in an underestimation of cupping and other topographic changes.

Nerve-fiber layer examination

The fundamental pathological process occurring in the glaucomatous optic nerve is a loss of retinal ganglion cells and their axons. This loss of nerve fibers follows the pattern of their structural arrangement in the retina and defines the sequence of the natural course of the disease. A normal NFL has a striated appearance radiating from the optic disc and is more prominent in the superior and inferior poles of the nerve, where the nerve bundles have a larger diameter. Temporal and nasal fibers are thinner and tightly arranged, giving the peripapillary retina a more uniform appearance. Thus, focal NFL loss will show a radiating wedge-shaped defect of variable width on the surface of the retina. Diffuse NFL loss will show a uniform decrease in the NFL pattern, being more difficult to identify in its early stages or when both types of defects coexist.

Biomicroscopy

Even though large NFL defects can often be seen with white light, more subtle defects require special variations in technique and instrumentation. A better view is obtained at the slit lamp after pupillary dilation using a red-free (green) filter and good illumination. Being a subjective examination, the potential for interobserver variability is always present.

Photography

Different photographic techniques have been described and attempts have been made to enhance visibility of the NFL. It appears that the use of blue or green filters with proper focusing gives the best results. A high-contrast, fine-grain, black-and-white film is currently recommended. Even though NFL photographic analysis has been greatly improved, it remains a technically challenging (subjective and qualitative) examination with variable results depending on the experience of the examiner (Fig. 6.13). False positive results can be obtained since localized defects can occur in normal patients.

Recording the optic nerve examination

Drawings

Careful, standardized drawing of the optic disc appearance is a useful clinical endeavor that requires the clinician to be meticulous and pay attention to small but important details. While several systems have been proposed, no uniform drawing system has been widely accepted. Detailed, written descriptions of the observed changes complement a drawing and provide valuable additional information. Interobserver variation, different drawing styles and the general availability of fundus photography make this a less than ideal method to document and follow the progression of the disease. This becomes critical when multiple observers are providing care. When no other method of recording the appearance of the discs is available, detailed and descriptive drawings are necessary.

Photography

Color fundus photography is widely available and as of today represents the standard to document and follow ONH morphology. While monoscopic color disc photos examined by a meticulous clinician can yield useful and reliable information, it is most desirable to obtain a stereo pair of photographs. High magnification can be achieved and 3D analysis of subtle features such as color, surface and vascular patterns can be performed with appropriate techniques. A standard fundus camera can be used to obtain sequential optic nerve images from two different angles by varying the position of the camera. A similar result can be obtained by using the Allen Stereo Separator, a glass plate that pivots right to left around its vertical axis. Photos are taken in two positions to obtain dissimilar images and create a stereoscopic effect. Images obtained by these two methods are then simultaneously viewed and a near-stereoscopic view is obtained. Simultaneous stereophotographs require a special camera with beam-splitting prisms to image the ONH. Stereo fundus cameras

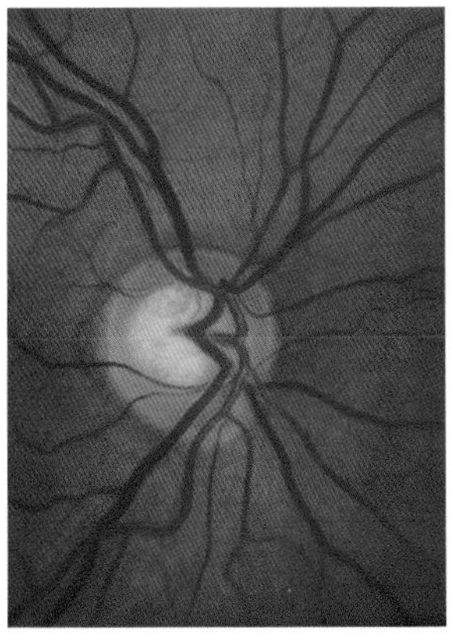
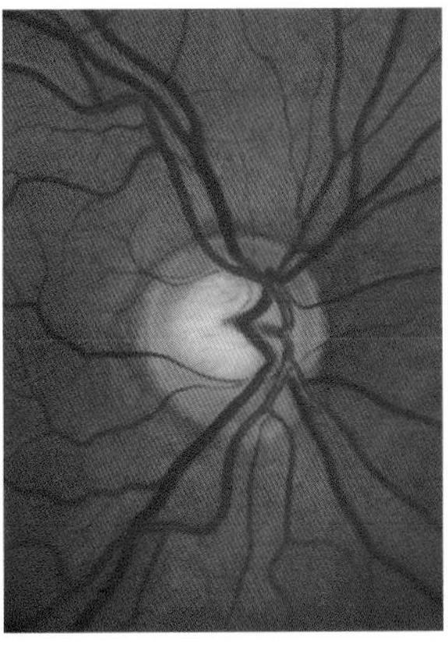

Figure 6.17 Simultaneous stereoscopic color disc photographs
Simultaneous stereoscopic color disc photographs taken with a Nidek camera. This technique gives the best stereoscopic view of the ONH currently available. (Courtesy of Jamie Brandt, MD.)

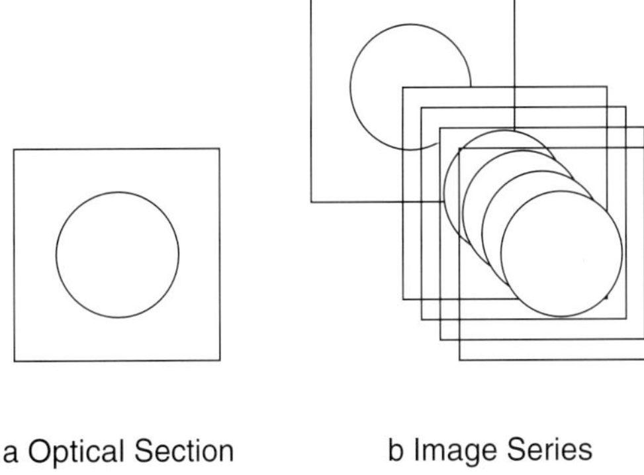

Figure 6.18 ONH multiple scans
Diagram showing how the multiple scans of the ONH are taken. Thirty-two images are obtained at different depths by the confocal laser ophthalmoscope. The computer will then reconstruct these images into a 3D representation of the optic disc surface.

are specifically designed for this purpose and resulting images produce the most consistent 3D view of the fundus.

Currently available cameras place two images in a single frame, resulting in less magnification than the sequential stereotechniques (Fig. 6.17). Stereophotography is the ideal photographic technique to document the appearance of the ONH in patients with glaucoma. The subjective component of this technique is determined by the experience and expertise of the observer, resulting in variable outcomes in some cases. Careful review of high-quality photos may reveal subtle findings not appreciated during clinical examination.

Computer-assisted analysis

Computer-assisted analysis has facilitated the design of new ways of exploring and measuring a variety of parameters in ophthalmology. The two most important target tissues in glaucoma (optic nerve head and retinal fiber layer) have been studied with the assistance of these techniques.

Optic nerve analysis

As mentioned and emphasized before, changes in the structure of the ONH and NFL may occur before detectable visual field loss. The several techniques previously discussed above are largely subjective with substantial intra- and interobserver variability. A number of computer-assisted techniques have emerged in an effort to detect early changes in an objective, quantitative manner. The analysis of the ONH surface (topographic analysis) has been the object of extensive effort in recent years. With the help of computer-assisted analysis to process real-life data acquisition, several devices have been developed. The following techniques are currently in use and development.

Confocal scanning laser ophthalmoscopy (cSLO)

This technique creates a true 3D map of the ONH by obtaining multiple optical sections at different depths. These sections are obtained by confocal imaging. The concept of confocal imaging is based on the focusing of a light beam on a specific point in space at a specific plane depth. Light returning from points outside this specific plane is greatly attenuated by the pinhole system, therefore allowing a selective ‘slicing’ of a structure in sections, illustrated in Figure 6.18. This is similar to the way computerized axial tomography works in radiology. Each section is scanned in the x and y co-ordinates. By manipulation of these co-ordinates, multiple sections at increasing depths are obtained and then ‘assembled’ by the processing system in what becomes a 3D reconstruction of the topography of the ONH. The reflected light is then analyzed, the signals are digitized and stored in a microcomputer. Quantitative analysis of these data can then be performed to determine multiple

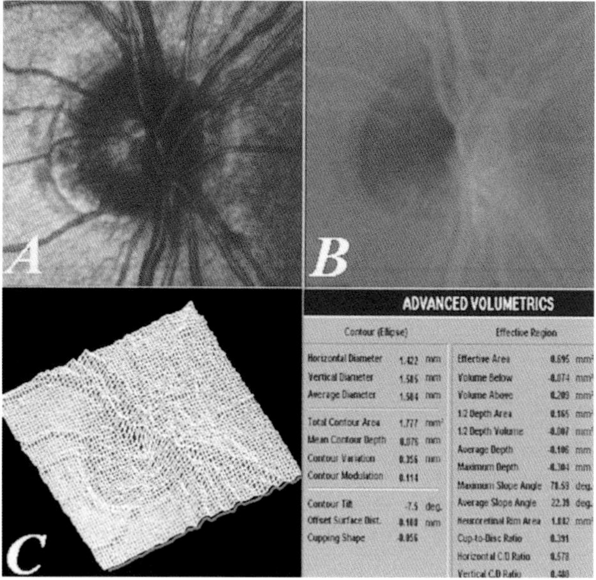

Figure 6.19 Topographic analysis of a normal ONH using confocal scanning laser ophthalmoscopy (cSLO)
(a) Image of the ONH as seen on the screen of the scanner. (b) Further computer processing reconstructs the multiple images into a single image as shown here. (c) Surface of the disc and peripapillary area enhanced by the grid pattern available from the wire-frame mode. The table shows topographic parameters derived from the multiple scans performed by the ophthalmoscope.

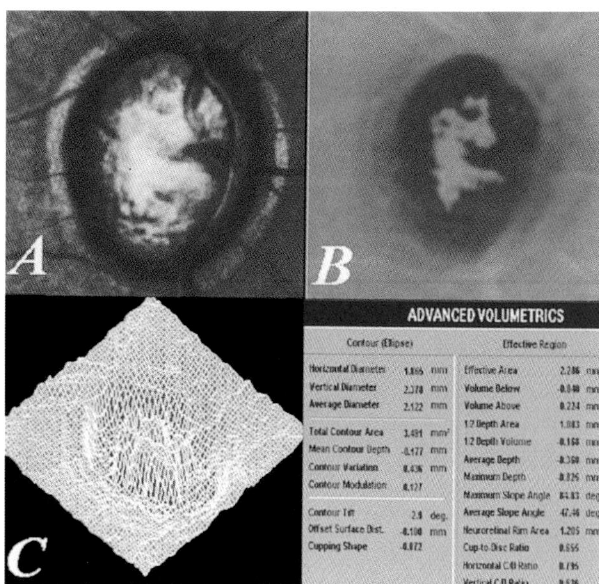

Figure 6.20 Topographic analysis of a glaucomatous ONH using cSLO
In addition to the extensive excavation note that this disc is larger than the disc in Fig. 6.19. The parameters show a decreased neuroretinal rim area and increased maximum depth. Note the marked vascular attenuation on the grid-enhanced view (C).

topographic parameters such as area, volume, depth and contour. All measurements are made relative to a reference surface or plane of reference.

Two instruments that incorporate this principle are currently in use. One is the Heidelberg Retinal Tomograph (HRT, Heidelberg Engineering, Heidelberg, Germany) which utilizes as source of illumination a diode laser (670 nm). The second device is the Topographic Scanning System (Top-SS, Laser Diagnostic Technologies Inc., San Diego, CA), which uses a near-infrared diode laser (780 nm). Figures 6.19 and 6.20 are examples of images from the Top-SS. While hardware and software differences exist, both systems use the same principles of confocal scanning.

These confocal imaging systems can obtain images through pupils as small as 1.5 mm, although 2.5 mm is considered ideal. Additionally, the system allows ONH examination despite moderate media opacities. These features represent significant advantages over previous ONH analyzers. Major issues in determining the utility of these devices in clinical practice are their reproducibility, accuracy and cost.

Nerve-fiber layer polarimetry

Direct and photographic examinations of the NFL have been discussed previously. Both are subjective qualitative techniques that, despite significant improvements, remain difficult to standardize. Quantitative analysis of the NFL is being performed with a scanning laser polarimeter (SLP), the Nerve Fiber Analyzer (NFA, Laser Diagnostic Technologies, San Diego, CA). This technique is based on the premise that the NFL has bi-refringent properties which change the polarization state of a beam of polarized light passing through it. This change is termed 'retardation' and is considered directly proportional to the thickness of the NFL.

In the NFA, a beam of polarized laser light penetrates the NFL and the retardation of the reflected light is detected and measured by a polarimeter. The electrical signal is then digitized and stored in a computer for analysis. The system then determines the corresponding retardation at that location. The NFA uses a near-infrared polarized diode laser (780 nm). The retardation is thus determined at multiple points in a 15 × 15 degree

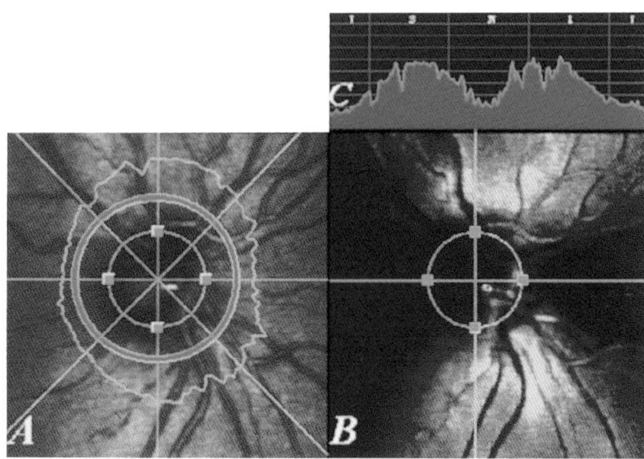

Figure 6.21 Nerve fiber layer analysis of a normal patient by scanning laser polarimetry
(a) The NFL thickness is measured along the thick green circle placed 1.5 disc diameters from the center of the disc. The thin, outer tracing represents the relative NFL thickness at each point of the 360-degree circumference. (b) This printout is a color-coded representation of the NFL thickness. The yellow-red areas represent thicker NFL measurements whereas the blue areas represent a thinner NFL. (c) This display shows the linear representation of the different NFL heights, known to be greater superiorly (S) and inferiorly (I). This morphologic feature results in the classic 'two humps' of a healthy NFL pattern. The indentations seen in these humps represent the large retinal vessels.

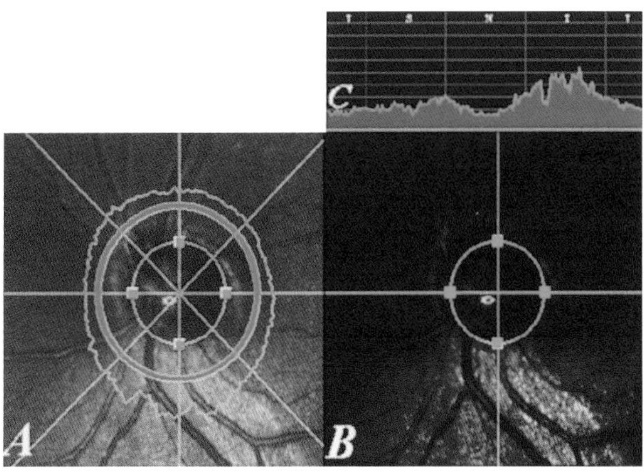

Figure 6.22 NFA image from a patient with glaucoma
This shows severe attenuation of the NFL affecting the superior portion of the ONH. (b) The color-coded printout shows a loss of the healthy yellow-red pattern superiorly. The blue color represents a diminished NFL height, almost indistinguishable from the nasal and temporal NFL. (c) This tracing shows significant flattening of the superior 'hump', indicating a considerable loss of nerve fibers entering the superior pole of the ONH. The visual field shows a dense inferior arcuate defect that correlates with the NFA findings.

grid centered on the optic nerve, yielding approximately 65 000 data points. These measurements are then converted into thickness units. The scanning time is about 0.7 seconds and an image is obtained with a total of 256 × 256 pixels in about 15 seconds. In contradistinction to topographic analysis, a plane of reference is not needed to obtain the measurements. Reproducibility of measurements is approximately 5–8 μm, and preliminary work has suggested that the measurements may be useful for detecting early glaucomatous damage, even in glaucoma suspects with normal visual fields. Examples of SLP images are given in Figures 6.21 and 6.22.

Summary

Most if not all clinical signs and symptoms seen in the most common types of glaucoma appear to result from an injury to the axons of the ganglion cells that constitute the optic nerve head. The precise pathophysiologic mechanisms and anatomic substrate of this injury are not completely understood. Intraocular pressure remains as the single most widely recognized risk factor linked to the development of GON. Additional proposed factors include genetic, circulatory, neurochemical and other mechanisms of disease. Early diagnosis of ONH damage and prompt detection of disease progression remain as critical goals. Towards these objectives, multiple diagnostic techniques can assist but not take the place of a careful clinical examination. To this date no single technique has proven to be clearly superior to others; instead they complement each other. New therapeutic approaches other than lowering of IOP are being considered as diverse pathogenic mechanisms are investigated. Assessing the status of the optic nerve head remains a crucial tool in the diagnosis, therapy and follow-up of patients with glaucoma.

FURTHER READING

Airaksinen PJ, Drance SM, Douglas GR et al., Diffuse and localized nerve fiber loss in glaucoma, *Am J Ophthalmol* (1984) **98**:566–71.

Airaksinen PJ, Nieminen H, Retinal nerve fiber layer photography in glaucoma, *Ophthalmology* (1985) **92**: 877–9.

Airaksinen PJ, Tuulonen A, Werner EB, Clinical evaluation of the optic disc and retinal nerve fiber layer. In: Ritch R, Shields MB, Krupin T, eds. *The Glaucomas*, 2nd edn. (St Louis, MO: Mosby-Year Book, 1996), 617–57.

Anatomy and physiology of the optic nerve. In: Miller NR, ed. *Walsh and Hoyt's Clinical Neuro-Ophthalmology*, 4th edn. (Baltimore, MD: Williams & Wilkins, 1982), Vol. 1, 41–59.

Anderson DR, Ultrastructure of human and monkey lamina cribrosa and optic nerve head, *Arch Ophthalmol* (1969) **82**:800–14.

Armaly MF, Genetic determination of cup/disc ratio of the optic nerve, *Arch Ophthalmol* (1967) **78**:35–43.

Bishop KI, Werner EB, Krupin T, et al., Variability and reproducibility of optic disk topographic measurements with the Rodenstock Optic Nerve Head Analyzer, *Am J Ophthalmol* (1988) **29**:1294–8.

Brown GC, Differential diagnosis of the glaucomatous optic disc. In: Varma R, Spaeth GL, eds. *The Optic Nerve in Glaucoma* (Philadelphia, PA: Lippincott, 1993), 99–112.

Caprioli J, Prum B, Zeyen T, Comparison of methods to evaluate the optic nerve head and nerve fiber layer for glaucomatous change, *Am J Ophthalmol* (1996) **121**:659–67.

Carpel EF, Engstrom PF, The normal cup-disk ratio, *Am J Ophthalmol* (1981) **91**:588–97.

Chauhan BC, Le Blanc RP, McCormick TA, Rogers JB, Re-test variability of topographic measurements with confocal scanning laser tomography in patients with glaucoma and control subjects, *Am J Ophthalmol* (1994) **118**:9–15.

Chi T, Ritch R, Stickler D, Pitman B, Tsai C, Hsieh FY, Racial differences in optic nerve head parameters, *Arch Ophthalmol* (1989) **107**:836–9.

Cioffi GA, Robin AL, Eastman RD, et al., Confocal laser scanning ophthalmoscope: reproducibility of optic nerve head topographic measurements with the confocal scanning laser ophthalmoscope, *Ophthalmology* (1993) **100**:57–62.

Cioffi GA, Van Buskirk EM, Vasculature of the anterior optic nerve and peripapillary choroid. In: Ritch R, Shields MB, Krupin T, eds. *The Glaucomas.* 2nd edn. (St Louis, MO: Mosby-Year Book, 1996), 177–88.

Cioffi GA, Van Buskirk EM, Anatomy of the ocular microvasculature, *Surv Ophthalmol* (1994) **38**:S107–16.

Colenbrander A, Principles of ophthalmoscopy. In: Tasman W, Jaeger EA, eds. *Duane's Clinical Ophthalmology.* Revised edn. (Philadelphia, PA: Lippincott-Raven, 1995), Vol. 1, 1–21.

Dandona L, Quigley HA, Jampel HD, Reliability of optic nerve head topographic measurements with computerized image analysis, *Am J Ophthalmol* (1989) **108**:414–21.

Drance SM, Fairclough M, Butler DM, Kottler MS, The importance of disc hemorrhage in the prognosis of chronic open angle glaucoma, *Arch Ophthalmol* (1977) **95**:226–8.

Dreher AW, Reiter KR, Retinal laser ellipsometry: a new method for measuring the retinal nerve fiber layer thickness distribution, *Clin Vision Sci* (1992) **7**:481–8.

Dreher AW, Reiter K, Scanning laser polarimetry of the retinal nerve fiber layer, *Proc SPIE Int Soc Opt Eng* (1992) **1746**:34–8.

Dreher AW, Tso PC, Weinreb RN, Reproducibility of topographic measurements of the normal and glaucomatous optic nerve head with the laser tomographic scanner, *Am J Ophthalmol* (1991) **32**:2992–6.

Dreyer EB, Zurakowski D, Schumer RA, Podos SM, Lipton SA, Elevated glutamate in the vitreous body of humans and monkeys with glaucoma, *Arch Ophthalmol* (1996) **114**:299–305.

Fechtner RD, Reproducibility of topographic measurements of the normal and glaucomatous optic nerve head with a new confocal laser scanning system, *Proc Am Acad Ophthalmol 1992. Annual meeting, Dallas.*

Fechtner RD, Ikram F, Essock EA, Advances in quantitative optic nerve analysis. In: Burde R, Slamovitz TL eds. *Advances in Clinical Ophthalmology* (St Louis, MO: Mosby-Year Book, 1996), 203–24.

Fechtner RD, Weinreb RN, Examining and recording the appearance of the optic nerve head. In: Starita RJ, ed. *Clinical signs in ophthalmology. Glaucoma Series.* Vol. XII, no. 5 (St Louis, PA: Mosby-Year Book, 1991), 2–15.

Fechtner RD, Weinreb RN, Mechanisms of optic nerve damage in primary open angle glaucoma, *Surv Ophthalmol* (1994) **39**:23–42.

Hayreh SS, Blood supply of the optic nerve head and its role in optic atrophy, glaucoma, and oedema of the optic disc, *Br J Ophthalmol* (1969) **53**:721–48.

Herschler J, Osher RH, Baring of the circumlinear vessel: an early sign of optic nerve damage, *Arch Ophthalmol* (1980) **98**:865–9.

Hitchings RA, Spaeth GL, The optic disc in glaucoma. I. Classification, *Br J Ophthalmol* (1976) **60**:778–85.

Johnson BM, Miao M, Sadun AA, Age-related decline of human optic nerve axon populations, *Age* (1987) **10**:5–9.

Jonas FB, Dichtl A, Evaluation of the retinal nerve fiber layer, *Surv Ophthalmol* (1996) **40**:369–78.

Jonas JB, Fernandez MC, Naumann GOH, Glaucomatous parapapillary atrophy. Occurrence and correlations, *Arch Ophthalmol* (1992) **110**:214–22.

Jonas JB, Zach F, Gusek GC, Naumann GOH, Pseudoglaucomatous physiologic large cups, *Am J Ophthalmol* (1989) **107**:137–44.

Katz LJ, Optic disc drawings. In: Varma R, Spaeth GL, eds. *The Optic Nerve in Glaucoma* (JB Lippincott Co., Philadelphia, 1993) 147–58.

Kruse FE, Burk ROW, Volcker GE, Zinser G, Harbart U, Reproducibility of topographic measurements of the optic nerve head with laser tomographic scanning, *Ophthalmology* (1989) **96**:1320–4.

Law FU, The origin of the ophthalmoscope, *Ophthalmology* (1986) **93**:140–1.

Levin LA, Louhab A, Apoptosis of retinal ganglion cells and anterior ischemic optic neuropathy, *Arch Ophthalmol* (1996) **114**:488–91.

Lichter PR, Variability of expert observers in evaluating the optic disc, *Trans Am Ophthalmol Soc* (1976) **74**:532–72.

Maumenee AE, Causes of optic nerve damage in glaucoma, *Ophthalmology* (1983) **90**:741–52.

Mikelberg FS, Drance SM, Schulzer M, Yidegiligne HM, Weis MM, The normal human optic nerve, *Ophthalmology* (1989) **96**:1325–8.

Mikelberg FS, Parfitt CM, Swindale NV, Graham SL, Drance SM, Gosine R, Ability of the Heidelberg retina tomograph to detect early glaucomatous visual field loss, *J Glaucoma* (1995) **4**:242–7.

Mikelberg FS, Wijsman K, Schulzer M, Reproducibility of topographic parameters obtained with the Heidelberg retina tomograph, *J Glaucoma* (1991) **2**:101–3.

Minckler DS, Optic nerve damage in glaucoma. 1. Obstruction to axoplasmic flow, *Surv Ophthalmol* (1981) **26**:128–36.

Motolko M, Drance SJ, Features of the optic disc in preglaucomatous eyes, *Arch Ophthalmol* (1981) **99**:1992–4.

Netland PA, Chaturvedi N, Dreyer EB, Calcium channel blockers in the management of low tenson and open-angle glaucoma, *Am J Ophthalmol* (1993) **115**:60–8.

Nicolela MT, Drance SM, Various glaucomatous optic nerve appearances. Clinical correlations, *Ophthalmology* (1996) **103**:640–9.

O'Connor DJ, Zeyen T, Caprioli J, Comparison of methods to detect glaucomatous optic nerve damage, *Ophthalmology* (1993) **100**:1498–503.

Orgul S, Cioffi GA, Bacon DR, Van Buskirk EM, Sources of variability of topometric data with a scanning laser ophthalmoscope, *Arch Ophthalmol* (1996) **113**:161–4.

Orgul S, Cioffi GA, Wilson DJ, Bacon DR, Van Buskirk EM, An endothelin-1 induced model of optic nerve ischemia in the rabbit, *Invest Ophthalmol Vis Sci* (1996) **37**:1860–9.

Orgul S, Meyer P, Cioffi A, Physiology of blood flow regulation and mechanisms involved in optic nerve perfusion, *J Glaucoma* (1995) **4**:427–43.

Osher RH, Herschler J, The significance of baring of the circumlinear vessel: a prospective study, *Arch Ophthalmol* (1981) **99**:817–18.

Pederson JE, Anderson DR, The mode of progressive disc cupping in ocular hypertension and glaucoma, *Arch Ophthalmol* (1980) **98**:490–5.

Peli E, Hedges TR, Schwartz B, Computerized enhancement of retinal nerve fiber layer, *Acta Ophthalmol* (1986) **64**:113–22.

Pendergast SD, Shields MB, Reproducibility of optic nerve head topographic measurements with the Glaucoma-scope, *J Glaucoma* (1994) **4**:170–6.

Pickard R, A method of recording disc alterations and a study of the growth of normal and abnormal disc cups, *Br J Ophthalmol* (1923) **80**:81–90.

Quigley HA, Addicks EM, Regional differences in the structure of the lamina cribrosa and their relation to glaucomatous optic nerve damage, *Arch Ophthalmol* (1981) **99**:137–43.

Quigley HA, Addicks EM, Green WR, Optic nerve damage in human glaucoma. III. Quantitative correlation of nerve fiber loss and visual field defect in glaucoma, ischemic neuropathy, papilledema and toxic neuropathy, *Arch Ophthalmol* (1982) **100**:135–46.

Quigley HA, Dunkelberger GR, Green WR, Retinal ganglion cell atrophy correlated with automated perimetry in human eyes with glaucoma, *Am J Ophthalmol* (1989) **107**:453–64.

Quigley HA, Katz J, Derick R, Gilbert D, Sommer A, An evaluation of optic disc and nerve fiber layer examinations in monitoring progression of early glaucoma damage, *Ophthalmology* (1992) **99**:19–28.

Quigley HA, Miller NR, George T, Clinical evaluation of nerve fiber layer atrophy as an indicator of glaucomatous optic nerve damage, *Arch Ophthalmol* (1980) **98**:1564–71.

Quigley HA, Nickells RW, Kerrigan LA, Pease ME, Thibault DJ, Zack DJ, Retinal ganglion cells death in experimental glaucoma and after axotomy occurs by apoptosis, *Invest Ophthalmol Vis Sci* (1995) **36**:774–86.

Rankin SJA, Drance SM, Buckley AR, Walman BE, Visual field correlations with color Doppler studies in open angle glaucoma, *J Glaucoma* (1996) **5**:15–21.

Repka MX, Quigley HA, The effect of age on normal human optic nerve fiber and diameter, *Ophthalmology* (1989) **96**:26–32.

Saheb NE, Drance SM, Nelson A, The use of photogrammetry in evaluating the cup of the optic nerve head for a study in chronic simple glaucoma, *Can J Ophthalmol* (1972) **7**:466–71.

Schumer RA, Podos SM, The nerve of glaucoma! *Arch Ophthalmol* (1994) **112**:37–44.

Schwartz JT, Reuling FH, Garrison RJ, Acquired cupping of the optic nerve head in normotensive eyes, *Br J Ophthalmol* (1975) **59**:216–22.

Shaffer RN, Ridgway WL, Brown R, Kramer SG, The use of diagrams to record changes in glaucomatous disks, *Am J Ophthalmol* (1975) **80**:460–4.

Sharma NK, Hitchings RA, A comparison of monocular and 'stereoscopic' photographs of the optic disc in the identification of glaucomatous visual field defects. *Br J Ophthalmol* (1983) **67**:677–80.

Sommer A, Intraocular pressure and glaucoma, *Am J Ophthalmol* (1994) **118**:1–8.

Sommer A, D'Anna SA, Kues HA, George T, High-resolution photography of the retinal fiber layer, *Am J Ophthalmol* (1983) **96**:535–9.

Sommer AS, Katz J, Quigley HA, et al., Clinically detectable nerve fiber atrophy precedes the onset of glaucomatous field loss, *Arch Ophthalmol* (1991) **109**:77–83.

Sommer A, Miller NR, Pollack I, Maumenee AE, George T, The nerve fiber layer in the diagnosis of glaucoma, *Arch Ophthalmol* (1977) **95**:2149–56.

Sommer A, Quigley HA, Robin AL, Miller NR, Katz J, Arkell S, Evaluation of nerve fiber layer assessment, *Arch Ophthalmol* (1984) **102**:1766–71.

Snead, MP, Rubinstein MP, Jacobs PM, The optics of fundus examination, *Surv Ophthalmol* (1992) **36**:439–45.

Spaeth GL, Optic nerve damage in glaucoma. 2. Insufficiency of blood flow, *Surv Ophthalmol* (1981) **26**:128–48.

Spaeth GL, Development of glaucomatous changes of the optic nerve. In: Varma R, Spaeth GL, eds. *The Optic Nerve in Glaucoma* (Philadelphia, PA: Lippincott, 1993), 63–81.

Spaeth GL, Hitchings RA, The optic disc in glaucoma: pathogenic correlation of five patterns of cupping in chronic open angle glaucoma, *Trans Am Acad Ophthalmol Otolaryngol* (1976) **81**:217–23.

Tielsch JM, Katz J, Quigley HA, Miller NR, Sommer A, Intraobserver and interobserver agreement in measurement of optic disc characteristics, *Ophthalmology* (1988) **95**:350–6.

Trobe JD, Glaser JS, Cassady JC, Optic atrophy. Differential diagnosis by fundus observation alone, *Arch Ophthalmol* (1980) **98**:1040–5.

Trobe FD, Glaser JS, Cassady J, Herschler J, Anderson DR, Nonglaucomatous excavation of the optic disc, *Arch Ophthalmol* (1980) **98**:1046–50.

Van Buskirk EM, Cioffi GA, Glaucomatous optic neuropathy, *Am J Ophthalmol* (1992) **113**:447–52.

Varma R, Minckler DS, Anatomy and pathophysiology of the retina and optic nerve. In: Ritch R, Shields MB, Krupin T eds. *The Glaucomas*. 2nd edn. (St Louis, MO: Mosby-Year Book, 1996), 139–75.

Varma R, Steinmann WC, Scott IU, Expert agreement in evaluating the optic disc for glaucoma, *Ophthalmology* (1992) **99**:215–21.

Varma R, Tielsch JM, Quigley HA, et al., Race-, age-, gender, and refractive error-related differences in the normal optic disc, *Arch Ophthalmol* (1994) **112**:1068–76.

Weinreb RN, Why study the ocular microcirculation in glaucoma? *J Glaucoma* (1992) **1**:145–7.

Weinreb RN, Diagnosing and monitoring glaucoma with confocal scanning laser ophthalmoscopy, *J Glaucoma* (1995) **4**:225–7.

Weinreb RN, Lusky M, Bartsch DU, Morsman D, Effect of repetitive imaging on topographic measurements of the optic nerve head, *Arch Ophthalmol* (1993) **111**:636–8.

Weinreb RN, Shakiba S, Zangwill L, Scanning laser polarimetry to measure the nerve fiber layer of normal and glaucomatous eyes, *Am J Ophthalmol* (1994) **119**:627–36.

Wiegner SW, Netland PA, Optic disc hemorrhages and progression of glaucoma, *Ophthalmology* (1996) **103**:1014–24.

Wilensky JT, Kolker AE, Peripapillary changes in glaucoma, *Am J Ophthalmol* (1976) **81**:341–5.

Wisman RL, Asseff DF, Phelps CD, Podos SM, Becker B, Vertical elongation of the optic cup in glaucoma, *Trans Am Acad Ophthalmol Otolaryngol* (1973) **77**:157–61.

Zeyen TG, Caprioli J, Progression of disc and field damage in early glaucoma, *Arch Ophthalmol* (1993) **111**:62–5.

7 Psychophysical and electrophysiological testing in glaucoma: visual fields and other functional tests

Neil T Choplin

Introduction

The detection of nerve fiber loss and prevention of its development and progression is the ultimate goal of the ophthalmologist in the diagnosis and management of patients with glaucoma. At the present time, there is no proven reliable and consistent way to 'count' optic nerve fibers, compare the 'count' to known normals to determine the presence or absence of glaucomatous disease, and accurately determine if the 'count' is changing over time. As axons are lost through the disease process, visual function declines in relation to the loss of fibers serving the region of the loss. Therefore, tests of optic nerve function are integral to the management of glaucoma patients as an indirect measure of the number of axons remaining.

Tests of optic nerve function can be objective or subjective. A variety of different test modalities have been investigated, looking for the ideal test that would be

1) easy to administer;
2) mostly objective (requiring minimal decision-making or other efforts on the part of the patient);
3) highly sensitive to early loss or minimal change in the disease state; and
4) specific for glaucoma.

No objective test meeting these criteria has been found. Clinical functional testing for glaucoma consists mostly of 'psychophysical' tests, which by their very nature are highly subjective and susceptible to the short-comings of human subjects. These tests require the patients to perceive something, intellectually interpret what was perceived, remember the instructions regarding what is supposed to be said or done if the correct 'something' was perceived, and effect some type of verbal or motor response. Perception, memory, interpretation and action thus characterize such psychophysical tests, and can all (individually, collectively or in some combination) lead to variability in the results. This can sometimes lead to false conclusions regarding the state of the disease process and inappropriate treatment.

Functional tests in glaucoma

(Table 7.1)

There is good evidence that chronic glaucoma selectively damages large optic nerve fibers, although fibers of all sizes are damaged. Functional testing, therefore, should be directed at the visual tasks subserved by these axons in an attempt to identify early damage. Some investigators have shown associated functional changes attributable to the loss of large optic nerve fibers, including declines in contrast sensitivity at high spatial frequencies, loss of pattern-evoked electroretinographic responses (PERG) after death of ganglion cells, and attenuation of PERG responses for high temporal frequencies of stimulation, supporting the idea that some part of glaucoma damage involves loss of the function of these large-diameter nerve fibers. Other investigators have suggested that the PERG may be helpful in identifying patients with ocular hypertension who will develop signs of glaucoma.

Table 7.1 Functional tests other than standard visual fields that have been used for glaucoma. Many different electrophysiological and psychophysical tests have been investigated in glaucoma, particularly in an attempt to identify early damage or risk factors for development or progression of damage. This table lists the various modalities that have been investigated, how they are performed, what they measure and what the findings are in glaucoma patients.

Test name	Objective or subjective	How performed	What it measures	Findings in glaucoma	Reference
Central contrast sensitivity	Subjective	Low-contrast flickering stimuli presented to the central four degrees	Minimum difference in luminance between stimulus and background of a flickering stimulus	Mean thresholds were lower than normal controls. Some ocular hypertensive patients also show reduction in threshold	Atkin et al., 1979; 1980
Temporal contrast sensitivity	Subjective	Stimulus of increasing frequency of flicker presented to the fovea	Intensity of stimulus required to perceive flicker at each presented flicker frequency	Frequency-specific loss at 15 Hz, nonfrequency specific mean sensitivity loss greater in glaucoma patients than suspects	Breton et al., 1991
Pattern-evoked electro-retinographic responses (PERG)	Objective	Reversing checkerboard pattern presented on a television screen at varying contrast while standard ERG measurements are obtained	Waveform generated, latencies of responses and amplitudes for each wave component	Second negative wave selectively depressed in patients with glaucoma. Some ocular hypertensives showed similar responses	Trick, 1985; Weinstein et al., 1988
Contrast sensitivity	Subjective	Patient views figures of decreasing contrast at multiple spatial frequencies and identifies orientation of stripe pattern	Ability to detect correct orientation of stripe pattern as contrast decreases	Decreased contrast acuity in glaucoma patients, particularly at high spatial frequencies	Nadler et al., 1990
Color vision	Subjective	Farnsworth–Munsell 100 Hue Test, Farnsworth D-15 Test, Nagel or Pickford–Nicholson anomaloscope	Defects in color vision	Blue-yellow defects may occur early in glaucoma, red-green defects appear with advanced optic neuropathy	Sample et al., 1986
Color contrast sensitivity	Subjective	Computer-driven color television system	Color contrast threshold as a fraction of the maximum color available for color combinations on each color axis	Sensitivity to blue and red lights (relative to green) significantly less than controls	Gunduz et al., 1988
Scotopic retinal sensitivity	Subjective	Patient dark adapted then presented with flickering stimulus increasing in luminance until seen	Sensitivity of dark-adapted retina to a flashing light	Reduction in absolute whole-field retinal sensitivity	Glovinsky et al., 1992
Flicker perimetry	Subjective	Static visual field testing performed with target flickering at 25 flashes/second	Threshold for target luminance against constant background	Flicker threshold elevated in glaucoma patients compared to normals but not compared to nonflickering stimulus	Feghali et al., 1991

Test name	Objective or subjective	How performed	What it measures	Findings in glaucoma	Reference
Flicker visual-evoked potential	Objective	Standard VEP recording while viewing a flickering stimulus of varying frequency	Amplitude and phase responses of VEP	Glaucoma patients showed amplitude loss at high flicker frequencies, correlating with visual field damage	Schmeisser et al., 1992
Color pattern-reversal visual-evoked potential	Objective	Standard VEP recording while viewing a reversing checkerboard of black-white, black-red or black-blue	P1-wave peak time and amplitude for each pattern	Glaucoma and ocular hypertensives showed significant decreases in the measured parameters compared to normal, especially to the black-red and black-blue checkerboards	Shih et al., 1991
Visual-evoked potentials after photostress	Objective	Standard VEP measure-ment before and following 30 seconds of photostress	Time for VEP recording to return to prestress baseline	Longer VEP recovery time required for glaucoma patients with intermediate values in ocular hypertensives compared to normals	Parisi and Bucci, 1992
High-pass resolution perimetry	Subjective	Rings of varying size presented to peripheral retina, patient indicates seen or not seen	'Ring' threshold, peripheral visual acuity	Similar to standard perimetry except that target size, rather than luminance, is the variable	Sample et al., 1992
Blue-on-yellow perimetry (Short-wavelength automated perimetry or SWAP)	Subjective	Modified automated static threshold perimeter with yellow background and blue projected stimuli	Visual field thresholds to blue stimuli on a yellow background	Abnormalities to blue-on-yellow may precede those to standard white-on-white and may predict which patients will develop loss or progress	Johnson et al., 1993a; 1993b

Damage to the optic nerve is not limited only to loss of large-diameter axons. There is considerable evidence that axonal loss occurs in bundles which may be visible ophthalmoscopically. Typical glaucomatous loss favors the superior and inferior poles of the disc. Areas of retina which have lost bundles of nerve fibers will manifest a loss of sensitivity compared to surrounding areas. Such areas of decreased sensitivity are detectable on visual field testing; these scotomas and other defects in the midperipheral portion of the visual field begin to emerge as large numbers of axons are lost. Diffuse loss of axons may occur early in certain types of glaucoma or late in uncontrolled and progressive cases, resulting in generalized reduction in visual sensitivity. Other visual functions affected by loss of nerve fibers include contrast sensitivity (Figs 7.1 and 7.2), temporal contrast sensitivity, color vision, scotopic retinal sensitivity, flicker perimetry, flicker visual-evoked potential, color pattern-reversal visual-evoked potentials, visual-evoked potentials following photostress, regional retinal visual acuity and foveal acuity. Loss of foveal acuity usually occurs late in the course of the disease but may occasionally occur early.

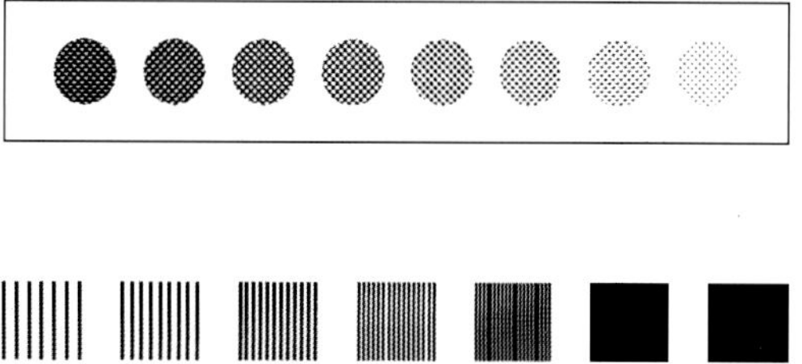

Figure 7.1 Testing contrast sensitivity
One method of testing contrast sensitivity requires the patient to discern the orientation of a pattern of stripes of increasing spatial frequency (more lines per unit area or degree of visual angle) and decreasing contrast. The top of the figure is an example of decreasing contrast between the test object and the background; the bottom of the figure illustrates a series of stimuli showing increasing spatial frequency, i.e. the pattern of stripes gets 'tighter' as the patient looks from left to right, making it harder to determine the orientation of the stripes. Tests involving these types of stimuli determine grating acuity.

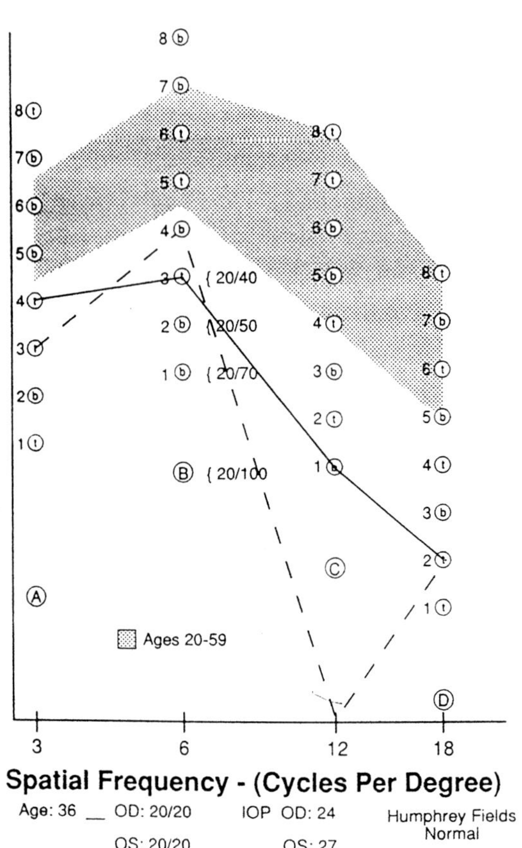

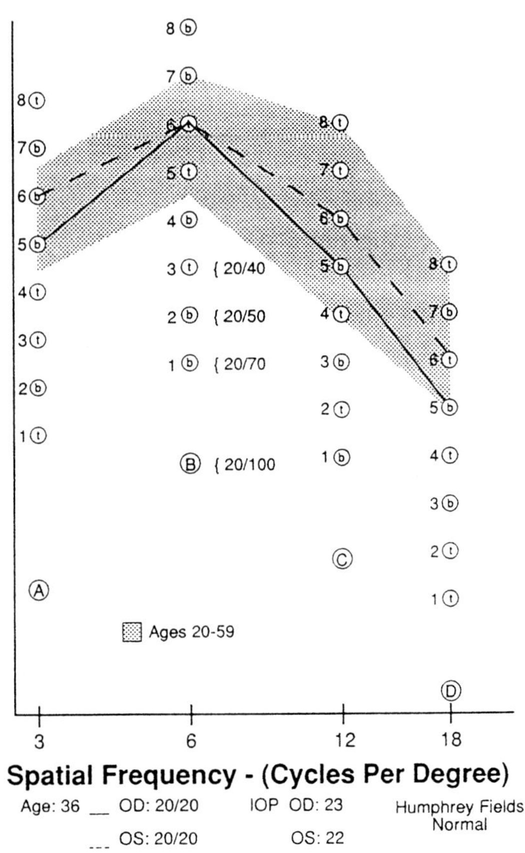

Figure 7.2 Decreased contrast sensitivity
Glaucoma may cause a decrease in contrast sensitivity in the absence of visual field defects or reduction in visual acuity. This figure is an example of decreased contrast sensitivity as determined by the Vectorvision system. The left side of the figure illustrates a reduction in sensitivity, particularly at the higher spatial frequencies (12 and 18 cycles per degree) in a patient with newly diagnosed open-angle glaucoma. The left eye, which has higher intraocular pressure, is worse. The gray area on the chart represents normal data. The right side of the figure illustrates normalization of the curves following institution of medical therapy and reduction in intraocular pressure.

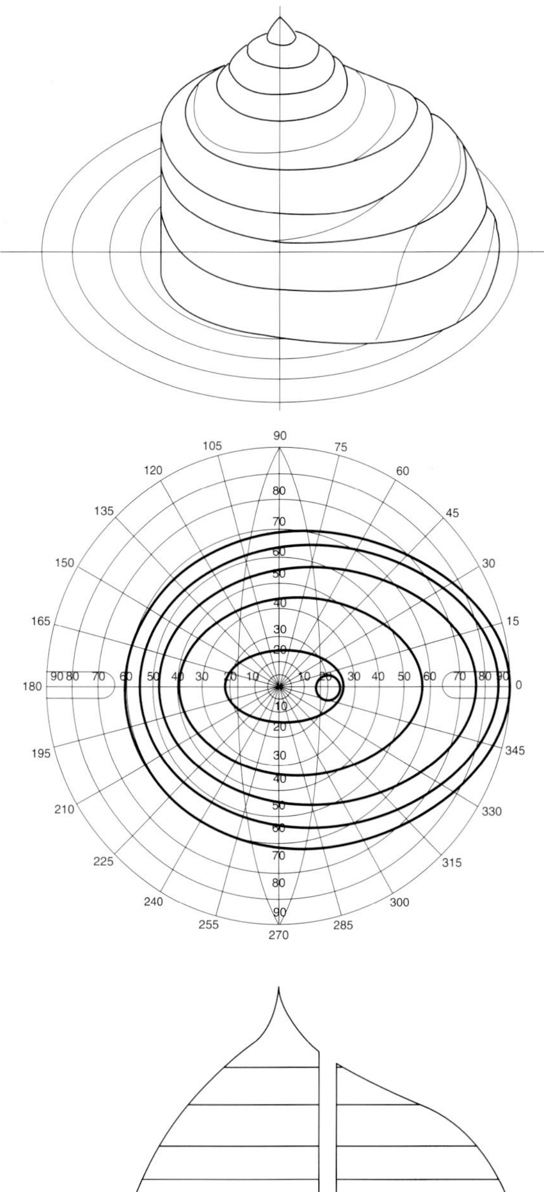

Figure 7.3 The normal visual field and methods to 'map' it

The visual field defines all that is visible to one eye at a given time. It has been likened to an 'island' or 'hill' of vision in a 'sea of blindness'. The job of visual field testing is to draw a map of the island of vision. The top of the figure represents the three-dimensional structure of a normal island of vision. The fovea is the 0,0 point on the *x* and *y* axes. The *z* axis represents the height of the island of vision at any point *x,y* above the 'sea', and is equivalent to the sensitivity of the retina at that point. Two different methods are available for drawing a map of the island. The middle of the figure represents the island as viewed from above as drawn by isopter perimetry, such as the tangent screen or Goldmann perimeter. An isopter may be thought of as the boundary of a retinal area within which all points have equal or greater sensitivity to those at the boundary. Each curved line, equivalent to the lines on the top figure, thus represent an isopter boundary. The lines are determined by moving test objects of fixed size and intensity from areas of nonseeing towards the center until the patient indicates it has been seen, thus giving this type of testing the name 'kinetic' perimetry. The smaller circles indicate areas determined by smaller and/or dimmer stimuli. By comparing the isopter locations and shapes to known normals, visual field defects can be determined. The bottom of the figure represents a 'slice', or profile of the island of vision through any meridian. It is determined by varying the intensity of a stimulus of fixed size at each point along the meridian until threshold has been determined. This type of testing has been termed 'static' perimetry, since the object does not move to determine threshold, and is typified by the Octopus perimeters and the Humphrey Field Analyzer (Zeiss-Humphrey Inc., San Leandro, CA). Testing multiple meridians and putting them together will give the three-dimensional picture of the island. Comparing the measured sensitivities to known normals allows for the detection of defects. Since quantitative information is generated (i.e. sensitivity values), statistical techniques can be applied for determining abnormalities and significant changes over time.

Table 7.2 **Visual field defects in glaucoma**

Visual field defects in glaucoma are well known. None of the defects that can occur in glaucoma is 100% specific; any defect that respects the horizontal meridian may occur in any optic nerve disorder. The interpretation of any visual field defect with regards to a differential diagnosis of disorders that can produce it must be made with regard to the entire clinical picture of the patient—intraocular pressure level, optic nerve appearance, family history and other risk factors, etc. This table lists the visual field defects that occur in glaucoma, and indicates the frequency with which those defects have been observed to be initial defects.

Type of defect	Glaucoma patients manifesting this as their initial defect (%)
Increasing scatter (fluctuation)	Probably all
Diffuse depression, i.e. increased threshold	
Paracentral defects	41
Nasal steps	54
Arcuate enlargement of the blind spot	30
Arcuate scotomata not connected to the blind spot	90
Nerve fiber bundle defects	
Altitudinal defects	
Temporal wedge defects	3
Central and temporal islands	
End-stage (temporal island only)	

Purely objective tests of visual function, such as electro-oculography, electroretinography and visual-evoked potentials lack specificity for glaucoma. Other objective tests, such as flicker visual-evoked potential, color pattern-reversal visual-evoked potentials and pattern-evoked electroretinographic responses, have so far proven to have limited clinical applicability due to equipment requirements (e.g. cost, complex engineering, lack of commercial availability), lack of familiarity to clinicians, complexity of interpretation and ease of performance.

Visual fields in glaucoma

(Figs 7.3–7.26)

Of the subjective tests currently available, visual field testing remains the mainstay, and the use of automated perimetry has allowed the development of standardized tests for obtaining quantitative measurements. Such measurements can be compared to known normal values to determine the presence of abnormalities, and can easily be followed over time for change. Statistical packages have been developed to help in the interpretation of quantitative visual field data, both for determining abnormality in a single visual field examination and for determining the significance of observed changes in a series of visual fields measured over time. Other researchers have investigated the combination of the known objective effects of optic nerve disease on color vision with the familiar types of subjective automated perimetry to determine if a blue stimulus on a yellow background will detect earlier defects than standard white-on-white perimetry. This has been named 'short-wavelength automated perimetry', or 'SWAP'. Visual field defects in glaucoma are summarized in Table 7.2.

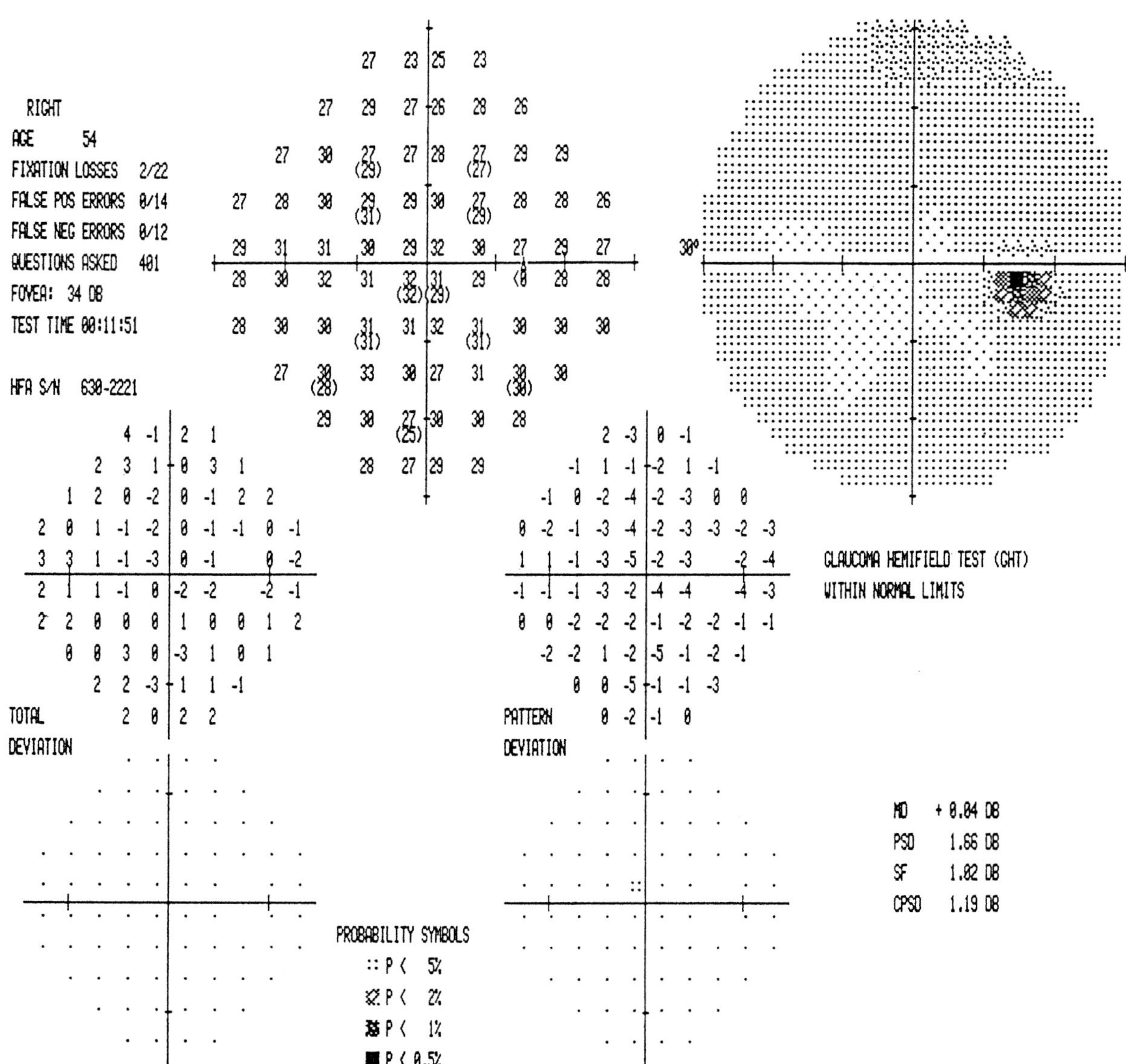

Figure 7.4 The visual field as measured by automated static perimetry

Modern automated static perimeters determine retinal threshold at an array of points and can display the results in a variety of ways. The user determines what points to test and what strategy to use to test them. This figure displays the results of a 30-2 threshold test from the Humphrey Field Analyzer. The test consists of an array of 76 points centered around the fovea with a spacing of six degrees and offset from the axes by three degrees. The numerical grid at the center top represents the retinal threshold expressed in decibels for each test point. Since the decibel scale is a relative scale representing attenuation of the maximum available stimulus intensity, high numbers (above 30 dB, depending upon age) represent good sensitivity (greater attenuation = dimmer stimulus = greater sensitivity). The 'graytone' display on the upper right is a graphical representation of the threshold values, with lighter symbols used for areas of better sensitivity and progressively darker symbols used to represent decreasing sensitivity. The plot on the middle left, labeled 'total deviation', is an array of the differences of the patient's measured threshold values from those exhibited by age-corrected normals, and the lower plot symbolically shows the probability of obtaining the value exhibited by the patient in the reference population. The pattern deviation plot represents a software correction applied to the field for any factors that affect all the points, allowing focal defects to be more readily displayed. A probability plot is displayed for the pattern deviation as well. This figure is an example of a visual field displaying no defects in a patient with mild elevation of intraocular pressure and normal-appearing optic nerves.

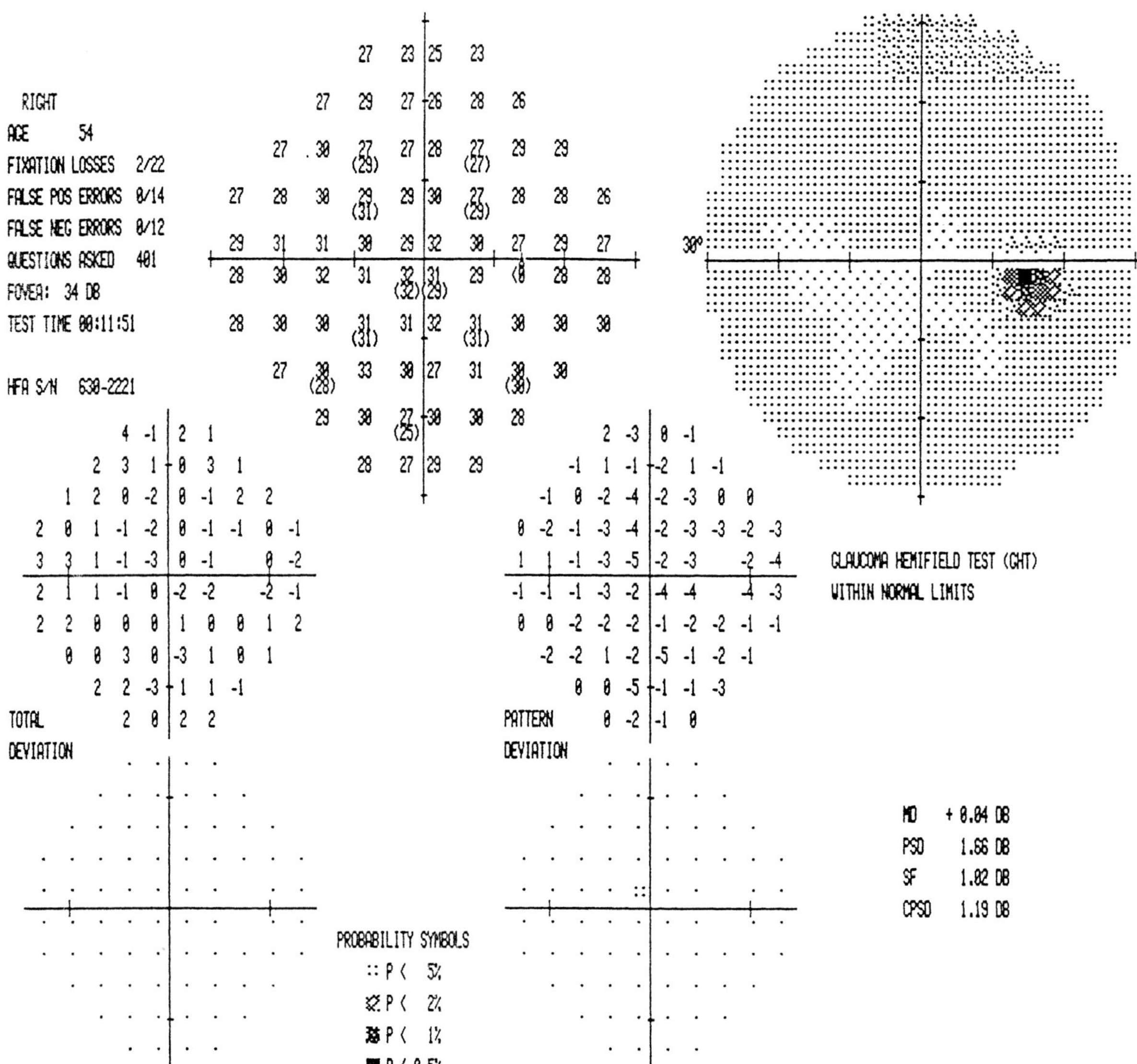

Figure 7.5 Asymmetrical visual field loss
Visual field loss occurs in two ways. The entire visual field may be diffusely affected, causing a loss of sensitivity at all points, manifested as lower threshold values. Many factors acting on the field can produce diffuse loss, including incorrect refraction at the time of the test so that the patient was not properly focused on the bowl, media opacities such as cataract which reduce the amount of light entering the eye, small pupils, inattentiveness and false negative responses, and diffuse optic nerve damage. This set of visual fields illustrates a difference in mean sensitivity between the two eyes, indicative of asymmetric damage.

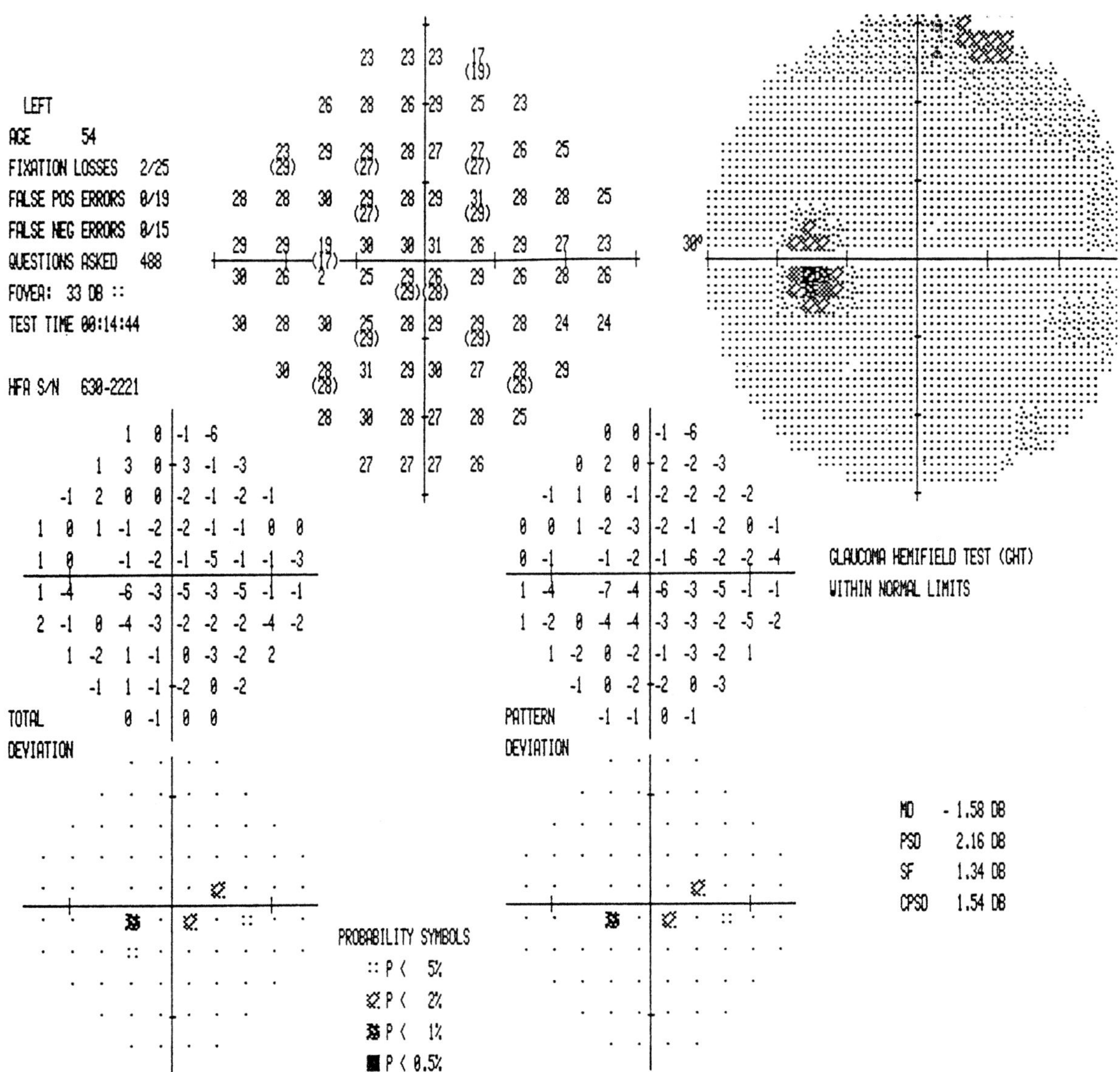

The right eye, the same as Figure 7.4, shows no defect and the mean deviation when compared to age-corrected normals is +0.04 dB. The left eye shows no significant focal defect, but a mean deviation of –1.58 dB, indicating a mild overall reduction in sensitivity, not only compared to the reference population but also more importantly when compared to the fellow eye. The intraocular pressures were 16 mmHg in the right eye and 23 mmHg in the left. In addition, there was a mild increase in the cup to disc ratio in the left eye. This mild reduction in sensitivity in the left eye would not usually be considered clinically significant, except when all the data are considered. It is consistent with mild diffuse depression and with early glaucomatous damage and consequently therapy was started in the left eye.

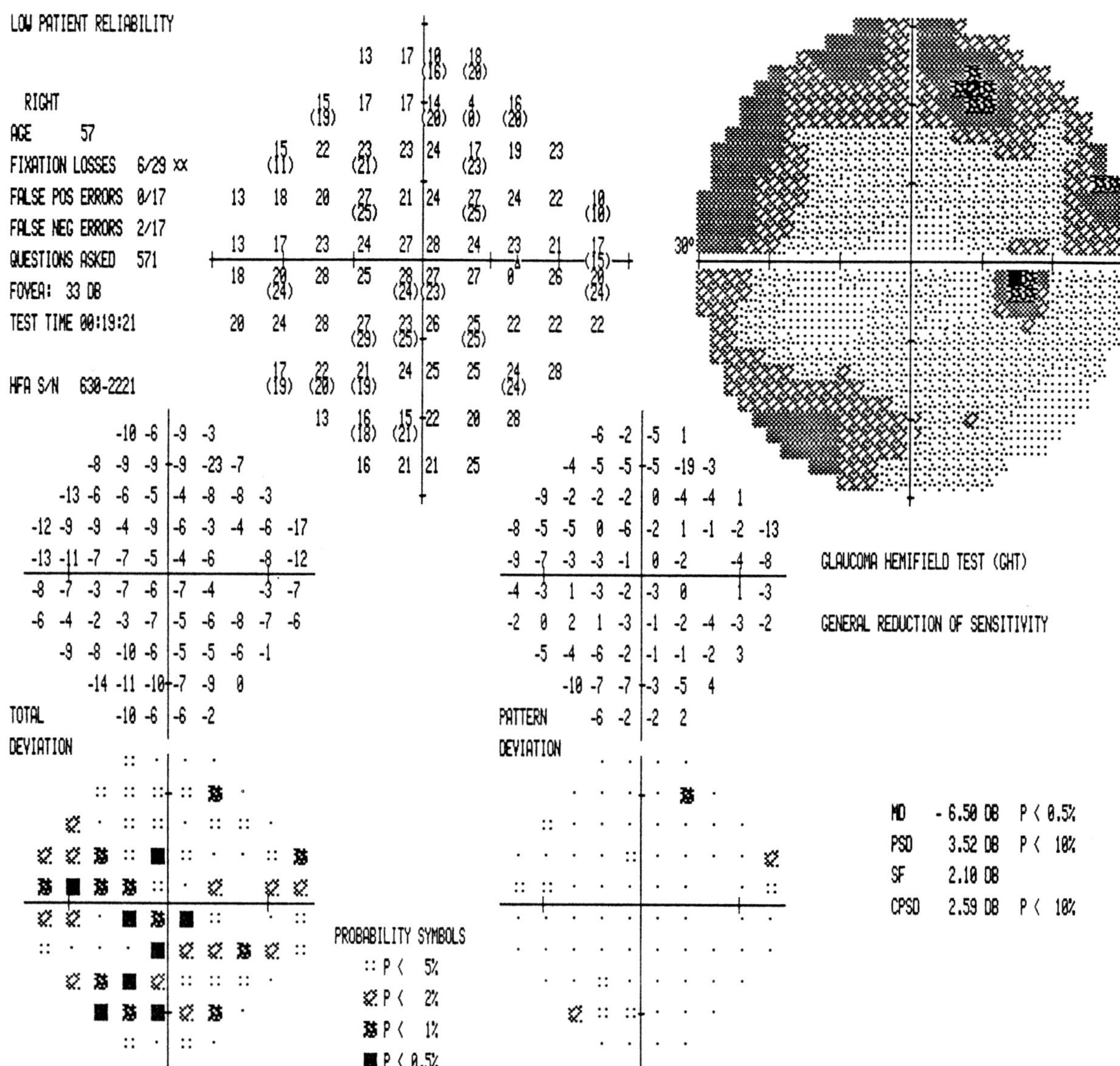

Figure 7.6 Diffuse depression
This is another example of diffuse depression occurring in a patient followed for many years with increased intraocular pressure which had been under treatment. The ocular media are clear, the patient's pupils were dilated for the examination, he was refracted following dilatation to insure the proper distance lens, and the full +3.00 add was used to make sure he was properly focused at the test distance. The mean deviation is –6.50 dB, a value expected to occur in less than 0.5% of the age-corrected normals (i.e. 99.5% of the normals had higher values than this patient), consistent with diffuse optic nerve damage.

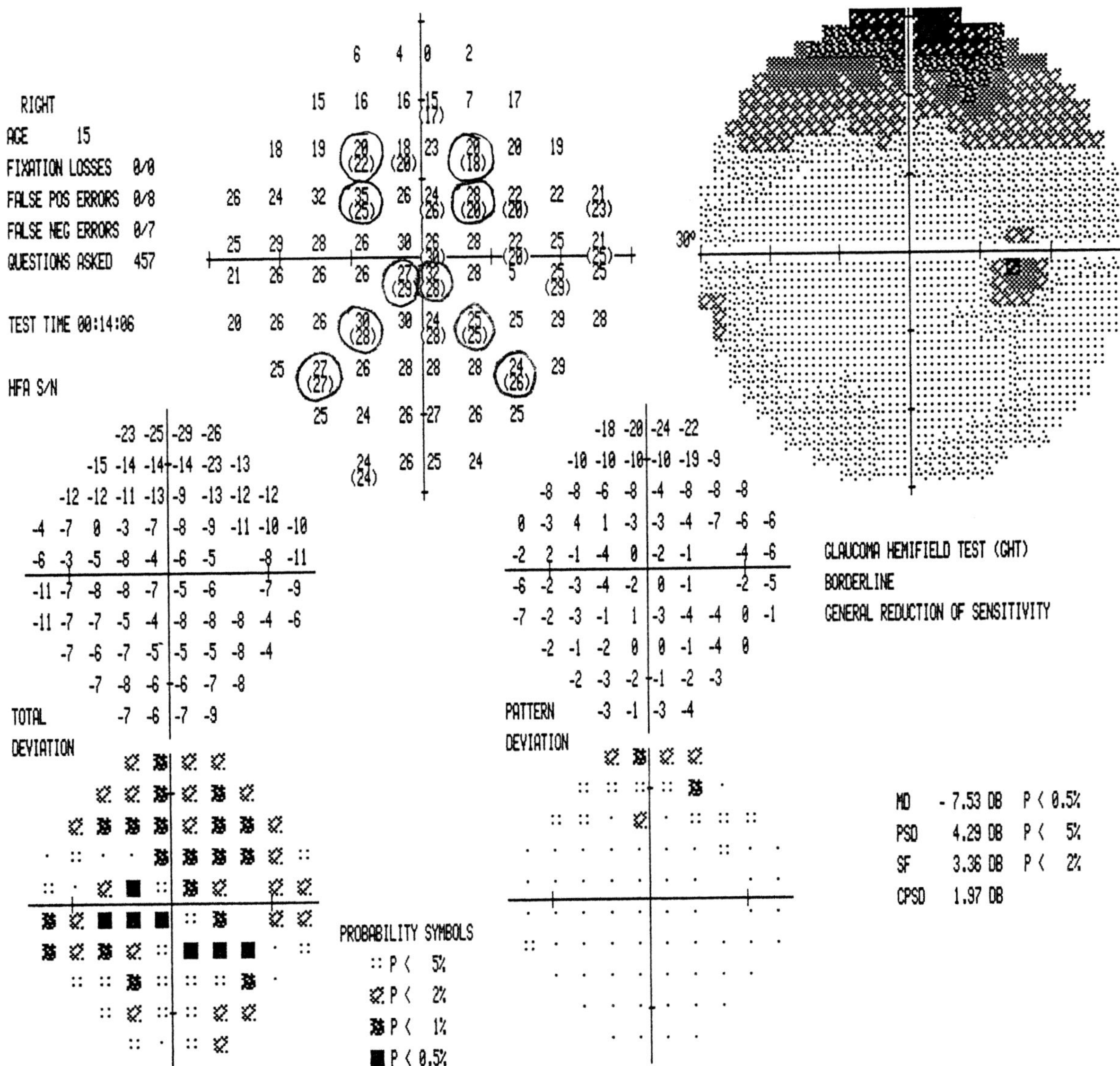

Figure 7.7 Fluctuation
The results of psychophysical tests, such as visual field testing, are subject to a certain degree of variability. Indeed, threshold is defined as that stimulus intensity that has a 50% probability of being seen. This in itself will give rise to varying results as points are retested. Test–retest variability in static perimetry is measurable, has known normal values and has clinical significance. Although an unreliable patient who does not know how to perform the test will show variability in results, unreliability is measured in other ways (i.e. fixation losses, false positive and false negative responses), and a large spread in repeat measures in an otherwise reliable field has other significance. It has been shown that as retinal sensitivity decreases, the variability of threshold in that region increases. It has also been shown that increasing fluctuation may precede the development of a visual field defect, thus giving its measurement particular clinical importance. This figure illustrates ten points (circled) that always have threshold measured twice. The difference of each measurement from the average value is squared, then the squares are summed, averaged across the field and the square root taken. Other factors are applied to account for point location in the field, and the result expressed as the short-term fluctuation value, or 'sf'. This patient has angle-recession glaucoma with intraocular pressure in the low 30s. The field demonstrates diffuse depression, but more importantly an increased sf value of 3.36, expected in less than 2% of the reference population. The high value is derived from two points in the superior arcuate area—one showing measurements of 35 and 25 dB and the other 28 and 20 dB. These large differences in repeat measurements (10 and 8 dB respectively) point to disturbed portions of the visual field that will most likely go on to develop paracentral and arcuate defects.

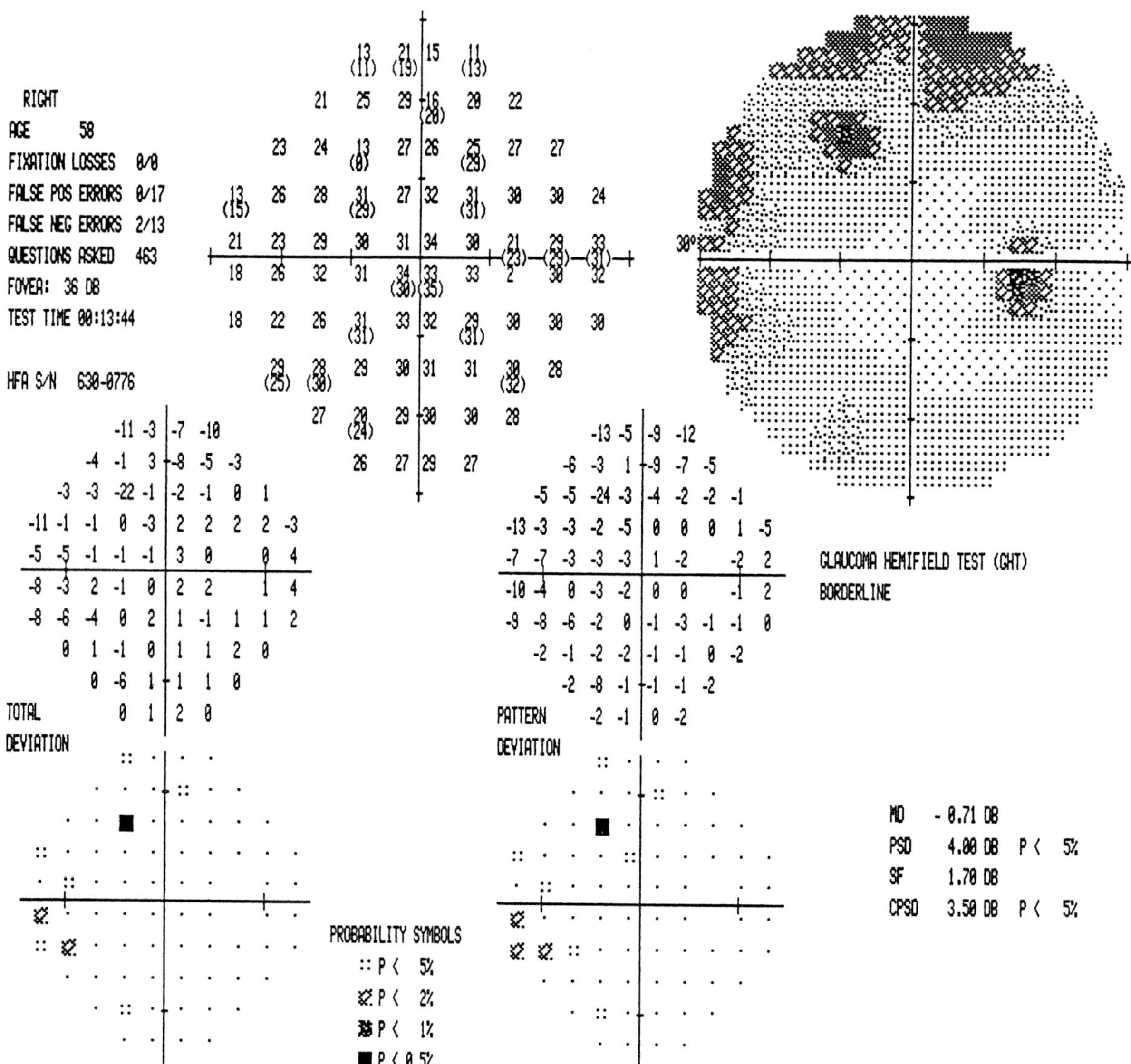

Figure 7.8 Isolated paracentral defects
As indicated in Table 7.2, isolated paracentral defects occur as the initial glaucoma defect in about 40% of patients. This patient shows an isolated defect in the superior paracentral region of 22 dB below normal. Note also the wide fluctuation in repeat measurements of this point (13 dB and then 0 dB). Untreated intraocular pressure was in the upper 20s in this eye.

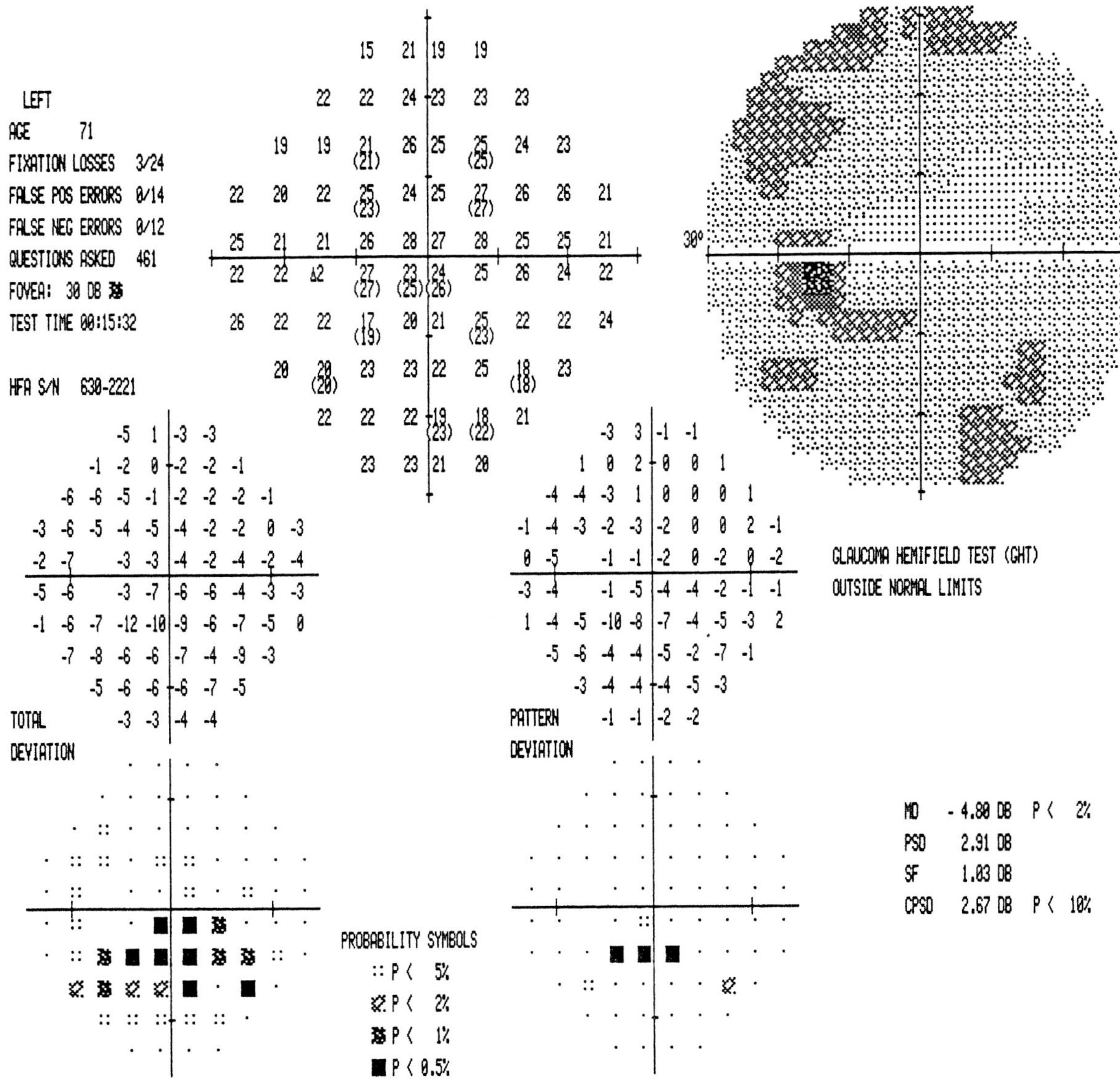

Figure 7.9 Asymmetry across the horizontal meridian Asymmetry across the horizontal meridian is an important sign of optic nerve disease. The glaucoma hemifield test is a software option as part of the statistical analysis package for the Humphrey Field Analyzer that compares the differences of mirror-image clusters of points on opposite sides of the horizontal from the reference population to determine asymmetry. This is an example of an asymmetric disturbance in the inferior portion of the visual field of a glaucoma patient with an abnormal glaucoma hemifield test. This patient shows an early inferior arcuate enlargement of the blind spot. Note also from the probability map of the pattern deviation that threshold values of 19 dB (or more) occur in the periphery of the superior hemifield in 95% of the age-corrected normals, but a value of 19 dB would be expected in the inferior arcuate area less than 0.5% of the time.

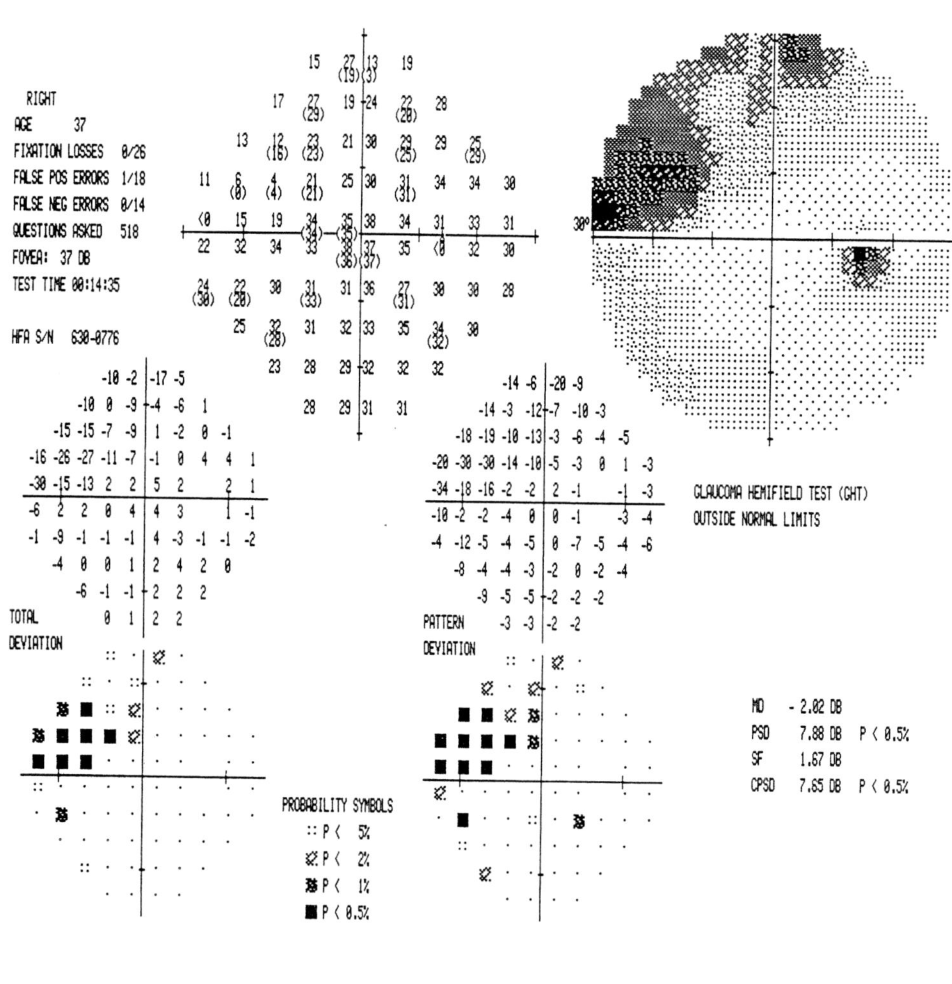

Figure 7.10 Nasal steps
Nasal steps are very common in glaucoma, representing an asymmetry in threshold across the horizontal midline at the nasal periphery of the measured field. They are the first defects in about half the glaucoma patients. This patient shows a dense superior nasal step.

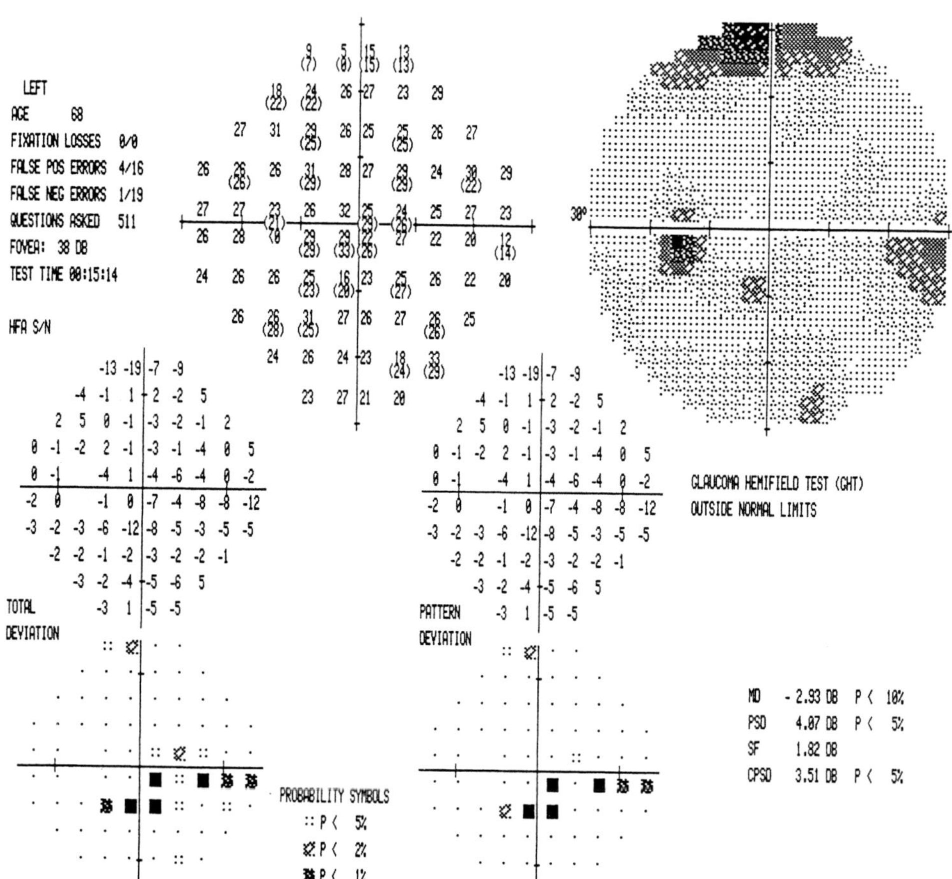

Figure 7.11 Early glaucomatous damage in the inferior hemifield
This is another example of early glaucomatous damage in the inferior hemifield. An inferior nasal step combined with inferior paracentral defects indicate damage to the superior arcuate nerve fibers.

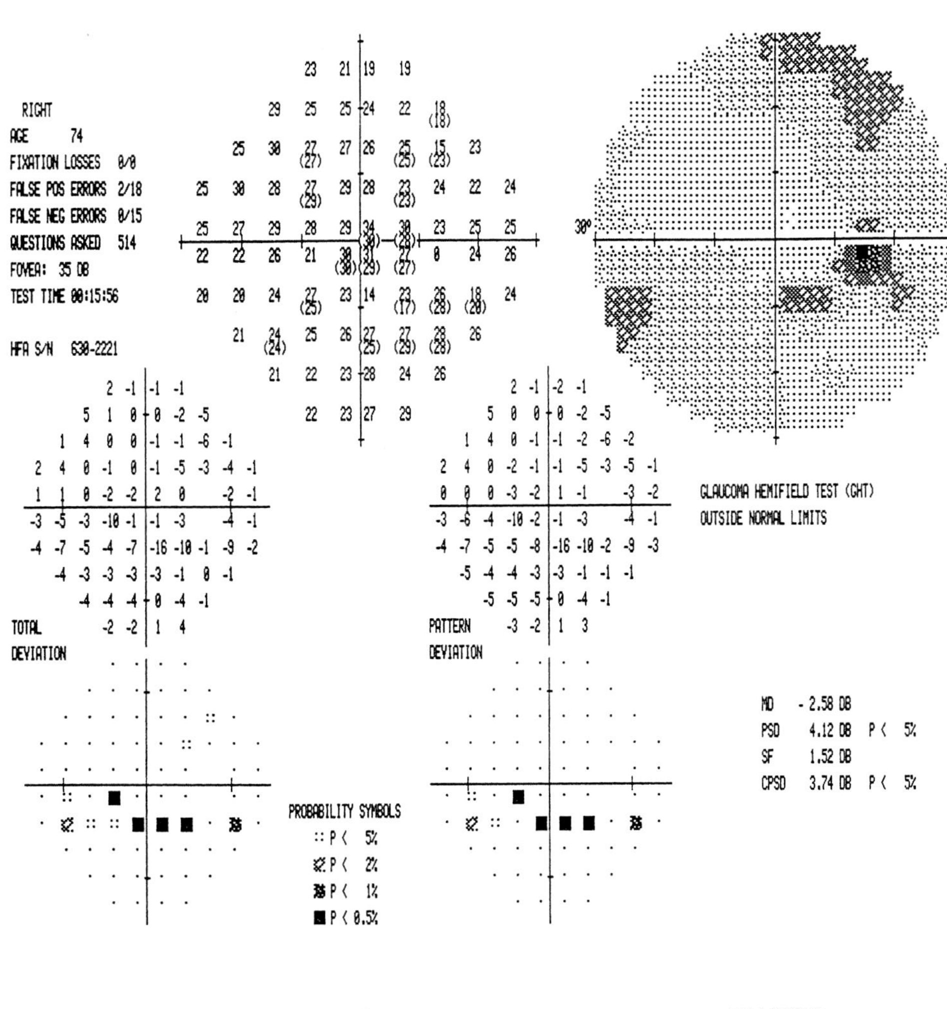

Figure 7.12 An inferior arcuate scotoma
This example of early glaucoma damage shows an inferior arcuate scotoma which does not reach the nasal periphery.

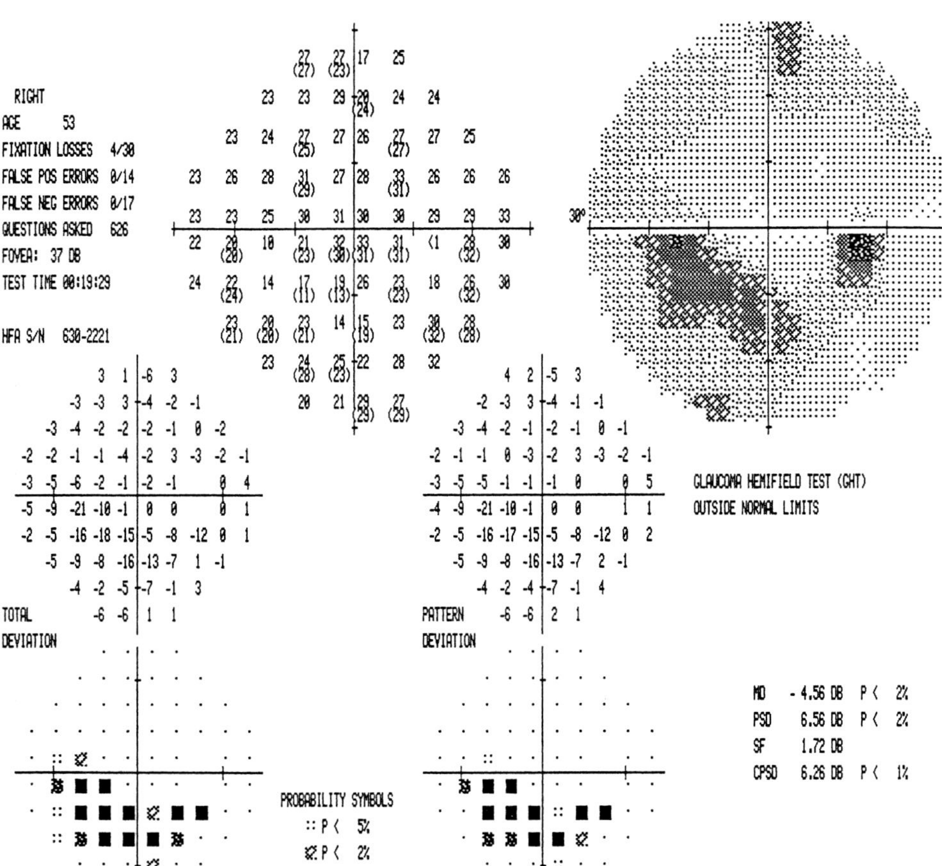

Figure 7.13 A broad inferior arcuate scotoma
This patient has had open-angle glaucoma for many years. He has extensive damage in the fellow eye and has lost fixation. This is an example of a broader inferior arcuate scotoma (compared to Fig. 7.12) which connects to the blind spot.

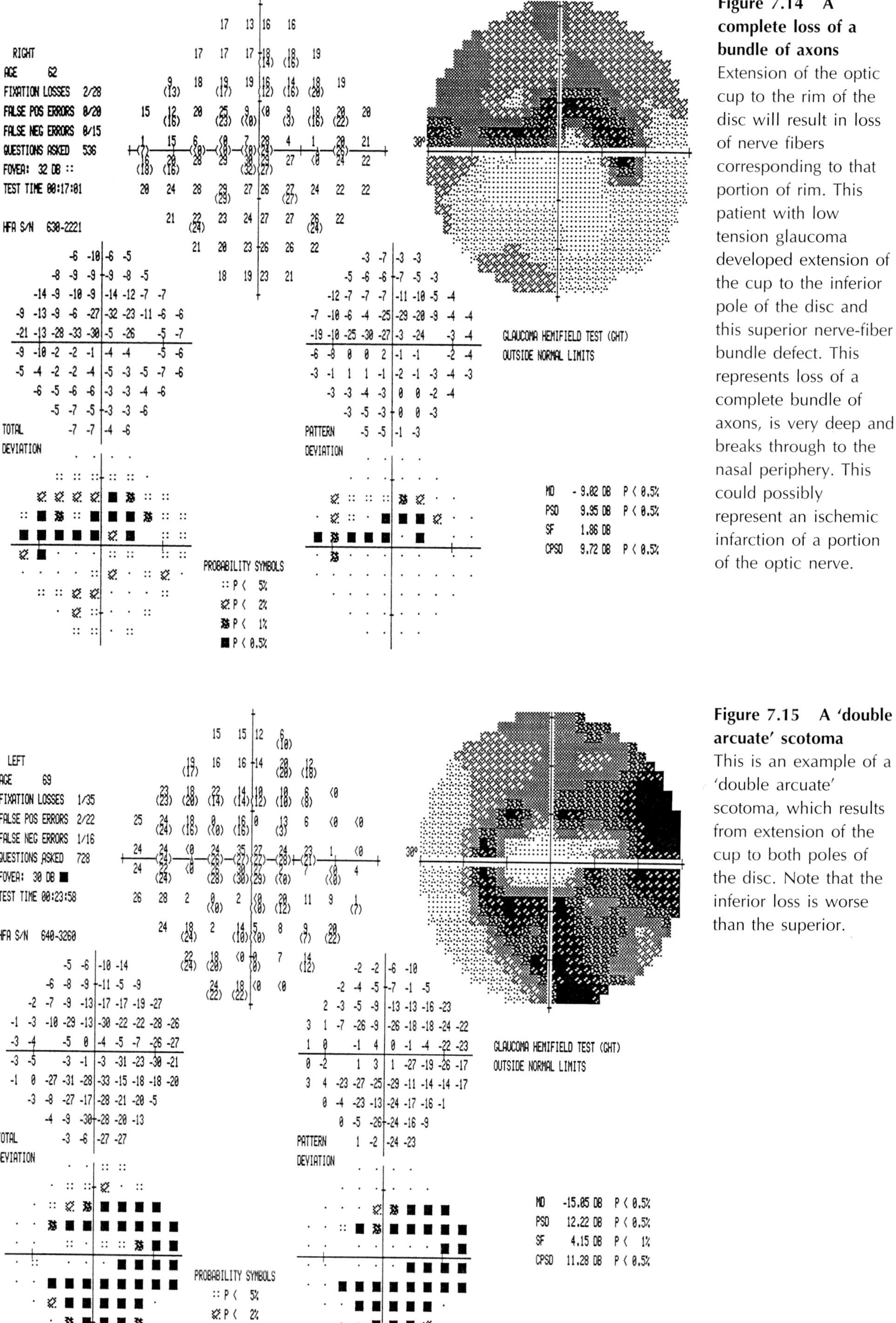

Figure 7.14 A complete loss of a bundle of axons
Extension of the optic cup to the rim of the disc will result in loss of nerve fibers corresponding to that portion of rim. This patient with low tension glaucoma developed extension of the cup to the inferior pole of the disc and this superior nerve-fiber bundle defect. This represents loss of a complete bundle of axons, is very deep and breaks through to the nasal periphery. This could possibly represent an ischemic infarction of a portion of the optic nerve.

Figure 7.15 A 'double arcuate' scotoma
This is an example of a 'double arcuate' scotoma, which results from extension of the cup to both poles of the disc. Note that the inferior loss is worse than the superior.

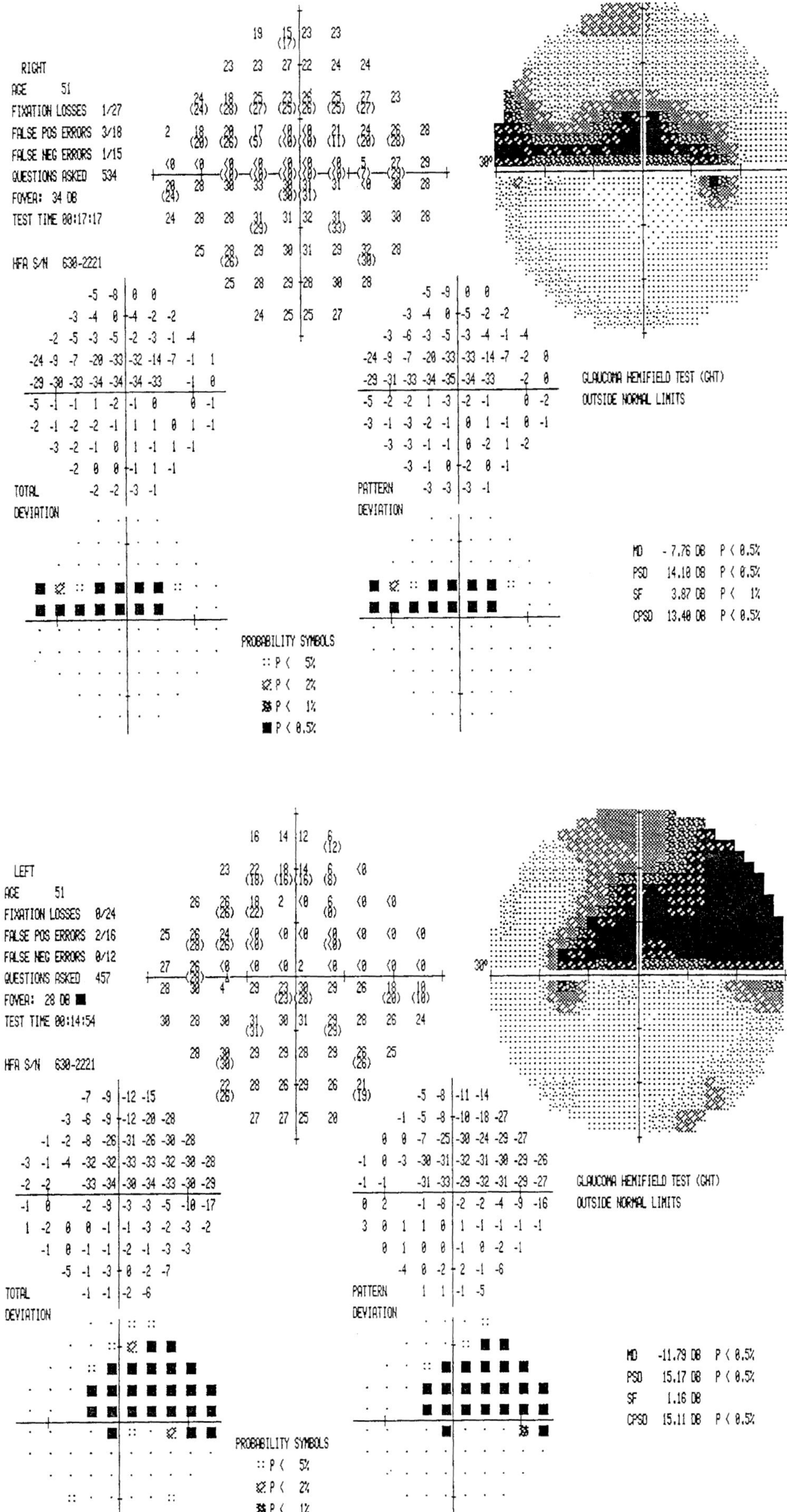

Figure 7.16 Complete nerve-fiber bundle defects
Complete nerve-fiber bundle defects are not common as the initial defects in glaucoma patients. This pair of visual fields from the right and left eyes of this 51-year-old African-American female were the patient's first visual fields. Initial pressures were in the upper 20s. Note the asymmetry, with the left eye worse than the right.

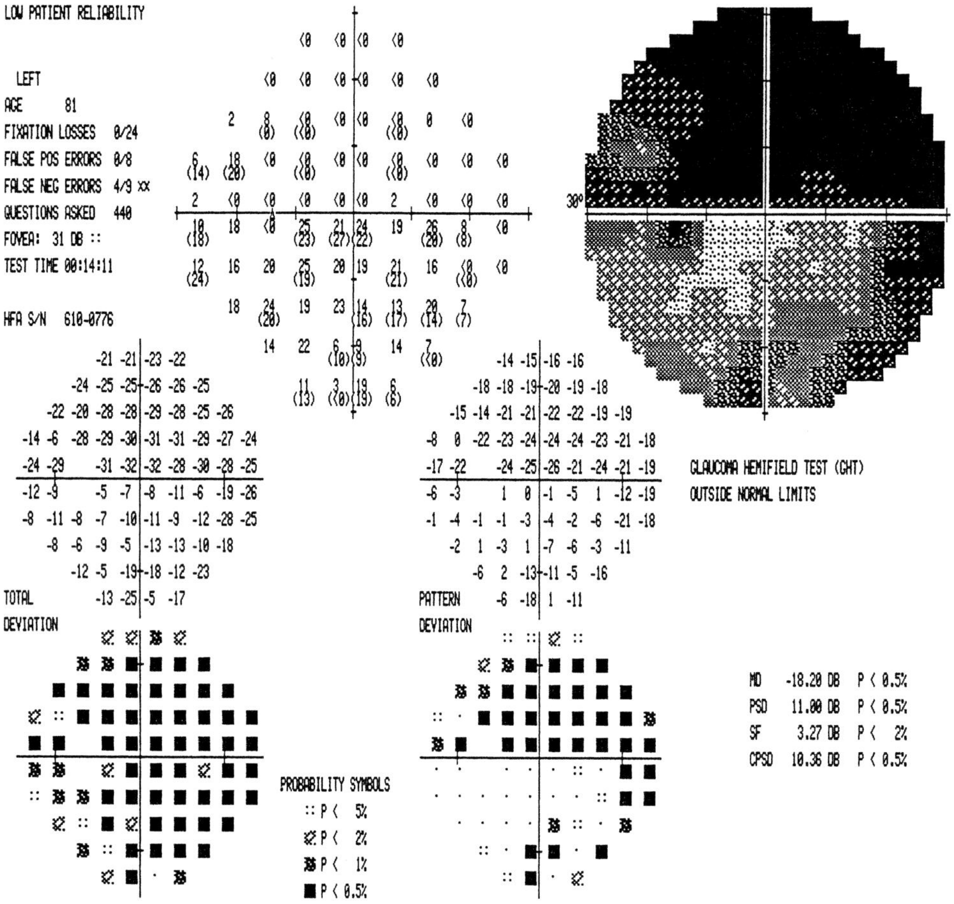

LOW PATIENT RELIABILITY

LEFT
AGE 81
FIXATION LOSSES 0/24
FALSE POS ERRORS 0/8
FALSE NEG ERRORS 4/9 xx
QUESTIONS ASKED 440
FOVEA: 31 DB ::
TEST TIME 00:14:11

HFA S/N 610-0776

TOTAL DEVIATION

PATTERN DEVIATION

PROBABILITY SYMBOLS
:: P < 5%
P < 2%
P < 1%
P < 0.5%

GLAUCOMA HEMIFIELD TEST (GHT)
OUTSIDE NORMAL LIMITS

MD -18.20 DB P < 0.5%
PSD 11.00 DB P < 0.5%
SF 3.27 DB P < 2%
CPSD 10.36 DB P < 0.5%

Figure 7.17 Superior altitudinal defect Complete loss of the inferior pole of the nerve will give rise to a superior altitudinal defect, illustrated here. Although commonly seen following ischemic optic neuropathy, this defect gradually enlarged over time in this patient with low-tension glaucoma (see Fig. 7.26).

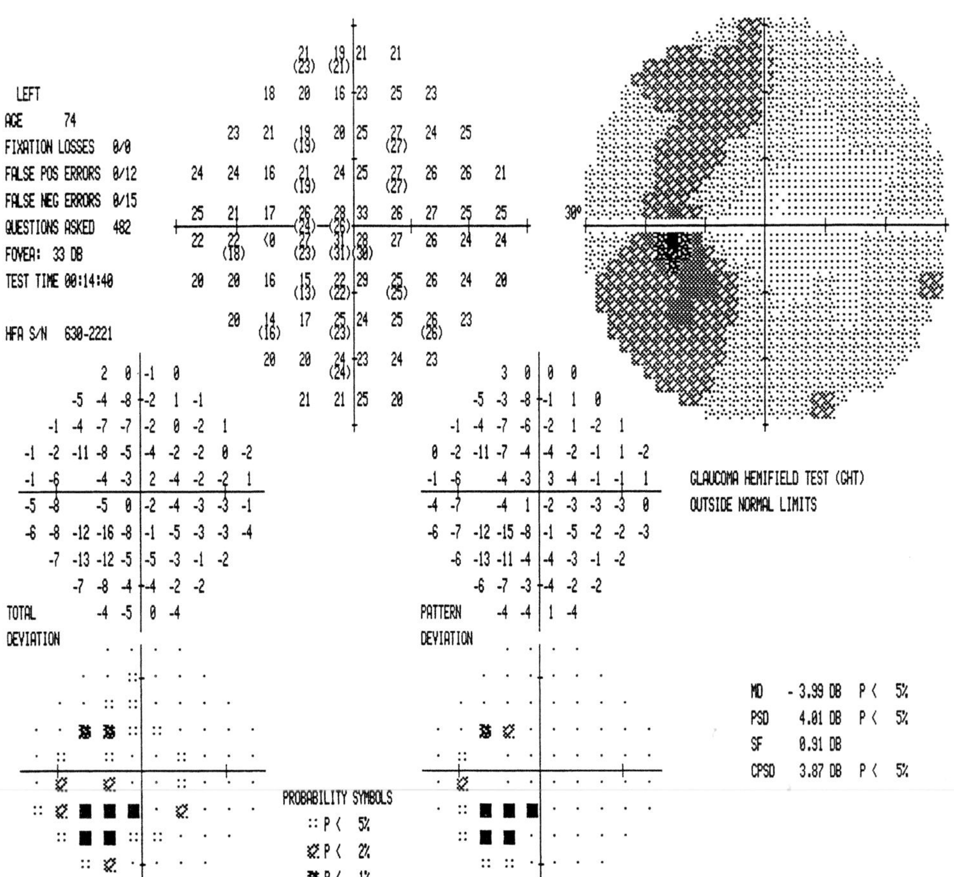

Figure 7.18 Isolated temporal defects Isolated temporal defects occur about 3% of the time as initial glaucoma defects. This patient shows temporal defects above and below the horizontal midline. Note that the statistical software gives more significance to the inferior disturbances, indicating that some depressions in the superior field of older people is not unusual.

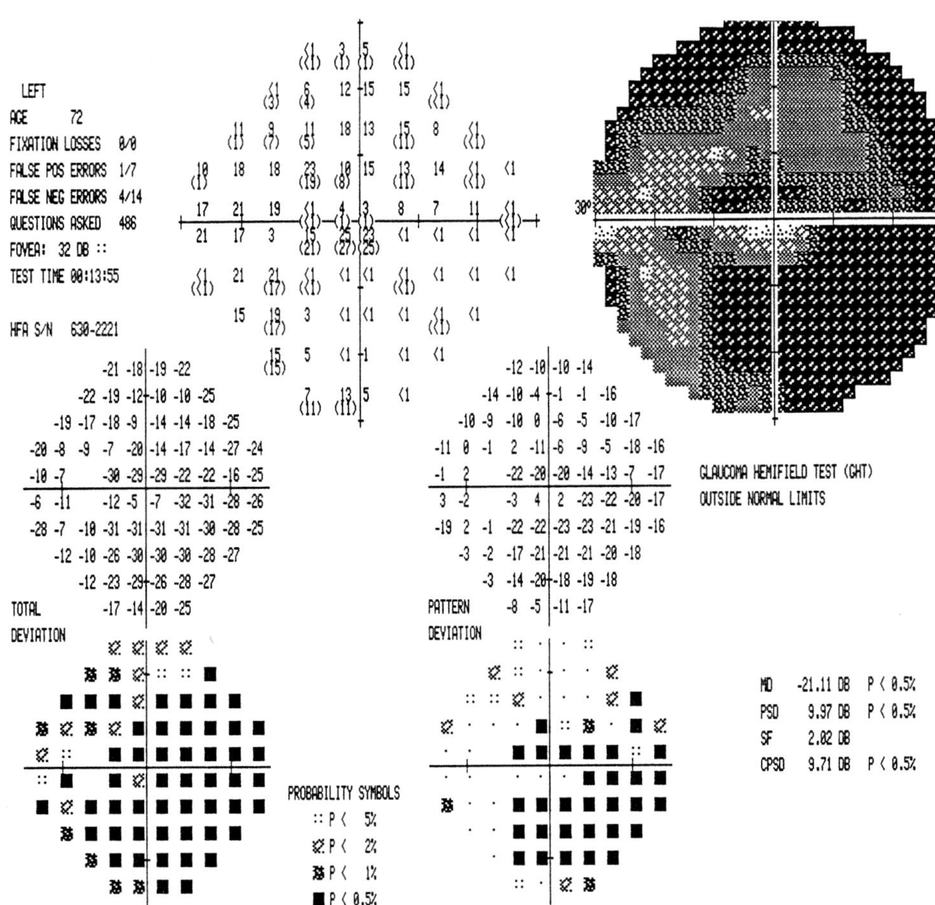

Figure 7.19 Far-advanced glaucomatous optic neuropathy Progressive loss of nerve fibers results in greater visual field loss, usually affecting the macular fibers and the nasal retina last, leaving central and temporal islands as the end-stage before complete visual loss. This is an example of a patient with far-advanced glaucomatous optic neuropathy, with small islands remaining centrally, temporally and in the superior arcuate area.

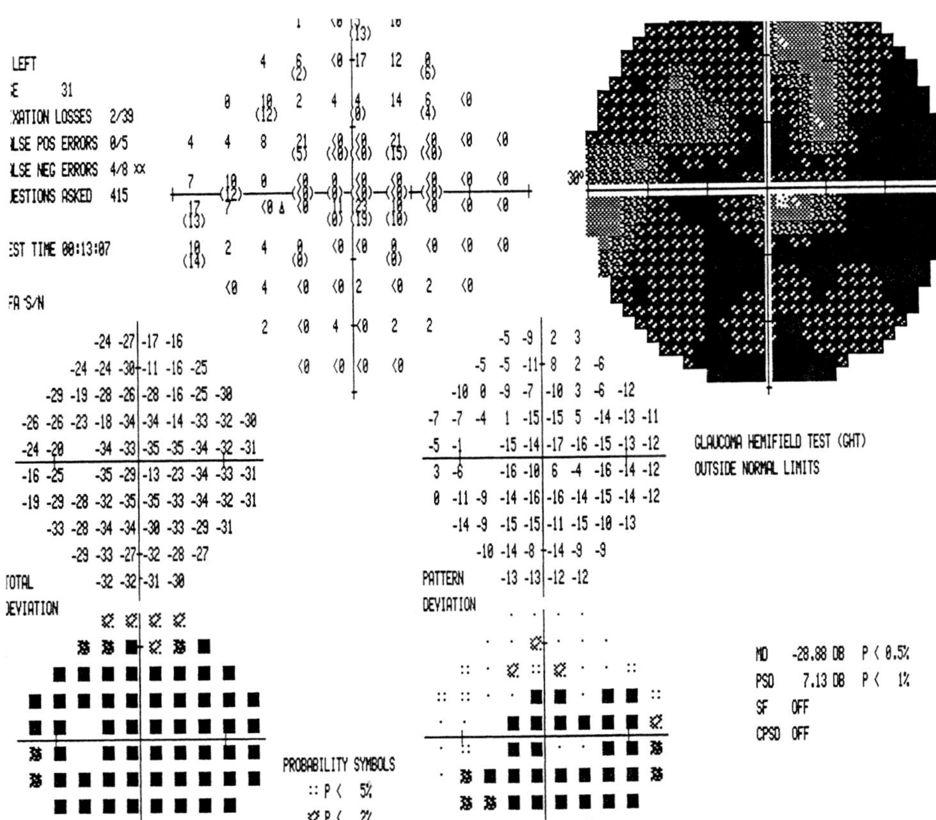

Figure 7.20 High intraocular pressure Very high intraocular pressure can lead to extensive loss which may become symptomatic. This visual field showing extensive damage was obtained upon initial presentation of a young male with intraocular pressure in the 50s. He noted visual loss and went for an eye examination. His visual acuity was reduced to 20/70. The fellow eye had minimal loss with pressures in the 30s and 20/20 vision. He was found to have abnormal anterior chamber angles, indicating a juvenile-onset type of glaucoma. Following filtering surgery, his visual acuity returned to 20/25 and some of the visual field loss returned.

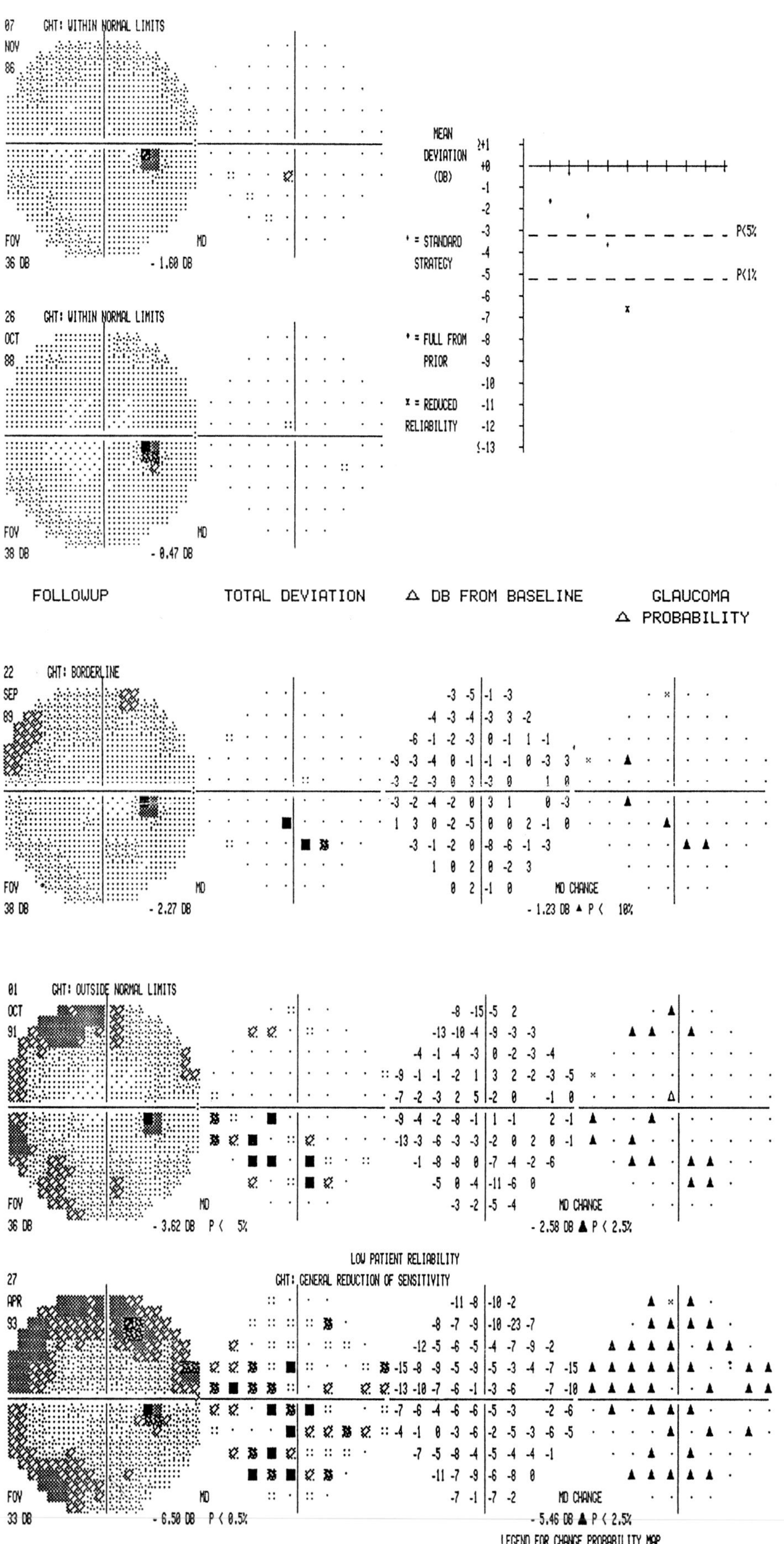

Figure 7.21 The progression of visual field defects
Visual fields may show progression over time in a variety of ways. If initially normal, they may go on to diffuse loss or the development of isolated depressions. This series of fields over a 7-year period was obtained in an African-American man with ocular hypertension which was under treatment. It shows a gradual but steady decrease in retinal sensitivity affecting the field uniformly (the last field is the same as Fig. 7.6). A review of optic nerve photographs (particularly comparing the earliest to the latest) shows a concentric enlargement of the cup over time with the neuroretinal rim still intact.

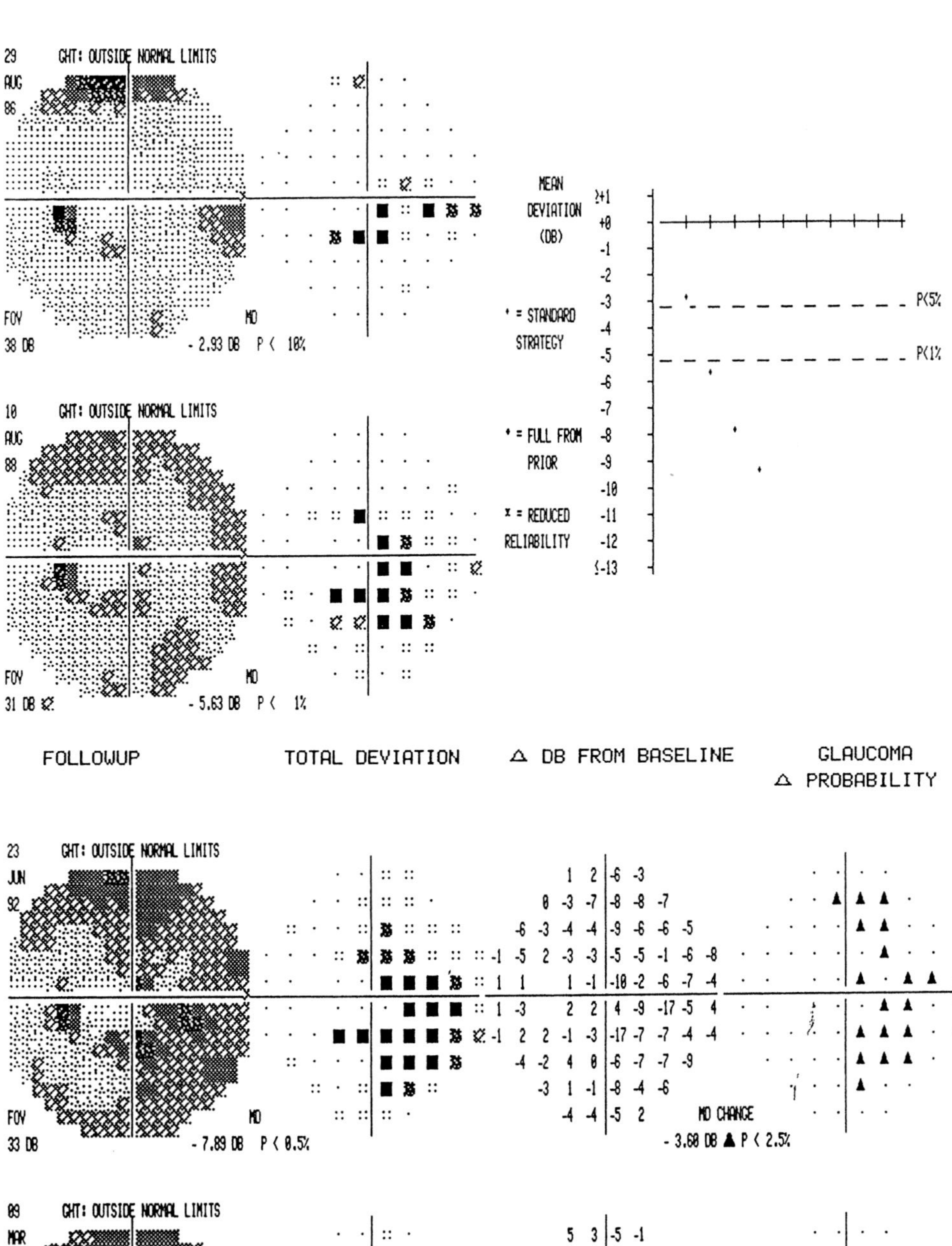

Figure 7.22 The development of new defects
Fields initially with defects may show the development of new defects. This series of fields in a patient with open-angle glaucoma shows completion of an inferior nerve-fiber bundle defect as well as the development of new defects in the superior field. Part of the diffuse change in the latter fields is due to the development of cataract.

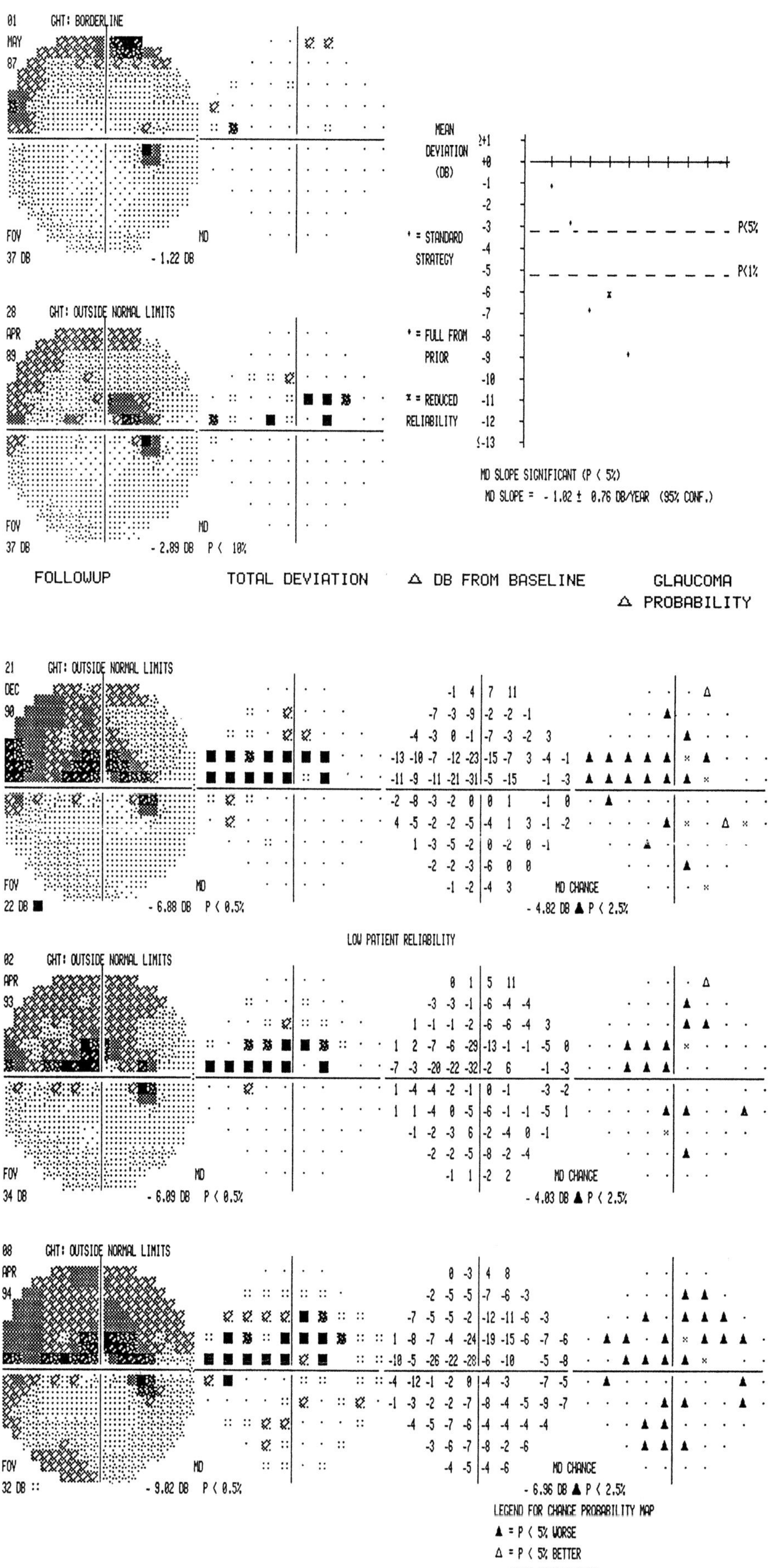

Figure 7.23 Widening and deepening of single nerve-fiber bundle defects
Visual fields may progress by widening and deepening of single nerve-fiber bundle defects. This series of visual fields is from the patient in Fig. 7.14. Initially the field was normal and then she developed disturbances in the superior arcuate area. These coalesced and extended over time to involve the entire bundle of axons and a good portion of the superior field.

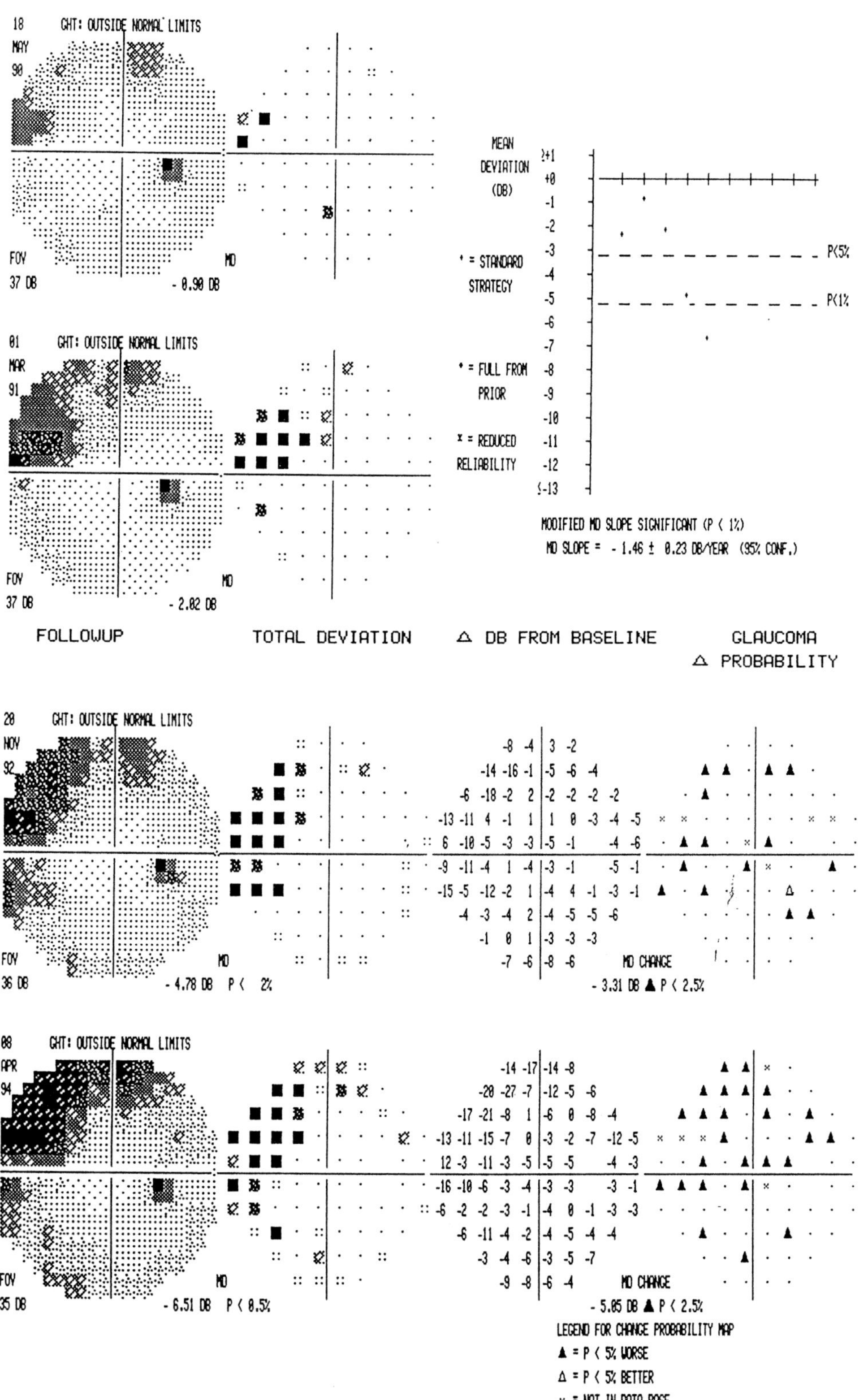

Figure 7.24 Gradual enlargement of the superior nasal step This series of visual fields was obtained from the fellow eye of the same patient in Fig. 7.20. Note the gradual enlargement of the superior nasal step. He has undergone filtering surgery in this eye as well.

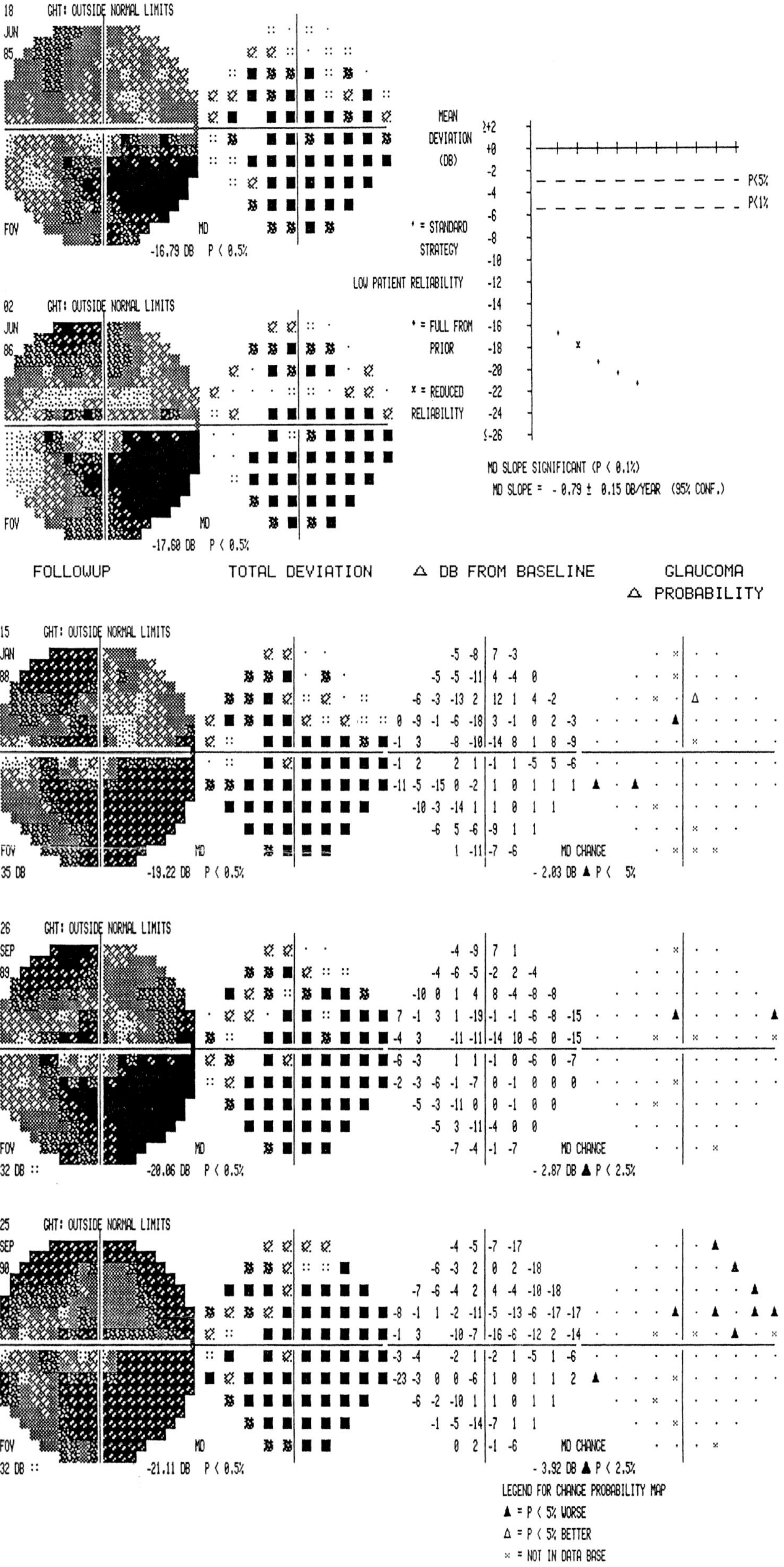

Figure 7.25 A steady decline of 1 dB per year
This is the series of visual fields of the patient in Fig. 7.19. Note the extension of the inferior nerve-fiber bundle defect and the development of new defects in the superior hemifield. The statistical software plots the mean deviation over time as a graph on the right side of the top of the printout, and performs statistical tests for significant change over time. This series shows a steady decline of about 1 dB per year, which was highly significant.

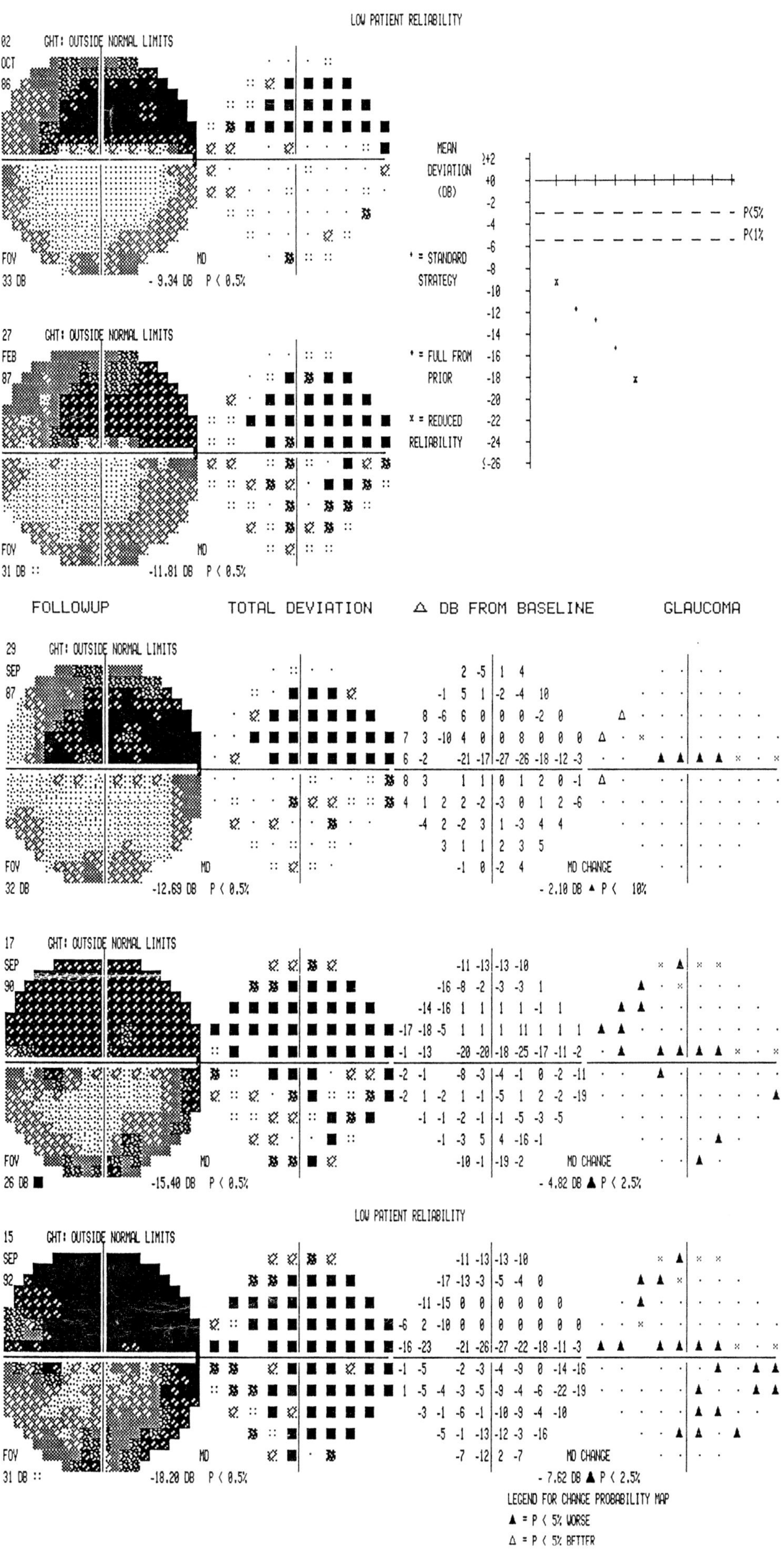

Figure 7.26 Extension of a dense superior nerve-fiber bundle defect
This series illustrates the extension of a dense superior nerve-fiber bundle defect to a complete altitudinal defect over a 6-year period.

FURTHER READING

Anctil JL, Anderson JR, Early foveal involvement and generalized depression of the visual field in glaucoma, *Arch Ophthalmol* (1980) **102**:363.

Atkin A, Bodis-Wollner I, Wolkstein M, et al., Abnormalities of central contrast sensitivity in glaucoma. *Am J Ophthalmol* (1979) **88**:205–11.

Atkin A, Wolkstein M, Bodis-Wollner I, et al., Interocular comparison of contrast sensitivity in glaucoma patients and suspects, *Br J Ophthalmol* (1980) **64**:858–62.

Aulhorn E, Harms H, Early visual field defects in glaucoma. In: Leydhecker W, ed. *Glaucoma: Tutzing symposium (1966)* (Basel: S Karger, 1967), 151.

Austin D, Acquired colour vision defects in patients suffering from chronic simple glaucoma, *Trans Ophthalmol Soc UK* (1974) **94**:880.

Breton ME, Wilson TW, Wilson RP, et al., Temporal contrast sensitivity loss in primary open-angle glaucoma and glaucoma suspects, *Invest Ophthalmol Vis Sci* (1991) **32**:2931–41.

Caprioli J, Automated perimetry in glaucoma, *Am J Ophthalmol* (1991) **112**:235–9.

Choplin NT, Edwards RP. *Visual Field Testing with the Humphrey Field Analyzer*, Thorofare, NJ, SLACK, Inc. 1995

Drance SM, The glaucomatous visual field, *Br J Ophthalmol* (1972) **56**:186.

Drance SM, et al., Acquired color vision changes in glaucoma: use of a 100-hue test and Pickford anomaloscope as predictors of glaucomatous field change, *Arch Ophthalmol* (1981) **99**:829.

Feghali JG, Bocquet X, Charlier J, et al., Static flicker perimetry in glaucoma and ocular hypertension. *Curr Eye Res* (1991) **10**:205–12.

Glovinsky Y, Quigley HA, Brum B, et al., A whole-field scotopic retinal sensitivity test for the detection of early glaucoma damage, *Arch Ophthalmol* (1992) **110**:486–90.

Gunduz K, Arden GB, Perry S, et al., Color vision defects in ocular hypertension and glaucoma: quantification with a computer-driven color television system. *Arch Ophthalmol* (1988) **106**:929–35.

Harrington DO, The Bjerrum scotoma. *Am J Ophthalmol* (1965) **59**:646.

Hart WM Jr, et al., Quantitative visual field and optic disc correlates early in glaucoma. *Arch Ophthalmol* (1978) **96**:2206.

Heijl A, Lindgren G, Olsson J, A package for the statistical analysis of visual fields. In: Greve and Heyl eds. *Seventh International Visual Field Symposium* (Dordrecht: Minitinus Nijoff/Dr W Junk Publishers, 1987), 153–68.

Hitchings RA, Spaeth GL, The optic disc in glaucoma. I. Classification, *Br J Ophthalmol* (1976) **60**:778.

Iwata K, Retinal nerve fiber layer, optic cupping, and visual field changes in glaucoma. In: Bellows JG, ed. *Glaucoma: contemporary international concepts* (New York: Masson, 1979), 139.

Johnson CA, Adams AJ, Casson EJ, et al., Blue-on-yellow perimetry can predict the development of glaucomatous visual field loss. *Arch Ophthalmol* (1993) **111**:645–50.

Johnson CA, Adams AJ, Casson EJ, et al., Progression of glaucomatous visual field loss as detected by blue-on-yellow and standard white-on-white perimetry. *Arch Ophthalmol* (1993) **111**:651–6.

Kirsch RE, Anderson DR, Clinical recognition of glaucomatous cupping. *Am J Ophthalmol* (1973) **75**:442.

Maffei L, Fiorentini A, Electroretinographic response to alternating gratings before and after section of the optic nerve. *Science* (1981) **211**:953.

Motolko M, Drance SM, Douglas GR, The early psychophysical disturbances in chronic open-angle glaucoma: a study of visual functions with asymmetric disc cupping. *Arch Ophthalmol* (1982) **100**:1632.

Nadler MP, Miller D, Nadler DJ, eds., *Glare and contrast sensitivity for clinicians* (New York: Springer-Verlag, 1990).

Parisi V, Bucci M, Visual evoked potentials after photostress in patients with primary open-angle glaucoma and ocular hypertension. *Invest Ophthalmol Vis Sci* (1992) **33**:436–42.

Pederson JE, Anderson JR, The mode of progressive disc cupping in ocular hypertension and glaucoma. *Arch Ophthalmol* (1980) **102**:1689.

Phelps CD, Remijan RW, Blondeau P, Acuity perimetry. *Doc Ophthalmol Proc Ser* (1981) **26**:111.

Quigley HA, Addicks EM, Green W, Optic nerve damage in human glaucoma. III. Quantitative correlation of nerve fiber loss and visual field defect in glaucoma, ischemic optic neuropathy, disc edema, and toxic neuropathy. *Arch Ophthalmol* (1982) **100**:135.

Quigley HA, Homan RM, Addicks EM, et al., Morphologic changes in the lamina cribrosa correlated with neural loss in open-angle glaucoma. *Am J Ophthalmol* (1983) **95**:673.

Quigley HA, Sanchez RM, Dunkelberger GR, et al., Chronic glaucoma selectively damages large optic nerve fibers. *Invest Ophthalmol Vis Sci* (1987) **28**:913–20.

Sample PA, Ahn DS, Lee PC, et al., High-pass resolution perimetry in eyes with ocular hypertension and primary open-angle glaucoma. *Am J Ophthalmol* (1992) **113**:309–16.

Sample PA, Weinreb RM, Boynton RM, Acquired dyschromatopsia in glaucoma, *Surv Ophthalmol* (1986) **31**:54–64.

Schmeisser ET, Smith TJ, Flicker visual evoked potential differentiation of glaucoma. *Optometry and Vis Sci* (1992) **69**:458–62.

Shih Y, Huang Z, Chang C, Color pattern-reversal evoked potential in eyes with ocular hypertension and primary open-angle glaucoma, *Documenta Ophthalmologica* (1991) **77**:193–200.

Stamper RL, Hsu-Winges C, Sopher M, Arden contrast sensitivity testing in glaucoma, *Arch Ophthalmol* (1982) **100**:947.

Trick GL, Retinal potentials in patients with primary open angle glaucoma: physiological evidence for temporal frequency tuning defect. *Invest Ophthalmol Vis Sci* (1985) **26**:1750.

Weinstein GW, Arden GB, Hitchings RA, et al., The pattern electroretinogram (PERG) in ocular hypertension and glaucoma. *Arch Ophthalmol* (1988) **106**:923–8.

8 Primary open-angle glaucoma

Paul P Lee

Introduction

The 1996 revision to the American Academy of Ophthalmology's (AAO) Preferred Practice Pattern (PPP) for primary open-angle glaucoma (POAG) defines the disease as a multifactorial optic neuropathy in which there is a characteristic acquired loss of optic nerve fibers. It is a 'chronic, generally bilateral and often asymmetrical disease, which is characterized (in at least one eye) by all of the following: [1] evidence of glaucomatous optic nerve damage from either or both . . . the appearance of the disc or retinal nerve fiber layer . . . or . . . the presence of characteristic abnormalities in the visual field; [2] adult onset; [3] open, normal-appearing anterior chamber angles; [and 4] absence of known other (e.g. secondary) causes of open-angle glaucoma'. Since practice guidelines (particularly those of the American Academy of Ophthalmology with regards to ophthalmic disease) are likely to carry significant legal weight, if not necessarily scientific heft, this is now the standard definition of POAG. What is clearly new, almost revolutionary, is that intraocular pressure is no longer part of the definition, and that the presence of both optic nerve and visual field abnormalities is no longer required. Rather, the diagnosis of open-angle glaucoma is now based on the presence of optic nerve damage, as manifested by either disc or field abnormalities. As such, this represents a significant departure from historical associations of glaucoma with intraocular pressure.

Epidemiology

Prevalence

Several population-based studies conducted over the last 20 years have illuminated our understanding of the incidence and prevalence of POAG within defined populations in the USA and abroad. Yet, it is important to read the reports from the studies in keeping with the definition of glaucoma used in the study reports relative to the new AAO definition. A diagnosis of glaucoma in the Beaver Dam Eye Study required that at least two of three criteria were met: abnormal visual field, optic disc, or intraocular pressure. The importance of such definitions to our understanding of the population prevalence rates of glaucoma can be seen if one reanalyzes the Beaver Dam findings. Adding those cases that had only a visual field abnormality or optic nerve finding (even with the requirement of a corresponding history of medical or surgical treatment of glaucoma with either abnormality) would raise the total prevalence of POAG in the study by 31%. The Rotterdam Study in The Netherlands defines glaucoma on the basis of a combination of visual field and optic nerve findings or an intraocular pressure greater than 21. In this study, however, more basic data were not given to allow one to reanalyze the rates. Without additional data, understanding the rates of POAG in this population, given the new definition of POAG, becomes problematic.

In the Barbados Eye Study of blacks, definite POAG required the presence of both optic disc and visual field abnormalities. Adding 'suspect OAG' participants defined as those with 'less complete' data (and thus potentially including those with only one of the two criteria or more equivocal findings in both criteria) would increase the rate of POAG in this population by 55%!

Only the Baltimore Eye Survey, in contrast, provides a definition based on either optic nerve head findings or visual field abnormalities, of varying strengths, consistent with the new AAO definition. Thus, readers and policy-makers should carefully read and understand how POAG is defined to understand its epidemiological magnitude. Using the new definition of glaucoma, estimates are that nearly 15 million Americans would be diagnosed as having

Table 8.1 **Effect of age on prevalence of POAG**

Study	Race	Age (years)	Prevalence rate (%)
Rotterdam	Not specified	55–59	0.2
		85–89	3.3
Baltimore Eye Survey	White	40–49	0.9
	White	>80	2.2
	Black	40–49	1.23
	Black	>80	11.26
Barbados	Black	40–49	1.4
		>80	23.2
Beaver Dam	White	43–54	0.9
		>75	4.7

glaucoma, not just the 1.6 million with some defined abnormality of visual function (generally fields).

Nevertheless, across each of these studies, certain general findings occur, regardless of the definition of glaucoma. First, the higher the age of the population, the more prevalent open-angle glaucoma was found to be. The relationship between age and prevalence of POAG from the four major prevalence studies mentioned above is summarized in Table 8.1. Secondly, comparing across the studies, blacks have a higher prevalence of glaucoma. Less well settled is the third issue of gender disparities in prevalence. In the Barbados and Rotterdam studies, men were noted to have a higher prevalence than women, as high as an average of 3.6% across all age groups in the Rotterdam study.

Risk factors

In subsequent analyses of many of these data sets as well as other independent studies, additional risk factors other than age and race (and perhaps gender) were identified. These include the presence of glaucoma in a primary relative of the patient or, sometimes, in any family member; family history has historically been thought to be one of the highest predictors of risk. In an analysis of the Barbados and Baltimore Eye Studies, age and race adjusted risk factors for a family history do reveal a high relative risk, but perhaps less than has traditionally been noted (again, keeping in mind the difference in definitions between the two studies). Table 8.2 summarizes the risk of positive family history on the prevalence of POAG from two major studies.

A widely acknowledged risk factor for primary open-angle glaucoma is the degree of elevation of the intraocular pressure. Recent work from the Baltimore Eye Survey has shown that even among normals, the higher the intraocular pressure the less nerve tissue (as measured by rim area) exists. Certainly, in every population-based study, the higher the intraocular pressure, the greater the rate of primary open-angle glaucoma.

Other conditions that have been implicated as increasing the risk of the development of POAG require additional analysis. Yet, an open mind and the performance of the appropriate studies will allow these other factors to be understood for their relative roles in POAG. Thus, other ocular conditions, such as high myopia, may also carry a higher risk of primary open-angle glaucoma. The presence of systemic medical conditions such as diabetes or hypothyroidism, may be associated with an increased risk for primary open-angle glaucoma.

Hypertension, which has been thought to be a risk factor for open-angle glaucoma in various studies, and has been equally forcefully rejected in others, may, according to findings from the Barbados study, be best understood by its relationship to perfusion pressure within the eye. Recent articles have identified that perfusion pressure differentials are an important risk factor for glaucomatous progression as well as for the presence of glaucoma. The effect of hypertension is thus confounded by the balance between perfusion pressure as reflected in the mean arterial pressure, the end diastolic pressure, and intraocular

Table 8.2 **Effect of positive family history on prevalence of POAG.**

Study	Adjustments	Risk factor	Odds ratio	95% confidence interval
Barbados	Age	Men	7.03*	4.33–11.41
		Women	3.43*	2.23–5.28
Baltimore	Age and race	POAG in parent	1.33	0.68–2.59
		POAG in sibling	2.89*	1.65–5.10
		POAG in child	1.14	0.26–5.03
		POAG in any first-degree relative	1.84*	1.21–2.80

Note:
*Statistically significant (P <0.05).

pressure, and the effects of medical treatment for hypertension. For example, Hayreh has shown that hypertensive patients on certain forms of antihypertensive medications have very low nocturnal arterial pressures, such that they were at greater risk of progression of optic neuropathy due, presumably, to nocturnal hypoxia or hypoperfusion of the optic nerve due to systemic hypotension. Seen in this light, our knowledge of hypertension as a potential risk factor encompasses a more complex and potentially more accurate understanding of the hemodynamic nature of vascular flow and its status in our larger understanding of the potential mechanisms underlying optic nerve damage.

Other associations have been found not to be significant, including alcohol intake, smoking, and migraine headache. Yet, as with hypertension in the past, further study may allow us to understand better the potential contributions of nutrition and environmental conditions to increasing or decreasing the risk of developing POAG.

Pathophysiology of glaucoma

Blood flow and hemodynamics

The work of Hayreh and others on systemic hypertension, as well as the effects of its medical treatment in causing night-time arterial hypotension, provides insight into potential mechanisms of damage to the optic nerve. Possibilities include: 1) direct damage to the optic nerve due to pressure effects on the connective tissue or the nerve fibers; 2) indirect effects of pressure in compromising vascular flow to the optic nerve; and 3) interaction between perfusion pressure and vascular supply (or on vascular supply itself), possibly ameliorated by the perfusion pressure relative to the intraocular pressure. However, these findings may not apply to many or most patients with POAG as defined today. Thus, there is a need for continued investigation and analysis in this area. An interesting implication of this finding is the potential role it opens for systemic conditions such as hypothyroidism and diabetes mellitus. Decreased cardiac output or reduced arterial pressure may make individuals more susceptible to perfusion deficit damage, while microvascular damage to capillaries and small blood vessels may act directly to heighten the likelihood of ischemia.

When additional issues relayed to vascular perfusion are examined, several other interesting studies add to our understanding. While many of these findings are controversial or have been at odds with other published studies, they offer interesting insights into potential factors. For example, Schulzer et al. identified two distinct groups of patients with glaucoma on the basis of hemodynamic and hematological characteristics. One group demonstrated some systemic sensitivity to stimuli causing vasospasm, while another demonstrated indirect indicators of vascular disease, including disturbed coagulation. Interestingly, the smaller former group (25% of study patients) demonstrated a correlation between peak intraocular pressure and severity of field defect, while the latter (75% of patients) did not. For reasons to be discussed below, peak intraocular pressure may not be the most accurate measure of the effect of intraocular pressure on the eye, yet this study suggests that studies that do not distinguish between these two (and perhaps more) possible subgroups in hemodynamic studies may be 'washing out' a true effect through cross-contamination of study populations. Indeed, an independent study from Japan found that 17–25% of patients with POAG also had a vasospastic response, a rate similar to the Schulzer study. However, even though 12 control patients had a similar 25% rate of vasospastic response, these patients were 4–8 years younger than the POAG subjects.

Other authors have also found deficits in the velocity of blood flow in various elements of the intraocular circulation, including the retinal, central retinal artery, and optic nerve head circulation. In a study of optic nerve head circulation, investigators demonstrated increased red blood cell aggregability due to decreased deformability, a finding similar to that of Schulzer et al. in the majority of their patients.

The structural characteristics of the vascular system have also been implicated in the development or worsening of POAG damage. In one review of optic disc photographs of 34 eyes with advanced field loss, the presence of a temporal cilioretinal artery was found to be protective in preserving central field and acuity. Investigators have postulated that defect areas in the microcirculation of the disc are associated with both ocular hypertension and POAG and with worsening of POAG status.

A fourth area of analysis has centered on understanding the pulsatile ocular blood flow through a variety of means. Since the vast majority of pulsatile flow travels through the choroidal (and thus ophthalmic artery) circulation (and the optic nerve head circulation derives from the ophthalmic as opposed to the retinal artery), measurements of flow are only rough measures of choroidal and ophthalmic artery flow. Nevertheless, while some studies have found deficits in such flow in patients with POAG, as well as differential effects on flow with different therapies, other studies have not found differences in flow in other samples. Yet, what is clear across studies is a wide variation across individuals in the ability to autoregulate pulsatile ocular blood flow, especially at night. Decreased nocturnal blood flow in some patients, or while supine in POAG patients (possibly due to increased intraocular pressure related to increased episcleral venous pressure in this position), may suggest particular susceptibility in certain patients or at certain times.

While partially clarifying the role played by vascular factors in the pathogenesis of glaucomatous optic neuropathy, the above studies also point out its complexity. It is now more apparent that understanding ocular perfusion requires an understanding of not only ocular blood flow parameters and its autoregulation (or lack thereof) but also an appreciation of systemic vascular factors and systemic diseases and the potential role played by ocular and systemic medications. Vascular factors are only part of the equation in our understanding of ocular perfusion. While such factors may be especially important in the 50% of patients with glaucoma who will have an intraocular pressure reading within the normal range on any one pressure examination, it is clear that intraocular pressure is also critical, since it generates much of the resistance to flow and perfusion.

Intraocular pressure

Intraocular pressure retains a critical role in the pathogenesis of glaucoma, since it is one part of the equation that determines the relative health of the optic nerve. Traditional work regarding the trabecular meshwork remains important, since impaired outflow associated with elevated intraocular pressure may result in the optic nerve damage that characterizes glaucoma, either structurally from direct pressure effects or indirectly through compromised perfusion.

Evidence is mounting that the most important characteristic of intraocular pressure for the development of glaucoma or for its progression is not the peak or average intraocular pressure, but the variation in intraocular pressure. For example, David et al. found that the diurnal variation in intraocular pressures was higher in ocular hypertensives and those with glaucoma than in normal patients, confirming the findings of a series of studies from Drance, Katavisto, and Kitazawa.

Studies of progression after intervention also found an important role for the variation of pressure. For example, Elsas et al. found that the variation in intraocular pressure was significantly greater in eyes prior to laser trabeculoplasty than it was after trabeculoplasty, with variation decreasing from 33% of the average intraocular pressure to less than 10% afterwards. In another study, Saiz et al. found that those patients who underwent successful trabeculectomy had lower peak intraocular pressures and also significantly lower amplitudes of diurnal variation in intraocular pressure than they did before surgery.

From a biophysical standpoint, it is reasonable that variation in intraocular pressure may be responsible for mechanical effects in the optic nerve head leading to glaucomatous optic atrophy. The human body is amazingly adaptable to static pressure loads, but it is the repeated loading and unloading of stress that causes breakdowns in structural properties (as in metal fatigue in airliners subject to repeated takeoffs

Table 8.3 **Recommendations for the initial assessment of a glaucoma patient.**

Elements of history	Elements of examination
Review family, ocular, and systemic history	Best corrected visual acuity
Review any available old records (old visual fields, disc photographs, etc.)	Pupillary examination with attention to afferent pupillary defect
Ocular and systemic medications being used	Intraocular pressure measurement prior to gonioscopy and dilatation
Previous ocular surgery, if any	Complete anterior segment slit-lamp examination
Previous medications used and review known systemic and local reactions	Gonioscopy
Time of last use of glaucoma medications	Evaluation of the optic disc and nerve fiber layer, with documentation of the optic nerve appearance
Severity of glaucoma in family members, including history of visual loss from glaucoma	Evaluation of the fundus for other abnormalities that might account for any visual field defects
Assessment of the impact of visual function on activities of daily living	Visual field examination by automated static threshold technique or by manual technique using a combination of kinetic and static techniques

and landings and pressurizations). Such variation may be important in leading to repeated episodes of stress that may, over time, cause injury to the optic nerve fibers that ultimately results in glaucomatous damage. The preferential loss of larger ganglion cells early in glaucoma may reflect the influence of this factor as well as others. Lamina cribrosa pores are larger in the polar regions of the optic nerve head (where the larger axons pass), with thinner septae between pores than in other areas of the nerve head. The repeated stress of changing intraocular pressure (causing mechanical deformation of the laminar plates) may lead to breakdown of the septae, loss of support for the axons, and axon damage. Alternatively, such variation may lead to episodes of relative ischemia that may, over time, cause injury to the optic nerve fibers resulting in glaucomatous damage.

New research areas

Two new areas of research may be of particular promise. First, the pursuit of localizing the gene(s) that are related to POAG proceeds apace. The chromosome for familial juvenile open-angle glaucoma has already been localized by several investigators. With the promise of molecular genetics, a greater grasp of the elements that cause POAG to develop may follow. Secondly, several investigators are now working on the concept that apoptotic mechanisms reflecting preprogrammed cell death may underlie much of glaucomatous nerve fiber and cell loss. Cell death may be triggered by certain environmental conditions, or the cell may be made more susceptible to environmental conditions. Indeed, genetic analysis may one day identify genotypic susceptibility to such death as a major factor in the development of POAG. As such, not everybody with the gene will necessarily develop glaucoma, but may be at higher risk.

Making the diagnosis of POAG

As noted in the definition of POAG, four elements are needed to make the diagnosis in a patient: 1) the

(a)

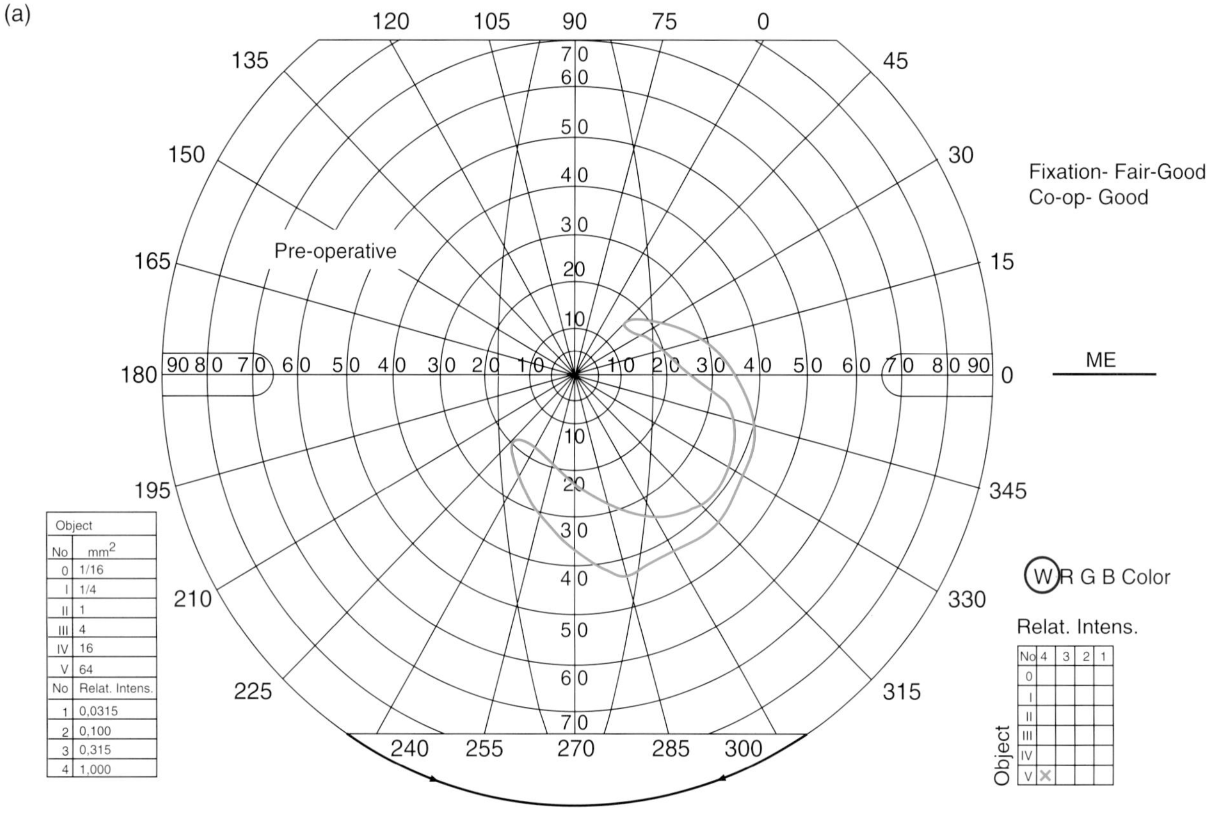

(b)

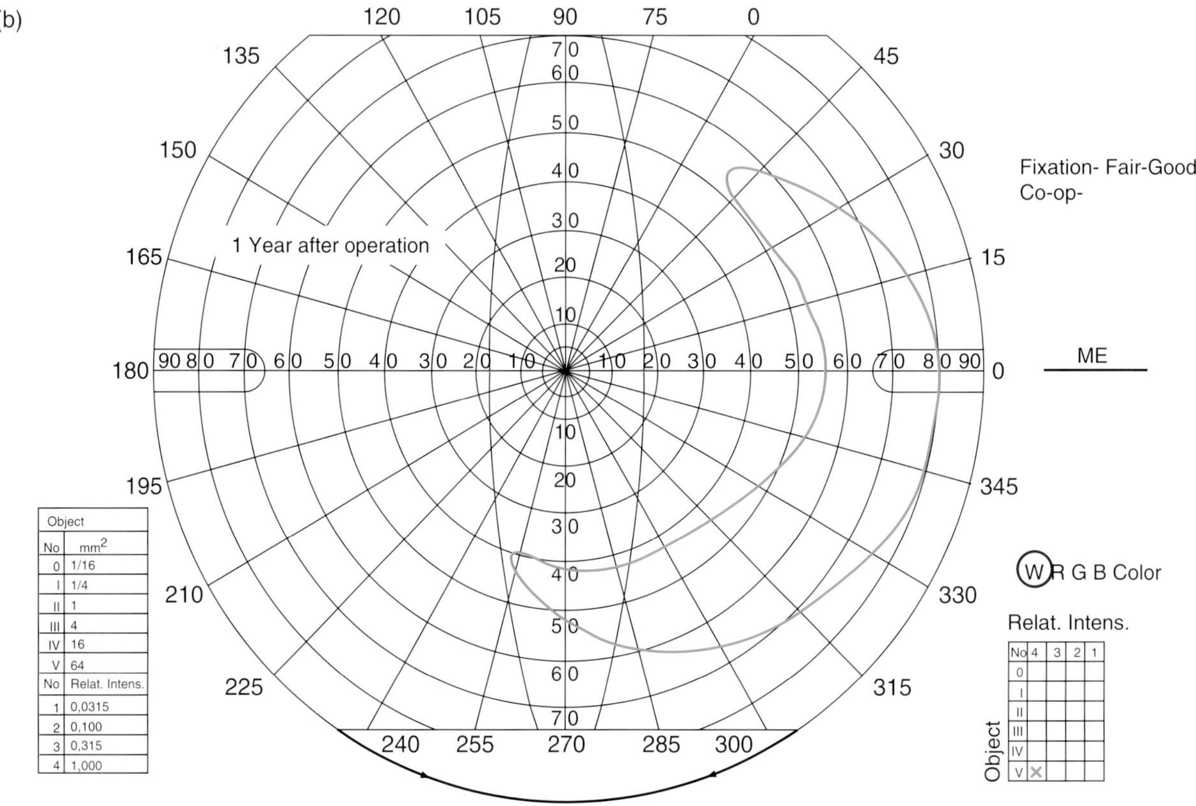

Figure 8.1 Series of visual fields in a glaucoma patient
The visual field of this patient taken just prior to filtration surgery is shown in (a). The subsequent fields ((b)–(e)) show considerable improvement attributed to the excellent intraocular pressure control obtained by the surgery.

(c)

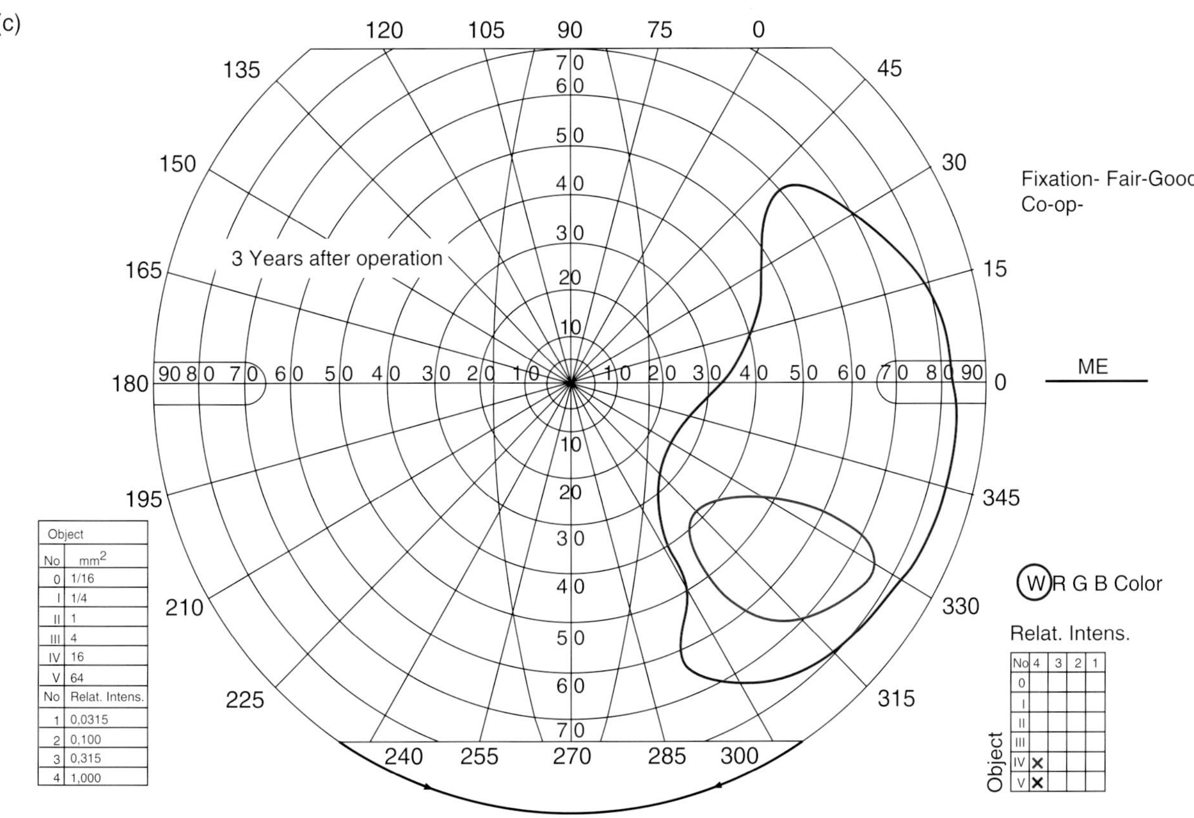
3 Years after operation
Fixation- Fair-Good
Co-op-
ME
W R G B Color
Relat. Intens.
Object
No mm2
0 1/16
I 1/4
II 1
III 4
IV 16
V 64
No Relat. Intens.
1 0,0315
2 0,100
3 0,315
4 1,000

(d)

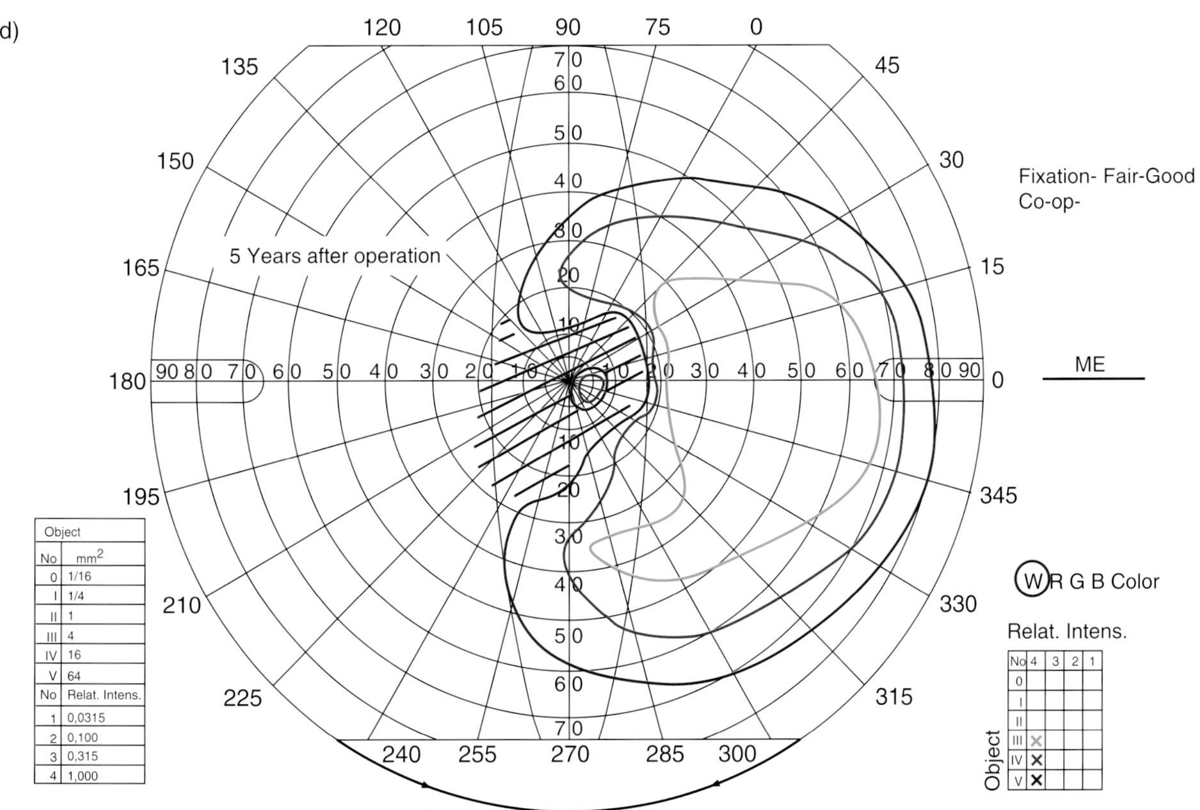
5 Years after operation
Fixation- Fair-Good
Co-op-
ME
W R G B Color
Relat. Intens.
Object
No mm2
0 1/16
I 1/4
II 1
III 4
IV 16
V 64
No Relat. Intens.
1 0,0315
2 0,100
3 0,315
4 1,000

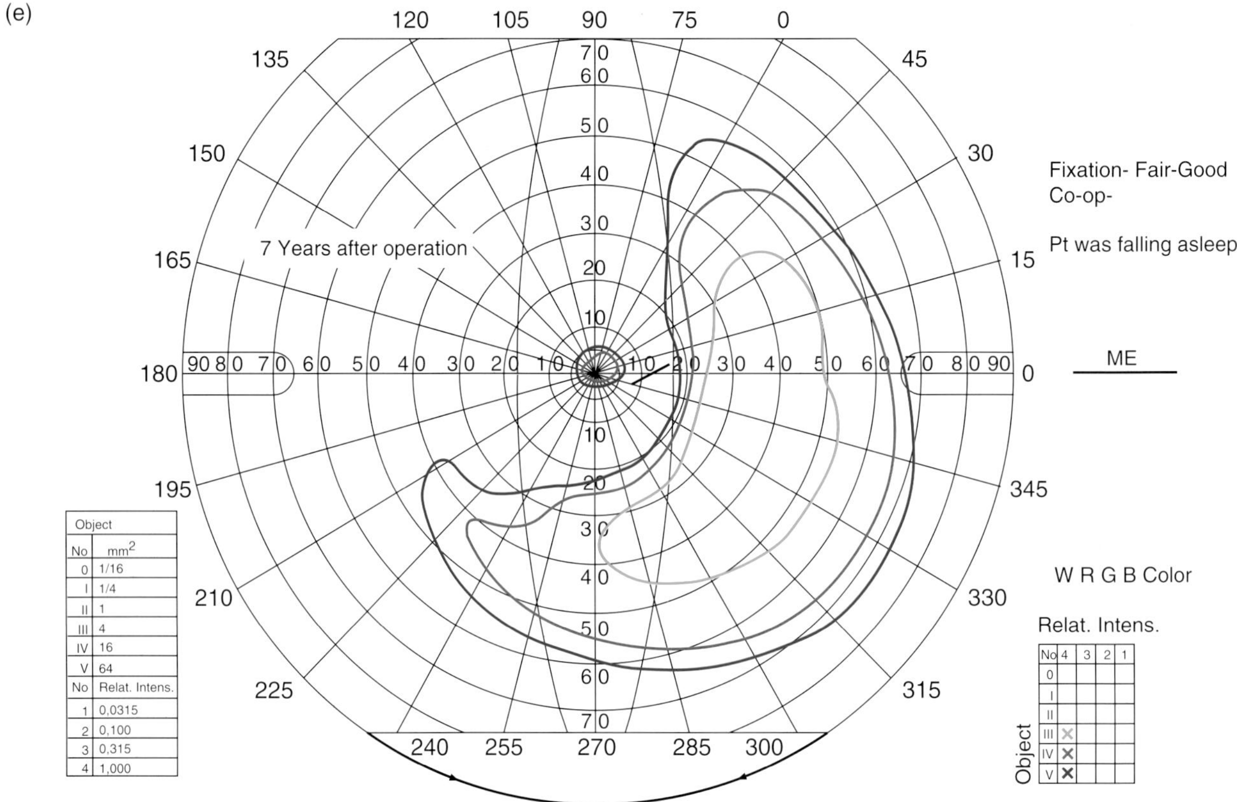

patient must be of adult age (with younger patients defined as having juvenile-onset glaucoma, though without necessarily any significant differences in treatment philosophy); 2) the anterior chamber angles must be 'open' by gonioscopy (see Chapter 5); 3) there must be no known cause (i.e. a secondary cause) for the glaucoma (see Chapter 9); and 4) there must be optic nerve damage, manifested by either optic disc or nerve fiber layer changes consistent with glaucoma (see Chapter 6) or characteristic visual field abnormalities (see Chapter 7). To assist the clinician in determining what changes are 'characteristic' or 'consistent with' POAG, the AAO provides illustrative examples of each. For visual fields, the definition explicitly encompasses arcuate defects, nasal steps, paracentral scotomata, or generalized depression. For disc or retinal nerve fiber layer appearance, the AAO explicitly includes thinning or notching of the disc rim, progressive change over time, and nerve fiber layer defects. For a full discussion and illustrations of these and other characteristics, please refer to the appropriate chapter.

Patients with POAG typically present with either no symptoms referable to the glaucoma (perhaps coming in for a visit due to cataract or macular degeneration or for a check-up) or with advanced loss in one or both eyes. Because the initial assessment requires that POAG be a diagnosis of exclusion, the history and examination should be carefully oriented towards eliminating other causes of glaucomatous loss. Thus, issues such as use of steroids of any kind, history of trauma (which can often appear normal on gonioscopy unless both eyes are carefully examined for the full 360 degrees and small asymmetries within an eye or across eyes noted), and symptoms of uveitis (looking for even one keratitic precipitate in the angle), should be asked of the patient and signs looked for on the examination.

To assist physicians in using the new definition and to meet the practice guideline requirements, the AAO Preferred Practice Patterns for POAG lists elements of history and examination that should be included in the initial assessment of glaucoma patients. These are summarized in Table 8.3.

Treatment principles

General goals

The traditional goal of glaucoma therapy is to stabilize optic nerve damage and to prevent additional damage. Occasionally, following adequate lowering of intraocular pressure, reversal or improvement in optic disc cupping has been reported by several authors, particularly in early cases of glaucoma among younger patients. Figure 8.1 demonstrates a case of significant recovery of visual field following aggressive treatment of POAG. Pre and postoperative fields of a patient with POAG with advanced cupping who underwent a successful trephination with postoperative intraocular pressures of between 6 and 8 mmHg are illustrated (courtesy of Pei-Fei Lee, MD). Thus, the real goal of glaucoma treatment should be to improve and perhaps to restore significant amounts of visual functioning, as measured through a variety of means.

It is vital that treatment be tailored to the needs of the individual patient, in partnership with the physician. Issues including compliance with therapy, patient understanding of the disease, cost of treatment, potential side-effects, and impact of therapy on patient's quality of life should be explicitly incorporated into the patient's care plan. It is not sufficient to limit discussions to intraocular pressure, visual field, and optic nerve status; discussions about the implications of POAG and its care need to be raised and addressed with the patient.

Lowering of intraocular pressure

Considering the new definition of POAG, our current ability to modulate the course of the disease is still relatively limited. At present, the only available treatment for POAG is to reduce the intraocular pressure. Whether this functions to improve perfusion or ocular blood flow, or has a direct mechanical benefit on the optic nerve, or both, is not clear. The evidence that lower intraocular pressure is more effective in preventing visual field loss can be indirectly seen in the results of the Moorfields Primary Treatment Trial and the Scottish Glaucoma Trial, in which initial trabeculectomy lowered intraocular pressure more than medicine and was also associated with less loss of field on follow-up. Similarly, the lower intraocular pressure obtained with initial laser trabeculoplasty in the Glaucoma Laser Trial was associated with less visual field loss than in the medication first group.

Once a diagnosis is made, the AAO PPP states that a 'target pressure' should be defined—i.e. the upper limit of what would be considered an 'acceptable' pressure for that eye for that patient. As such, this target pressure is only an estimate and subject to revision based on the clinical course of the patient. In selecting the target pressure, it should be **at least** 20% lower than the baseline intraocular pressure range, and should be set lower for those eyes which have more pre-existing damage, or if the top is quite high. Additional factors to consider, which may argue for an even lower target intraocular pressure, are the presence of strong risk factors (see above), the history of loss in the fellow eye at certain intraocular pressure ranges, and the rapidity of damage (if known).

In order to determine whether the target pressure is appropriate, patients need periodic monitoring of their optic nerve status, directly through evaluation of the disc and nerve fiber layer and indirectly through the performance of periodic visual fields. Where damage has occurred at or below target pressures, then the target pressure must be reset, again starting with **at least** an additional 20% drop off the current intraocular pressure. The timing of the follow-up assessment depends on the patient and the severity of the glaucoma.

The interval between follow-up visits to the physician is determined by attainment of the target intraocular pressure (or failure to attain the pressure) and presence or absence of disease progression. For example, if the target intraocular pressure has been achieved and no progression is noted, control for longer than 6 months suggests that follow-up every 3–12 months should be sufficient. For more recent control (<6 months) follow-up in 1–6 months is warranted. However, if the target intraocular pressure needs to be reset because of progression at or below the initial target, follow-up should occur in 1 week to 3 months. For those eyes in which the target has not yet been achieved, follow-up should occur between 1 day and 1 month (for progression) or 3 months (if no progression).

During follow-up visits, the history should include interval ocular and systemic medical history, an inquiry into local or systemic problems with medication, verification of the appropriate use of medications, and general assessment of the impact of the condition and treatment on daily living. Each examination should include a visual acuity, intraocular pressure in both eyes, and a slit-lamp examination. For periodic optic nerve evaluations, if the target intraocular pressure has been achieved and no progression is noted, control for longer than 6 months suggests that follow-up disc evaluations every 6–18 months should be sufficient. For more recent control (<6 months) follow-up in 6–12 months is warranted. However, if the target intraocular pressure needs to be reset because of progression at

Table 8.4 **Recommendations for follow-up.**

Progression of disease	Status	Duration of control	Recommended interval
Progressive optic nerve and/or visual field damage	Not at target pressure	n/a	1 day to 1 month
No	Not at target pressure	n/a	1 day to 3 months
Progressive optic nerve and/or visual field damage	At initial target pressure, requires resetting target	n/a	1 week to 3 months
Progression documented at prior visit	New target recently achieved	Less than 3 months	1 to 3 months
No	At target pressure	Less than 6 months	1 to 6 months
No	At target pressure	More than 6 months	3 to 12 months

or below the initial target, follow-up disc evaluation should occur in 2–6 months. For those eyes in which the target has not yet been achieved, follow-up should occur between 1 and 6 months (for progression) or 2–6 months (if no progression).

For interval visual fields, if the target intraocular pressure has been achieved and no progression is noted, control for longer than 6 months suggests that follow-up every 6–24 months should be sufficient. For more recent control (<6 months) follow-up in 6–24 months is warranted. However, if the target intraocular pressure needs to be reset because of progression at or below the initial target, follow-up fields should occur in 3–12 months. For those eyes in which the target has not yet been achieved, follow-up should occur also between 3 and 12 months. These recommendations are summarized in Table 8.4.

The AAO makes clear that these are ranges which need to be adjusted to fit the needs of individual patients. Thus, for example, if acceptable compliance is lacking, then physicians need to adjust the treatment regimen to enhance the utility of the therapy to the patient. Similarly, if problems develop with certain medications, switching patients to new medications will necessitate more frequent follow-up, just as if a new target pressure was being acquired.

While the PPP takes no position on the performance of diurnal curves as an aid to understanding progression or the likelihood of developing glaucoma, just as it takes no position on the utility of ocular hemodynamic assessments, these are potentially useful adjuncts to guiding therapy.

New approaches

The recent introduction of three new classes of topical therapy for POAG (see Chapter 13) heralds a fertile area in new and potentially more effective therapies for glaucoma. Yet, at root, therapeutic approaches are needed that directly address the pathophysiological basis of POAG. From recent work on understanding how glaucomatous damage occurs, several intriguing approaches and possibilities exist.

Renewed interest in the transport capabilities of the endothelial cells of the trabecular meshwork now offers new insights and potentially new classes of drugs for reducing the abnormal outflow resistance that underlies the mechanism for elevated pressure in many patients with POAG. Similarly, work that targets neuronal damage and ischemia has begun to offer hope that at least part of glaucomatous damage can potentially be reversed, through classes of drugs as diverse as glutamate receptor blockers (such as phencyclidine), calcium channel blockers, nitric oxide synthase inhibitors, nerve growth factors, and free-radical scavengers and antioxidants. Research on apoptosis and mechanisms of cell death provides hope that one day 'neuroprotective' drugs will become available to prevent the death of retinal ganglion cells initiated by uncontrolled intraocular pressure or whatever the underlying causative agent may be.

Summary

Our understanding of primary open-angle glaucoma and all forms of glaucoma has grown enormously in the past 20 years. Perhaps nowhere is this more evident than in how we view what primary open-angle glaucoma is. Today, it is a multifactorial optic neuropathy. It has been said by many authors that POAG most likely represents a spectrum of conditions that, today, we label with one name. From the work on ocular perfusion and hemodynamic characteristics, to intraocular pressure diurnal variation, to gene analysis, to optic nerve head structure, it is the diversity present in the population that often contributes to our still fuzzy thinking about POAG. From a scientific viewpoint, the future looks enormously promising for new understanding and new treatments.

From a clinical standpoint, care today is much more defined. The American Academy of Ophthalmology's Preferred Practice Pattern lays out specific recommendations to assist physicians in caring for their patients with POAG. Even more importantly, care today reflects modern notions of a physician–patient partnership. No longer are intraocular pressure, field, and disc status the holy grail of patient relationships. Rather, understanding and addressing the condition of POAG within the context of a patient's life are now the central focus.

FURTHER READING

American Academy of Ophthalmology, *Preferred practice pattern: primary open-angle glaucoma* (San Francisco, CA: AAO, 1996).

Bosem ME, Lusky M, Weinreb RN, Short-term effects of levobunolol on ocular pulsatile flow, *Am J Ophthalmol* (1992) **114**:280–6.

Claridge KG, Smith SE, Diurnal variation in pulsatile ocular blood flow in normal and glaucomatous eyes. *Surv Ophthalmol* (1994) **38 (Suppl)**:S198–S205.

David R, Zangwill L, Briscoe D, et al., Diurnal intraocular pressure variations: an analysis of 690 diurnal curves, *Br J Ophthalmol* (1992) **76**:280–3.

Dielemans I, Vingerling JR, Wolfs RCW, et al., The prevalence of primary open-angle glaucoma in a population-based study in The Netherlands, *Ophthalmology* (1994) **101**:1851–5.

Drance SM, The significance of the diurnal tension variations in normal and glaucomatous eyes, *Arch Ophthalmol* (1960) **64**:494–501.

Elsas T, Junk J, Johnsen H, Diurnal intraocular pressure after successful primary laser trabeculoplasty, *Am J Ophthalmol* (1991) **112**:67–9.

Epstein DL, Will there be a remedy to reverse the changes in the trabecular meshwork and the optic nerve? A personal point-of-view on glaucoma therapy, *J Glaucoma* (1993) **2**:138–40.

Glaucoma Laser Trial Research Group, The Glaucoma Laser Trial (GLT) and Glaucoma Laser Trial Follow-up Study. 7. Results, *Am J Ophthalmol* (1995) **120**:718–31.

Hamard P, Jamard J, Dufaux J, Blood flow rate in the microvasculature of the optic nerve head in primary open angle glaucoma: a new approach, *Surv Ophthalmol* (1994) **38 (Suppl)**:S87–S94.

Harris A, *Non-invasive assessment of ocular hemodynamics in glaucoma: a review of the literature* (Bloomington, IN: Indiana University, 1995).

Hayreh SS, Zimmerman MB, Podhajsky P, Alward WLM, Nocturnal arterial hypotension and its role in optic nerve head and ocular ischemic disorders, *Am J Ophthalmol* (1994) **117**:603–24.

James CB, Effect of trabeculectomy on pulsatile ocular blood flow, *Br J Ophthalmol* (1994) **78**:818–22.

Jay JL, Allan D, The benefit of early trabeculectomy versus conventional management in primary open-angle glaucoma relative to severity of disease, *Eye* (1989) **3**:528–35.

Katavisto M, The diurnal variations of ocular tension in glaucoma, *Acta Ophthalmologica* (1964) **78**:1–30.

Kitzawa Y, Horie T, Diurnal variation in intra-ocular pressure in primary open-angle glaucoma, *Am J Ophthalmol* (1975) **79**:557–66.

Klein BEK, Klein R, Jensen SC, Open-angle glaucoma and older-onset diabetes, *Ophthalmology* (1994) **101**:1173–7.

Klein BEK, Klein R, Meuer SM, Goetz LA, Migraine headache and its association with open-angle glaucoma: the Beaver Dam Eye Study, *Invest Ophthalmol Vis Sci* (1993) **34**:3024–7.

Klein BEK, Klein R, Ritter LL, Relationship of drinking alcohol and smoking to prevalence of open-angle glaucoma, *Ophthalmology* (1993) **100**:1609–13.

Klein BEK, Klein R, Sponsel WE, et al., Prevalence of glaucoma: the Beaver Dam Eye Study, *Ophthalmology* (1992) **99**:1499–504.

Lee PP, The effect of Preferred Practice Patterns on malpractice actions, *J Glaucoma* (1992) **1**:286–9.

Lee SS, Schwartz B, Role of the temporal cilioretinal artery in retaining central visual field in open-angle glaucoma, *Ophthalmology* (1992) **99**:696–9.

Leske MC, Connell AMS, Schachat AP, Hyman L, The Barbados Eye Study Group, The Barbados Eye Study: prevalence of open-angle glaucoma, *Arch Ophthalmol* (1994) **112**:821–9.

Leske MC, Connell AMS, Wu S-Y, Hyman LG, Schachat AP, The Barbados Eye Study Group: Risk factors for open-angle glaucoma, *Arch Ophthalmol* (1995) **113**:918–24.

Mastropasqua L, Lobefalo L, Mancini A, Ciancaglini M, Palma S, Prevalence of myopia in open angle glaucoma, *Eur J Ophthalmol* (1992) **2**:33–5.

Migdal C, Gregory W, Hitchings R, Long-term functional outcome after early surgery compared with laser and medicine in open-angle glaucoma, *Ophthalmology* (1994) **101**:1651–7.

Quigley HA, Open-angle glaucoma, *N Engl J Med* (1993) **328**:1097–106.

Rankin SJA, Walman BE, Buckley AR, Drance SM, Color Doppler imaging and spectral analysis of the optic nerve vasculature in glaucoma, *Am J Ophthalmol* (1995) **119**:685–93.

Schultz JS, Initial treatment of glaucoma: surgery or medications. III. Chop or drop? *Surv Ophthalmol* (1993) **37**:293–305.

Schulzer M, Drance SM, Carter CJ, et al., Biostatistical evidence of two distinct chronic open angle glaucoma populations, *Br J Ophthalmol* (1990) **74**:196–200.

Schumer RA, Podos SM, The nerve of glaucoma, *Arch Ophthalmol* (1994) **112**:37–44.

Schwartz B, Circulatory defects of the optic disk and retina in ocular hypertension and high pressure open-angle glaucoma, *Surv Ophthalmol* (1994) **38 (Suppl)**: S23–S34.

Sharir M, Zimmerman TJ, Initial treatment of glaucoma: surgery or medications. II. Medical therapy, *Surv Ophthalmol* (1993) **37**:293–305.

Sheffield VC, Stone EM, Alward WLM, et al., Genetic linkage of familial open angle glaucoma to chromosome 1q21–q31, *Nat Genet* (1994) **4**:47–50.

Sherwood MB, Migdal CS, Hitchings RA, Initial treatment of glaucoma: surgery or medications. I. Filtration surgery, *Surv Ophthalmol* (1993) **37**:293–305.

Smith KD, Arthurs BP, Saheb J, An association between hypothyroidism and primary open-angle glaucoma, *Ophthalmology* (1993) **100**:1580–4.

Smith KD, Tevaarwerk GJM, Allen LH, Case reports: reversal of poorly controlled glaucoma on diagnosis and treatment of hypothyroidism, *Can J Ophthalmol* (1992) **27**:345–7.

Sommer A, Tielsch JM, et al., Relationship between intraocular pressure and primary open angle glaucoma among white and black Americans, *Arch Ophthalmol* (1991) **109**:1090–5.

Tielsch JM, Katz J, Sommer A, Quigley HA, Javitt JC, Family history and risk of primary open angle glaucoma, *Arch Ophthalmol* (1994) **112**:69–73.

Tielsch JM, Katz J, Sommer A, Quigley HA, Javitt JC, Hypertension, perfusion pressure, and primary open-angle glaucoma, *Arch Ophthalmol* (1995) **113**:216–21.

Tielsch JM, Sommer A, Katz J, Toyall RM, Quigley HA, Javitt J, Racial variations in the prevalence of primary open-angle glaucoma: the Baltimore Eye Survey, *JAMA* (1991) **266**:369–74.

Trew DR, Smith SE, Postural studies in pulsatile ocular blood flow: II. Chronic open angle glaucoma, *Br J Ophthalmol* (1991) **75**:71–5.

Usuai T, Iwata K, Finger blood flow in patients with low tension glaucoma and primary open-angle glaucoma, *Br J Ophthalmol* (1992) **76**:2–4.

Wiggs JL, Haines JL, Pagliniauan C, et al., Genetic linkage of autosomal dominant juvenile glaucoma to 1q21–q31 in three affected pedigrees, *Genomics* (1994) **21**:299–303.

Wolf S, Arend O, Sponsel WE, et al., Retinal hemodynamics using scanning laser ophthalmoscopy and hemorheology in chronic open-angle glaucoma, *Ophthalmology* (1993) **100**:1561–6.

9 Secondary open-angle glaucomas

Jonathan Myers and L Jay Katz

Introduction

The secondary open-angle glaucomas comprise a number of conditions in which intraocular pressure (IOP) becomes elevated through a variety of mechanisms other than primary dysfunction of the trabecular meshwork. Often the term 'glaucoma' is applied even in the absence of optic nerve damage. The glaucoma is often characterized by the addition of the descriptive term referring to the condition responsible for the elevated IOP. Primary open-angle glaucoma is discussed in Chapter 8, and the angle-closure glaucomas are discussed in Chapter 10.

Pigmentary glaucoma

Pigmentary glaucoma is a secondary open-angle glaucoma in which released iris pigment interferes with trabecular meshwork function leading to elevated intraocular pressure. A flaccid peripheral iris, bowing posteriorly, is believed to rub against the zonular fibers damaging the iris pigment epithelium. Radial, slit-like iris transillumination defects are typical (Fig. 9.1). Risk factors for development of pigmentary dispersion syndrome include myopia, male sex, white race and young age. Blacks and Asians rarely develop pigmentary dispersion; this

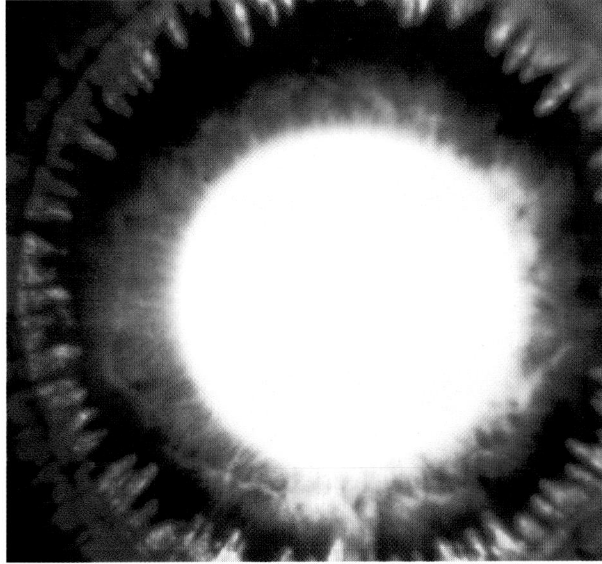

Figure 9.1 Transillumination defects seen using the red reflex
Characteristically in the peripheral half of the iris, they correspond to the location and orientation of the zonular fibers. Mild cases may have very few transillumination defects; these may increase or decrease with time.

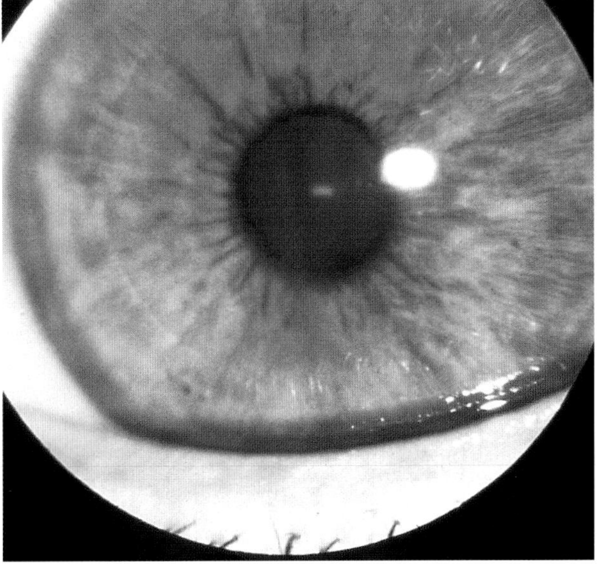

Figure 9.2 The Krukenberg spindle
The Krukenberg spindle, a vertical deposition of pigment in the lower central cornea, is apparently shaped by convection currents in the anterior chamber.

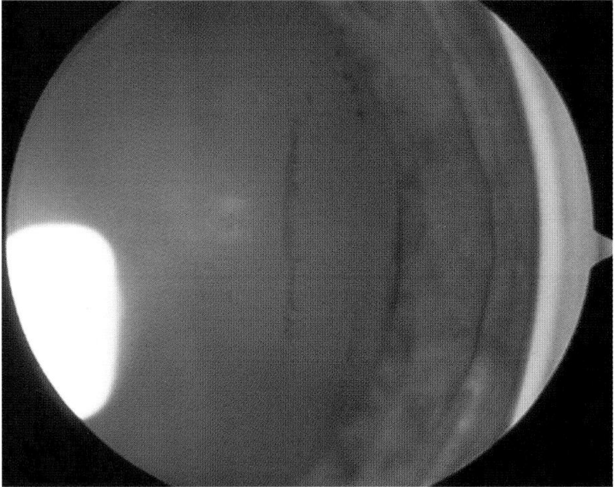

Figure 9.3 Pigment deposition
Pigment deposition on the posterior surface of the lens is highly suggestive of PDS and PG.

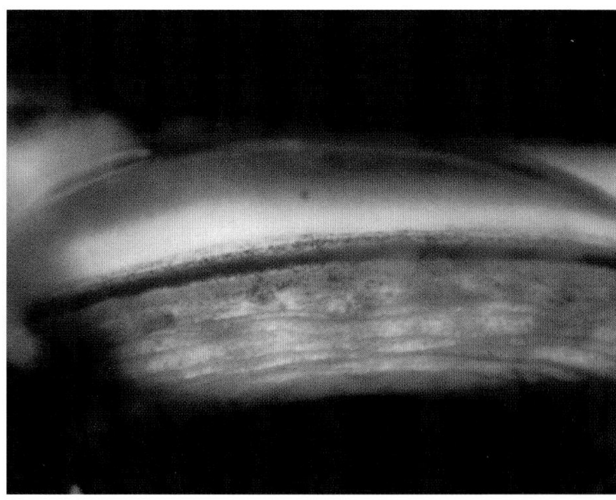

Figure 9.4 Heavy pigmentation
Heavy pigmentation of the trabecular meshwork and other angle structures is seen circumferentially. Typical 'Q' configuration (bowing posteriorly in the periphery) of the iris is also seen.

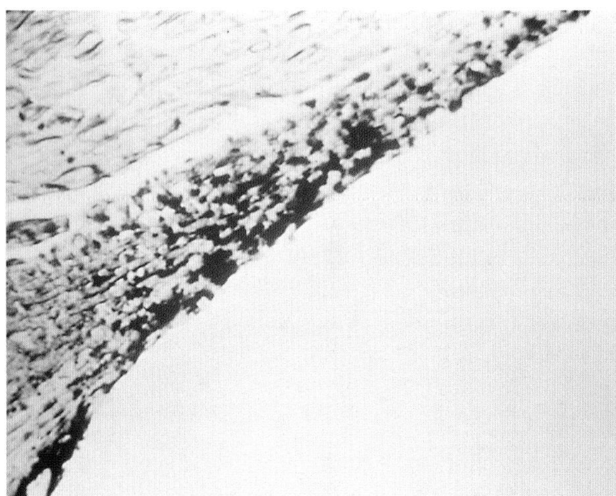

Figure 9.5 Histopathologic section showing trabecular meshwork laden with pigment
Endothelial cells coating the trabecular beams in the meshwork phagocytize the pigment. Experiments have shown that when enough pigment is released, overloaded endothelial cells move off the beams and disintegrate. Trabecular collapse with loss of filtering intratrabecular spaces follows leading to decreased facility of outflow and increased intraocular pressure.

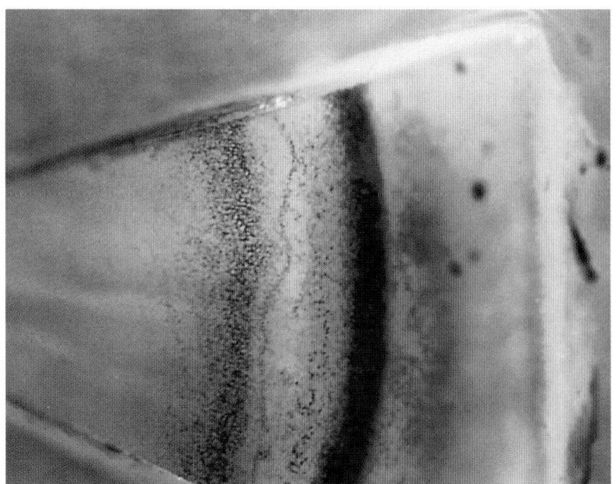

Figure 9.6 Pigment deposition on angle structures
Specimen showing pigment deposition on angle structures, including anterior to Schwalbe's line.

may be due to their thicker, less flaccid irides. With increasing age, increasing relative pupillary block may play a protective role as aqueous in the posterior chamber accumulates and keeps the peripheral iris away from the zonular fibers.

Released pigment is carried by aqueous flow into the anterior chamber. Pigment may be phagocytized by corneal endothelial cells, creating a Krukenberg spindle (Fig. 9.2). Pigment may also be deposited in circumferential iris furrows and on the posterior lens surface (Fig. 9.3). Aqueous flow carries the pigment to the trabecular meshwork which is typically heavily pigmented for 360 degrees (Figs 9.4 and 9.5). Pigment deposition anterior to Schwalbe's line is seen in the inferior 180 degrees (Fig. 9.6).

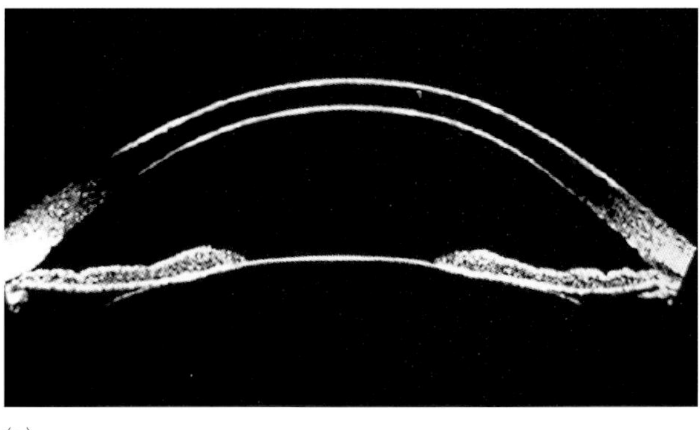

(a)

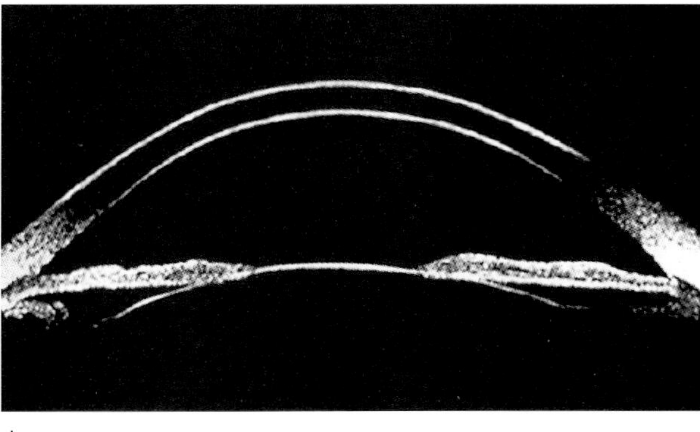

(b)

Figure 9.7 Ultrasound biomicroscopic images
Reverse pupillary block occurs when a blink forces a small amount of aqueous into the anterior chamber, past a floppy iris laying against the lens. This slight increase in anterior chamber volume and pressure bows the iris back against the lens and zonular fibers, increasing the block and increasing the contact which leads to pigment release. The iridotomy relieves this block allowing the iris to come forward from the lens (b). This *may* prevent further pigment release and the development of glaucoma if done early in the disease process.

Approximately one third of patients with pigment dispersion syndrome will go on to develop pigmentary glaucoma over 15 years. Treatment of pigmentary glaucoma includes the full spectrum of pharmacologic, laser and surgical modalities. Miotics work well to lower pressures both by opening the trabecular meshwork and by pulling the iris away from zonular fibers, reducing pigment release. However, many of these young patients are intolerant of miotic-induced headaches and blurred vision. Longer-release preparations, such as pilogel and ocuserts, reduce these symptoms adequately for some patients. These patients are also at increased risk for retinal detachment with miotics. For these reasons many clinicians start with aqueous suppressants such as beta blockers, and more recently apraclonidine and dorzolamide. Adrenergic agents are also effective.

Laser peripheral iridotomy has been advanced as a prophylactic therapy, although no studies have yet demonstrated its efficacy. This procedure relieves reverse pupillary block and may reduce iris chafe and pigment release (Fig. 9.7).

Argon laser trabeculoplasty has been shown to be very effective. Lower laser powers are sufficient as the trabecular meshwork pigment absorbs the energy well. However, long-term results show more than half of patients losing treatment effect within five years.

Conventional filtering surgery yields good results in pigmentary glaucoma. Results are similar to those obtained in patients with primary open-angle glaucoma. Antimetabolites should be used cautiously, as these young, myopic patients are more prone to hypotensive maculopathy.

Exfoliation syndrome

Exfoliation syndrome is a common cause of secondary open-angle glaucoma in many populations. Signs of exfoliation syndrome may be seen in over 20% of patients in Iceland and Finland, accounting for as much as half of the glaucomatous population. In the USA, the incidence is much lower but patients with exfoliation syndrome still make up about 10% of those with glaucoma, perhaps even more of the ocular hypertensives. With age, the incidence of exfoliation syndrome increases, and this may contribute to its association with female gender. Findings are more often unilateral in American studies, but bilaterality increases with longer follow-up.

The classic finding in exfoliation syndrome is the grayish-white flaky material on the anterior lens capsule (Figs 9.8 and 9.9). This material may also be seen at the pupil margin, corneal endothelium, trabecular meshwork, zonular fibers and ciliary body; after cataract extraction it appears on the posterior capsule, intraocular lens and vitreous face as well. This same material has been found in the conjunctiva, orbital blood vessels, skin, myocardium, lung, liver, gallbladder, kidney and cerebral meninges, usually localized to connective tissue.

Abrasive exfoliation material on the anterior lens capsule leads to the release of pigment from the posterior surface of the iris. Peripupillary transillumination

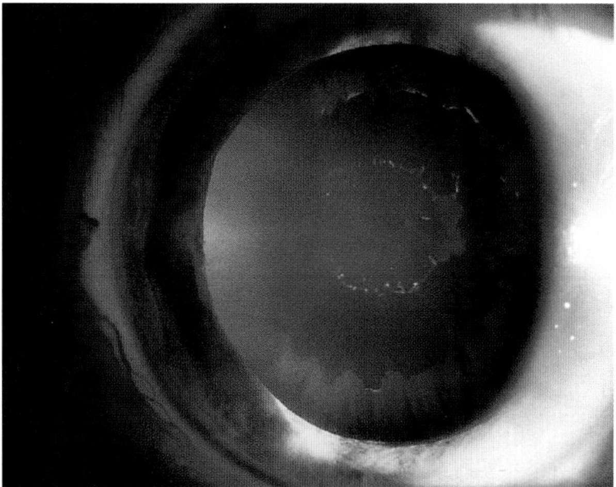

Figure 9.8 Exfoliation material on the anterior lens capsule
Deposition of exfoliative material is often in a bull's-eye configuration consisting of a central disc, midperipheral clearing and a more irregular peripheral ring of deposits.

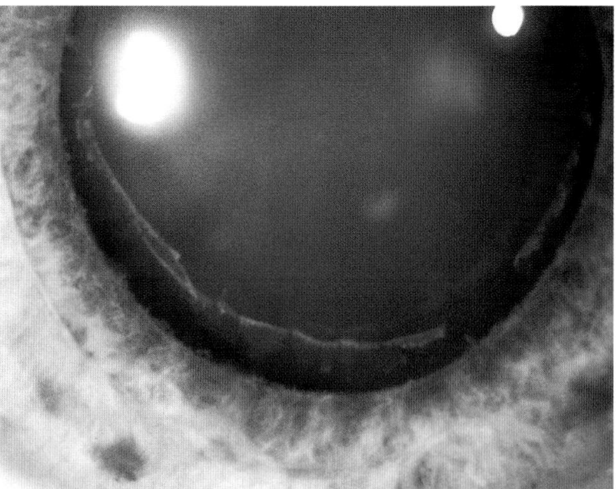

Figure 9.9 Exfoliation material
Seen on dilatation only; central disc deposition absent.

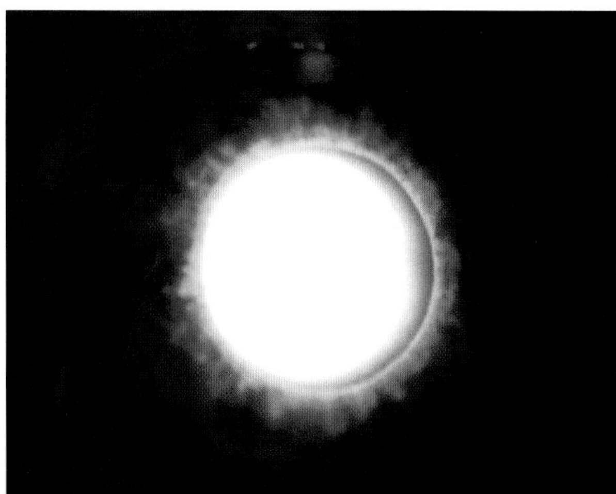

Figure 9.10 Transillumination defects
Transillumination defects in exfoliation syndrome are typically near the pupil margin.

defects and loss of the pigmented ruff may be evident (Figs 9.10 and 9.11). Pigment deposition is seen throughout the anterior chamber and angle (Fig. 9.12). Pigment and exfoliation material within the trabecular meshwork are thought to lead to the increased intraocular pressure associated with exfoliation syndrome.

Affected eyes show poor dilatation with mydriatics for a number of reasons. Iris ischemia leads to neovascularization and posterior synechiae. Chronic miotic therapy reduces mydriasis and allows the lens iris diaphragm to move forward, contributing to the formation of synechiae. Narrow angles are common and secondary angle closure may result. Exfoliation material deposition in the iris stroma may increase rigidity. Intraocular pressure spikes secondary to pigment dispersion are common with dilatation. Zonular fibers in affected eyes are weakened; lens dislocation may occur with minimal surgical manipulation or spontaneously (Fig. 9.13). These factors make cataract extraction more difficult, increasing the likelihood of vitreous loss.

Glaucoma in exfoliation syndrome is associated with higher intraocular pressures and increased treatment failures when compared to primary open-angle glaucoma. Miotic therapy increases trabecular meshwork outflow and may reduce pigment release, but also contributes to posterior synechiae and reduced dilatation. Argon laser trabeculoplasty is effective, but transient intraocular pressure spikes following treatment may be more common and more severe compared to primary open-angle glaucoma. Some patients show reduced intraocular pressures following lens extraction; this is thought to be secondary to reduced pigment release since the exfoliation material is still produced. The success with trabeculectomy is similar to that seen in primary open-angle glaucoma.

Aphakic and pseudophakic glaucomas

Increased intraocular pressure is a well-known complication of cataract extraction. Reported

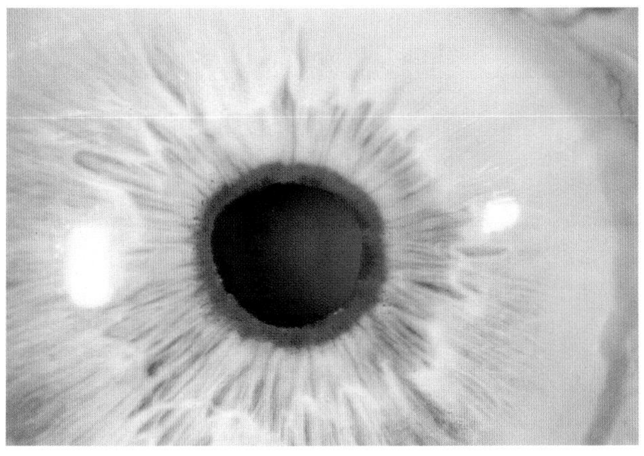
(a)

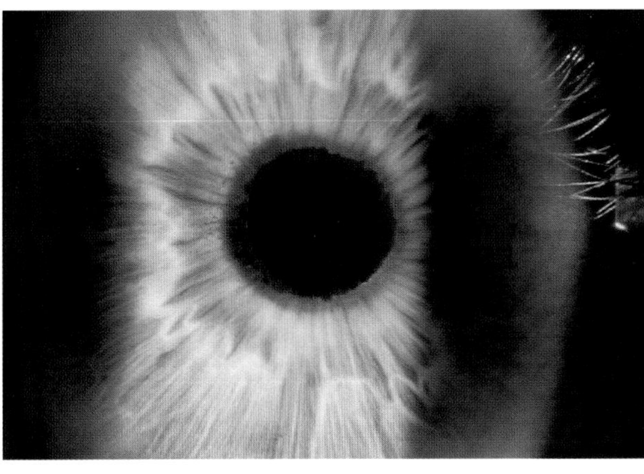
(b)

Figure 9.11 Clinically unilateral exfoliation syndrome and glaucoma
This patient with clinically unilateral exfoliation syndrome and glaucoma shows absence of the pigmented ruff at the pupil margin in the affected eye (a) and a normal ruff in the unaffected eye (b).

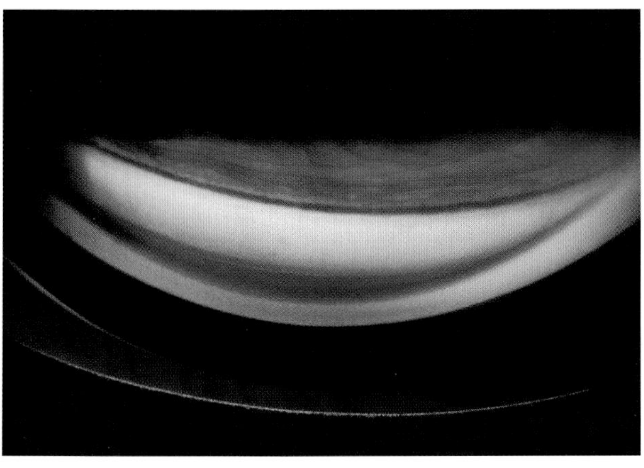
(a)

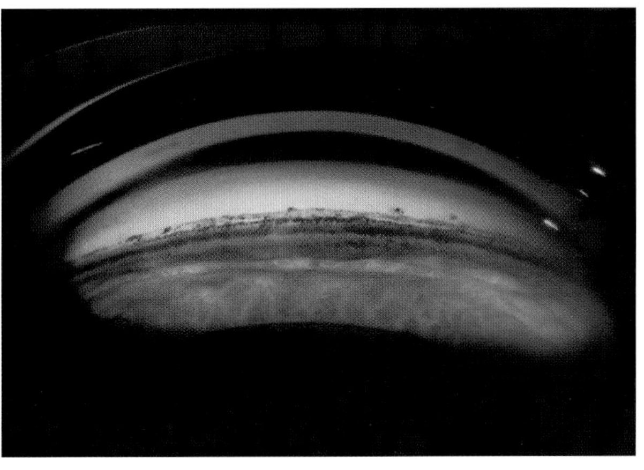
(b)

Figure 9.12 Anterior chamber angle with pigment deposition in exfoliation syndrome
Pigment is unevenly deposited over angle structures (a) in the superior angle. Sampaolesi's line, a wavy line of pigment anterior to Schwalbe's line, is present inferiorly (b). This pattern of pigmentation differs from that seen in pigmentary glaucoma which is typically more homogeneous and often limited to the trabecular meshwork.

incidences vary depending on sample size and technique; increased intraocular pressures may be less common with extracapsular cataract extraction and phacoemulsification than with intracapsular approaches. Many etiologies lead to postoperative pressure elevations and are best considered by time of onset.

Within the first week, many of the materials dispersed during surgery can lead to elevated pressures. Alpha-chymotrypsin frequently results in reduced facility of outflow in the first two days following intracapsular cataract extraction. Retained viscoelastic material is a source of trabecular obstruction manifesting in the first postoperative day. Increased intraocular pressures are seen with all current viscoelastics; no definitive difference in incidence has been shown among them. The viscoelastic Orcolon was withdrawn from the market because of pressure spikes. Meticulous removal at time of surgery may reduce the frequency of this complication. Hyphema following surgery also blocks outflow and can lead to elevated intraocular pressure. Debris, inflammation and trabecular edema

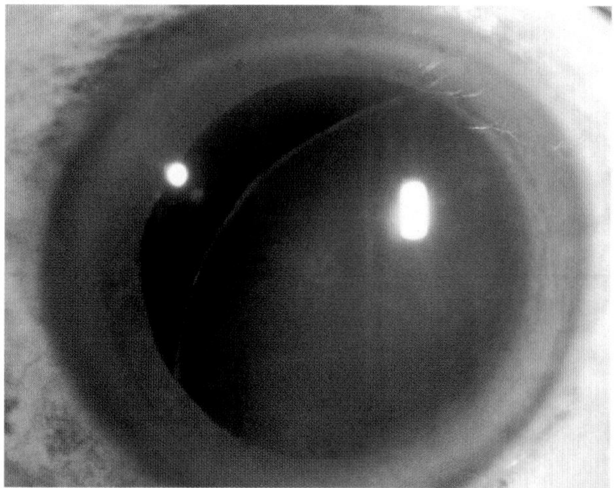

Figure 9.13 Spontaneously dislocated lens
This patient with exfoliation syndrome has a spontaneously dislocated lens in the absence of trauma.

may also play roles in acutely elevated pressures postoperatively. Pre-existing glaucoma increases the frequency and severity of acute postoperative pressure elevations. These complications are best treated medically with aqueous suppressants and topical steroids. Fibrin clots may be treated with intracameral injection of tissue plasminogen activator (Fig. 9.14). Surgical evacuation of viscoelastic or blood is reserved for pressures which do not respond to medical therapy and threaten the optic nerve.

After the first week, other factors may lead to glaucoma. Vitreous in the anterior chamber may reduce aqueous outflow. Hyphema, related to wound construction or intraocular lens position, may occur. Ghost-cell glaucoma results from long-standing hyphema or vitreous hemorrhage leading to degenerated erythrocytes which are less flexible and block trabecular channels. Retained lens particles become hydrated and more prominent, blocking the trabecular meshwork. Postoperative inflammation related to retained lens particles, intraocular lens position, vitreous traction and surgical trauma may become more manifest. Corticosteroid-induced glaucoma must be considered as a common source of increased intraocular pressure in postoperative patients on topical steroids. Discontinuation of steroids or a therapeutic challenge of the fellow eye with topical steroids will aid often in the diagnosis.

Late pressure elevations, occurring months to years following surgery, may also be secondary to inflammation and hemorrhage. *Propionibacterium acnes* endophthalmitis may lead to chronic inflammation with increased pressures. Intraocular lenses may be a source of inflammation and hyphema in the UGH (Uveitis, Glaucoma, Hyphema) syndrome (Figs 9.15 and 9.16). Anterior chamber lenses may directly damage the trabecular meshwork. Vitreous in the anterior chamber may still block outflow. Following YAG laser capsulotomy, inflammation may lead to quite significant pressure elevations, whose frequency is greatly reduced by pretreatment with a topical $alpha_2$ agonist, such as apraclonidine.

Angle-closure glaucoma related to intraocular lenses is discussed in Chapter 10.

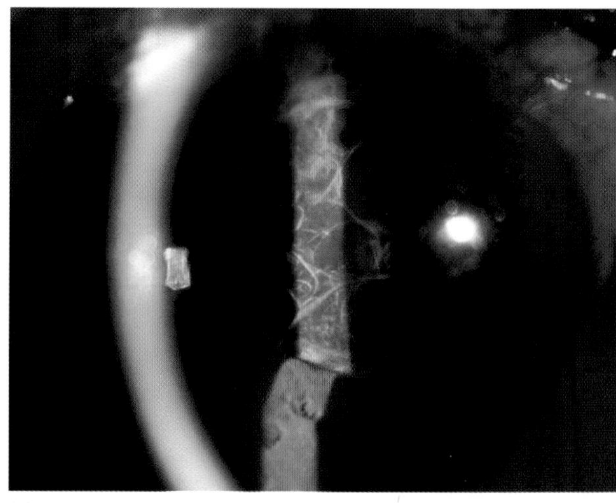

(a)

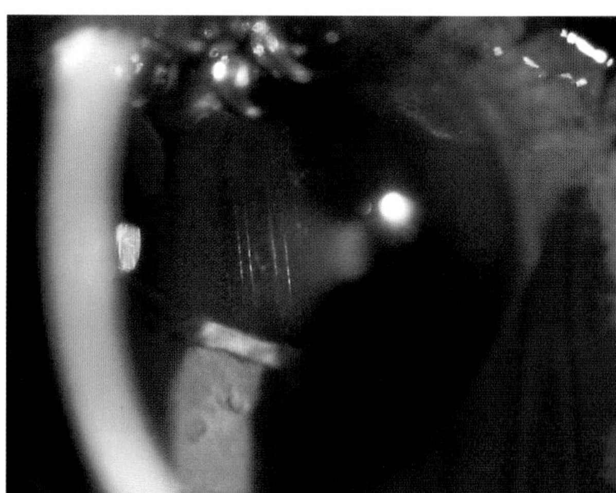

(b)

Figure 9.14 Fibrin clots
Fibrin clot over posterior chamber intraocular lens with elevated intraocular pressure following combined guarded filtration procedure and cataract extraction (a). Same eye (b) following intracameral injection of tissue plasminogen activator. Visual acuity improved dramatically, intraocular pressure dropped from 38 to 10, and remained well controlled.

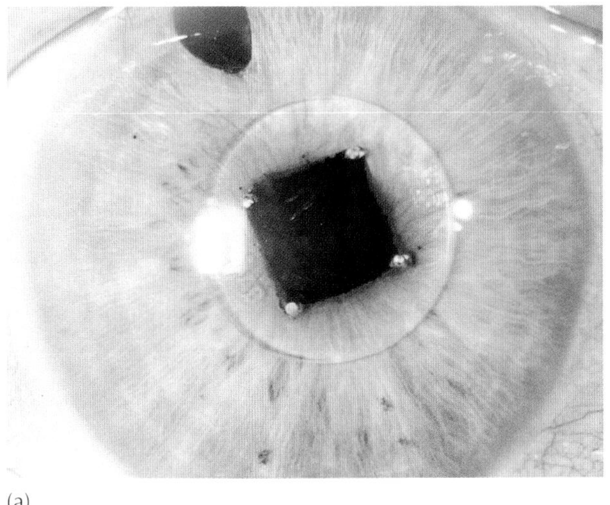

(a)

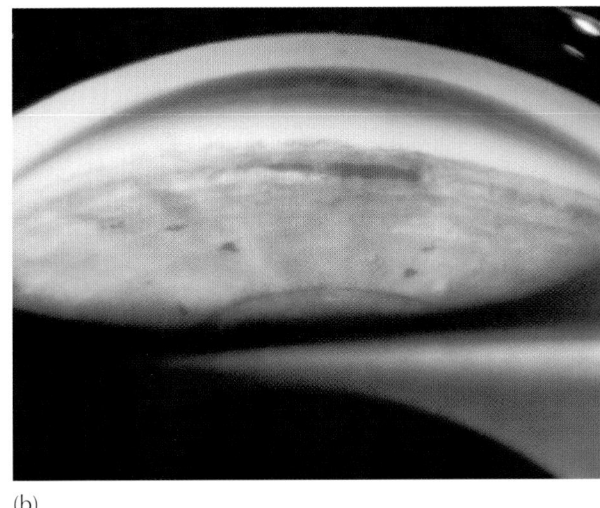

(b)

Figure 9.15

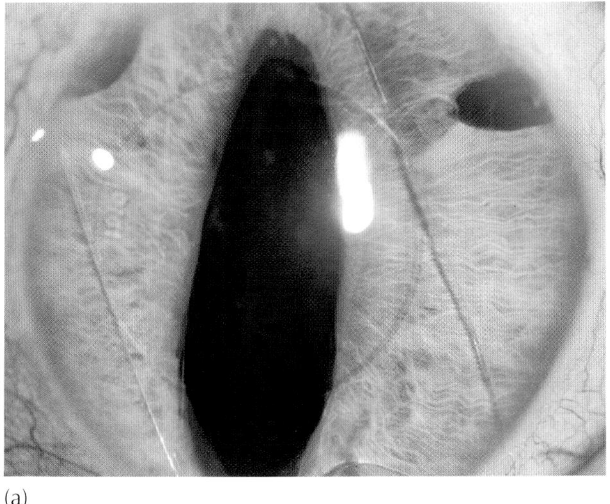

(a)

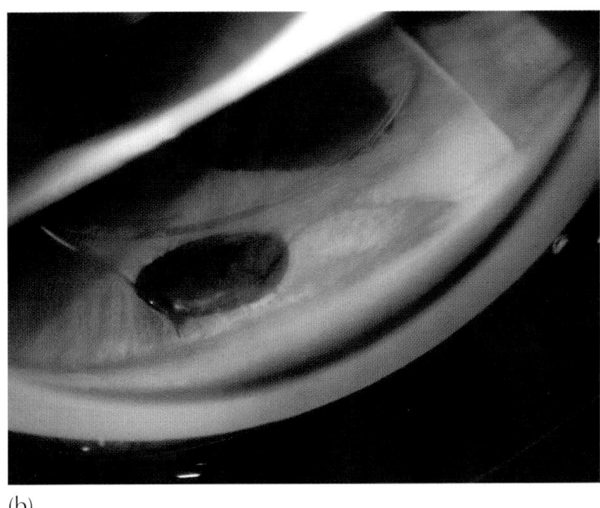

(b)

Figure 9.16

Figure 9.15 and **9.16** **UGH syndrome**
Right (Fig 9.15(a) and (b)) and left (Fig. 9.16(a) and (b)) eyes of a patient with intraocular lenses and the UGH syndrome in both eyes. This patient had multiple hyphemas over a period of years. In some instances the inflammation was readily apparent but the hyphema was only appreciated on gonioscopy. (a) shows the clinical appearance, while (b) is the goniophotograph.

Corticosteroid-induced glaucoma

The use of corticosteroids in any form may lead to the development of a secondary open-angle glaucoma. Increased intraocular pressure has been demonstrated with topical, periocular, inhalational and systemic steroids as well as with increased endogenous steroids in adrenal hyperplasia and Cushing's syndrome (Fig. 9.17). Past steroid use and glaucoma may simulate the presentation of normal-tension glaucoma, as the optic nerve damage and visual field loss may have occurred when the IOP was elevated when the steroids were being used and returned to normal levels once steroid use terminated.

Topical steroids are more likely to elevate intraocular pressure than systemic steroids. Intraocular pressures rise more frequently and more severely with the more potent steroids and with greater dosing. Pressure elevation typically manifests 2–6 weeks after the

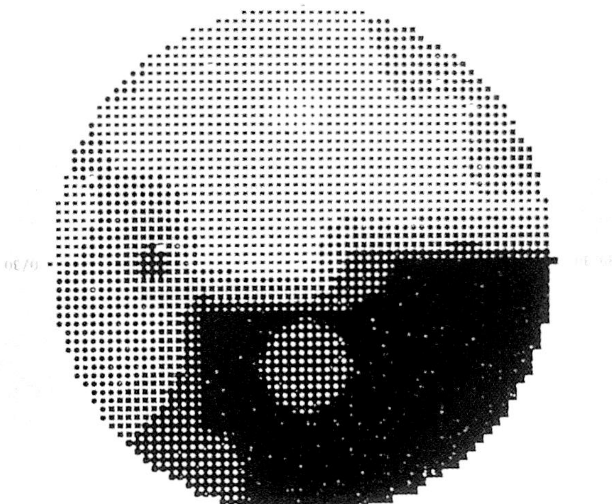

Figure 9.17 Advanced visual field loss
This doctor who self-prescribed topical steroids for vernal conjunctivitis for many years without eye examinations developed steroid glaucoma with advanced visual field loss.

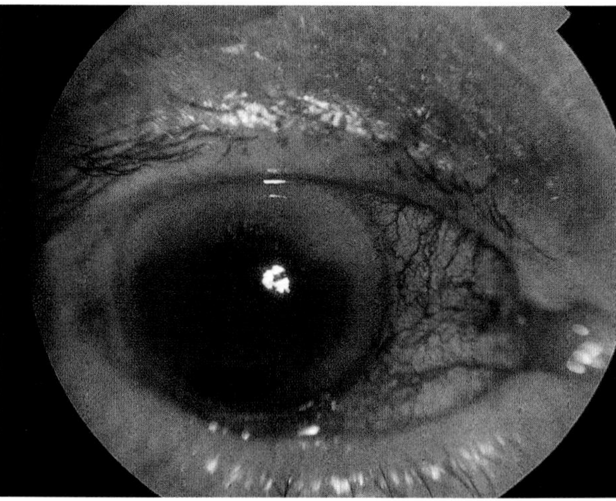

Figure 9.18 Traumatic hyphema
Two fluid levels exist as the red blood cells settle and clot.

initiation of steroids. Patients with primary open-angle glaucoma respond much more frequently and severely to steroids with elevated intraocular pressure. Depending on steroid dose, duration and diagnostic criteria, over 90% of patients with primary open-angle glaucoma may have pressure elevations with steroids compared to 5–10% of normals. Other risk factors for steroid responsiveness include ocular hypertension, angle-recession glaucoma (in either eye), primary relative of patient with primary open-angle glaucoma, pigmentary glaucoma, myopia, diabetes and history of connective tissue disease, but not exfoliative glaucoma.

Corticosteroids result in the accumulation of glycosaminoglycans in the trabecular meshwork, reducing outflow facility. Theories for the mechanism of this accumulation of glycosaminoglycans include increased production as well as reduced clearance, mediated either by nuclear steroid receptors or by membrane stabilization.

The diagnosis may be made either by withdrawing steroid therapy and observing reduced pressures or by challenging the fellow eye in topical steroid cases. Intraocular pressures usually return to baseline within 1–2 months, but may remain high in patients who have been on steroids for long periods of time. Elevated pressures following periocular injection of steroids may require the excision of depot steroids. Aqueous suppressants and miotics can be effective in treating the elevated pressure. Argon laser trabeculoplasty may be useful, although less effective than in primary open-angle glaucoma, pigmentary glaucoma and exfoliative glaucoma.

Post-traumatic glaucomas

Ocular trauma remains a common cause for emergency room visits and hospital admissions, being most frequent among young males. Causes vary with age: play-related accidents in young children, sports and assaults in young adults, and work and domestic accidents or abuse in older adults. The mechanism of trauma often dictates the specific injuries to the eye; almost all may lead to glaucoma. Nonpenetrating injuries of the eye secondary to blunt trauma are usually related to the anterior to posterior compression of the eye with secondary equatorial stretching. This stretching may result in pupil sphincter tears, iridodialysis, angle recession, cyclodialysis, trabecular dialysis, disruption of the zonules and retinal dialysis or detachment. Tears in the face of the ciliary body, usually between the circular and longitudinal muscles, may disrupt the major arterial circle of the iris and the arterial and venous connections of the ciliary body resulting in hyphema. Severity may range from a microhyphema, in which the slit lamp microscope is necessary to appreciate the presence of blood in the anterior chamber, to total hyphema, in which the anterior and posterior chambers are entirely filled with blood (Figs 9.18 and 9.19).

Following injury, intraocular pressure may be elevated or reduced, depending on the balance of several factors. Aqueous secretion may be acutely reduced; uveoscleral outflow may be increased by an accompanying cyclodialysis; blood may obstruct an injured and inflamed trabecular meshwork. Although red blood cells normally pass through the

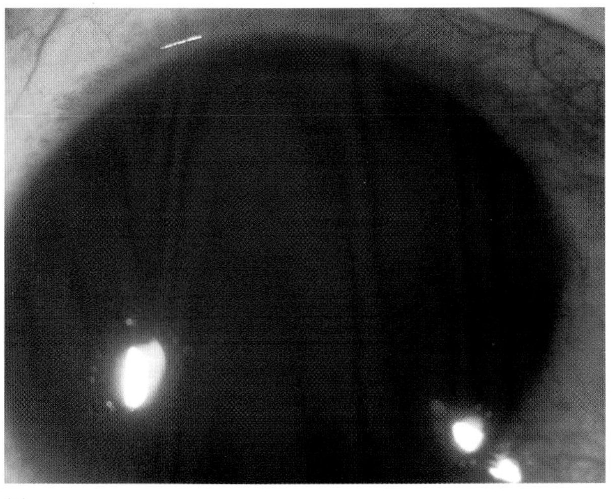
(a)

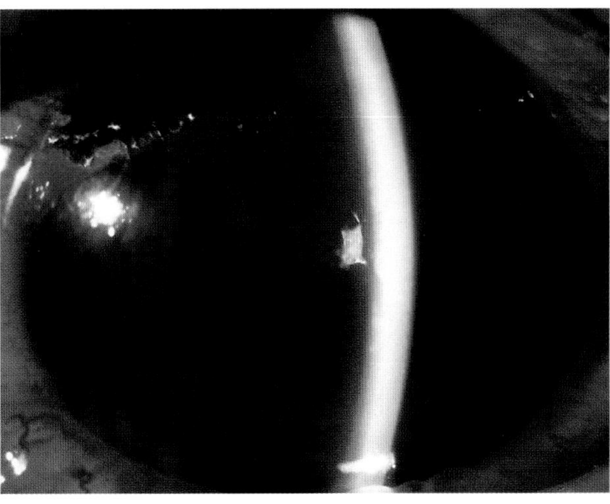
(b)

Figure 9.19 Total hyphema
(a) The incidence of elevated intraocular pressure increases with the amount of blood in the anterior chamber. More than half of those with total hyphemas have significant pressure elevations. (b) With 'blackball' or 'eight-ball' hyphemas, this approaches 100%. Patients with sickle-cell disease may suffer severe pressure elevations with relatively minor hyphemas.

pores in the meshwork, acute inflammation and swelling of the meshwork combined with excessive amounts of red blood cells and debris may overwhelm the meshwork's capacity. Aqueous suppressants are effective in many cases. Steroids help to reduce inflammation. Miotics are generally avoided as they may predispose to posterior synechiae, further compromise the blood–aqueous barrier and reduce uveoscleral outflow.

Patients with hyphema are generally kept at bedrest and treated with mydriatics and topical steroids. Aminocaproic acid, an antifibrinolytic agent, is also used in some centers to reduce the incidence of rebleeds, which may be severe. Prolonged elevation of intraocular pressure may require surgical evacuation of the blood. Timing is dependent on the ability of the nerve to withstand elevated pressures; otherwise healthy nerves may tolerate pressures of up to 50 mmHg for several days. Evacuation may also be necessary because of the development of blood staining of the cornea, especially in those at risk for amblyopia (Fig. 9.20). Surgical evacuation is ideally performed near the fourth day post-trauma. This is past the peak incidence of rebleed and allows time for the anterior chamber blood to clot and retract somewhat from ocular structures, facilitating removal.

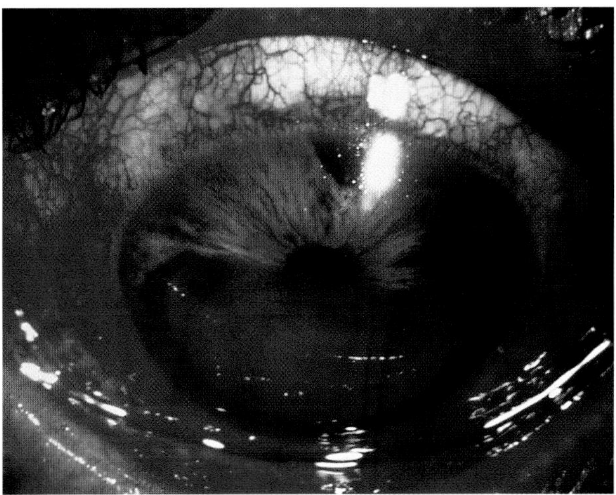

Figure 9.20 Corneal blood staining following a traumatic hyphema
These generally clear over weeks to months, starting at the periphery, following hyphema resolution. In patients in the age group capable of developing ambylophia, incipient blood staining may require surgical evacuation of the blood.

Patients with sickle-cell disease are at greater risk for complications from hyphemas. Significant intraocular pressure elevations may occur with even small hyphemas. Sickling has been demonstrated in the anterior chamber blood; this may reduce clearance and increase intraocular pressure. Central retinal arterial obstruction may occur at lower pressures following hyphemas in these patients. Carbonic anhydrase inhibitors are avoided in sickle-cell disease as they may worsen sickling and reduce clearance of blood by increasing aqueous ascorbic acid and by promoting systemic acidosis. African-American patients with hyphemas should be screened for sickle-cell hemoglobin, and positive

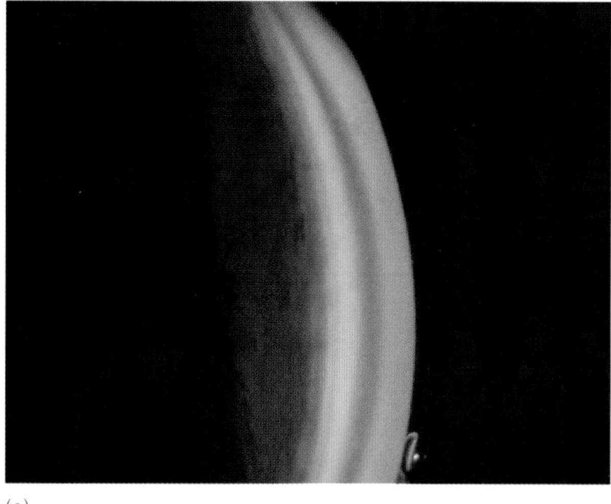

(a)

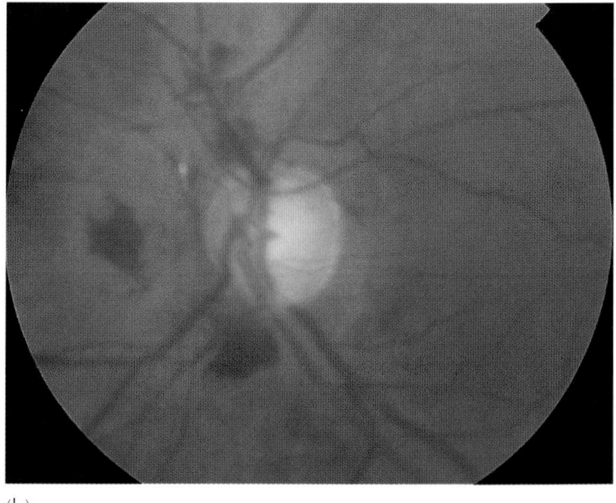

(b)

Figure 9.21 Angle recession
(a) An abnormally wide ciliary body band is seen, as well as bare sclera posteriorly. Fundoscopic examination (b) revealed a glaucomatous optic nerve with markedly increased cupping compared to the fellow eye. Traumatic scars of the retinal pigment epithelium are also seen.

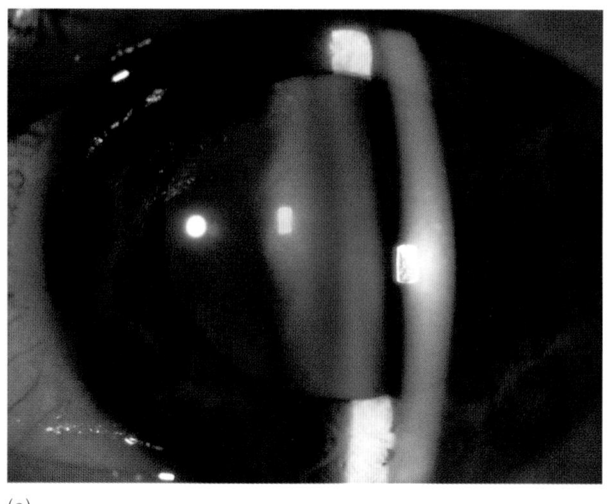

(a)

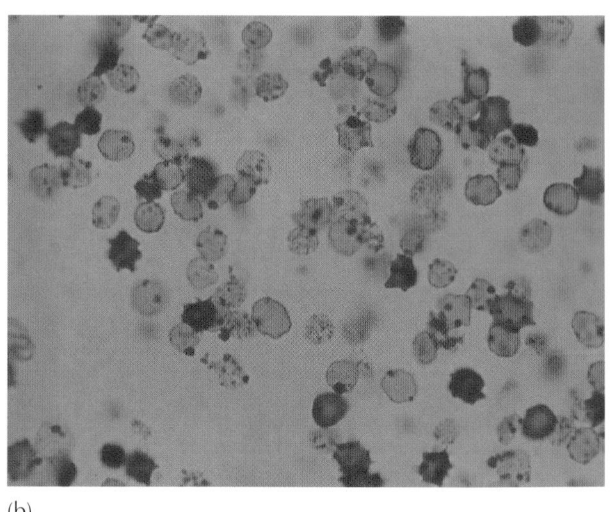

(b)

Figure 9.22 Ghost-cell glaucoma
This patient with ghost-cell glaucoma had 2+ anterior chamber khaki-colored cells and marked khaki-colored cells in the anterior vitreous (a). Vitrectomy specimen showed ghost cells (b).

patients should undergo hemoglobin electrophoresis. All available therapies should be used to keep intraocular pressures below 25 mmHg.

As also discussed elsewhere (see Chapter 10), trauma may also lead to angle-closure glaucoma through a variety of mechanisms. Clots may cover the pupil leading to pupillary block and angle closure. Dislocated lenses may cause pupillary block. Post-traumatic inflammation may lead to extensive peripheral anterior and posterior synechiae. Shallow anterior chambers with penetrating trauma also may create extensive anterior synechiae. Rarely, photoreceptors from a retinal detachment will cause a secondary open-angle glaucoma (Schwartz's syndrome).

Angle-recession glaucoma is an important late complication of ocular trauma. Intraocular pressures may remain normal for years to decades and then become severely elevated. Patients must be strongly advised of the need for lifelong, regular follow-up. Angle-recession glaucoma is more common in eyes with 180 degrees or more of angle recession, occurring in 6–20% over a 10-year period (Fig. 9.21). Angle recession must be considered in unilateral glaucomas. Patients often do not recall the long-past trauma. With time, angle recession also tends to scar, becoming less evident by gonioscopy in apparent severity and extent or even forming peripheral anterior synechiae. The affected areas, although reapproximated, still have nonfunctioning meshwork, secondary to scarring or their closure by a Descemet's-like membrane. Fellow eyes are at increased risk of developing open-angle glaucoma: 25% were affected in one study.

Angle-recession glaucoma may respond to aqueous suppressants. Miotics and argon laser trabeculoplasty are rarely effective. Long-term success rates for trabeculectomy are worse than in primary open-angle glaucoma; some surgeons use antimetabolites on primary procedures for this reason.

Ghost-cell glaucoma

Ghost cells are degenerated red blood cells whose leaky membranes have allowed much of the cell's hemoglobin to escape. Residual, degenerated hemoglobin precipitates on the inner cell walls in the form of Heinz bodies. These spherical cells are much less pliable than red blood cells and cannot pass through the intertrabecular spaces. Ghost cells in the anterior chamber result in elevated intraocular pressure much more readily than red blood cells. The formation of ghost cells requires the sequestration of red blood cells in the vitreous for several weeks. The source of vitreous hemorrhage does not matter: a bleed from diabetic neovascularization of the retina, hemorrhage secondary to trauma or a postsurgical hyphema with spill-over into the vitreous through a compromised vitreous face may evolve into a secondary glaucoma. After several weeks, the degenerated cells migrate into the anterior chamber through a defect in the vitreous face (surgical or traumatic) and obstruct the trabecular meshwork. Tan or khaki-colored cells are seen in the anterior chamber, anterior vitreous, on the trabecular meshwork, and may also form a pseudohypopyon (Fig. 9.22). If the vitreous face is intact, the ghost cells do not reach the anterior chamber and glaucoma does not develop.

Several other blood-related elevations of intraocular pressure may be differentiated from ghost-cell glaucoma. Hyphemas may result in acutely elevated pressure, especially in patients with sickle-cell disease. This is secondary to obstruction of the meshwork by red blood cells in the first days following the hyphema. Rarely, an eight-ball, total hyphema may persist long enough to contain ghost cells which add to the trabecular obstruction. Hemolytic glaucoma occurs when the contents of ruptured red blood cells are ingested by macrophages which then obstruct the meshwork. Hemolytic glaucoma is also typically seen in the first days to weeks following the initial hemorrhage. Hemosiderotic glaucoma, in which iron-containing blood breakdown products stain and poison the cells of the trabecular meshwork, occurs much later, often years after the hemorrhage.

Aqueous suppressants often control the intraocular pressure. Miotics are rarely helpful as the meshwork is obstructed; similarly, argon laser trabeculoplasty is not indicated. Anterior chamber lavage with balanced salt solution may resolve the glaucoma. If unsuccessful, or too great a reservoir of ghost cells remains in the vitreous, total vitrectomy, removing as much hemorrhagic material as possible, is usually effective in resolving the glaucoma.

Inflammatory glaucomas

Inflammation within the eye alters aqueous humor dynamics and can lead to increased intraocular pressure. Acute inflammation may reduce aqueous secretion and increase uveoscleral outflow, reducing intraocular pressure. However, inflammatory material, consisting of white blood cells, macrophages and proteins, may obstruct the trabecular meshwork. Chemical mediators of inflammation may further compromise trabecular function as may trabeculitis (inflammation of the trabecular meshwork itself). Trabecular dysfunction may be transient, clearing with resolution of the inflammation, or may persist with permanent structural changes reducing trabecular outflow facility. Additionally, inflammatory scarring may lead to peripheral anterior synechiae and posterior synechiae resulting in angle-closure glaucoma (see Chapter 10). Chronic uveitis may lead to neovascularization and neovascular glaucoma. Patients may manifest some or all of these findings, the balance dictating the nature of the glaucoma. For example, a patient may present acutely during a uveitic episode with uveitic hypotony, progress to a secondary open-angle glaucoma as white blood cells block the meshwork, develop an angle-closure component as synechiae form, and then be left with a chronic mixed-mechanism secondary glaucoma with residual synechiae and scarring of the meshwork.

Virtually all sources of ocular inflammation can lead to glaucoma. Idiopathic uveitis (Fig. 9.23), glaucomatocyclitic crisis (Fig. 9.24), Fuch's heterochromic cyclitis (Fig. 9.25), lens-related uveitis (Fig. 9.26),

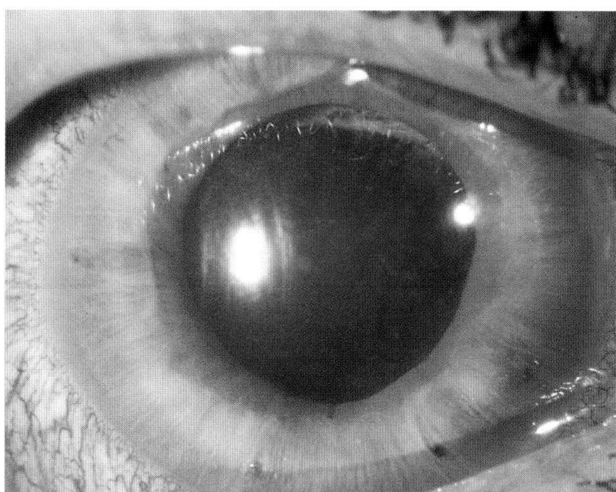

Figure 9.23 Idiopathic uveitis resulting in secondary glaucoma with closed and open-angle components
Note the multiple peripheral iridectomies for previous acute iris bombè. Following resolution of acute attacks the patient had persistent elevation of intraocular pressure in spite of large areas of anterior chamber angle on gonioscopy.

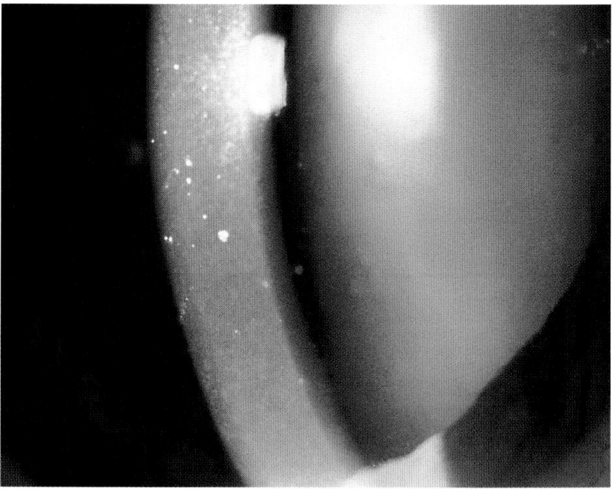

Figure 9.24 Glaucomatocyclitic crisis (Posner–Schlossman syndrome)
Unilateral involvement consisting of fine keratic precipitates in a patient with minimal anterior chamber reaction and markedly elevated intraocular pressure. Following multiple similar attacks, the patient developed chronically elevated intraocular pressure and optic nerve damage requiring trabeculectomy.

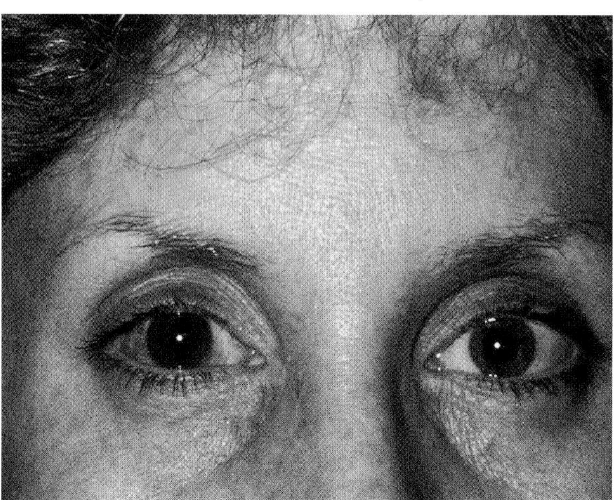

Figure 9.25 Fuch's heterochromic cyclitis
Note the much lighter iris color in the involved eye. The triad of heterochromia, uveitis and cataract typically appears in the third to fourth decade. The uveitis is asymptomatic. Open-angle glaucoma is common, increasing with duration of the disease. Friable angle vessels may bleed easily with surgery; however, frank neovascularization of the iris and neovascular glaucoma are uncommon.

herpes (Fig. 9.27) and sarcoidosis (Fig. 9.28) may all result in increased intraocular pressure. Other uveitic glaucomas include HLA-B27-related uveitides, pars planitis, sarcoidosis, juvenile rheumatoid arthritis, Behcet's disease, Crohn's disease, syphilis, toxoplasmosis, coccidiomycosis, mumps, rubella, leprosy, sympathetic ophthalmia, Vogt–Koyanagi–Harada syndrome and other less common entities.

Treatment strategies are similar for these entities. Resolution of inflammation is the first goal, which may require topical or systemic steroids, antibiotics for infectious diseases and lens extraction in lens-related conditions. Increased intraocular pressure secondary to steroid therapy or to increased aqueous production with resolving inflammation may confuse the clinical picture. Cycloplegics are effective through many mechanisms. Dilatation prevents the formation of a small secluded pupil and relieves the discomfort of ciliary spasm. Cycloplegics also improve uveoscleral outflow and stabilize the blood–aqueous barrier. Topical and systemic aqueous suppressants are effective. Miotics should be avoided as these agents cause increased breakdown of the blood–aqueous barrier, making the inflammation worse, and also reduce uveoscleral outflow. Argon laser trabeculoplasty is generally ineffective and increases inflammation. Filtering surgery is less successful in these patients, especially during acute attacks. Adjunctive use of antimetabolites such as 5-fluorouracil and mitomycin-C may improve results. Drainage tube implants may also be effective. Cyclodestructive procedures can be used in refractory cases, but add to intraocular inflammation and pose significant risks to vision.

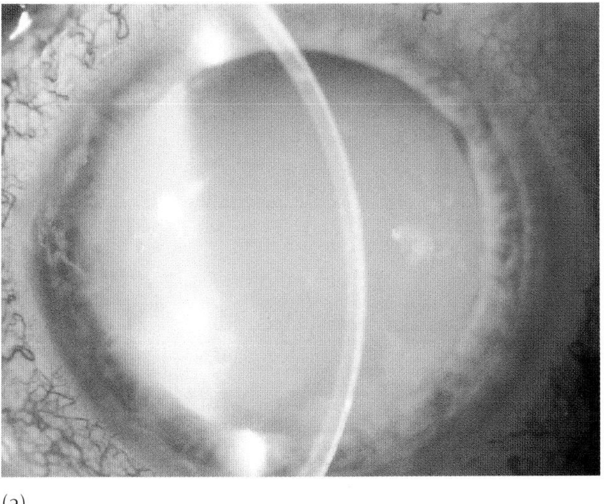

(a)

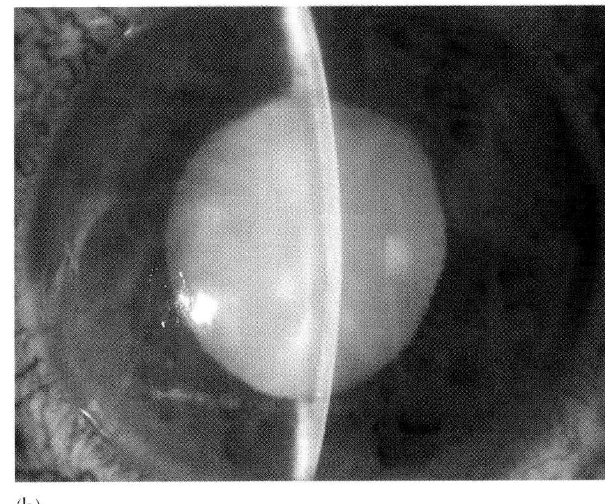

(b)

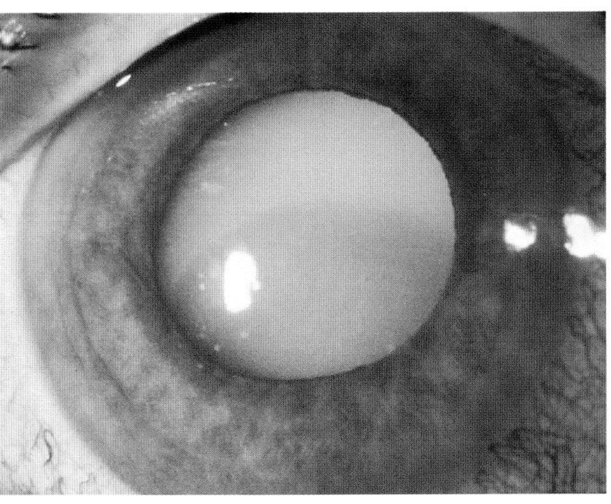

(c)

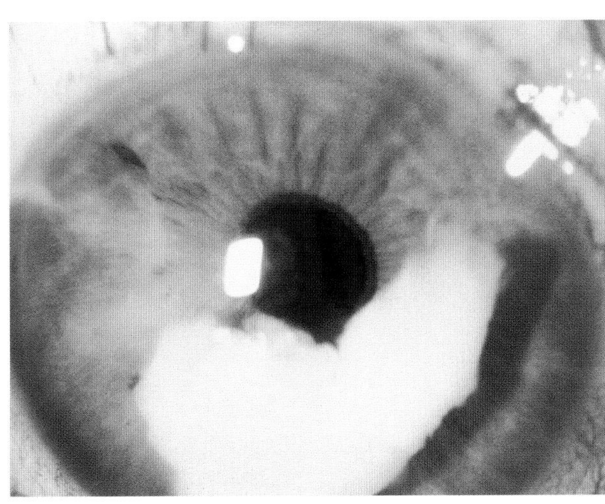

(d)

Figure 9.26 Lens-related glaucoma
In phacolytic glaucoma, a hypermature lens leaks proteins into the anterior chamber through a grossly intact capsule (a); these proteins and ingesting macrophages block the trabecular meshwork. A swollen, mature cataract may also lead to pupillary block in phacomorphic glaucoma; (b) note the narrow angle present in a patient with phacomorphic glaucoma. A hypermature cataract with liquefied cortex and dense nucleus may also lead to phacolytic glaucoma (c).

Retained lens cortex (d) following cataract extraction may increase in size with hydration and lead to glaucoma through trabecular obstruction by lens material. Phacoanaphylaxis exists when lens material is present outside the capsule following surgery or trauma and leads to granulomatous inflammation. A previous history of trauma to the lens or cataract surgery in the fellow eye is typical. Phacoanaphylaxis often leads to significant pressure elevation.

Glaucoma associated with ocular tumors

Benign and malignant intraocular tumors may cause glaucoma by a variety of mechanisms. Direct infiltration of the trabecular meshwork by the tumor can block aqueous outflow. Free-floating tumor cells may obstruct the meshwork. Hemorrhage may produce a secondary open-angle glaucoma. Tumor-related neovascularization of the iris and angle produces glaucoma in some cases. Large posterior masses sometimes press the iris and lens anteriorly, resulting in angle closure (Chapter 10). Tumor-related glaucomas are typically unilateral. Treatment of the glaucoma without diagnosis of the tumor may have serious consequences for the patient. A thorough examination will reveal most intraocular

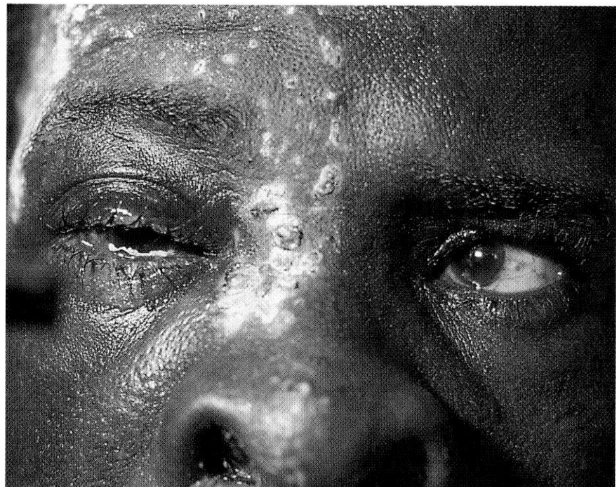

Figure 9.27 Herpes zoster ophthalmicus
Herpes zoster ophthalmicus with characteristic skin lesions affecting the dermatome of the first branch of the facial nerve. The tip of the nose is involved, a harbinger of ocular involvement (Hutchinson's sign). Marked conjunctival injection and a granulomatous uveitis are present. Glaucoma is a frequent complication in herpes zoster and herpes simplex uveitis.

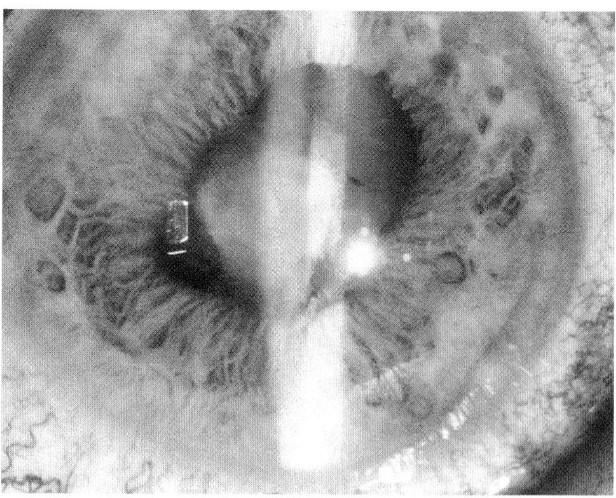

Figure 9.28 Sarcoid uveitis with posterior synechiae and cataract
Up to one half of patients with sarcoid suffer from uveitis at some point during the disease process. Granulomatous anterior uveitis is a common manifestation, frequently becoming bilateral, recurrent and chronic. Sarcoid nodules on the iris (Busacca's in the crypts, Koeppe's at the pupillary margin) may be seen. Secondary open and closed-angle glaucoma is common. As the disease is more common in blacks, clinicians must be wary of steroid-induced glaucoma as a complication of treatment.

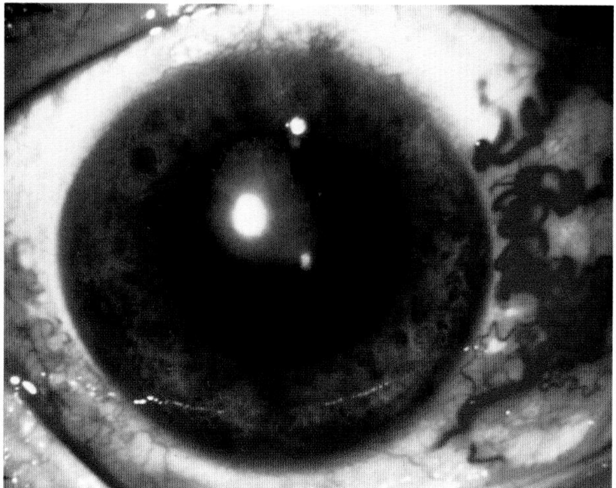

Figure 9.29 Uveal melanoma
Sentinel vessel overlying the sclera in a patient with uveal melanoma.

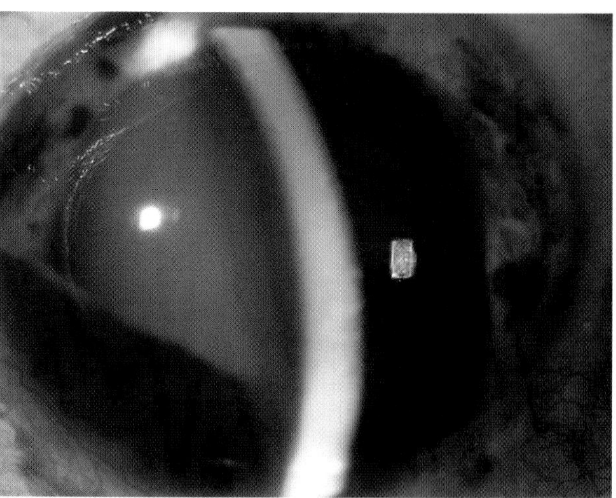

Figure 9.30 Iris melanoma
Hyphema in patient with iris melanoma producing a secondary open-angle glaucoma.

malignancies, especially for clinicians alert to such tip-offs as a sentinel vessel (Fig. 9.29).

Uveal melanoma is the most common intraocular malignancy in adults, and is the most common cause of tumor-related glaucoma. Iris melanomas may obstruct the trabecular meshwork by direct invasion or by hemorrhage (Fig. 9.30). Ciliary body melanomas may be more difficult to detect, remaining hidden until relatively large. Glaucoma most often results from the tumor pushing the iris anteriorly to close the anterior chamber angle. Glaucoma may also result because of direct extension of the tumor into the trabecular meshwork, iris neovascularization,

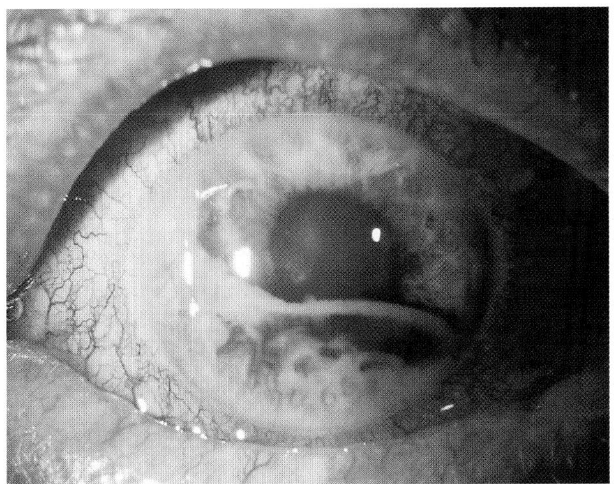

Figure 9.31 Metastatic tumor
Metastatic tumor to iris from lung.

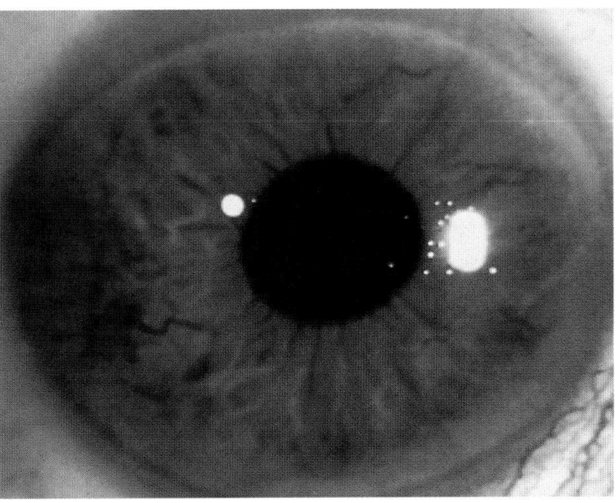

Figure 9.32 Multiple myeloma
Multiple myeloma of iris.

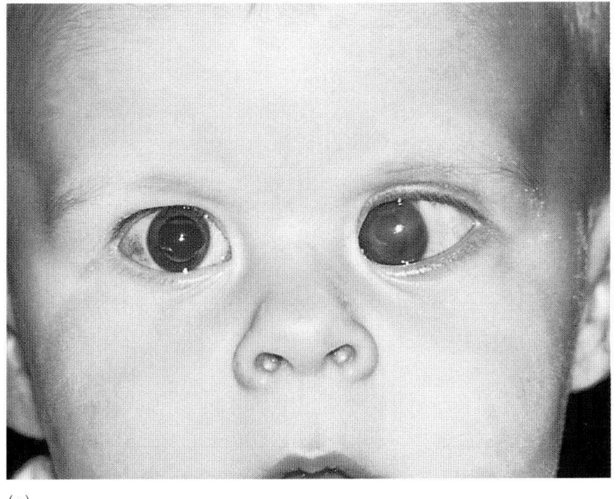

(a)

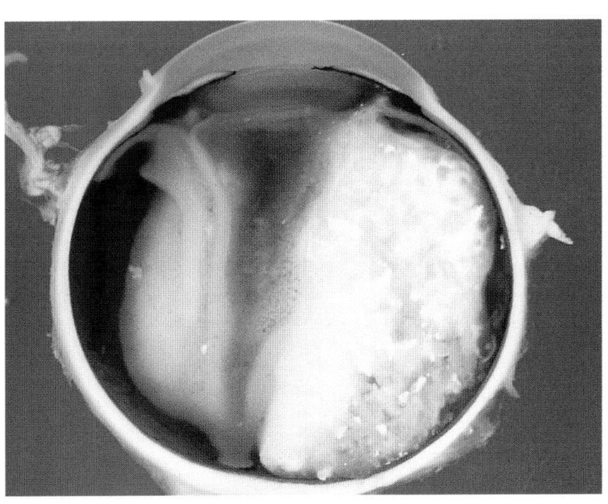

(b)

Figure 9.33 Retinoblastoma
Retinoblastoma causing glaucoma (a) (external photo) and (b) gross pathology.

hyphema or tumor necrosis causing obstruction of the meshwork by cells and debris. Choroidal melanoma less commonly causes glaucoma. Mechanisms of glaucoma in choroidal melanomas include iris and angle neovascularization most commonly, as well as angle closure, hemorrhage and necrosis.

Histologically benign tumors of the iris may also cause glaucoma. Diffuse uveal melanomas may block the meshwork with melanoma cells or pigment. Melanocytomas, most commonly found on the optic disc but also seen in the iris or ciliary body, can produce glaucoma. These tumors have a propensity to undergo necrosis and fragmentation, blocking the trabecular meshwork with debris, producing the so-called melanomalytic glaucoma. Differentiation of these tumors from their malignant counterparts is a crucial step in treatment, often requiring histopathologic study.

Intraocular metastases are typically to the uveal tissues. Glaucoma is found more frequently in metastases to the iris and ciliary body (64% and 67%, respectively) than in metastases to the choroid

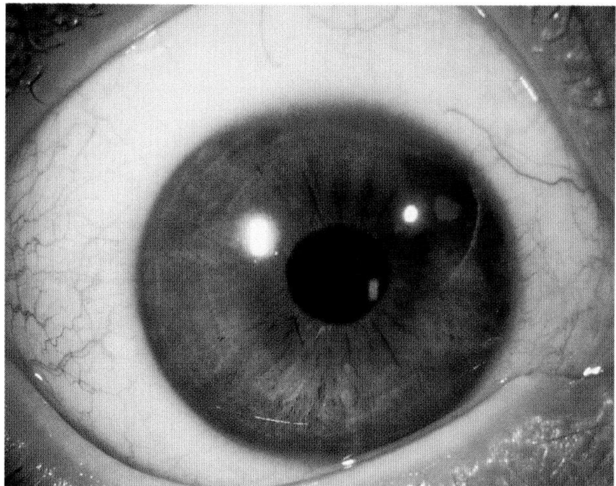

Figure 9.34 Neurofibromatosis type 1
Neurofibromatosis type 1 with Lisch nodules, most prominently superonasal. Lisch nodules, variably pigmented collections of melanocytic spindle cells, are seen bilaterally in all patients over age 16 with neurofibromatosis type 1. Nodules are rare and unilateral in neurofibromatosis type 2.

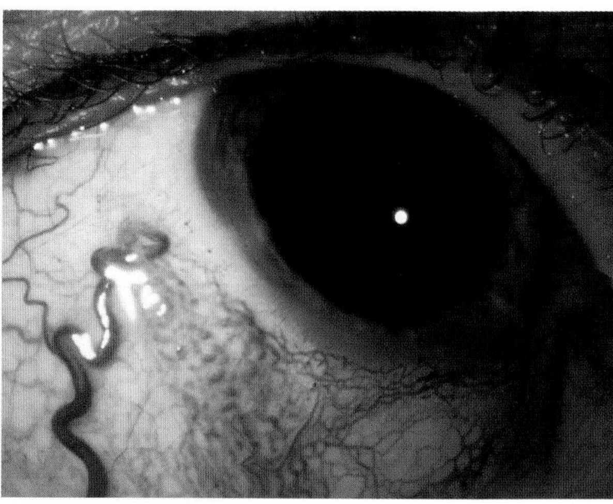

Figure 9.35 Sturge–Weber syndrome with glaucoma
Note dilated conjunctival vessel and episcleral hemangioma.

(2%). Common primary tumors include those of the breast and lung, as well as tumors of the gastrointestinal tract, kidney, thyroid and skin. Efforts to identify the primary neoplasm are not always successful. Friable metastases often seed the anterior chamber angle, obstructing the trabecular meshwork (Figs 9.31 and 9.32). Pseudohypopyons and ring infiltrates are sometimes seen.

Benign reactive lymphoid hyperplasia can directly invade the trabecular meshwork. Large cell lymphoma (reticulum cell sarcoma, histiocytic lymphoma) and leukemia may also infiltrate the meshwork and lead to glaucoma.

Retinoblastoma is the most common intraocular malignancy of childhood. Glaucoma is not uncommon, occurring in 17% of cases in one study (Shields). In that study of 303 eyes, the glaucoma was thought to be secondary to iris neovascularization with or without hemorrhage in 72%, angle closure in 26% and tumor seeding in 2% (Fig. 9.33). The less common but benign meduloepithelioma may also cause glaucoma secondary to iris neovascularization, as well as direct invasion of angle structures or obstruction of the meshwork by hyphema and tumor-related debris.

Various ocular tumors are manifested by the phakomatoses. Unilateral glaucoma, congenital or later onset, may be seen in neurofibromatosis of both types (Fig. 9.34). Half of all eyes with plexiform neuromas of the upper lid develop glaucoma. The glaucoma associated with encephalotrigeminal angiomatosis (Sturge–Weber syndrome) is discussed along with other causes of increased episcleral venous pressure below. Congenital glaucoma may also be seen. Oculodermal melanocytosis (nevus of Ota) has been reported to have an incidence of glaucoma of 10%, including angle-closure, open-angle and congenital varieties.

Increased episcleral venous pressure

The Goldmann equation, $Po = F/C + Pev$ (where Po is intraocular pressure, F is aqueous production, C outflow facility and Pev episcleral venous pressure), describes a direct relation of intraocular pressure to episcleral venous pressure. Normal episcleral venous pressure is between 9 and 10 mmHg. Increases in episcleral venous pressure lead to increases in intraocular pressure. Experimentally, this relationship is slightly less than 1 : 1, possibly due to decreased aqueous inflow or increased uveoscleral outflow with increased intraocular pressure. However, any cause of increased episcleral venous pressure may increase intraocular

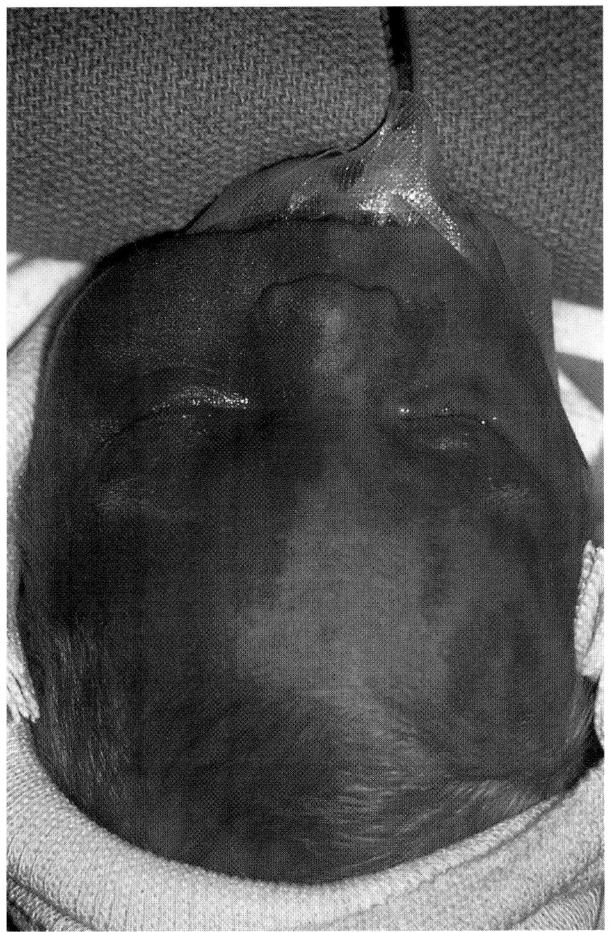

Figure 9.36 Sturge–Weber syndrome in an infant
Infant with Sturge–Weber syndrome undergoing examination under anesthesia. Intraocular pressure was normal. Glaucoma is more common with upper lid involvement by the hemangioma.

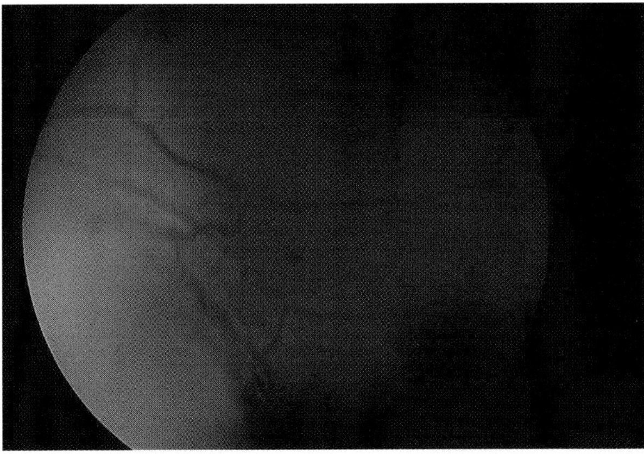

Figure 9.37 Resolving suprachoroidal hemorrhage following trabeculectomy in patient with Sturge–Weber syndrome
Although prophylactic partial-thickness scleral windows with full-thickness sclerostomies were performed, a large hemorrhage still occurred.

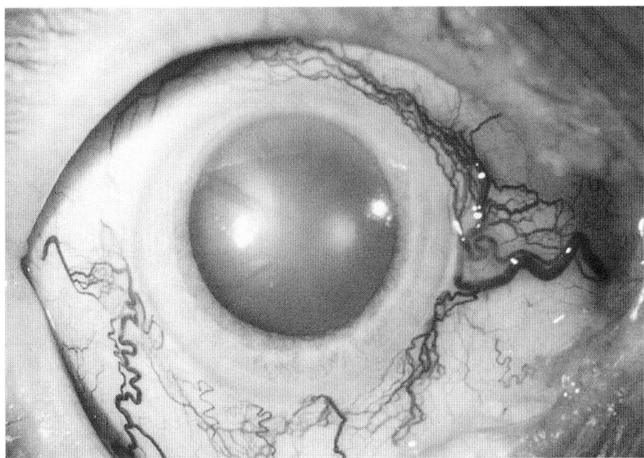

Figure 9.38 Dilated and tortuous episcleral vessels
In patient with carotid-cavernous fistula and increased intraocular pressure. These patients are also at risk for ocular ischemia leading to neovascular glaucoma, uveal effusions with angle closure, and central retinal arterial and venous obstruction.

pressure. Obstruction of venous drainage along any part of the outflow pathway may lead to increased episcleral venous pressure and increased intraocular pressure. Dilated vessels are seen beneath the conjunctiva that do not blanch with epinephrine. Blood may be seen in Schlemm's canal on gonioscopy. Orbital congestion in thyroid ophthalmopathy may increase episcleral and intraocular pressures; this may be responsive to steroids, radiation and decompression. Thrombosis of an orbital vein or the cavernous sinus can produce similar findings. Retrobulbar tumors, jugular vein obstruction and superior vena cava syndrome also lead to increased episcleral pressure.

Arteriovenous anomalies, by exposing the venous system to the greater pressures of the arterial system, result in increased episcleral venous pressure. Sturge–Weber syndrome (Figs 9.35–9.37), carotid cavernous fistulas (Fig. 9.38) and orbital varices can in this manner produce glaucoma. Idiopathic cases of increased episcleral venous pressure exist as well (Fig. 9.39).

Treatment of the underlying cause of increased venous pressure is ideal but not always possible or worth while. Embolization of carotid-cavernous fistulas carries significant risk of central nervous system vascular accident; many close spontaneously. Aqueous

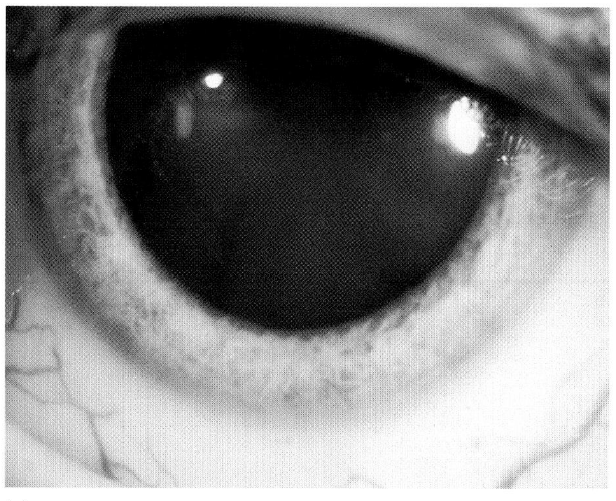

(a)

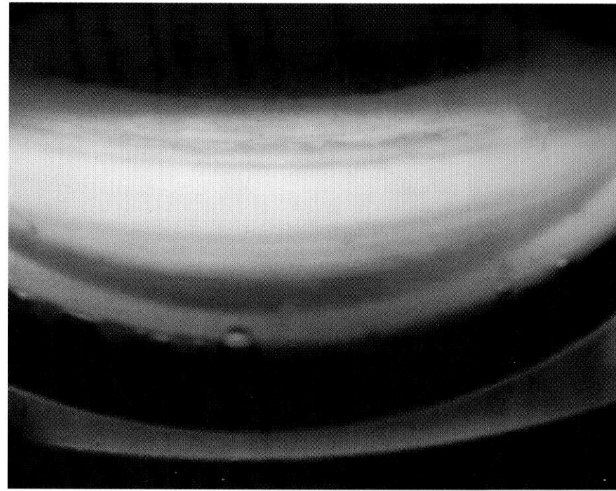

(b)

Figure 9.39 Sporadic, idiopathic elevated episcleral venous pressure
Patient with sporadic, idiopathic elevated episcleral venous pressure shows mildly dilated episcleral vessels (a) and blood in Schlemm's canal on gonioscopy (b). Familial forms of idiopathic elevated episcleral venous pressure exist as well.

suppressants often are helpful. Miotics and argon laser trabeculoplasty are not often useful given the typically normal facility of outflow. Trabeculectomy is effective as it bypasses the elevated episcleral venous pressure, but has a higher incidence in these patients of serous and hemorrhagic choroidal detachments. Prophylactic partial-thickness scleral flaps with full-thickness sclerostomies have been advocated.

FURTHER READING

Campbell DG, Schertzer RM, Pigmentary glaucoma. In: Ritch R, Shields MB, Krupin T, eds. *The glaucomas*, 2nd edn. (St Louis, MO: Mosby, 1996), 975–92.

Campbell DG, Schertzer RM, Ghost cell glaucoma. In: Ritch R, Shields MB, Krupin T, eds. *The glaucomas*, 2nd edn. (St Louis, MO: Mosby, 1996), 1277–88.

Epstein DL, *Chandler and Grant's glaucoma*, 3rd edn. (Philadelphia, PA: Lea & Febiger, 1986), 332–51.

Epstein DL, *Chandler and Grant's glaucoma*, 3rd edn. (Philadelphia, PA: Lea & Febiger, 1986), 391–5.

Epstein DL, *Chandler and Grant's glaucoma*, 3rd edn. (Philadelphia, PA: Lea & Febiger, 1986), 403–7.

Farrar SM, Shields MB, Current concepts in pigmentary glaucoma, *Surv Ophthalmol* (1993) **37**:233–52.

Folberg R, Parrish RK II, Glaucoma following trauma. In: Tasman W, Jaeger EA, eds. *Duane's clinical ophthalmology*, revised edn. (Philadelphia, PA: Lippincott, 1994), 54C, 1–7.

Krupin T, Feitl ME, Karalekas D, Glaucoma associated with uveitis. In: Ritch R, Shields MB, Krupin T, eds. *The glaucomas*, 2nd edn. (St Louis, MO: Mosby, 1996), 1225–58.

Lampink A, Management of the aphakic and pseudophakic patient with glaucoma. In: Higginbotham EJ, Lee DA, eds. *Management of difficult glaucoma* (Boston, MA: Blackwell Scientific, 1994), 144–54.

Mermoud A, Heuer DK, Glaucoma associated with trauma. In: Ritch R, Shields MB, Krupin T, eds. *The glaucomas*, 2nd edn. (St Louis, MO: Mosby, 1996), 1259–76.

Ritch R, Exfoliation syndrome. In: Ritch R, Shields MB, Krupin T, eds. *The glaucomas*, 2nd edn. (St Louis, MO: Mosby, 1996), 993–1022.

Shields JA, Shields CL, Shields MB, Glaucoma associated with intraocular tumors. In: Ritch R, Shields MB, Krupin T, eds. *The glaucomas*, 2nd edn. (St Louis, MO: Mosby, 1996), 1131–42.

Tomey KF, Traverso CE, Glaucoma associated with aphakia and pseudophakia. In: Ritch R, Shields MB, Krupin T, eds. *The glaucomas*, 2nd edn. (St Louis, MO: Mosby, 1996), 1289–324.

10 The angle-closure glaucomas

Jeffrey M Liebmann, Robert Ritch and David S Greenfield

Introduction

The angle-closure glaucomas are a diverse group of disorders characterized by apposition of the iris to the trabecular meshwork. This results in mechanical blockage of aqueous outflow, progressive trabecular dysfunction, synechial closure and elevated intraocular pressure (IOP).

Angle closure can be caused by one or a combination of the following:

1) Abnormalities in the relative sizes or positions of anterior segment structures.
2) Abnormalities in the absolute sizes or positions of anterior segment structures.
3) Abnormal forces in the posterior segment which alter the anatomy of the anterior segment.

Classification of angle closure by the anatomic level of the cause of the block, defined by the structure producing the 'forces' leading to the block, facilitates understanding of the various mechanisms, and appropriate treatment in any particular case becomes an exercise in deductive logic. Four levels of block, from anterior to posterior, have been defined. Each level of block may have a component of each of the levels preceding it. The appropriate treatment becomes more complex for each level of block, as each level may also require the treatments for lower levels of block. The four levels are I) block originating at the level of the iris (Figs 10.1–10.24); II) block originating at the level of the ciliary body (Figs 10.25–10.44); III) block at the level of the lens (Figs 10.45–10.56); and IV) block related to pressure posterior to the lens (Figs 10.57–10.65). Angle-closure glaucoma may also be associated with other ocular disorders (Figs 10.66–10.78).

With high-frequency, high-resolution, anterior segment ultrasound biomicroscopy (UBM), the structures surrounding the posterior chamber can be imaged, examination of which has been previously limited to histopathologic examination. UBM is ideally suited to the study of the angle-closure glaucomas because of its ability to image simultaneously the ciliary body, posterior chamber, iris–lens relationship and angle structures. In this chapter, the angle-closure glaucomas will be evaluated, with an emphasis on their anatomic basis.

FURTHER READING

Lowe RF, Ritch R. Angle-closure glaucoma. Clinical types. In: Ritch R, Shields MB, Krupin T, eds. *The glaucomas*, 2nd edn. (St Louis, MO: Mosby, 1996), 827.

Ritch R, Liebmann JM. Argon laser peripheral iridoplasty. *Ophth Surg Lasers* (1996) **27**:289–300.

Tello C, Chi T, Shepps G, Liebmann J, Ritch R, Ultrasound biomicroscopy in pseudophakic malignant glaucoma. *Ophthalmol* (1993) **100**:1330–4.

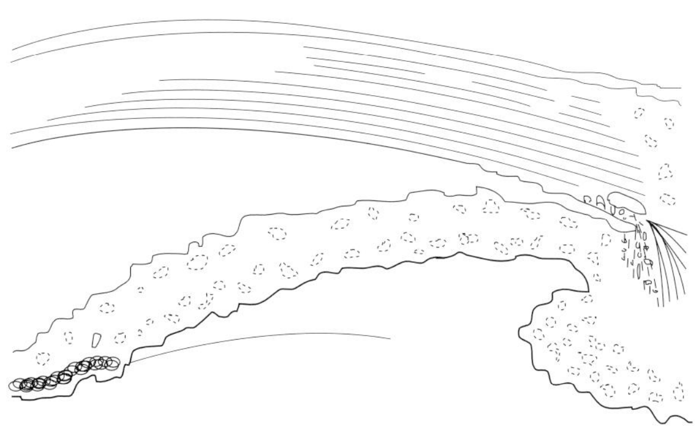

Figure 10.1 Relative pupillary block
Relative pupillary block is the underlying mechanism in approximately 90% of patients with angle closure. Relative pupillary block typically occurs in hyperopic eyes, which have a shorter than average axial length, a more shallow anterior chamber, a thicker lens, a more anterior lens position and a smaller radius of corneal curvature. In pupillary block, flow of aqueous from the posterior to the anterior chamber is impeded between the anterior surface of the lens and the posterior surface of the iris. Aqueous pressure in the posterior chamber becomes higher than that in the anterior chamber, causing anterior iris bowing, narrowing of the angle and acute or chronic angle-closure glaucoma.

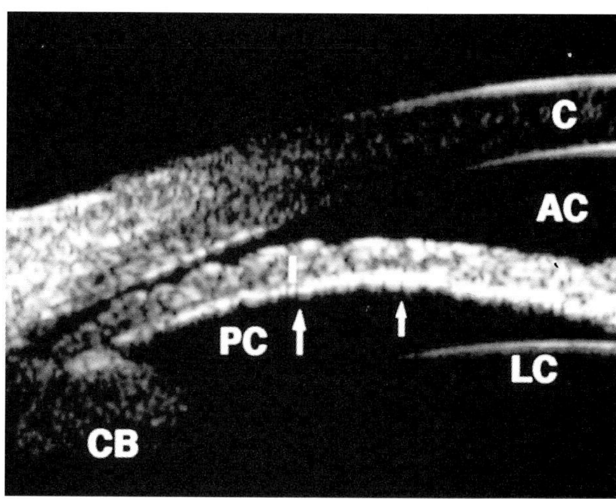

Figure 10.2 Relative pupillary block and angle closure (pupillary block angle closure), UBM
In phakic pupillary block angle closure, the iris (I) has a convex configuration (small white arrow) because of the relative pressure differential (large white arrows) between the posterior chamber (PC) (the site of aqueous production) and the anterior chamber (AC). The cornea (C), anterior lens capsule (LC) and ciliary body (CB) are visible.

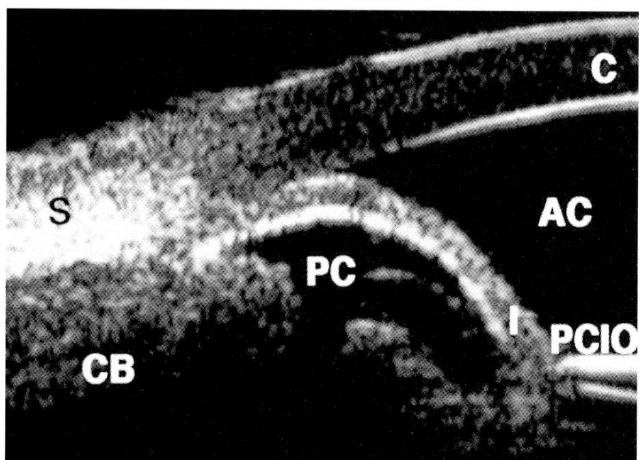

Figure 10.3 Pseudophakic pupillary block, UBM
In pseudophakic pupillary block, resistance to aqueous flow occurs because of posterior synechiae between the iris (I) and posterior chamber intraocular lens (PCIOL) which limit aqueous flow into the anterior chamber causing the iris in this patient to assume a bombè configuration. The angle is closed.

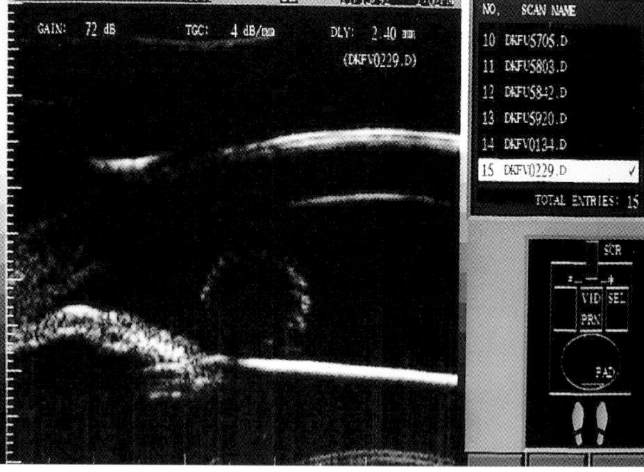

Figure 10.4 Iridovitreal block, UBM
Occasionally, aqueous access to the anterior chamber can be impeded by vitreous in the posterior or anterior chambers. In this illustration, the round bulge of vitreous prolapse into the anterior chamber is visible and the iris is convex. A posterior chamber intraocular lens is present.

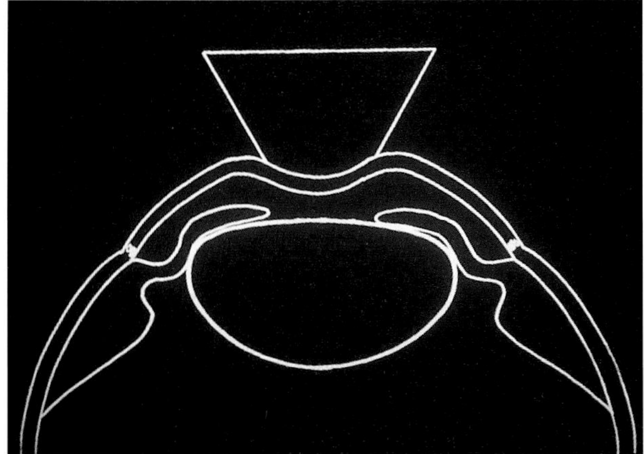

Figure 10.5 Indentation gonioscopy
Indentation gonioscopy is critical to accurate diagnosis of the angle-closure glaucomas. During indentation, the central corneal curvature is altered, forcing aqueous posteriorly. The iris is pushed against the lens, creating a flap valve effect, which prevents aqueous from moving through the pupil into the posterior chamber. Aqueous is then forced into the angle recess, which opens an appositionally closed angle. (See Chapter 5 for further discussion of the role of gonioscopy in the diagnosis and management of angle-closure glaucoma.)

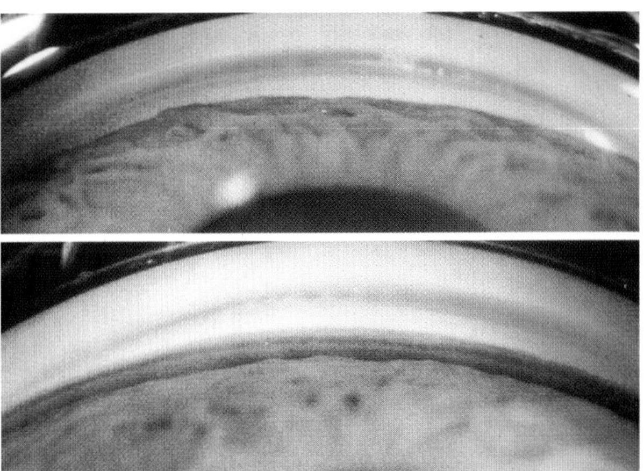

Figure 10.6 Indentation gonioscopy in relative pupillary block
In pupillary block, the peripheral iris is held in its anterior position because of the force of the aqueous behind it (top) (see also Fig. 10.1). During indentation, the peripheral iris can move posteriorly because of the minimal resistance of the aqueous behind the iris plane to the force of indentation (bottom). This is very different from other forms of angle closure, such as plateau iris syndrome.

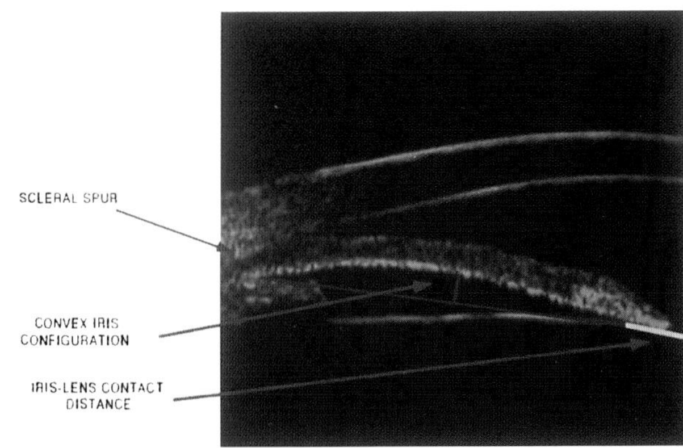

Figure 10.7 Iris–lens contact in pupillary block, UBM
The anatomy of relative pupillary block in a phakic, unoperated patient is illustrated in this ultrasound biomicrograph. Scleral spur is clearly visible, and the trabecular meshwork just anterior to it is in contact with the iris. Note the relatively short region of iris–lens contact. Although there is resistance to flow through the pupillary space, the increased pressure within the posterior chamber compared to the anterior chamber has lifted the remaining iris off the lens surface.

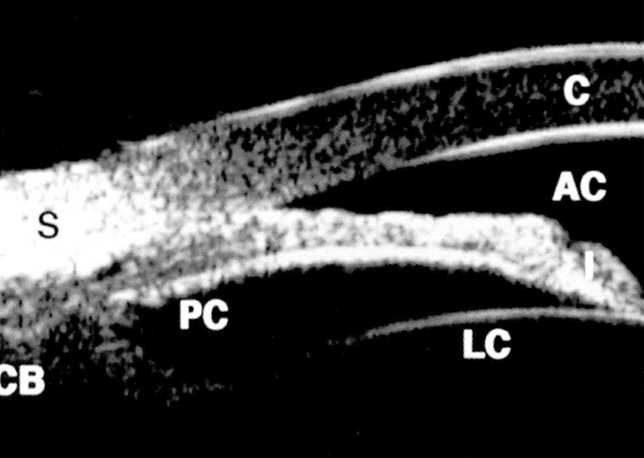

Figure 10.8 Synechiae formation, UBM
Iris apposition to the trabecular meshwork is an indication for laser iridotomy. In this patient, the iris is in contact with the trabecular meshwork. A small, clear, fluid-filled space is present immediately posterior to the region of iridotrabecular contact, indicating that the first location for appositional closure in this eye was in the mid or upper trabecular meshwork.

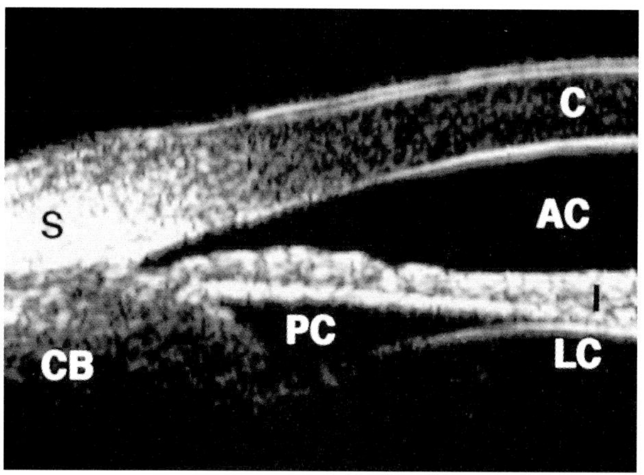

Figure 10.9 **Laser iridotomy, UBM**
Laser iridotomy is the definitive treatment for pupillary block, and allows aqueous pressures in the anterior and posterior chambers to equalize and the iris to assume a planar configuration. Following laser iridotomy in the patient shown in Fig. 10.8, the iris has flattened and the angle has opened. There are no peripheral anterior synechiae present.

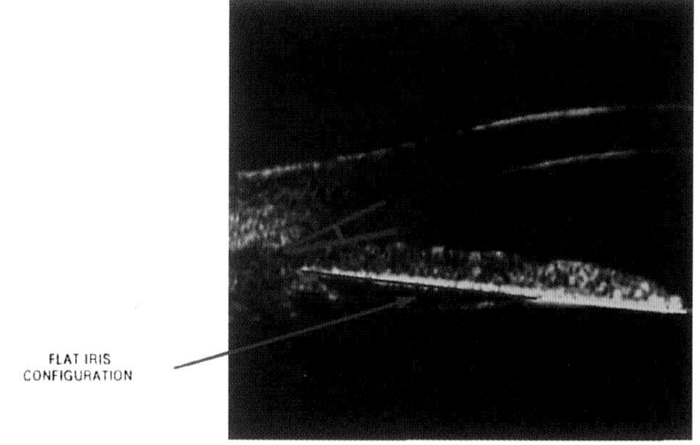

Figure 10.10 **Anatomy following laser iridotomy, UBM**
Following iridotomy, the angle in the patient shown in Fig. 10.7 has opened. Note the increase in iris–lens contact, as aqueous now bypasses the pupillary space and flows through the iridotomy.

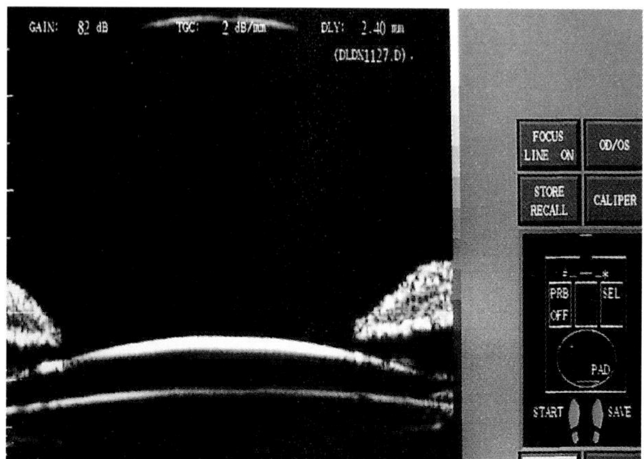

Figure 10.11 **Pseudophakic pupillary block, UBM**
An alteration in the relationship between the anterior surface of the posterior chamber intraocular lens and iris occurs following laser iridotomy for pseudophakic pupillary block. In pseudophakic pupillary block, aqueous flows between the posterior chamber intraocular lens and the iris into the anterior chamber and may lift the iris off the surface of the lens.

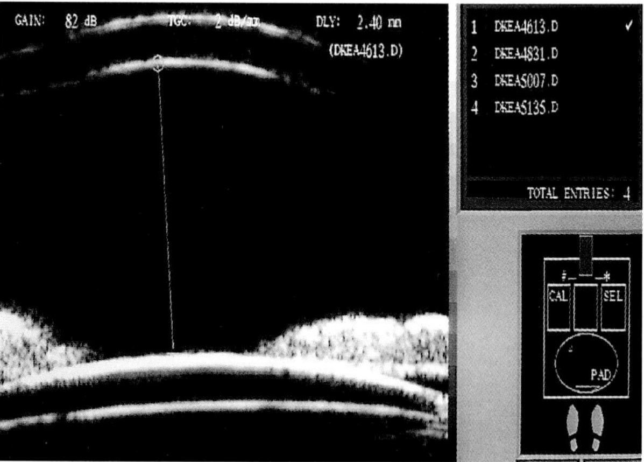

Figure 10.12 **Laser iridotomy for pseudophakic pupillary block, UBM**
Following laser iridotomy in the eyes shown in Fig. 10.11, the iris moves posteriorly against the intraocular lens as aqueous bypasses the pupil, flows through the iridotomy and allows the iris to flatten.

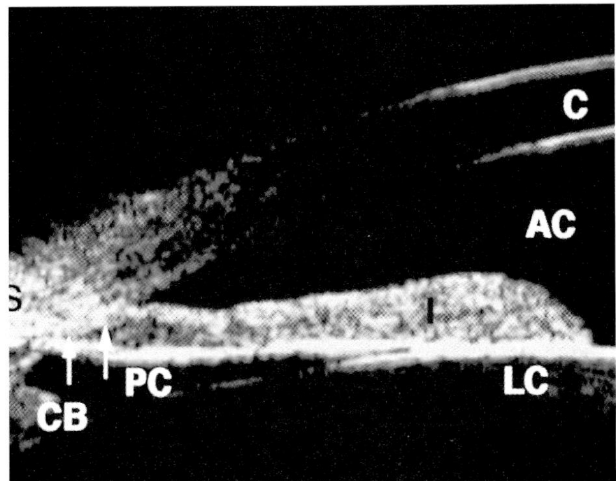

Figure 10.13 Chronic angle closure with synechiae, UBM
Following laser iridotomy for pupillary block angle-closure glaucoma in this patient, the iris has assumed a flat configuration, consistent with relief of pupillary block, but iridotrabecular apposition persists (arrows), indicating the presence of synechial closure.

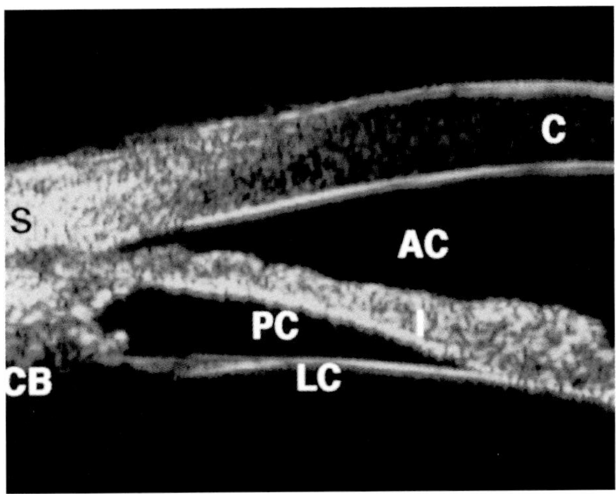

Figure 10.14 Dark-room provocation, UBM
When assessing a patient with a narrow angle for occludability, it is important to perform gonioscopy in a completely darkened room, using the smallest square of light for a slit beam, so as to avoid stimulating the pupillary light reflex. Miotics can also cause iris convexity by increasing resistance to aqueous flow through the pupillary space. This eye is being scanned under normal room illumination. The angle is open.

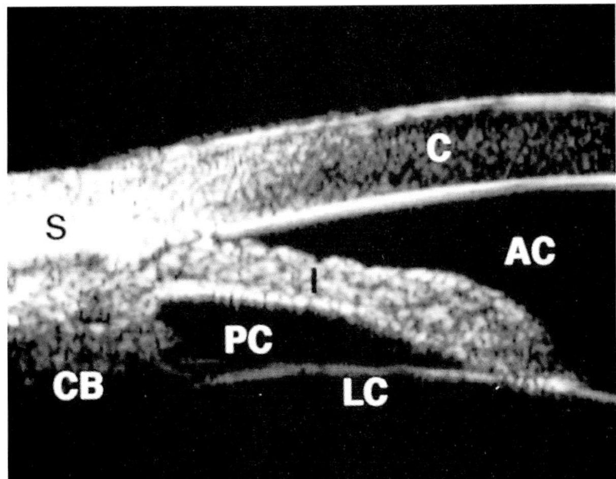

Figure 10.15 Dark-room provocation, UBM
Under dim illumination, the pupil dilates and the peripheral iris moves into the angle causing appositional angle closure. At least two minutes in total darkness should be allowed for the angle to close before assuming that it is not spontaneously occludable. If the angle closes under these conditions, opening the door of the examination room, turning on the light or increasing the size of the slit beam will allow the pupil to constrict once again, so that the angle configuration in any quadrant can be compared in a light–dark–light situation.

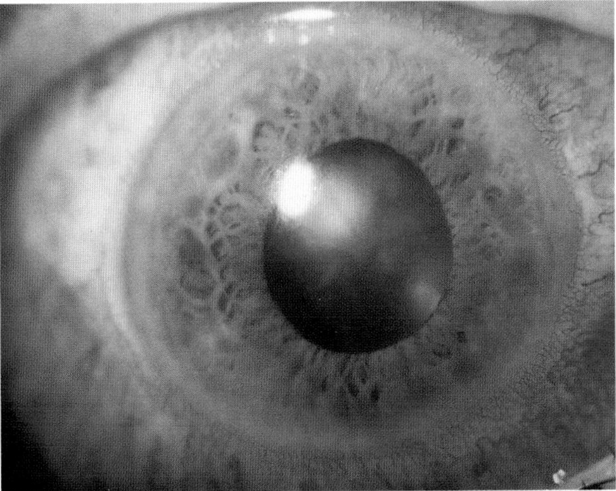

Figure 10.16 Acute angle-closure glaucoma, clinical photograph
Acute angle-closure glaucoma is often characterized by ocular injection, blurred vision and pain. The pupil is often fixed in a mid-dilated position.

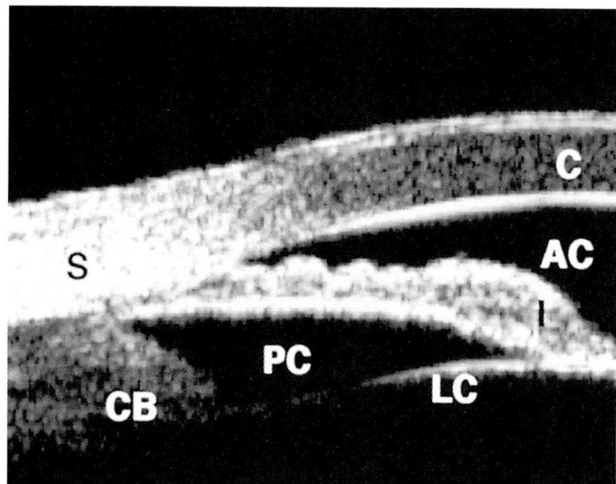

Figure 10.17 Acute angle-closure glaucoma, UBM
During an attack of acute angle closure, the length of iridolenticular contact is typically small, although the resistance to aqueous flow through the pupil is maximal.

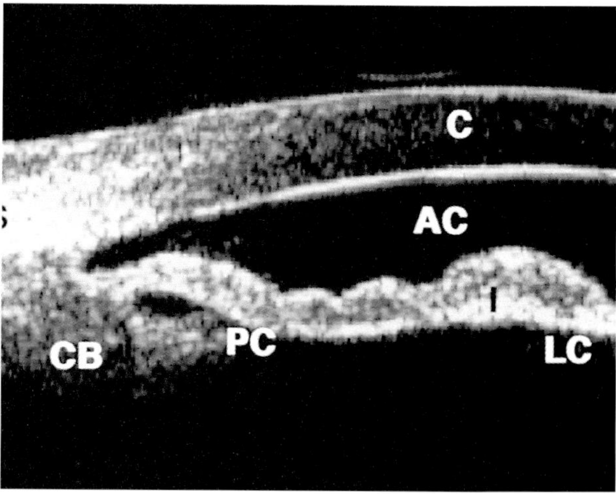

Figure 10.18 Peripheral anterior synechiae, UBM
Following laser iridotomy, the angle opens if peripheral anterior synechiae are not present. Following laser iridotomy in the patient described in Fig. 10.17, the iris remains in contact with the lens surface and assumes its curvilinear contour. The peripheral iris has flattened following the iridotomy.

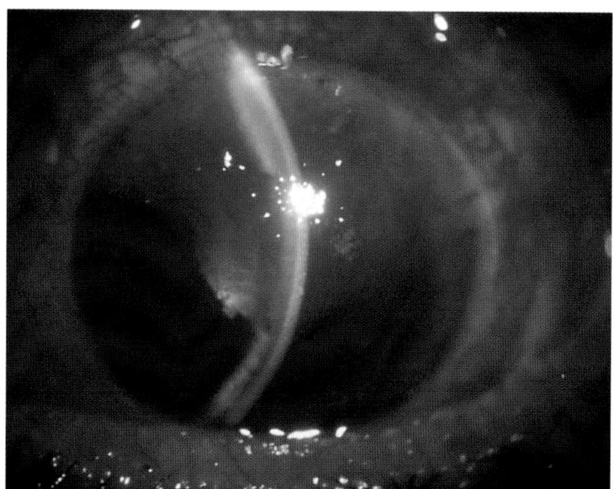

Figure 10.19 Acute pseudophakic pupillary block, clinical photograph
Prior to treatment in this patient with acute pseudophakic pupillary block, the anterior chamber is shallow and the cornea is edematous. The intraocular pressure is 65 mmHg.

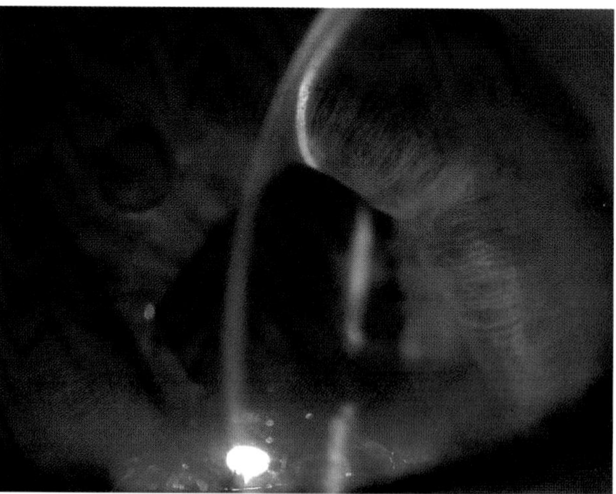

Figure 10.20 Acute pseudophakic pupillary block, clinical photograph
In this patient with an anterior chamber intraocular lens and pupillary block, the iris surrounding the intraocular lens has assumed a bombè configuration, while the portion of iris immediately posterior to the IOL remains held in its flat position by the implant itself.

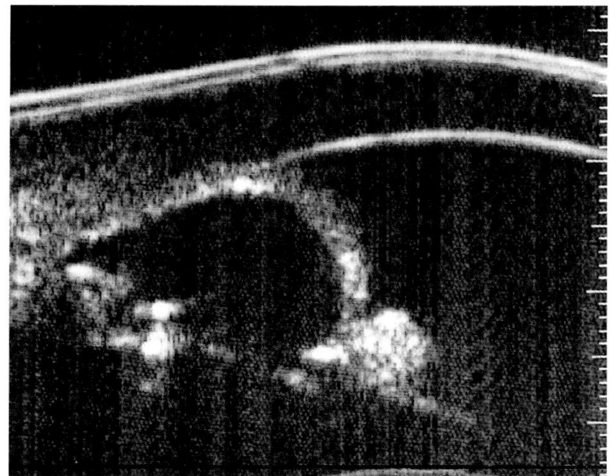

Figure 10.21 Pupillary block with anterior chamber pseudophakia, UBM
In this patient with acute pseudophakic pupillary block angle-closure glaucoma, iris bombè is present (small arrow) and the optic is in relatively normal position (large arrow). The end of the haptic is visible (arrowhead).

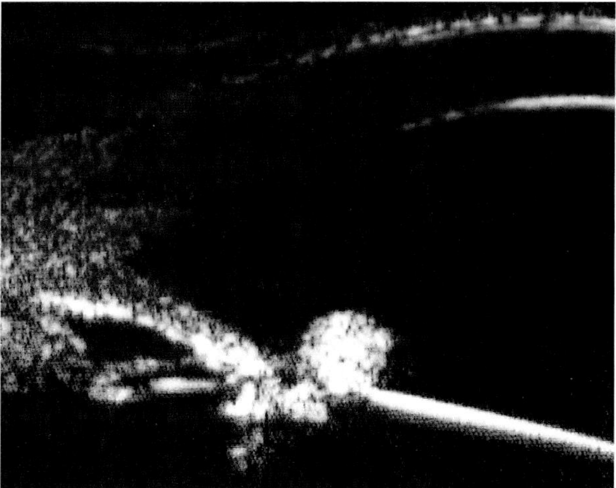

Figure 10.22 Acute angle-closure glaucoma, UBM
Following laser iridotomy, the iris configuration has returned to normal (small arrow) and the positions of the optic (large arrow) and haptic (arrowhead) are unchanged. The iridotomy (curved arrow) is partially visible. It was placed centrally because the peripheral iris was against the cornea when pupillary block was present.

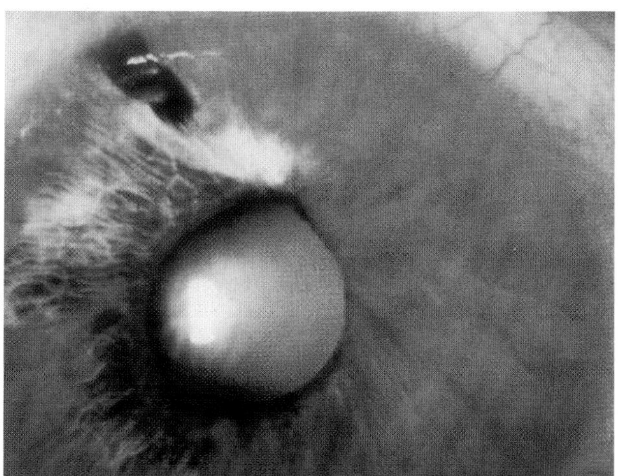

Figure 10.23 Sectoral iris atrophy, clinical photograph
Following the resolution of an attack of acute angle-closure glaucoma, sectoral iris atrophy may occur from pressure-induced iris ischemia.

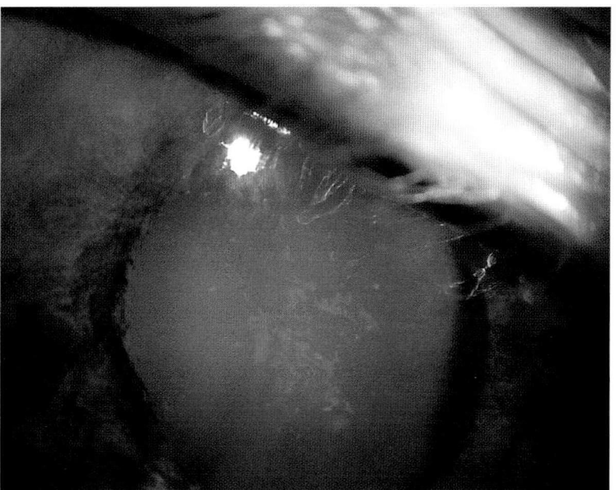

Figure 10.24 Glaukomflecken, clinical photograph
Subepithelial lens opacification may occur following acute angle-closure glaucoma and is termed glaukomflecken.

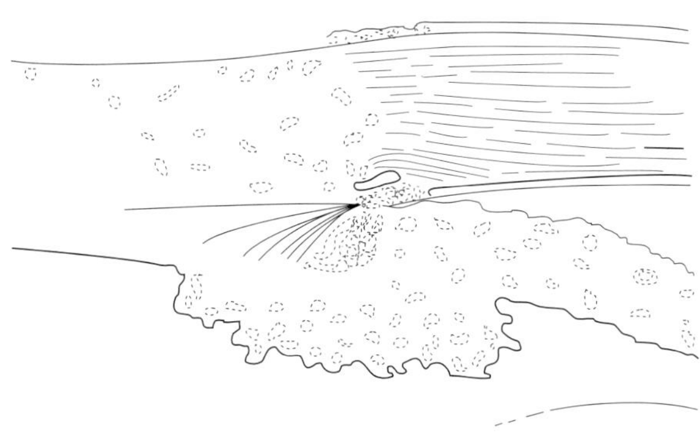

Figure 10.25 Plateau iris syndrome
A large or anteriorly positioned ciliary body can maintain the iris root in proximity to the trabecular meshwork, creating a configuration known as plateau iris.

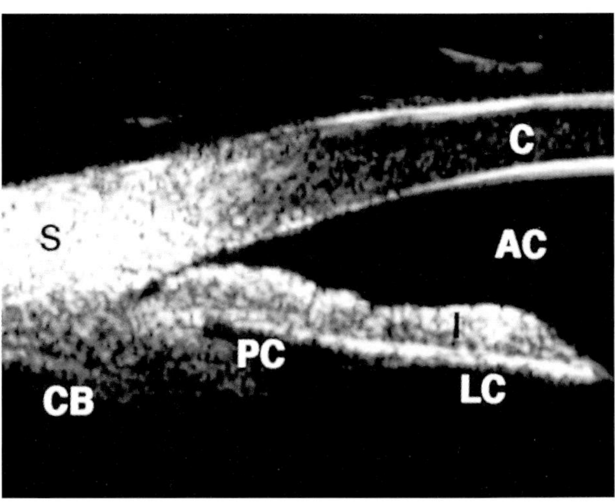

Figure 10.26 Plateau iris syndrome, UBM
In plateau iris syndrome, the physical presence of an anteriorly placed ciliary body (CB) forces the peripheral iris (I) into the angle. In this patient, iridotomy has relieved the contribution of pupillary block to the angle narrowing (the iris contour is planar in this patient), but not the closure related to the abnormal ciliary body position. The angle in this patient is barely open.

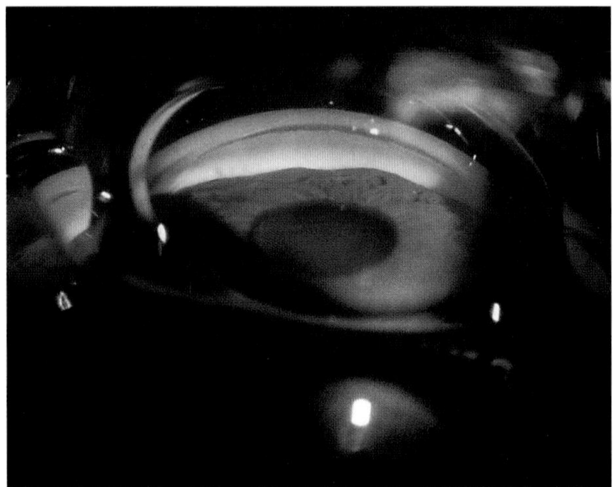

Figure 10.27 Gonioscopy in plateau iris
Gonioscopic appearance of the angle in plateau iris syndrome prior to indentation.

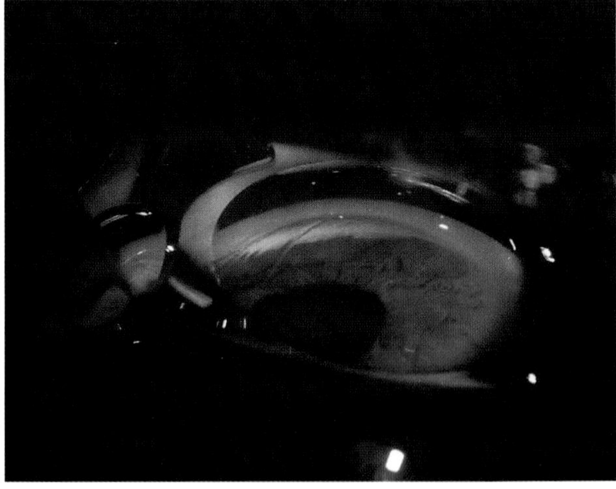

Figure 10.28 Indentation gonioscopy in plateau iris
The physical presence of the lens behind the iris plane holds the iris in position and tries to prevent posterior movement of the peripheral iris. As a result, a sinuous configuration results (sigma sign), in which the iris follows the curvature of the lens, reaches its deepest point at the lens equator, then rises again over the ciliary processes before dropping peripherally. Much more force is needed during gonioscopy to open the angle than in pupillary block because the ciliary processes must be displaced, and the angle does not open as widely.

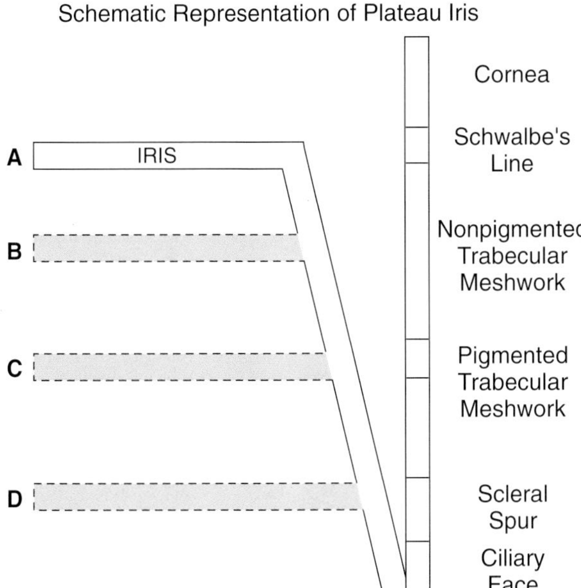

Figure 10.29 Degrees of plateau iris configuration
The extent, or the 'height' to which the plateau rises determines whether or not the angle will close completely or only partially. In the complete plateau iris syndrome, the angle closes to the upper meshwork or Schwalbe's line, blocking aqueous outflow and leading to a rise in IOP. This situation is far less common than the incomplete syndrome, in which the angle closes only partially, leaving the upper portion of the filtering meshwork open, so that IOP will not rise.

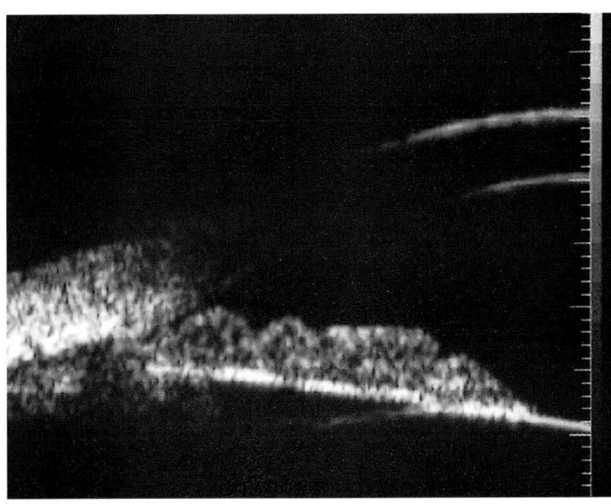

Figure 10.30 Angle closure in plateau iris, UBM
The angle is closed in this patient with plateau iris syndrome. The iris configuration is planar.

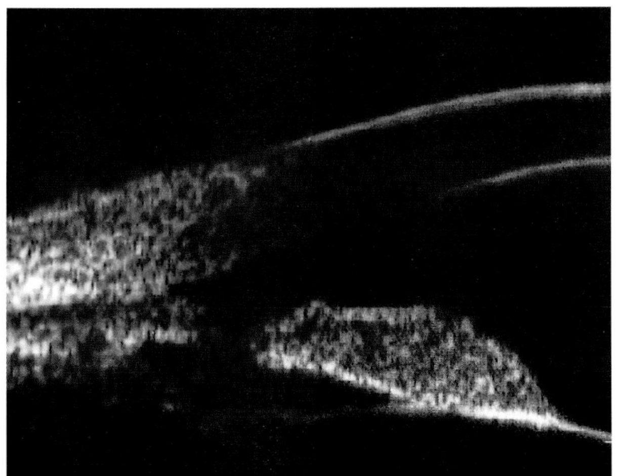

Figure 10.31 Laser iridotomy in plateau iris, UBM
patent laser iridotomy in the eye shown in the Fig. 10.30 with plateau iris syndrome and persistent appositional angle closure.

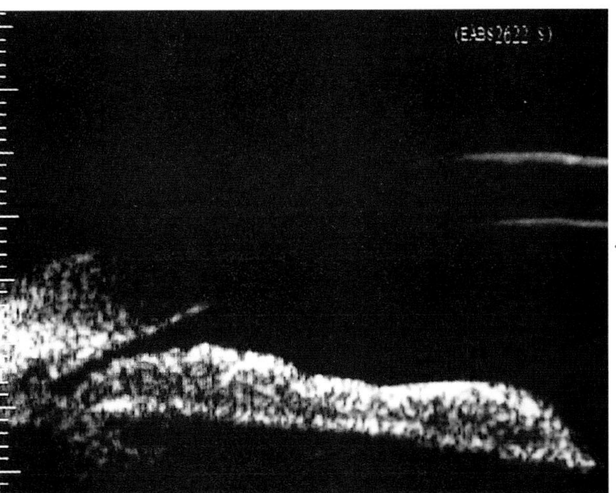

Figure 10.32 Dark-room provocation in plateau iris, UBM
Provocative testing in eyes with plateau iris configuration should be performed following laser iridotomy. Under normal room illumination, the angle in this patient with plateau configuration is narrow, but open.

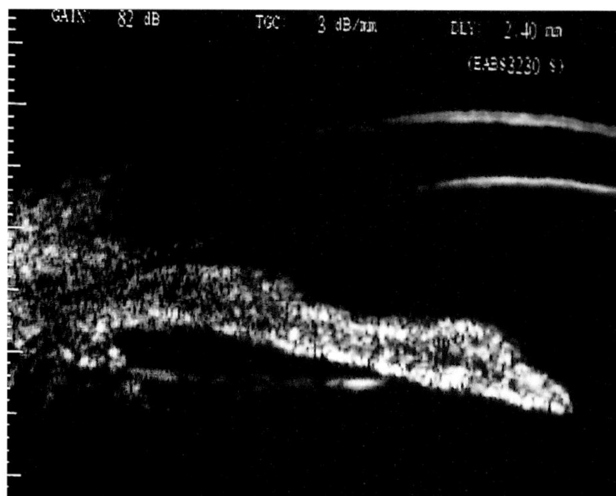

Figure 10.33 Dark-room provocation in plateau iris, UBM

During dark-room provocation and ultrasound scanning, the peripheral iris dilates and appositional angle closure develops.

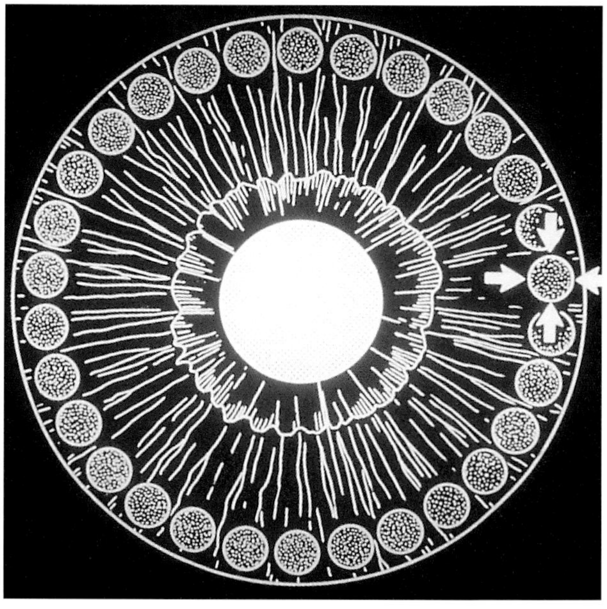

Figure 10.34 Location of laser iridoplasty

The treatment of angle closure secondary to plateau iris syndrome requires argon laser peripheral iridoplasty. Laser energy (long duration, low power, large spot size) is applied to the extreme iris periphery.

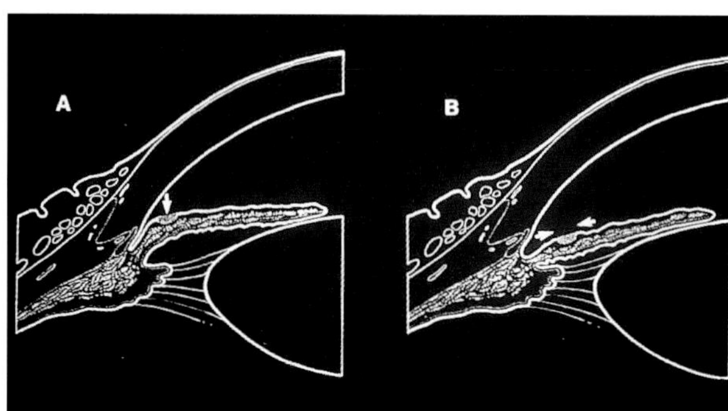

Figure 10.35 Effects of peripheral iridoplasty on the iris

Iridoplasty compacts the iris stroma and pulls it towards the site of the laser application. When the iris which is opposed to the meshwork (A) moves towards the burn, the angle opens (B).

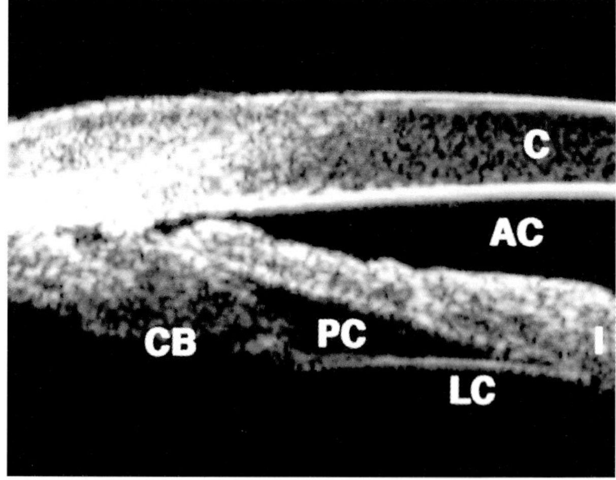

Figure 10.36 Peripheral iridoplasty (pretreatment), UBM

Angle closure caused by plateau iris syndrome prior to laser iridoplasty.

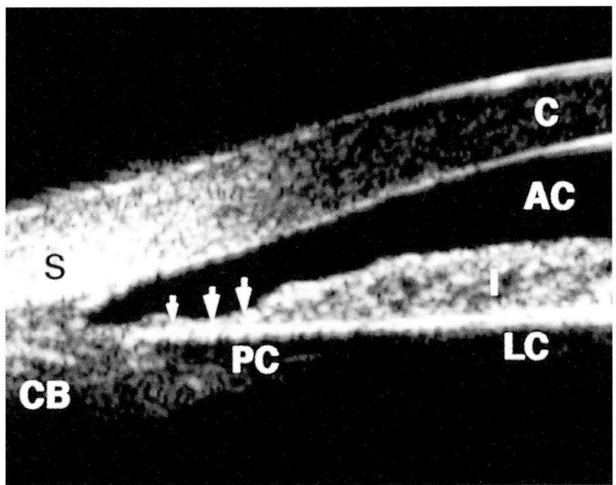

Figure 10.37 Laser iridoplasty (post-treatment), UBM Following argon laser peripheral iridoplasty, the site of the burn is visible (arrows). The iris stoma has been compacted and the angle is open.

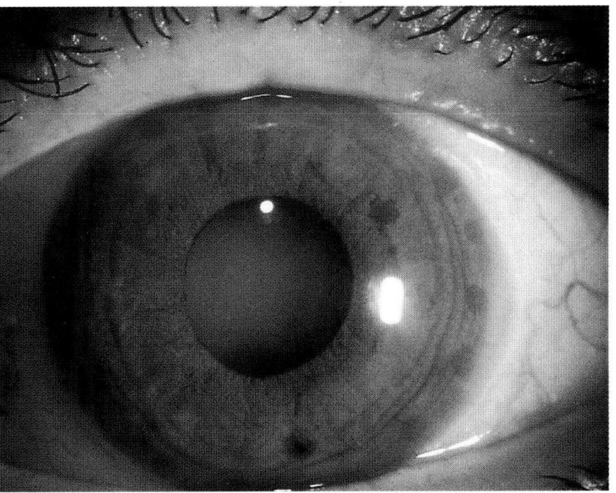

Figure 10.38 Laser iridoplasty, clinical photograph The key to iridoplasty, which can also be used during an acute attack of angle-closure glaucoma unresponsive to medical therapy or when iridotomy cannot be safely performed because of hazy media, is correct placement of the laser applications which, in this patient, has produced a ring of hyperpigmented spots corresponding to the treatment sites. This patient has an inferiorly placed laser iridotomy.

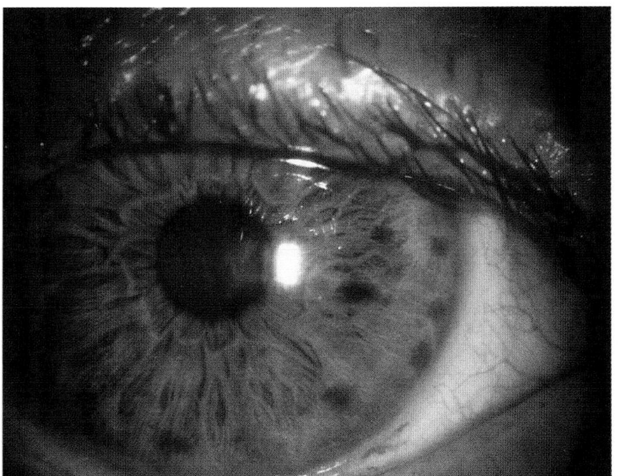

Figure 10.39 Laser iridoplasty, clinical photograph Iridoplasty in this patient was performed incorrectly, and laser application sites are visible in the midperipheral iris.

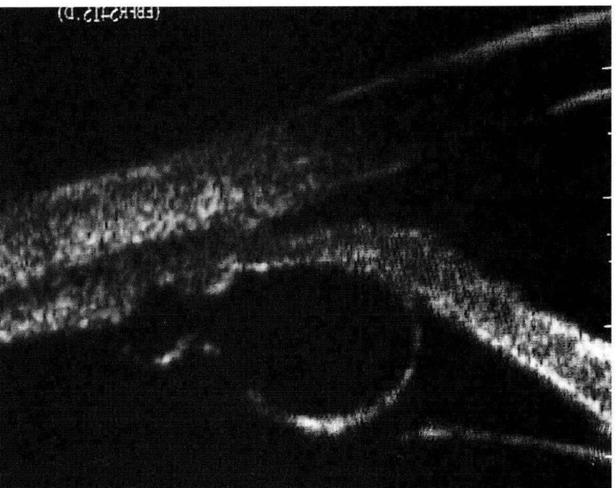

Figure 10.40 Pseudoplateau iris configuration, UBM Other abnormalities of ciliary body architecture may result in a condition termed pseudoplateau iris. This general term is nonspecific and does not differentiate between distinct entities as cyst, tumor or inflammation. These conditions are usually easily diagnosed, as the angle is closed either in one quadrant or, if cysts are multiple, intermittently. Focal forms of angle closure may be induced by cystic or solid masses involving the iris or the ciliary body. Iridociliary cysts are characterized by an echolucent interior. For example, a pigment epithelial cyst in this patient has caused focal narrowing of the anterior chamber angle in the region of the cyst.

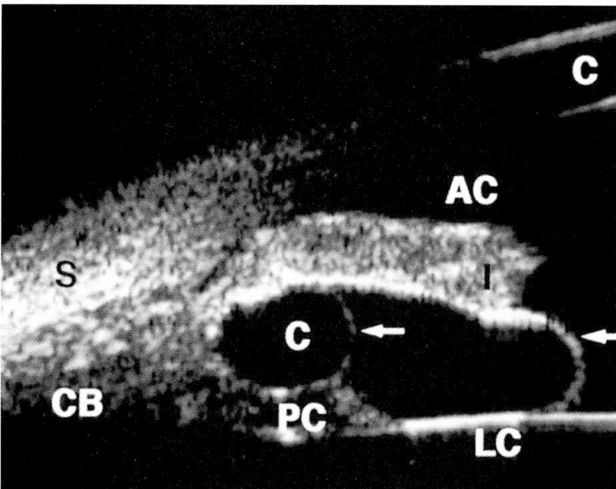

Figure 10.41 Loculated iridociliary cysts, UBM
Pigment epithelial cysts can arise from the pigment epithelium of the iris, the ciliary body or the junction between them. Iridociliary cysts are the most common form, and some have multiple loculations. The walls of these cysts are indicated (arrows).

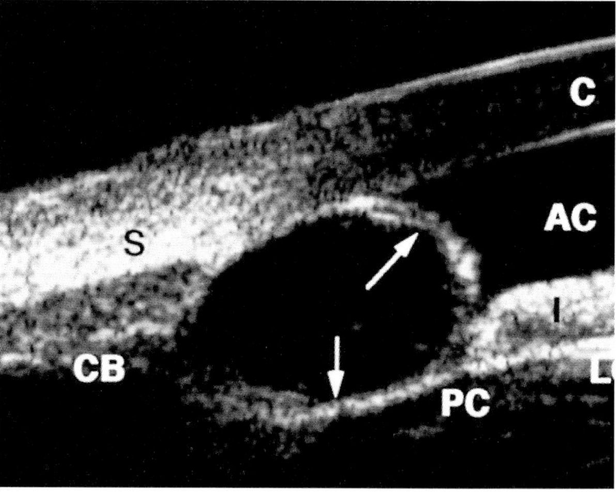

Figure 10.42 Ciliary body cyst, UBM
Abnormal embryogenesis can lead to focal angle closure by true cysts of the ciliary body stroma, as is present in this patient. The pigment epithelium is normal and the ciliary body architecture is distorted.

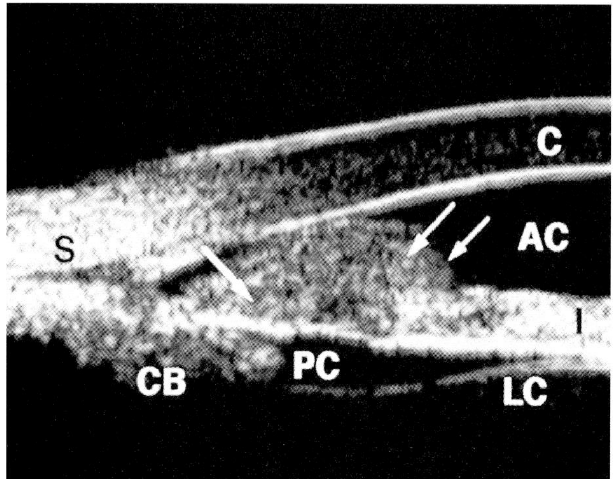

Figure 10.43 Anterior segment tumors, UBM
Primary or metastatic tumors of the iris and/or ciliary body can cause angle closure. This iris tumor is causing mechanical obstruction of the meshwork.

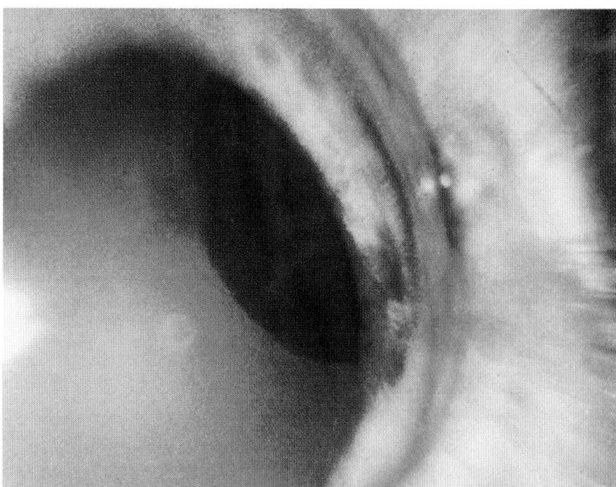

Figure 10.44 Ciliary body tumor, clinical photograph
Ciliary body enlargement can occur due to anterior segment inflammation as shown here.

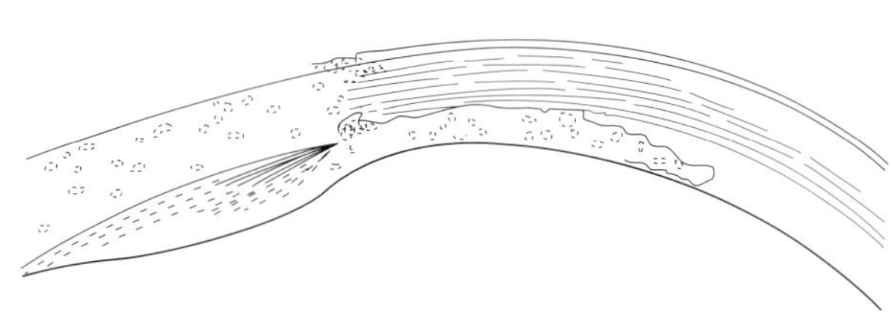

Figure 10.45 Lens-induced angle closure
Angle-closure glaucoma may be caused by an anteriorly subluxed, dislocated, intumescent lens. In this schematic, the physical presence of anteriorly positioned, enlarged lens is causing shallowing of the anterior chamber and angle closure.

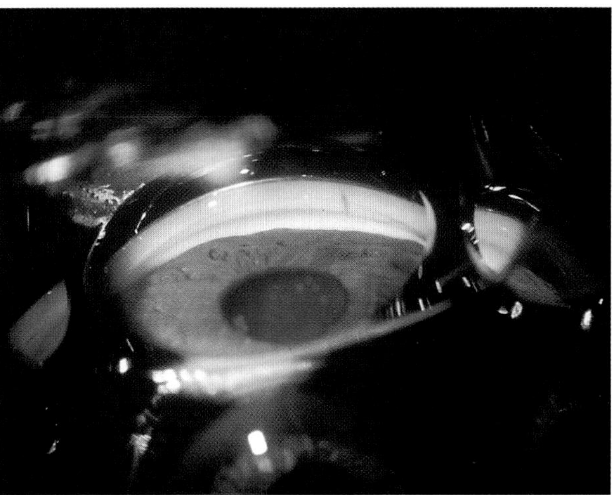

Figure 10.46 Gonioscopy in lens-induced angle closure
Prior to indentation in a patient with lens-induced angle closure, the angle is closed.

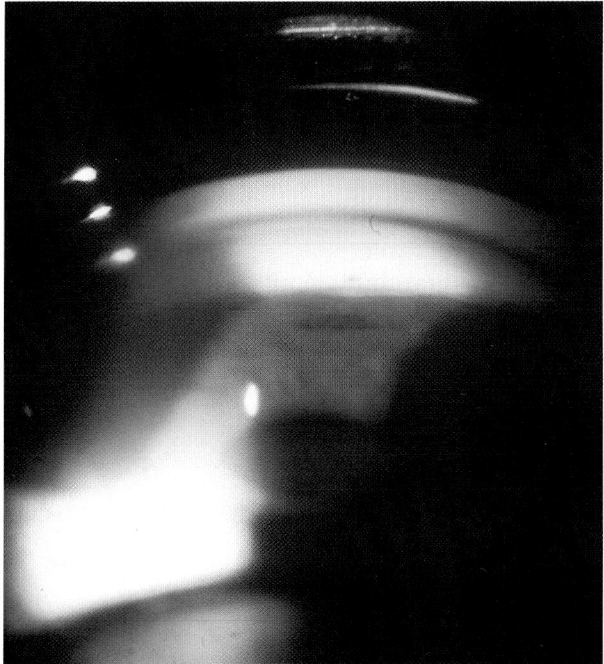

Figure 10.47 Indentation gonioscopy
Because of the enlarged lens, indentation permits only slight opening of the angle.

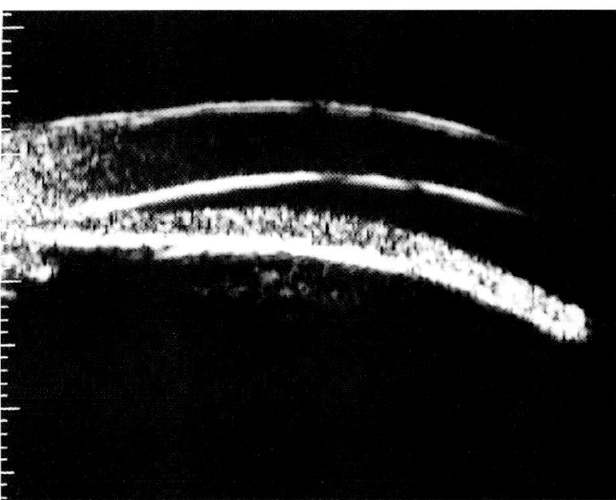

Figure 10.48 Laser iridotomy in lens-induced angle closure, UBM
Ultrasound biomicroscopy following laser iridotomy shows the iris to be in contact with the anterior lens surface, mechanically obstructing the angle.

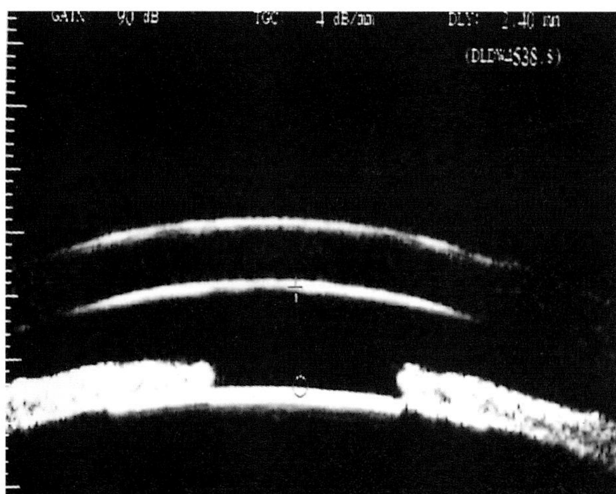

Figure 10.49 Central anterior chamber depth in lens-induced angle closure, UBM
The central anterior chamber is considerably shallower in eyes with lens-induced angel closure than in eyes with angle closure caused by pupillary block or plateau iris syndrome.

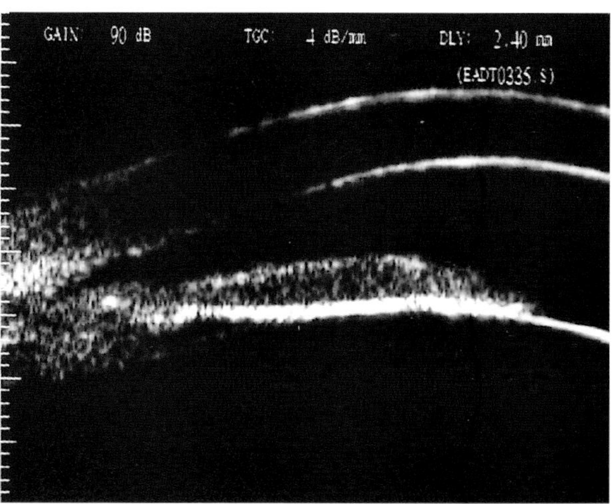

Figure 10.50 Peripheral iridoplasty in lens-induced angle closure, UBM
Following peripheral iridoplasty in the patient shown in Fig. 10.48, the angle widened.

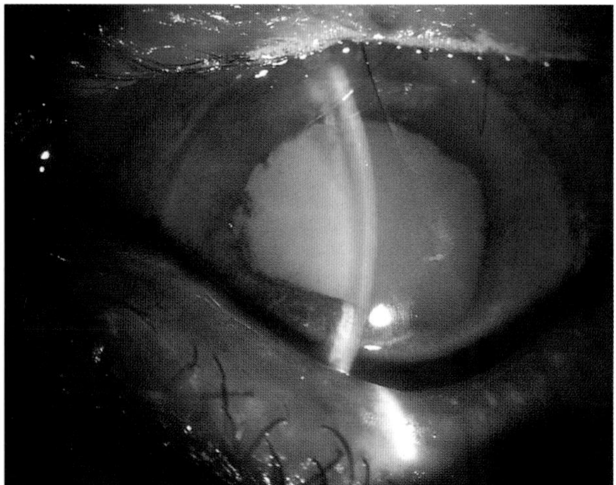

Figure 10.51 Lens intumescence, clinical photograph
Occasionally, the lens may become intumescent and cause crowding of the anterior segment.

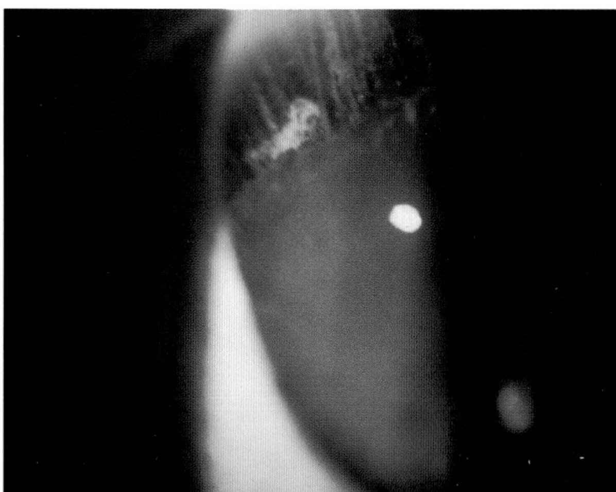

Figure 10.52 Lens subluxation, clinical photograph
Alterations in lens position can result in angle-closure glaucoma in a number of ways. Perhaps the most common and underdiagnosed cause of lens subluxation is exfoliation syndrome. In this disorder, zonular laxity permits the lens to move slightly anteriorly, increasing relative pupillary block and leading to angle closure. Eventually zonular dehiscence from the ciliary body may occur, and lead to lens dislocation. In this figure, dehisced zonules can be seen resting on the equatorial lens capsule.

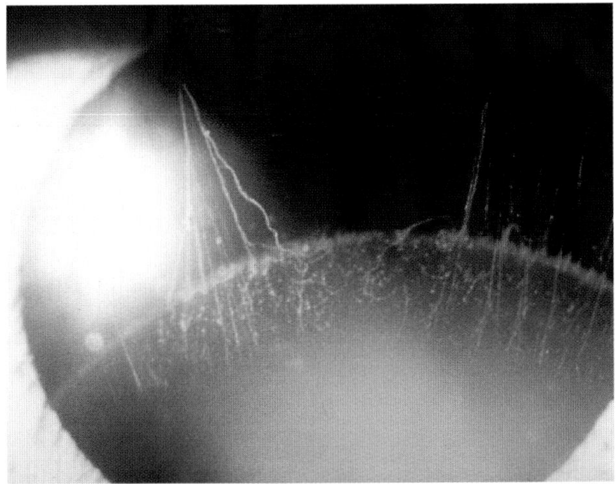

Figure 10.53 Lens dislocation in exfoliation syndrome, clinical photograph
In this patient with exfoliation syndrome, nearly complete superior zonular dehiscence has allowed the lens to move inferiorly.

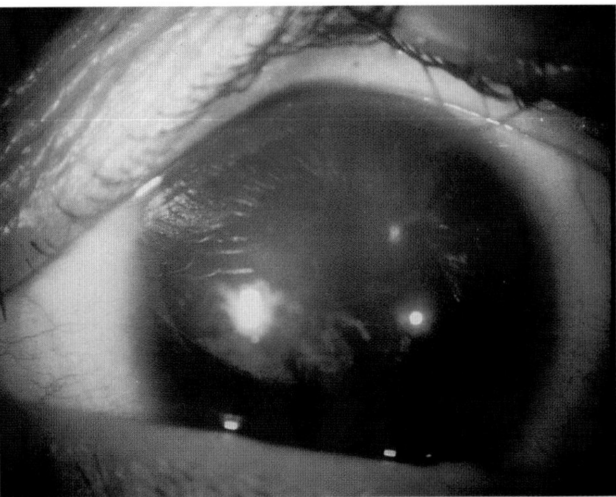

Figure 10.54 Marfan's syndrome, clinical photograph
Lens subluxation and dislocation are a common feature of Marfan's syndrome. The most common direction for lens movement is superotemporal. In homocystinuria, the subluxed lens tends to move inferonasally.

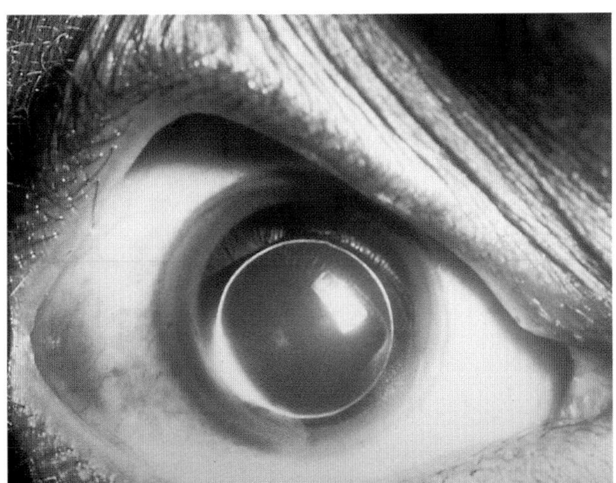

Figure 10.55 Microspherophakia, clinical photograph
In microspherophakia, the smaller lens can dislocate into the anterior chamber, where it can become entrapped.

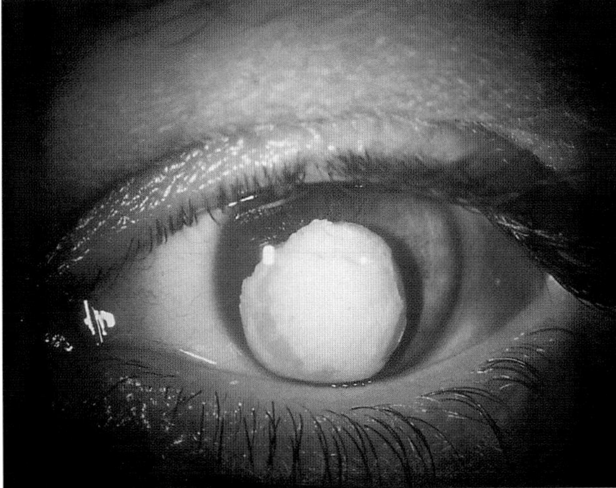

Figure 10.56 Traumatic lens dislocation
The lens in the anterior chamber can cause pupillary block and acute angle closure. Long-standing anterior dislocation can lead to progressive cataract formation.

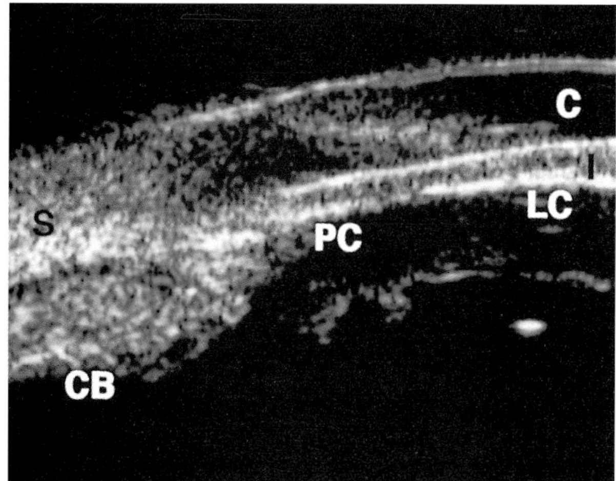

Figure 10.57 Malignant glaucoma, UBM
Malignant glaucoma (ciliary block glaucoma; aqueous misdirection) is a poorly understood clinical entity characterized by angle closure, normal posterior segment anatomy and failure of the angle to open following iridotomy. Most, but not all, cases occur postoperatively. In malignant glaucoma, the lens and iris are forced anteriorly by posterior pressure. In this eye, the anterior lens capsule (LC) is nearly against the corneal endothelium (C).

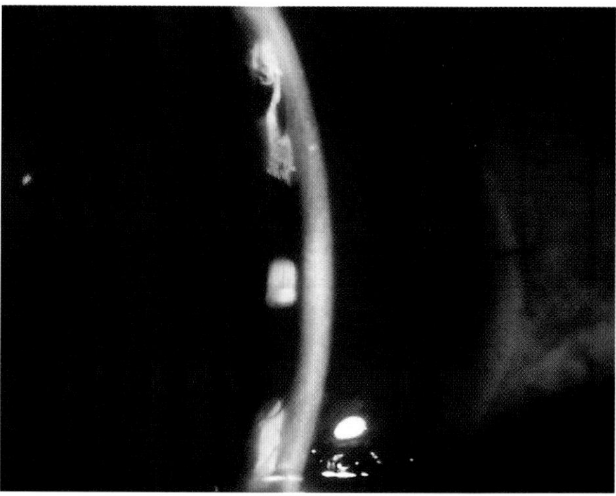

Figure 10.58 Pseudophakic malignant glaucoma, clinical photograph
Following uneventful cataract surgery in this patient with undiagnosed angle-closure glaucoma, the anterior chamber shallowed and the pressure rose. Multiple iridotomies failed to restore normal anatomic relationships.

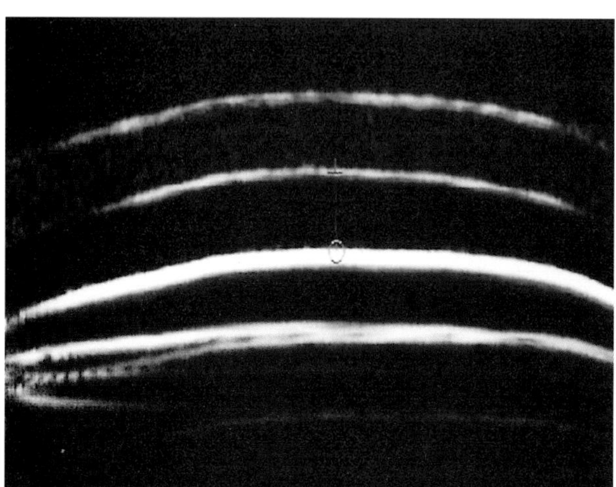

Figure 10.59 Pseudophakic malignant glaucoma, UBM
Ultrasound biomicroscopy prior to treatment. (The central anterior chamber is shallow.)

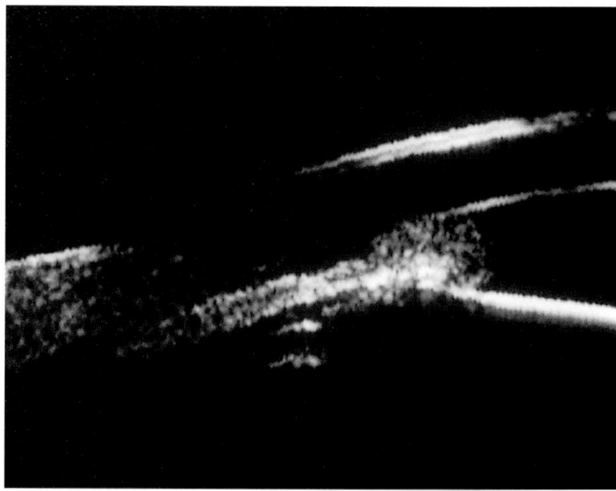

Figure 10.60 Pseudophakic malignant glaucoma, UBM
In the temporal angle, peripheral iridocorneal apposition is present (small arrows). The haptic is visible beneath the iris (large arrow).

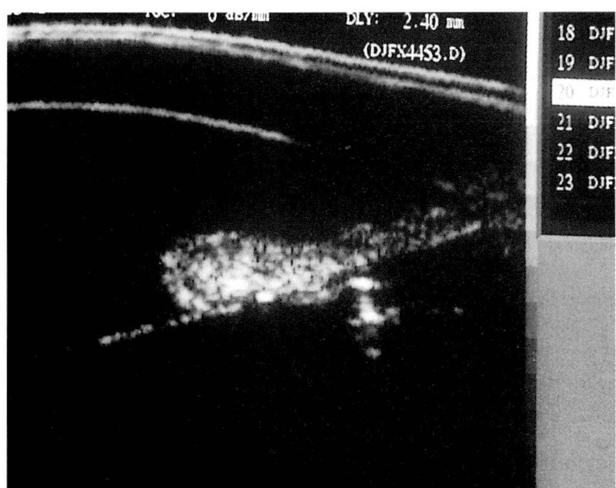

Figure 10.61 Pseudophakic malignant glaucoma, UBM Immediately following Nd:YAG laser capsulotomy/anterior hyaloidectomy, the angle is open (small arrow) and the haptic has moved posteriorly (large arrow).

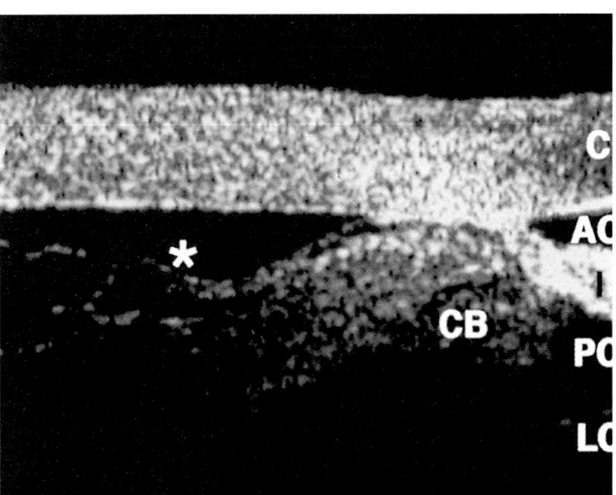

Figure 10.62 Phakic malignant glaucoma, UBM In this phakic patient with a clinical diagnosis of a malignant glaucoma, the angle has closed because of anterior rotation of the ciliary body due to annular ciliary body detachment (asterisk), rather than aqueous misdirection. This distinction is clinically important in as much as the treatment involves vigorous topical and occasional systemic steroids, intensive cycloplegia and possible drainage of the supraciliary fluid. It does not typically respond to Nd:YAG laser surgery.

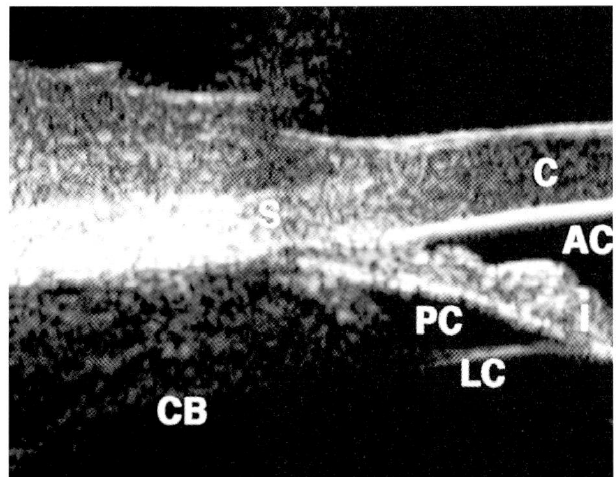

Figure 10.63 Scleritis and angle closure, UBM In a similar fashion, anterior rotation of the ciliary body may occur following panretinal photocoagulation, scleral buckling procedures, central retinal vein occlusion, contraction of retrolental tissue such as in retinopathy of prematurity or inflammation of adjoining tissues, such as this patient with anterior scleritis with secondary ciliary body edema. Note the overlying thickened conjunctiva.

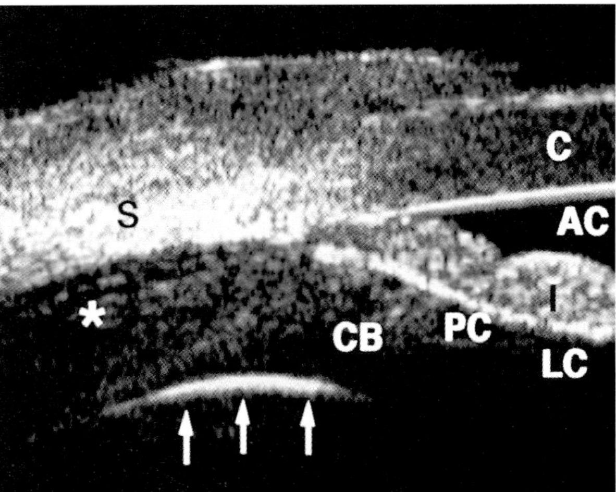

Figure 10.64 Intravitreal gas and angle closure, UBM Intravitreal expansile gas (arrows) may cause progressive angle closure following vitreoretinal surgery. In this particular case, the ciliary body, iris and lens have been forced anteriorly, closing the angle.

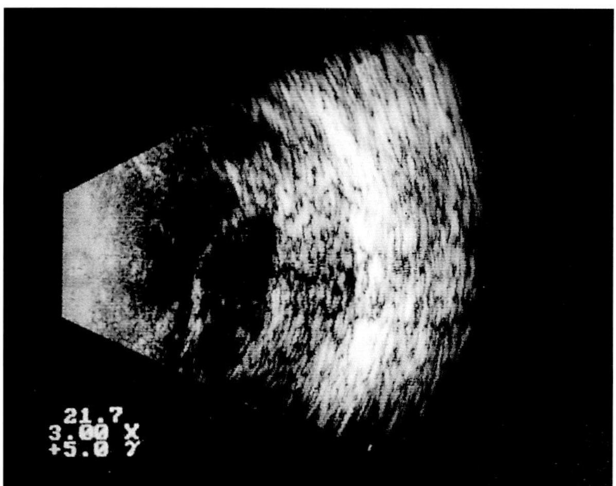

Figure 10.65 Choroidal hemorrhage, B scan ultrasound
Choroidal hemorrhage can result in forward movement of the lens–iris diaphragm and elevated intraocular pressure. Although intraoperative choroidal hemorrhage is relatively rare during glaucoma surgery, delayed choroidal hemorrhage in hypotonus eyes is not. The typical presenting complaint is the abrupt onset of pain, often associated with Valsalva maneuver, in an eye with known hypotony and choroidal effusion.

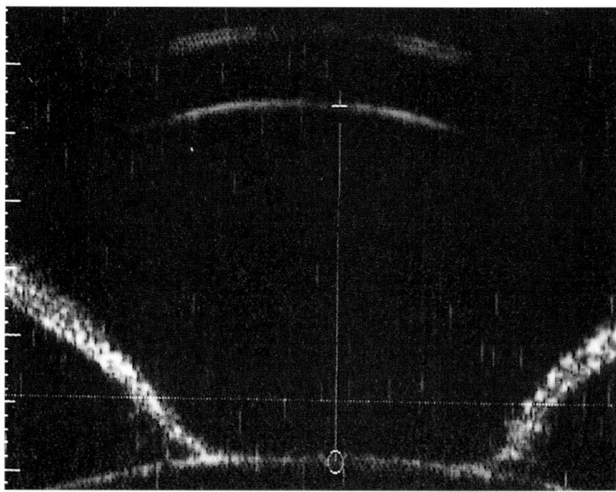

Figure 10.66 Uveitis and glaucoma, UBM
Intraocular inflammation can cause angle closure by a variety of mechanisms. In this patient acute angle closure has developed because of a pupil secluded by posterior synechiae. The iris is adherent at the pupillary border, and has assumed a bombè configuration elsewhere.

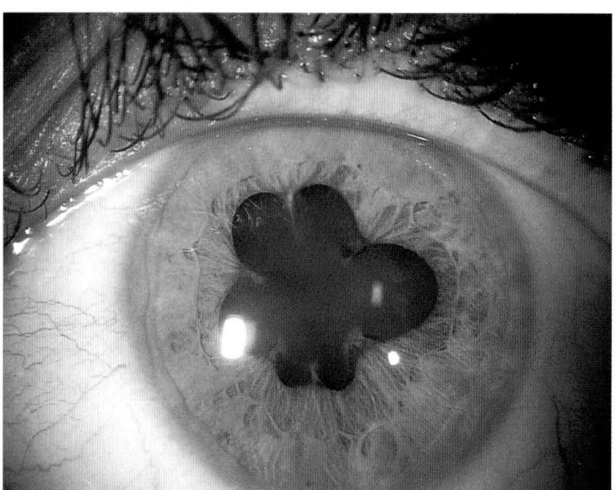

Figure 10.67 Posterior synechiae due to uveitis, clinical photograph
Early posterior synechias formation often presage the development of increased pupillary block. Frequent dilatation may prevent complete pupillary block.

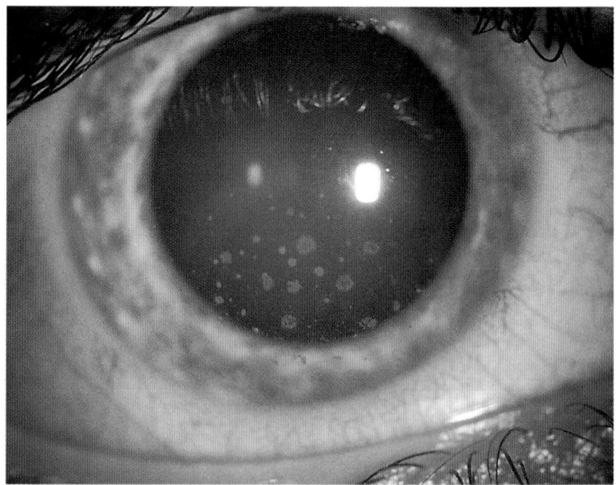

Figure 10.68 Keratic precipitates, clinical photograph
When peripheral anterior synechiae are present without pupillary block, other evidence of prior intraocular inflammation should be sought. In this patient with multiple synechiae but an otherwise wide-open angle, old keratic precipitates provide evidence of prior anterior uveitis.

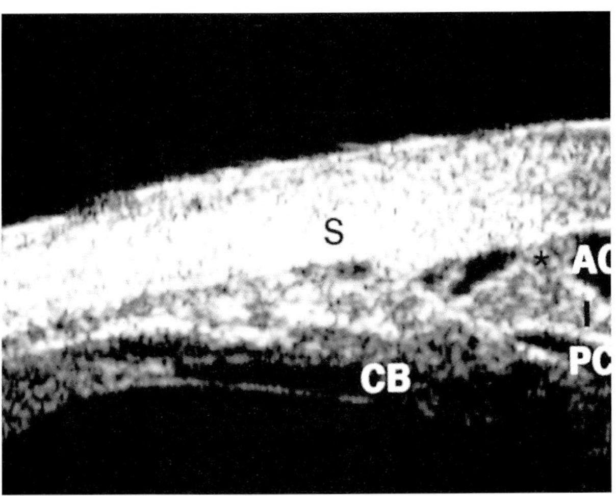

Figure 10.69 Uveitis-related anterior synechiae, UBM
In this patient with sarcoid uveitis, peripheral anterior synechiae have formed in angle.

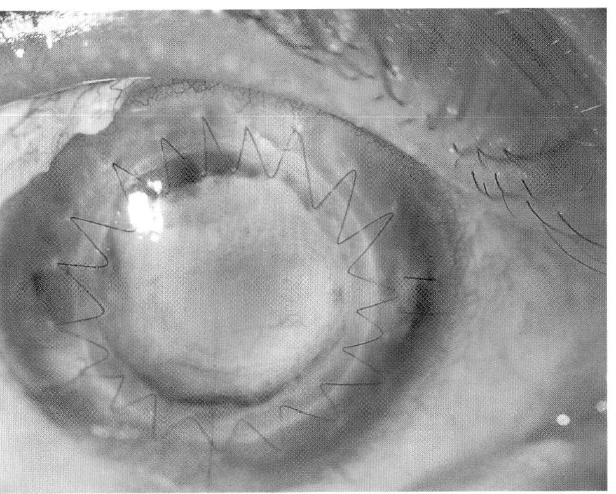

Figure 10.70 Anterior chamber fibrin, clinical photograph
Severe inflammatory reactions, such as this fibrin mass on the anterior surface of a recently implanted intraocular lens, may result in pupillary block.

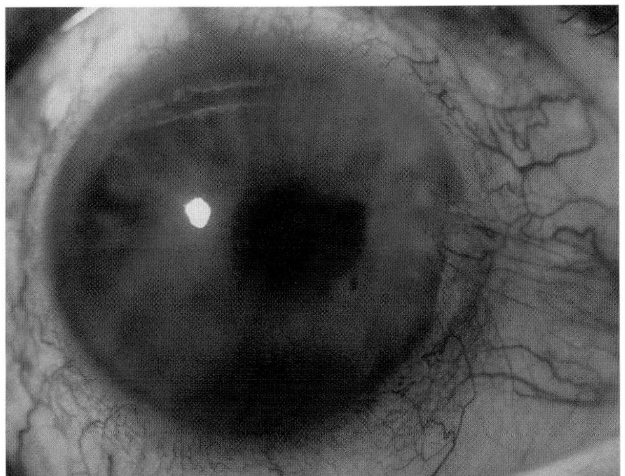

Figure 10.71 Neovascular glaucoma, clinical photograph
Neovascularization of the anterior segment causes glaucoma by direct obstruction of the trabecular meshwork by the proliferating neovascular membrane. Neovascular glaucoma, which may be recalcitrant to therapy, is often associated with high intraocular pressures and spontaneous hyphema.

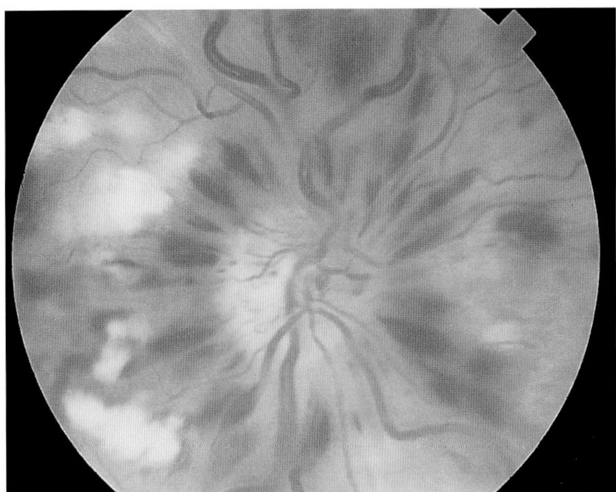

Figure 10.72 Central retinal vein occlusion, fundus photograph
The most common cause of iris neovascularization is retinal ischemia. Ischemic central retinal vein occlusion (shown here) and proliferative diabetic retinopathy are the two most common disorders associated with rubeosis iridis.

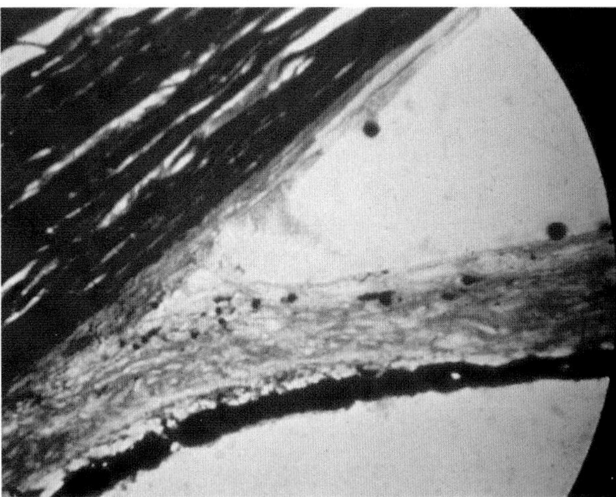

Figure 10.73 Angle neovascularization, histopathology
As the neovascular membrane proliferates, it slowly covers the angle structures.

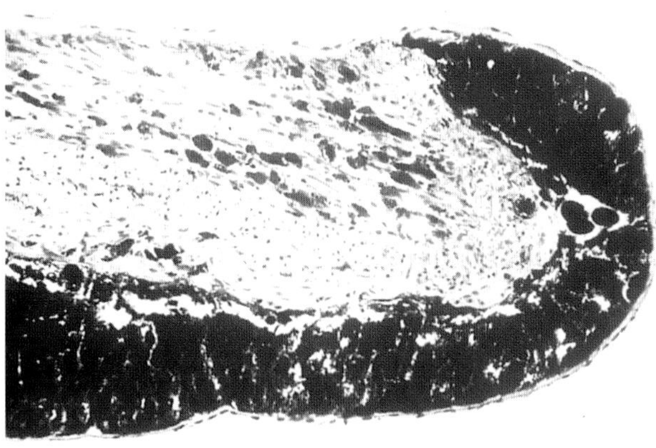

Figure 10.74 Ectropion uveae, histopathology
Contraction of the membrane pulls the iris into the angle, and may cause ectropion uveae, as shown in this figure.

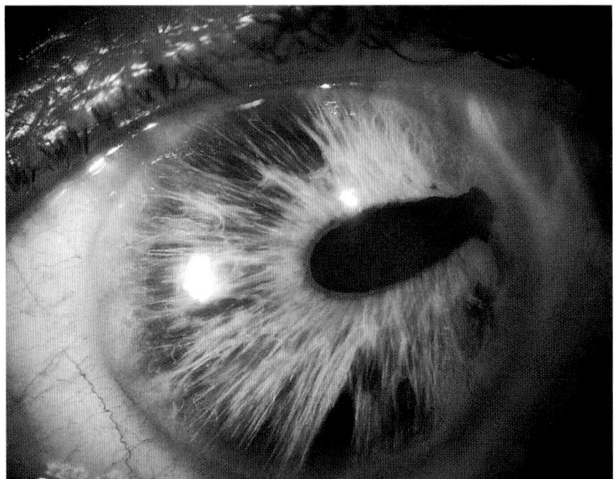

Figure 10.75 Iridocorneal endothelial syndrome, clinical photograph
Iridocorneal endothelial syndrome is also associated with a proliferating anterior segment membrane. In this disorder, migration of corneal endothelial and associated basement membrane cause obstruction of the trabecular meshwork and iris abnormalities. Essential iris atrophy, shown here, is characterized by corectopia, melting holes and stretching holes caused by membrane contraction.

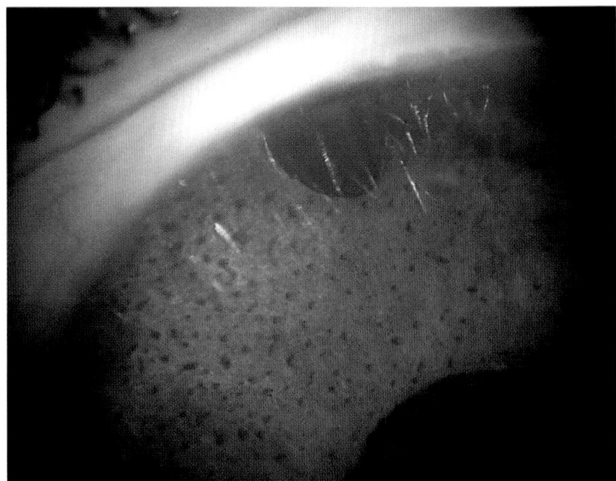

Figure 10.76 Iris–nevus syndrome, clinical photograph
Another variant of iridocorneal endothelial syndrome, the iris–nevus syndrome.

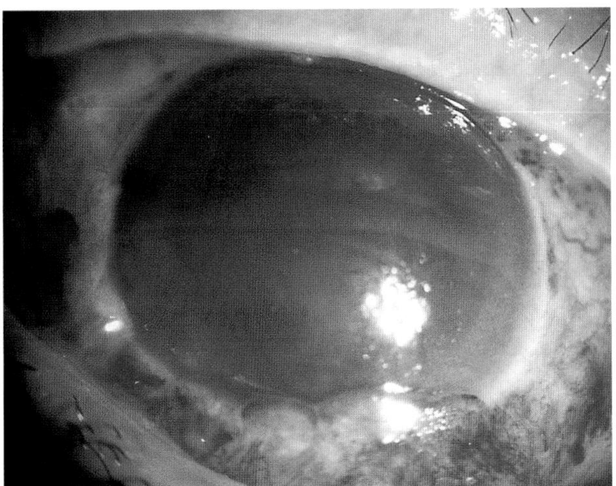

Figure 10.77 Hyphema, clinical photograph
Anterior segment trauma can cause angle closure because of uveitis or lens subluxation. In this patient with hyphema, pupillary block caused by the obstruction to aqueous flow by the anterior segment clotted blood is part of the differential diagnosis of the elevated intraocular pressure.

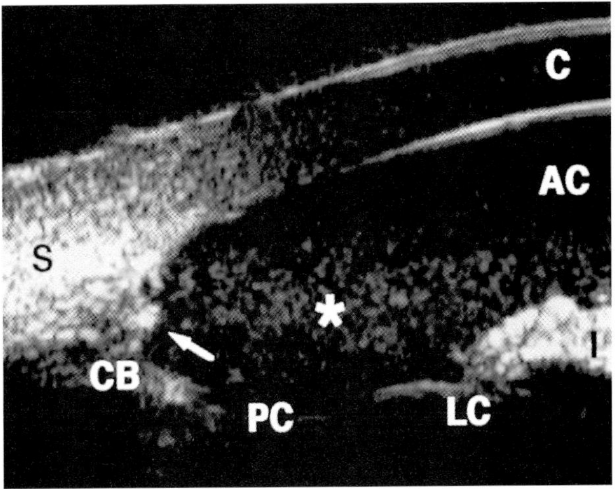

Figure 10.78 Iridodialysis and angle recession, UBM
Blood within the anterior chamber (asterisk) may mask other forms of angle injury, such as iridodialysis and angle recession.

11 Normal-tension glaucoma

Louis B Cantor and Darrell WuDunn

Introduction

Von Graefe first described the condition we now recognize as normal or low-tension glaucoma in the 1850s. Glaucoma as a disease entity associated with elevated intraocular pressure had only been recognized for approximately 40 years; the notion of glaucoma without elevated intraocular pressure was not well received and still remains an enigma to this day. With the development of tonometry in the early 1900s and increased use of ophthalmoscopy to examine the optic disc, normal-tension glaucoma became a more widely recognized and accepted clinical entity. Many names were applied to this condition including pseudoglaucoma, amaurosis with excavation, cavernous optic atrophy, paraglaucoma, arteriosclerotic optic atrophy, low-tension glaucoma, and others. The variety of terms applied to this disease entity or group of entities which we have come to call normal-tension glaucoma underscores our lack of understanding of their pathophysiology.

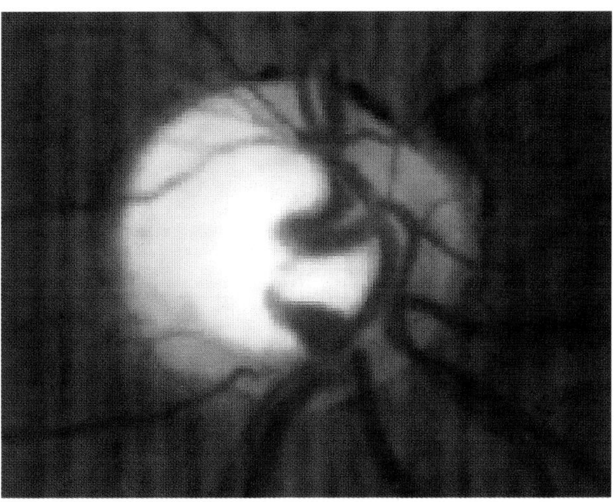

Figure 11.1 Concentric thinning of the neuroretinal rim
Optic disc cupping with concentric thinning of the neuroretinal rim in primary open-angle glaucoma. (*Note:* The striped pattern is projected on the fundus in this image to enhance topographic analysis.)

Definition

Since little is known of the etiology and pathophysiology of primary open-angle glaucoma (not to mention normal-tension glaucoma), the definitions of these conditions remain elusive. Several authors have proposed that we begin to think of the glaucomas in new ways and that we not base our understanding and definitions on levels of intraocular pressure. Perhaps the clinical appearance of the optic nerve head or pathogenesis of damage to the eye should be of primary consideration. Unfortunately, such assessment is not easy and may even be impossible given our current level of understanding. However, it is important that we seek to define glaucoma based on characteristics of the optic neuropathy and functional visual loss rather than the level of intraocular pressure. We also need to define the glaucomas based on the pathogenesis of the optic nerve damage, although at present our knowledge in this area is very incomplete. Current technology should allow us to begin to describe more accurately (and therefore define) the glaucomas based upon such things as the optic disc, the retinal nerve fiber layer, deficits in visual function, or other physiologic and anatomic characteristics.

Normal-tension glaucoma may thus be defined as an optic neuropathy which has certain characteristics that are within the spectrum of the disease we recognize as glaucoma. The hallmark of glaucomatous nerve damage is 'cupping' although this characteristic is highly variable and may take many forms (Fig. 11.1). The level of intraocular pressure

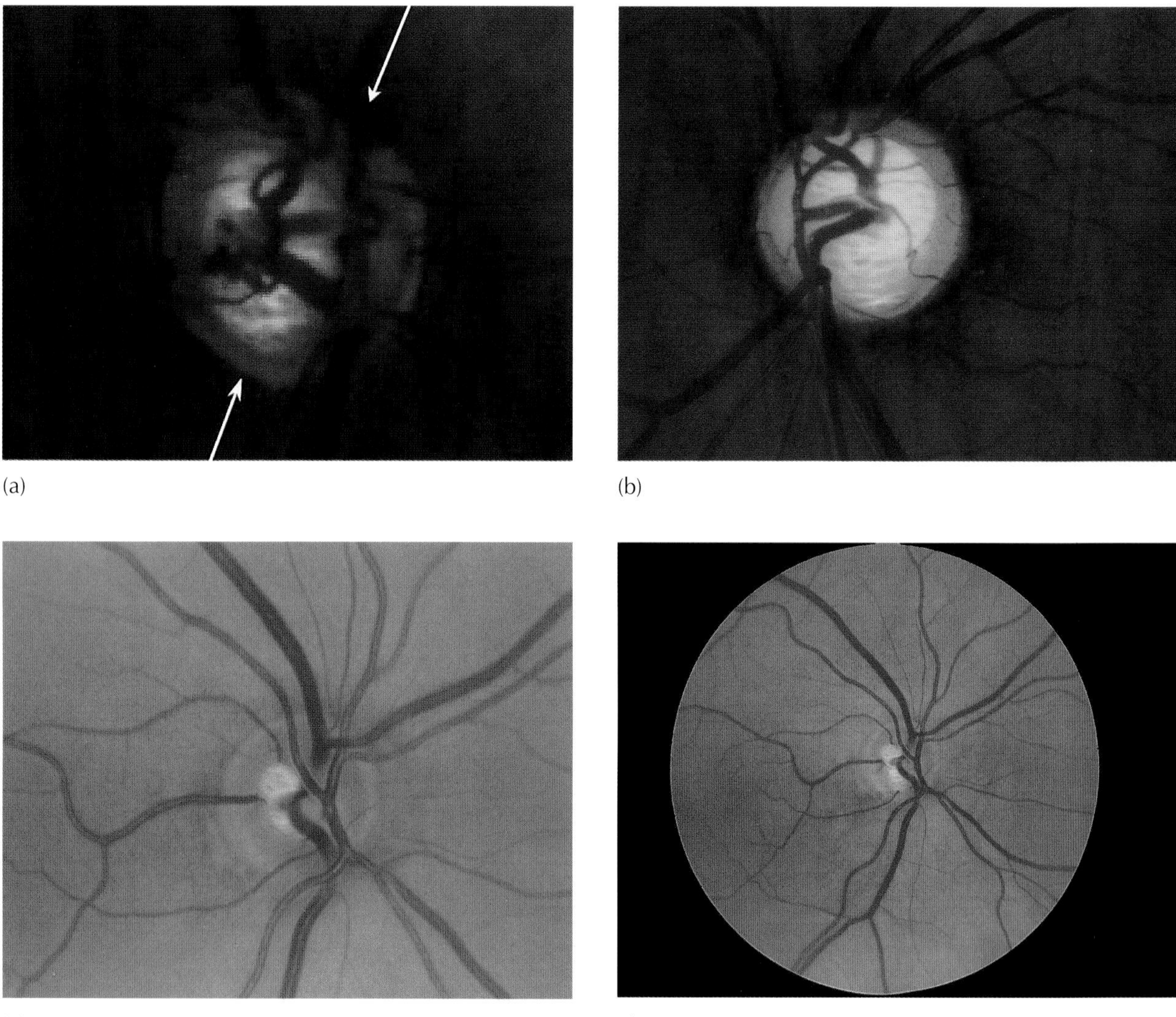

Figure 11.2 Notching of the rim
(a) 'Focal glaucoma' with typical notching of the neuroretinal rim often found in younger individuals with normal-tension glaucoma. Also note development of collateral shunt vessels. (b) Another example of a large focal notch in the neuroretinal rim, giving a typical 'keyhole' cup. (c) and (d). Development of a focal notch in a normal-tension glaucoma patient over a 15-year period. Note in (c) the vertical extension of the cup towards the 5:30 position (d) 15 years later, the cup has extended to the disc margin obliterating the rim and the patient has developed a corresponding superior arcuate scotoma (e). (Figures 11.2 ((b)–(e)) courtesy of Neil T Choplin, MD.)

may be considered just one of the possible risk factors for this disease process similar to current definitions for primary open-angle glaucoma, although it appears that intraocular pressure plays less of a role in normal-tension glaucoma than it may in primary open-angle glaucoma. As shall be discussed, the optic disc and visual field changes in normal-tension glaucoma may be different from those occurring in primary open glaucoma. There is conflicting evidence in this regard which is due in part to our inability to define appropriate study populations and therefore to discriminate accurately between the various glaucomas. It may also be that we are describing a disease process with a broad spectrum which would defy discrimination. Historically, different authors have used various benchmarks for the intraocular pressure in defining their study populations, none of which has proven to be satisfactory. This has gradually led to a change in terminology from low-tension glaucoma to normal-tension glaucoma implying less emphasis on intraocular pressure while still

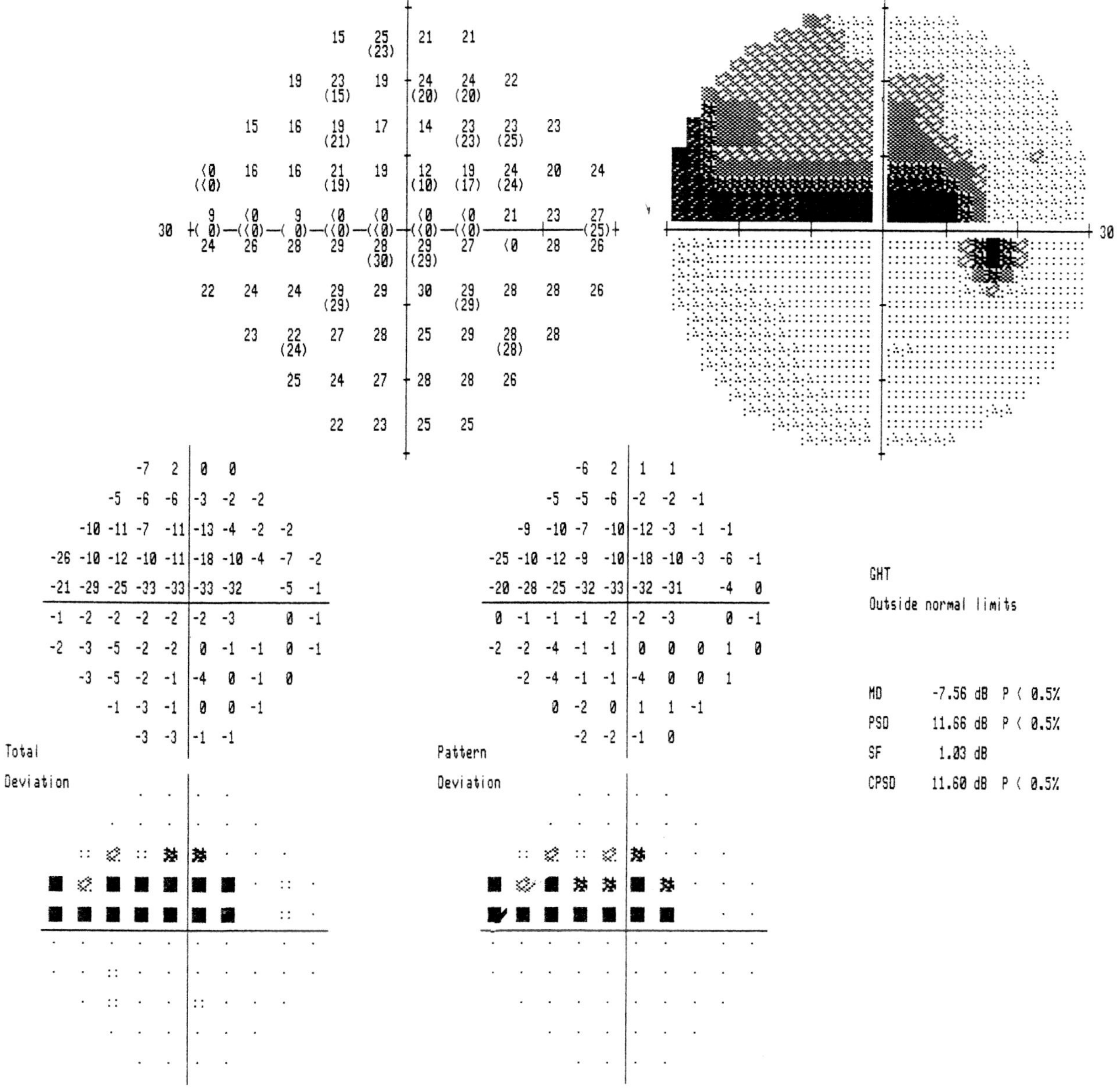

(e)

attempting to described the clinical features of a type of glaucoma where the level of intraocular pressure is not statistically elevated based on population norms, although the pressure may still play a role in some individuals. Despite all these limitations in our ability to define normal-tension glaucoma accurately, it is still a worthwhile exercise to review the clinical and epidemiological findings which have been described in normal-tension glaucoma compared to primary open-angle glaucoma.

Epidemiology

'Hardness of the eyeball' has been attributed to glaucoma for over a century. Leydhecker et al. described the intraocular pressure in the general population. Utilizing Schiotz tonometry in 20 000 individuals they observed that the mean pressure in their population was 15.5 ± 2.57 mmHg (see Chapter 4). At that time anyone with an intraocular pressure more than two standard deviations above the mean

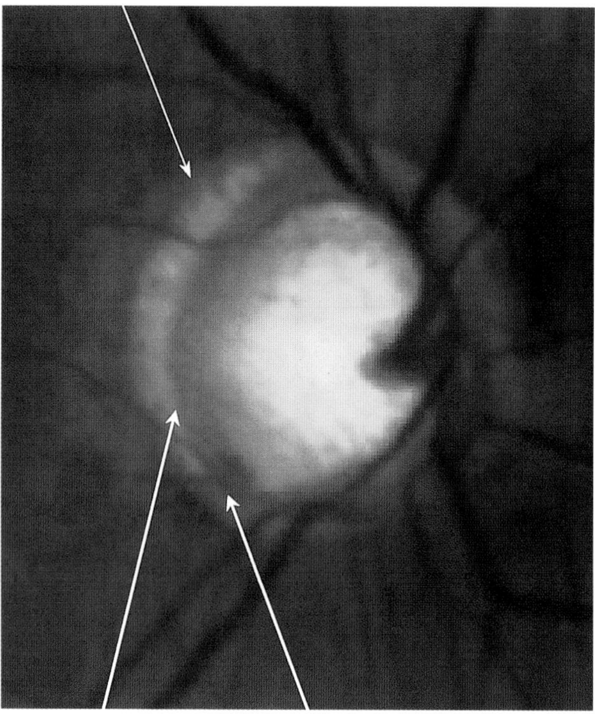

Figure 11.3 Loss of inferotemporal rim
Low-tension glaucoma with greatest loss of temporal and inferior rim. Also note peripapillary atrophy and resolving disc hemorrhage at the 6:30 position.

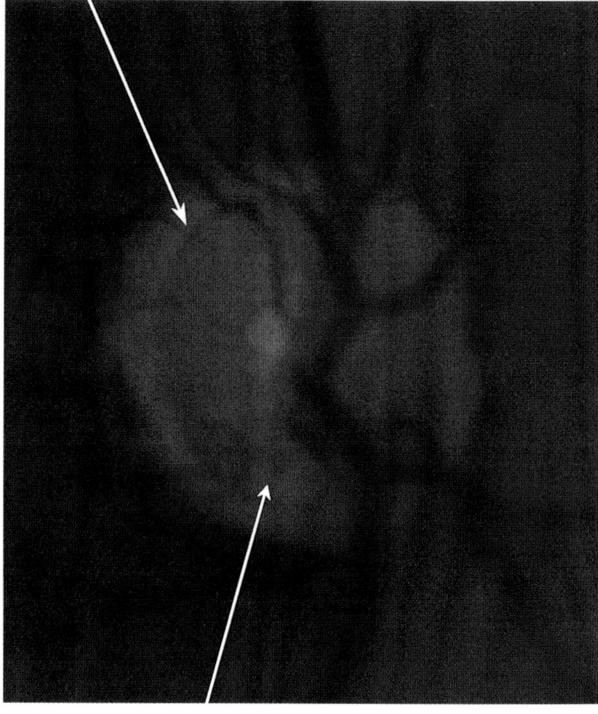

Figure 11.4 Loss of inferotemporal rim
Loss of temporal and inferior rim with especially deep inferior cupping of the optic disc in normal-tension glaucoma.

(20.5 mmHg) was considered suspect for glaucoma, and an intraocular pressure above three standard deviations (24 mmHg) was felt to be diagnostic for glaucoma. Many investigators have provided ample evidence that elevated intraocular pressure and glaucoma are not synonymous. Continuing epidemiological studies provide additional evidence. Intraocular pressure is known to be distributed in a non-Gaussian fashion and to be skewed towards higher pressures. Clinical evidence indicates that there are many exceptions to the commonly held notions linking intraocular pressure and glaucoma, both in eyes with high pressure that do not have glaucoma damage and in eyes with low or normal pressures that do have glaucomatous optic nerve atrophy or visual field loss. Recent population-based prevalence studies suggest that perhaps 40–60% of individuals with either optic disc changes consistent with glaucoma, characteristic visual function loss, or both, have intraocular pressures within two standard deviations of the population mean. Therefore the entity we call normal-tension glaucoma appears to have at least an equal if not greater prevalence than primary open-angle glaucoma.

Epidemiologic evidence of other risk factors for normal-tension glaucoma compared to primary open-angle glaucoma is incomplete. Age, race, and family history are known risk factors for primary open-angle glaucoma. Age is thought to be a factor in some cases of normal-tension glaucoma. Senile sclerotic glaucoma, described by Greve and others, occurs mostly in older individuals and is characterized by relatively low intraocular pressures, peripapillary atrophy, and choroidal sclerosis. However, the entity of focal glaucoma based on focal notching of the disc described by Spaeth is characteristically seen in younger individuals than what has been described for primary open-angle glaucoma (Fig. 11.2). The role of race remains undefined in normal-tension glaucoma. A positive family history may be noted for normal-tension glaucoma and primary open-angle glaucoma, although it is not clear if the risk is similar between the different entities.

Optic disc

A wide variety of optic disc changes may occur in normal-tension glaucoma. Controversy exists as to whether these changes differ from those seen in primary open-angle glaucoma. The call for a new classification system for glaucoma based on the appearance of the optic disc by Spaeth and others includes descriptions of clinical entities for which a low intraocular pressure may be characteristic.

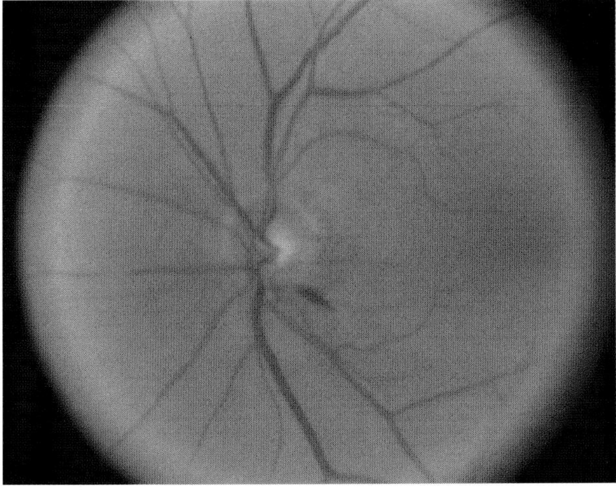

Figure 11.5 Disc hemorrhage
Typical splinter hemorrhage at the disc margin in a patient with normal-tension glaucoma. This hemorrhage was an incidental finding in this patient, being followed with a congenital optic nerve pit in the fellow eye. Shortly after this photograph was taken she was diagnosed with biopsy-proven giant cell arteritis. Over the course of 12 years, she developed significant progressive cupping in each eye, with superior altitudinal hemianopias in each eye despite intraocular pressure never documented over 18 mmHg. The visual fields are depicted in Figs 7.7 snf 7.26.

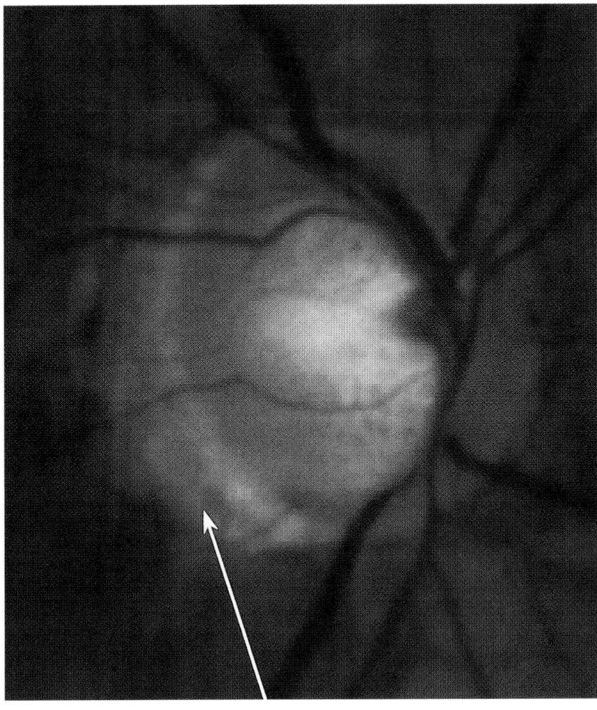

Figure 11.6 Peripapillary atrophy in normal-tension glaucoma (arrow)
This change is typical of what has been termed 'senile sclerotic glaucoma'.

Nicolela and Drance have also described certain disc appearances that may be characteristic of specific glaucoma entities, some of which are characterized by low intraocular pressure. Lewis et al. could not distinguish normal-tension glaucoma from primary open-angle glaucoma by disc appearance when attempting to predict visual field loss. Miller and Quigley also could not distinguish between the two glaucoma entities in a retrospective review of disc photographs, except they did comment that the connective tissue bundles within the lamina cribrosa were less apparent in normal-tension glaucoma. Levene felt there were similar disc changes in normal-tension glaucoma and primary open-angle glaucoma, although there may be a disproportionate degree of cupping relative to the extent of the visual field loss in eyes with lower pressures and glaucoma. Tuulonen and Airaksinen concluded from their study that eyes with normal-tension glaucoma had larger discs than primary open-angle glaucoma, where large and small discs were approximately equal. Jonas and Sturmer, however, concluded that glaucomatous optic neuropathy was not related to disc size.

The amount of cupping and the topography of the disc rim have also been evaluated in normal-tension glaucoma. Caprioli and Spaeth determined that the disc rim in eyes with normal-tension glaucoma is thinner than in eyes with primary open-angle glaucoma (matched for visual field loss), especially along the inferior and temporal margins (Figs. 11.3 and 11.4). This is consistent with the suggestion by Levene that there was disproportionate cupping relative to the extent of visual field loss in normal-tension glaucoma. Fazio et al., utilizing computerized disc analysis, concluded that the cupping in normal-tension glaucoma is more broadly sloping with less disc volume alteration than in primary open-angle glaucoma.

Another interesting finding in normal-tension glaucoma is focal notching or 'acquired pits' in the neuroretinal rim (Fig. 11.4). Javitt et al. found a higher prevalence of acquired pits in normal-tension glaucoma compared to primary open-angle glaucoma eyes with similar degrees of visual field loss. Spaeth has referred to this type of disc change as perhaps one of the characteristic types of glaucomatous optic atrophy and suggested that this type of finding be used to develop new ways of classifying glaucoma. This is more common in females, and individuals with this pattern of disc change tend to have lower intraocular pressures and tend to be younger.

Disc hemorrhages have also been frequently described as occurring more frequently in normal-tension

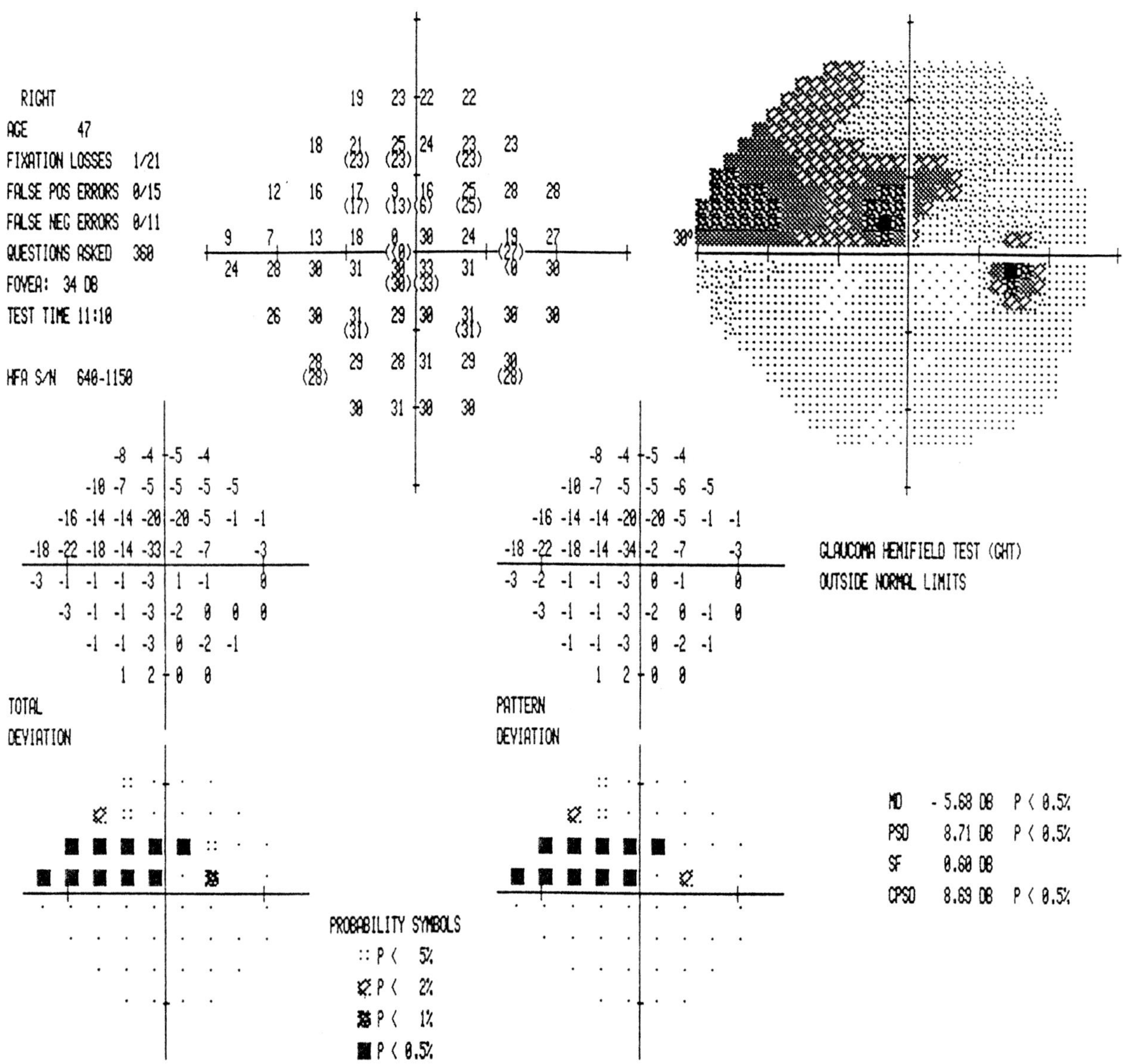

Figure 11.7 Superonasal visual field defect near fixation
This typical low-tension glaucoma defect involves loss of inferotemporal nerve fibers. It is very dense and comes close to fixation.

glaucoma (Fig. 11.5). Kitazawa et al. noted a prevalence of disc hemorrhage of 20.5% in individuals with normal-tension glaucoma. Recurrent disc hemorrhage occurred in 64% of these eyes which was much higher than the other groups studied. Drance noted that disc hemorrhages are not rare events. The closer the disc is followed and the disc appearance recorded, the more hemorrhages will be noted. He estimated the prevalence to be about 20% in normal-tension glaucoma. In addition, Drance felt there were possibly two groups of patients: those who hemorrhage and those who do not. Disc hemorrhages were also felt to precede retinal nerve fiber layer loss, topographic changes of the optic disc, and visual field loss. Hendricks et al., however, felt the cumulative incidence of disc hemorrhages was similar in ocular hypertension, primary open-angle glaucoma, and normal-tension glaucoma. With treatment, however, they noted that the incidence of disc hemorrhages decreased in ocular hypertension and primary open-angle glaucoma but not in normal-tension glaucoma. In addition, recurrent disc hemorrhages tended to be scattered all over the disc in normal-tension glaucoma but tended to occur at the same site in primary open-angle glaucoma and ocular hypertension, perhaps implying a different etiology for the disc hemorrhage in the different conditions.

Peripapillary atrophy also has been reported to occur more frequently in normal-tension glaucoma than in

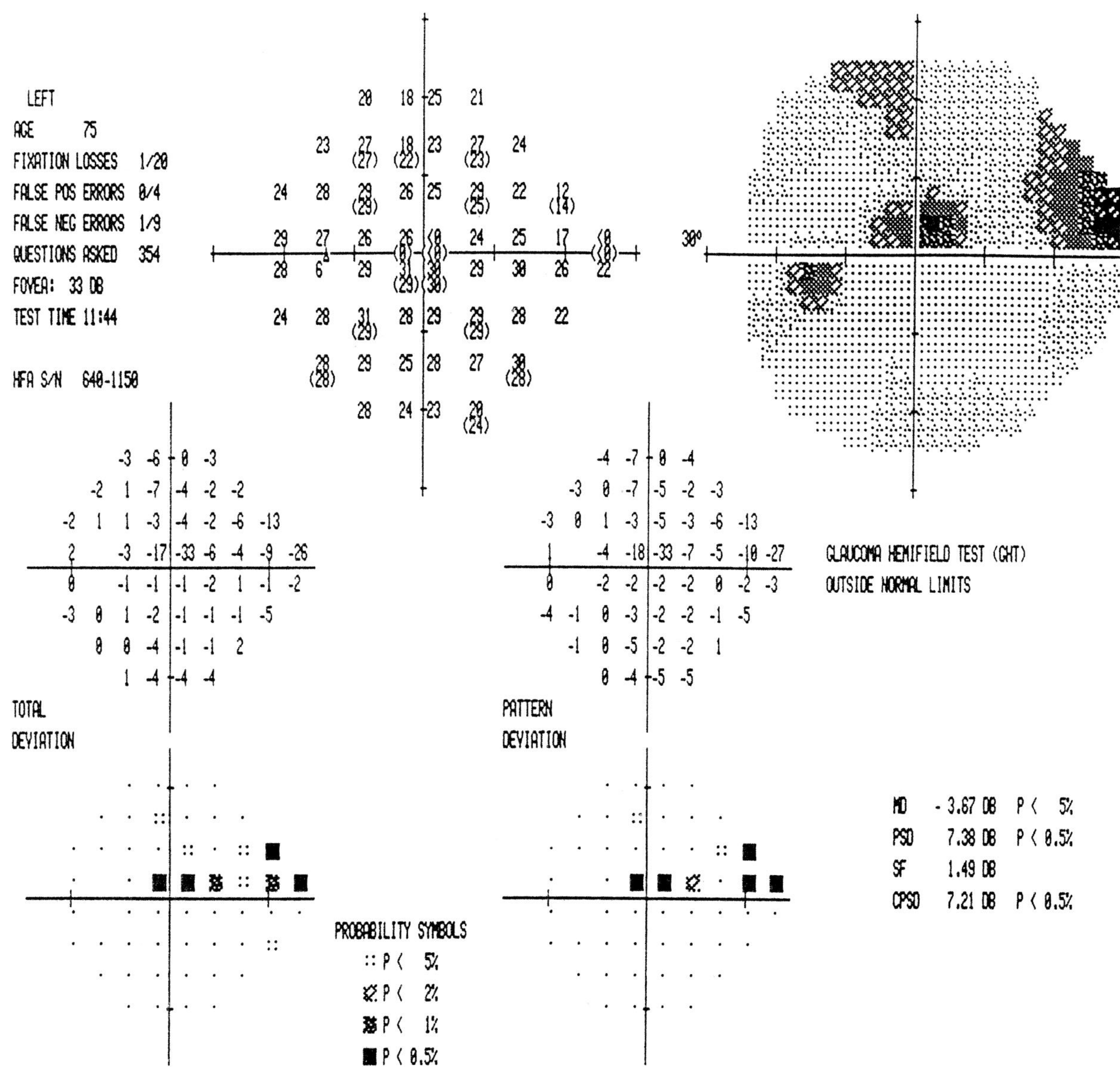

Figure 11.8 Example of a visual field defect near fixation
Note the depth of the defect and the sharp drop off between defect and the surrounding points.

primary open-angle glaucoma (Fig. 11.6). Buus and Anderson reported that peripapillary crescents correlated with disc damage and were therefore more common in normal-tension glaucoma than in ocular hypertension. Geijssen and Greve noted peripapillary atrophy in the entity of senile sclerotic glaucoma. However, Jonas and Xu felt that there were similar degrees of peripapillary atrophy between normal-tension glaucoma and primary open-angle glaucoma in their study population.

It therefore becomes problematic to define what, if any, features of the optic disc are characteristic of normal-tension glaucoma. Our inability to do so undoubtedly reflects on our inability to define what are likely to be the many entities which may result in glaucomatous optic atrophy, the complexities of attempting to study and analyze the optic disc, and the tremendous physiologic variability which is typical of the eye and optic nerve.

Visual fields

The diagnosis of normal-tension glaucoma is made on the basis of progressive visual field loss and/or optic changes in the absence of elevated intraocular pressure. For the most part, visual field defects in normal-tension glaucoma are similar to defects found in high-tension glaucoma. Nasal steps, paracentral

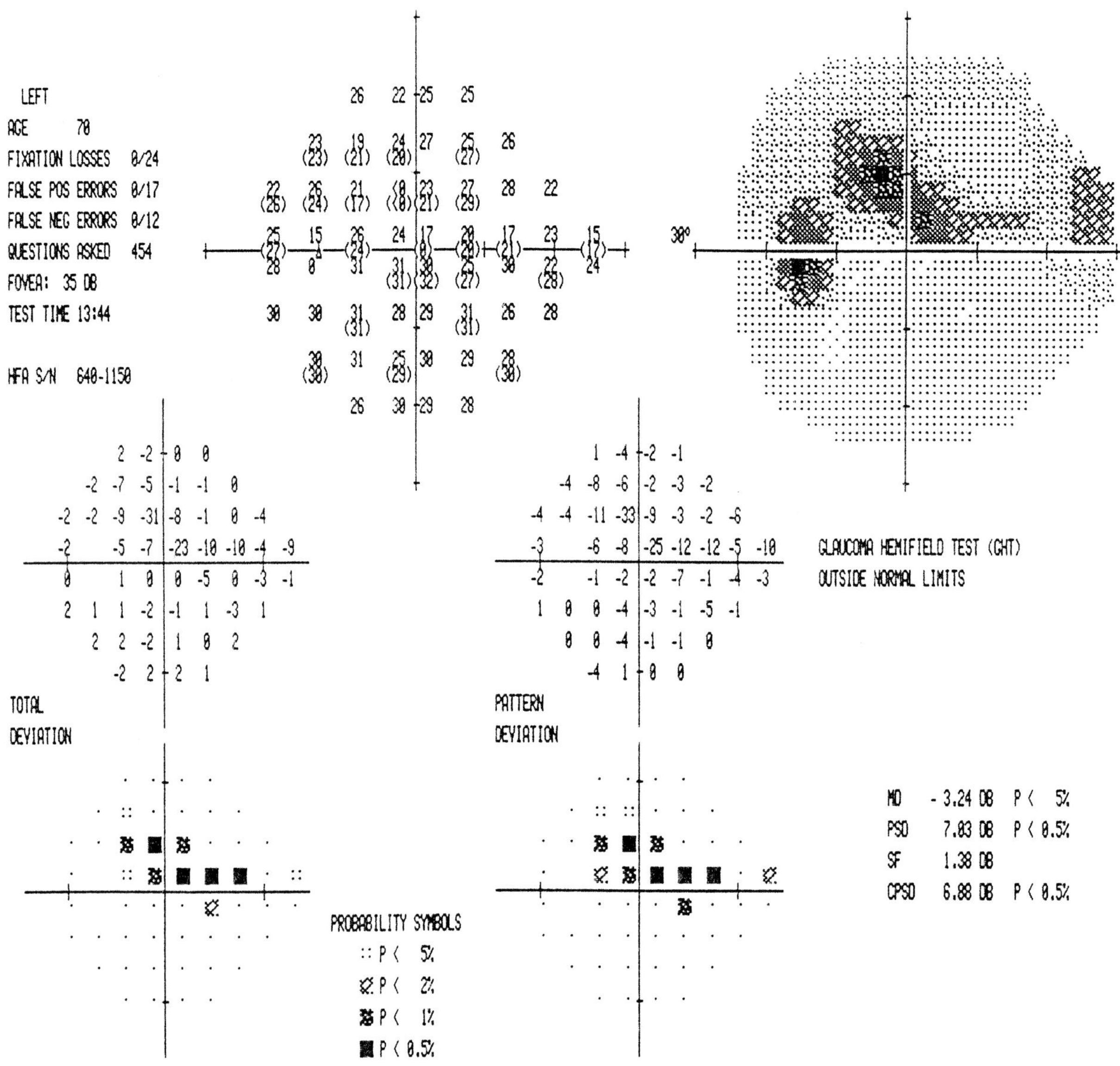

Figure 11.9 Another example of a defect near fixation
Note the overall pattern is that of a nerve fiber layer defect.

scotomas, and arcuate defects predominate. As reported in numerous studies, subtle differences between visual fields of normal-tension and high-tension glaucoma patients appear to exist. Anderton and Hitchings, as well as Caprioli and Spaeth, found a higher incidence of defects near fixation, especially superonasally, in normal-tension glaucoma (Fig. 11.7). In addition, Caprioli and Spaeth noted that these defects had greater depth and steeper slope than the defects of high-tension glaucoma subjects (Figs 11.8 and 11.9). Other studies, however, do not support these findings. Motolko and others, and Greve and Geijssen, found no significant difference in the proximity of field defects to fixation between the normal-tension and high-tension glaucoma groups. King et al. even found that defects in high-tension glaucoma tended to be closer to fixation.

The assertion that normal-tension glaucoma field defects are 'deep, steep, and creep' towards fixation in comparison to high-tension glaucoma fields is still being debated. Phelps et al. attributed the disparate findings of the various studies to the different methodologies used.

Most studies have found that the superior hemifield and particularly the superonasal quadrant are the most frequent locations for normal-tension glaucoma defects. Furthermore, Araie et al. reported that the inferior hemifield just below fixation may be

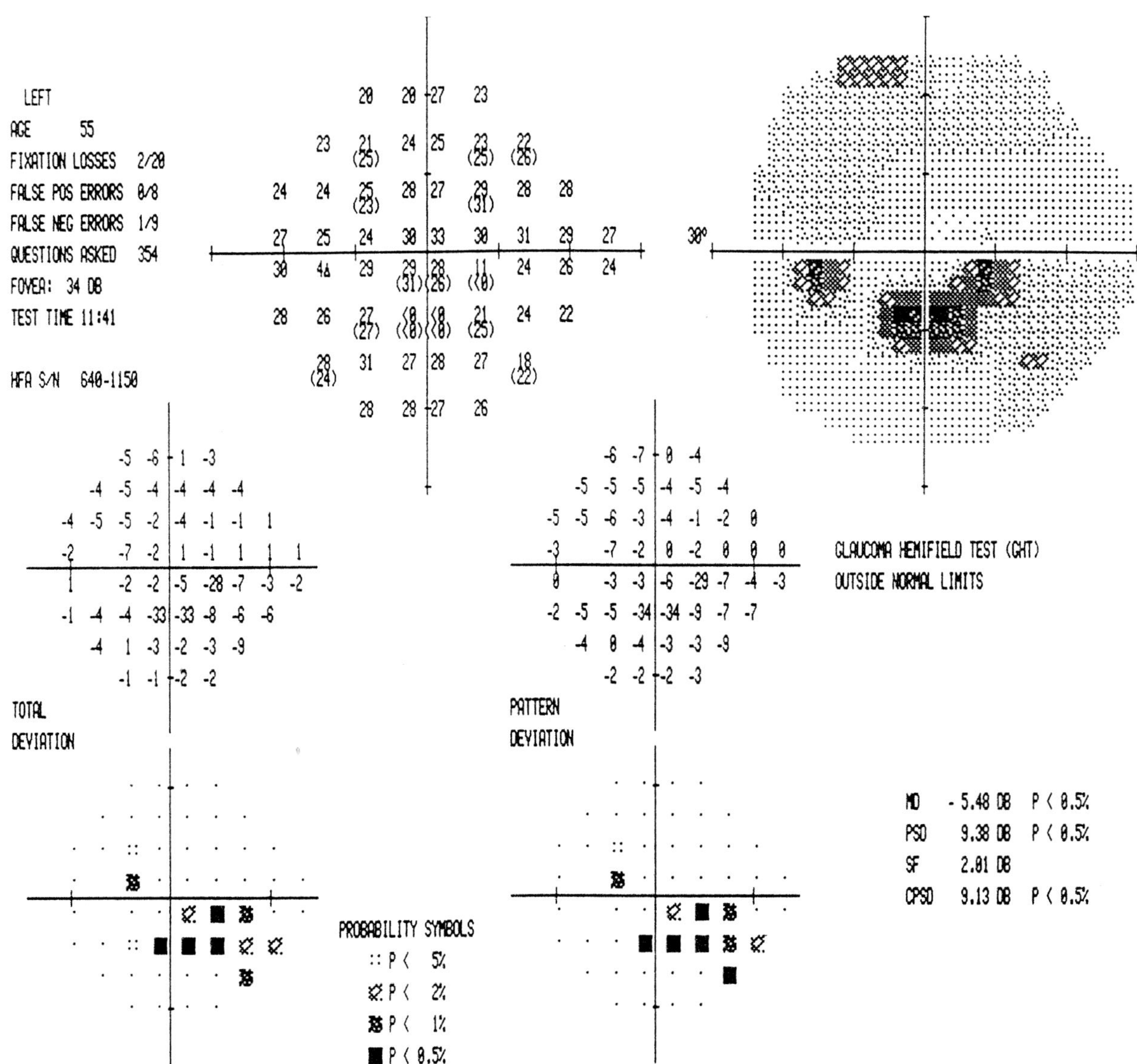

Figure 11.10 Inferior field defect
Although less common than superior defects, inferior defects also tend to be deep and steep and may be close to fixation.

relatively spared. Inferior defects that do occur are also typically deep with steep slopes (Fig. 11.10).

Other differences between fields in normal-tension glaucoma and high-tension glaucoma have been shown. Several groups, including Araie et al., Chauhan et al., and Drance et al., have shown that diffuse visual field loss is more common in the high-tension group. This finding is based on the decreased overall sensitivity of the 'spared' hemifield (no local defect) in high-tension glaucoma (Fig. 11.11). Araie et al. concluded that, even in the late stages of disease, diffuse depression may be more common in high-tension glaucoma. Zeiter and others reported that localized defects in the inferior hemifield may be more common in normal-tension glaucoma. The difference between normal-tension and high-tension glaucoma with respect to diffuse versus local field loss may be attributable to the difference in intraocular pressure rather than some other intrinsic difference between normal-tension and high-tension glaucoma. Instead of comparing normal-tension with high-tension glaucoma groups, several studies compared glaucoma subjects (both low tension and high tension) having diffuse visual field loss with those having localized field defects. Caprioli et al., Glowazki and Flammer, and Samuelson and Spaeth all found significantly higher intraocular pressures in subjects with diffuse field loss than in subjects with localized field loss.

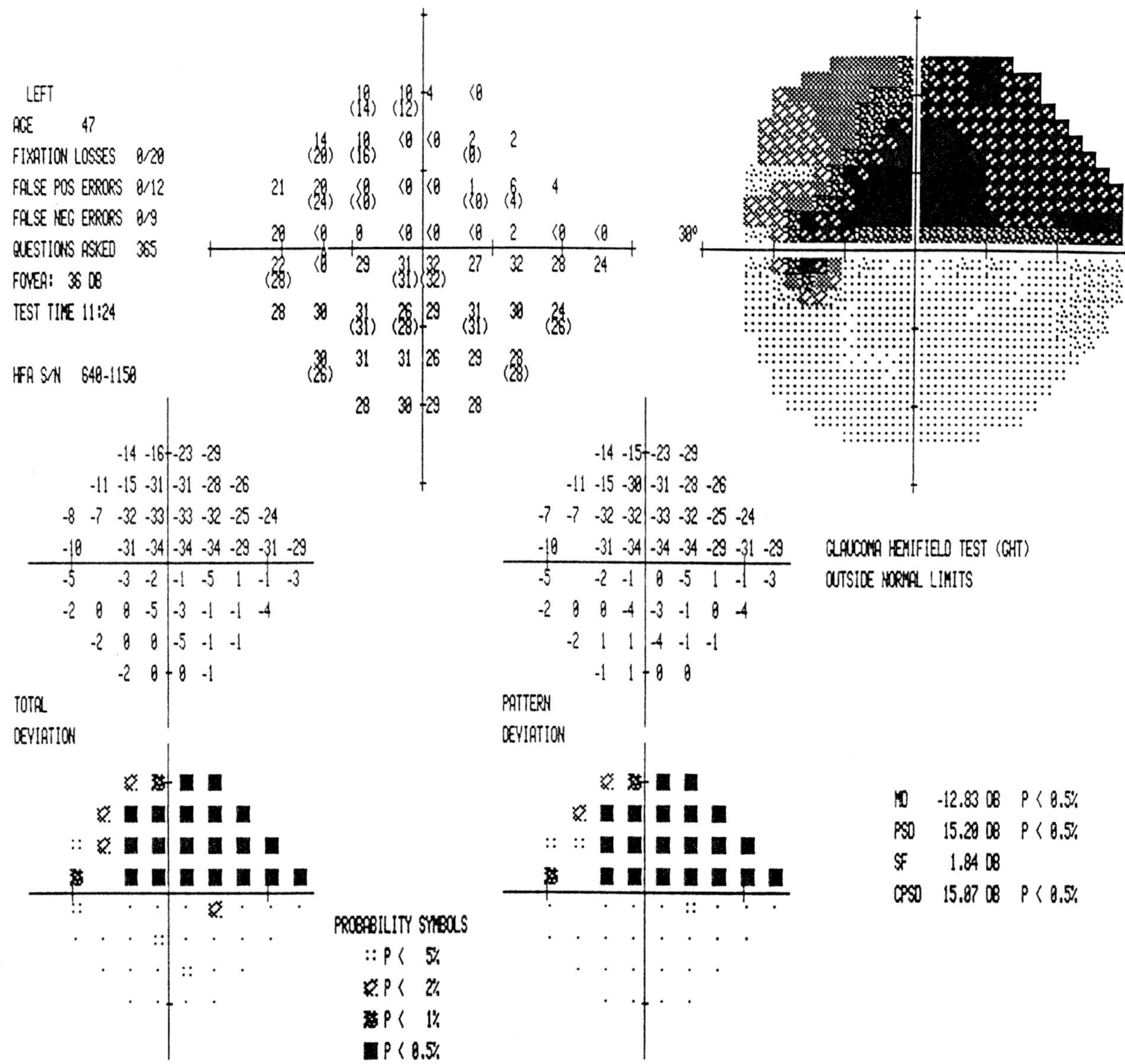

Figure 11.11 Superior hemifield loss

The 'spared' inferior hemifield exhibits minimal overall sensitivity loss.

While these differences between normal-tension and high-tension glaucoma fields are no doubt important to our scientific understanding of normal-tension glaucoma, the clinical significance is less clear. Distinguishing between normal-tension and high-tension glaucoma is obviously not based on the visual field defects. However, we should be aware that defects near fixation may be quite common in persons with normal-tension glaucoma. Defects near fixation are clearly more worrisome than more peripheral ones. In monitoring for the progression of disease, we must realize that the existing defects may deepen rather than enlarge so particular attention should be paid to the total deviation at each point (Fig. 11.12).

Several studies have addressed the rate of progression of visual field loss in normal-tension glaucoma. Two retrospective analyses found a rather alarming rate of progression. Gliklich et al. found progression in 53% of eyes at three years and 62% at five years. Noureddin et al. found progression in 37% of eyes with a mean follow-up of 28 months. A very high rate of progression was initially seen in the Normal Tension Glaucoma Study in which a duplicate field determination was necessary to confirm a change. However, by statistical analysis of the field data, the study group find a very high false-positive rate of progression. The criteria for progression were revised to include two sets of duplicate fields (four total) spaced three months apart that show the same change

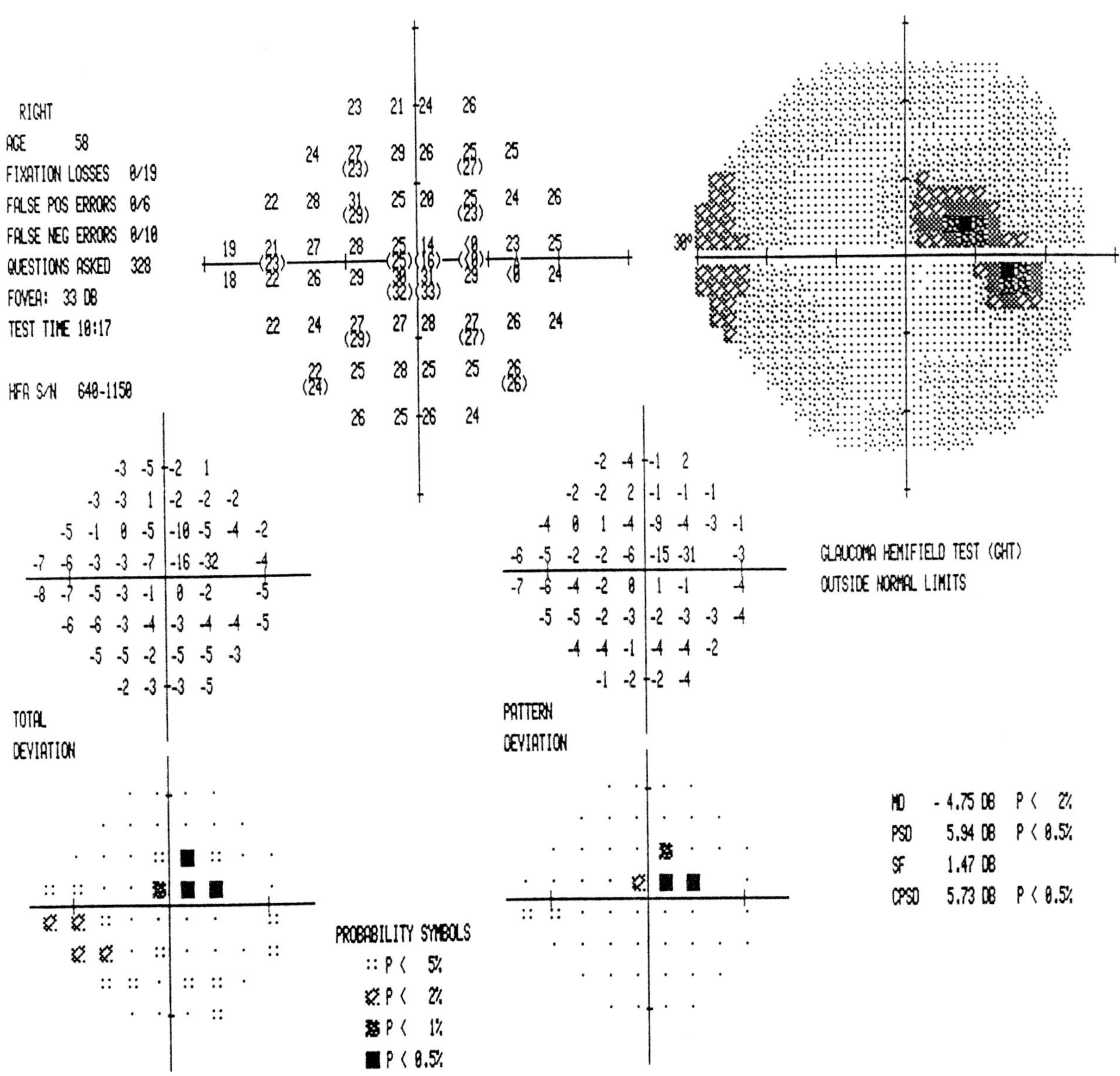

Figure 11.12 Paracentral scotoma
The field defect has encroached fixation and should be monitored closely for further deepening of the defect.

of at least ten decibels. This increased testing reduced the false-positive rate to only 2%. The estimated rate of progression by the revised criteria was only 1.3% per patient per three-month period. In light of the findings of the Normal Tension Glaucoma Treatment Trial, we may need to repeat visual field testing several times before concluding that progression has occurred in a person with normal-tension glaucoma.

Treatment of low-tension glaucoma

The treatment of low-tension glaucoma remains as much an enigma as the disease itself. Evidence from long-term controlled studies regarding the role of medical, laser, or surgical therapy in the management of low-tension glaucoma is lacking. In general, the accepted clinical treatment of low-tension glaucoma parallels that for primary open-angle glaucoma. Individuals are usually initially treated with medical therapy designed to lower their intraocular pressure to a level at least 30% lower than pretreatment levels, and may undergo laser or glaucoma filtering surgery with pressures of 8–12 mmHg as the target goal. However, therapy for low-tension glaucoma is always being critically re-evaluated and novel approaches to therapy in some individuals are being considered. Based on studies which suggest a role for vascular autoregulatory dysfunction or vasospasm in low-tension glaucoma, some individuals have recommended therapy specific for these proposed pathophysiologic abnormalities. In addition, there is increasing interest in agents that may have neuroprotective effects. At this time, however, there is no generally agreed upon, proven, or effective therapy for low-tension glaucoma.

Medical therapy for low-tension glaucoma is usually initiated with beta blockers. The beta-1 antagonist, betaxolol, may improve blood flow or help preserve visual function and may, therefore, be of benefit in low-tension glaucoma. However, long-term studies addressing the efficacy of betaxolol, although suggestive, are not complete. Nonselective beta blockers generally lower pressure more than a selective beta blocker; however, there are concerns regarding potential vasoconstriction related to the pharmacologic properties of these agents. Although direct evidence of clinically significant vasospasm in low-tension glaucoma has been suggested, the evidence for such an effect is yet to be defined.

Adrenergic agonists may also be considered for therapy in low-tension glaucoma. Today the use of nonselective adrenergic agonists such as epinephrine and dipivefrin is decreasing in favor of an alpha-2-agonist such as apraclonidine or brimonidine. The use of apraclonidine long term is limited due to its ocular allergic complications and tachyphylaxis. In addition, apraclonidine is a known potent vasoconstrictor. Brimonidine tartrate is a more highly selective alpha-2-agonist with a much lower rate of allergy and tachyphylaxis. In addition, this drug has been shown to be nonvasoconstrictive in animal and human studies. Brimonidine lowers intraocular pressure in a manner that is comparable to the nonselective beta blockers. In addition, brimonidine has demonstrated neuroprotective effects in several animal models, which may be of theoretic benefit in low-tension glaucoma.

The new prostaglandin analog, latanoprost, may also be a useful therapeutic agent for low-tension glaucoma. Some individuals may obtain very significant lowering of their intraocular pressure with this agent, even below that of episcleral venous pressure. However, there is a relatively high rate of individuals in whom the drug may not lower the intraocular pressure significantly. In addition, concerns regarding changes in iris stromal pigmentation, potential retinal complications in at-risk individuals (such as cystoid macular edema), ocular inflammation, and other unknown ocular or systemic complications of this new agent are still being addressed. Despite these concerns, latanoprost may be a useful adjunct in the medical therapy of low-tension glaucoma.

Carbonic anhydrase inhibitors are also agents to be considered for low-tension glaucoma. This class of drugs has been shown to be vasodilatory in addition to decreasing intraocular pressure. The use of systemic carbonic anhydrase inhibitors is limited because of their side-effects and the topical carbonic anhydrase inhibitor, dorzolamide, has become more widely used. However, concerns still remain about potential sulfonamide-related or other types of side-effects from these drugs and the amount of intraocular lowering with dorzolamide may not be sufficient to reach target pressures.

The cholinergic agonists, such as pilocarpine, may also be considered. However, use of these drugs may be limited due to ocular side-effects and the frequent dosing regimens which are required.

Newer therapeutic approaches directed at improving blood flow to the optic nerve have also been considered. Calcium channel blockers have received the most interest and study. Although some suggestive indirect evidence exists that individuals on calcium channel blockers may have better visual field survival, these studies are open to criticism and there is still much work to be done. In addition, these agents can be associated with serious systemic side-effects, such as hypotension and a reported increased risk of myocardial infarction. The search for other novel approaches to treating low-tension glaucoma goes on and will, it is hoped, lead to more satisfactory medical approaches in the future.

Argon laser trabeculoplasty may be used for low-tension glaucoma; however, the intraocular pressure lowering is generally only modest, at best, and is usually only temporary. However, when trying to reach a target pressure, it is considered a relatively safe option to consider in some individuals.

Most clinicians agree that in the face of progressive low-tension glaucoma, aggressive surgical therapy should be considered. Several studies have suggested that with aggressive surgery and intraocular pressure lowering to the low teens or lower, visual field progression can be slowed or halted in many individuals. Long-term controlled studies on the effect of surgery are being carried out in individuals with low-tension glaucoma and those results are still pending. When considering glaucoma filtering surgery for low-tension glaucoma many clinicians and glaucoma specialists will consider the use of an antimetabolite such as 5-FU or mitomycin. Although the use of antimetabolites increases the likelihood of obtaining low intraocular pressures, one must also deal with the short-term complications of hypotony, choroidal effusions, and flat anterior chamber, as well as the potential long-term complications of cataract progression, bleb leaks, and endophthalmitis.

Unfortunately, despite what might be considered optimal therapy, many patients with low-tension glaucoma seem to progress. Our lack of understanding of the etiology of low-tension glaucoma undoubtedly contributes to our therapeutic failures. Further research is necessary to define the underlying causes that predispose to low-tension glaucoma so that future therapy may be directed at specific pathophysiologic abnormalities.

FURTHER READING

Anderton S, Hitchings RA, A comparative study on visual fields of patients with low-tension glaucoma and those with chronic simple glaucoma, *Doc Ophthalmol Proc Series* (1983) **35**:97–9.

Araie M, Hori J, Koseki N, Comparison of visual field defects between normal-tension and primary open-angle glaucoma in the late stage of the disease, *Graefe's Arch Clin Exp Ophthalmol* (1995) **233**:610–16.

Araie M, Yamagami J, Suziki Y, Visual field defects in normal-tension and high-tension glaucoma, *Ophthalmology* (1939) **100**:1808–14.

Armaly MF, Ocular pressure and visual fields: a ten year follow-up study, *Arch Ophthalmol* (1969) **81**:25–40.

Bankes JLK, Perkins ES, Tsolokis S, et al., Bedford glaucoma survey, *Br Med J* (1968) **1**:791–6.

Buus DR, Anderson DR, Peripapillary crescents and halos in normal-tension glaucoma and ocular hypertension, *Ophthalmology* (1989) **2**:16–19.

Caprioli J, Sears M, Miller JM, Patterns of early visual field loss in open-angle glaucoma, *Am J Ophthalmol* (1987) **103**:512–17.

Caprioli J, Spaeth GL, Comparison of the optic nerve head in high- and low-tension glaucoma, *Arch Ophthalmol* (1985) **5**:1145–9.

Caprioli J, Spaeth GL, Comparison of visual field defects in the low-tension glaucomas with those in the high-tension glaucomas, *Am J Ophthalmol* (1984) **97**:730–7.

Chauhan BC, Drance SM, Douglas GR, Johnson CA, Visual field damage in normal-tension and high-tension glaucoma, *Am J Ophthalmol* (1989) **108**:636–42.

Drance SM, Disc hemorrhages in the glaucomas, *Surv Ophthalmol* (1989) **19**:331–7.

Drance SM, The visual field of low-tension glaucoma and shock-induced optic neuropathy, *Arch Ophthalmol* (1977) **95**:1359–61.

Drance SM, Douglas GR, Airaksinen PJ, Schulzer M, Hitchings RA, Diffuse visual field loss in chronic open-angle and low-tension glaucoma, *Am J Ophthalmol* (1987) **104**:577–80.

Duke-Elder S, Jay B, *Disease of the lens and vitreous: glaucoma and hypotony* (London: Kimpton, 1969).

Fazio P, Krupin T, Feitl M, Werner EB, Carre DA, Optic disc topography in patients with low-tension and primary open angle glaucoma, *Arch Ophthalmol* (1990) **5**:705–8.

Geijssen HC, Greve EL, The spectrum of primary open-angle glaucoma. 1. Senile sclerotic glaucoma versus high tension glaucoma, *Ophthalmic Surg* (1987) **13**:297–313.

Gliklich RE, Steinmann WC, Spaeth GL, Visual change in low-tension glaucoma over a five-year follow-up, *Ophthalmology* (1989) **96**:316–20.

Glowazki A, Flammer J, Is there a difference between glaucoma patients with rather localized visual field damage and patients with more diffuse visual field damage? *Doc Ophthalmol Proc Series* (1987) **49**:317–20.

Greve EL, Geijssen HC, Comparison of glaucomatous visual field defects in patients with high and with low intraocular pressures, *Doc Ophthalmol Proc Series* (1983) **35**:101–5.

Hendricks KH, van den Enden A, Rasker MT, Hoyng PFJ, Cumulative incidence of patients with disc hemorrhages in glaucoma and the effect of therapy, *Ophthalmology* (1994) **2**:1165–72.

Hitchings RA, Anderton SA, A comparative study of visual field defects seen in patients with low-tension glaucoma and chronic simple glaucoma, *Br J Ophthalmol* (1983) **67**:818–21.

Javitt JC, Spaeth GL, Katz LJ, Poryzees E, Addiego R, Acquired pits of the optic nerve: increased prevalence in patients with low-tension glaucoma, *Ophthalmology* (1986) **2**:1038–44.

Jonas JB, Sturmer J, Papastathopoulos K, Meier-Gibbons F, Dichtl A, Optic disc size in normal pressure glaucoma, *Br J Ophthalmol* (1995) **4**:1102–5.

Jonas JB, Xu L, Parapapillary chorioretinal atrophy in normal-pressure glaucoma, *Am J Ophthalmol* (1993) **6**:501–5.

King D, Drance SM, Gouglas G, Schulzer M, Wijsman K, Comparison of visual field defects in normal-tension glaucoma and high-tension glaucoma, *Am J Ophthalmol* (1986) **101**:204–7.

Kitazawa Y, Shirato S, Yamamoto T, Optic disc hemorrhages in the glaucomas, *Ophthalmology* (1986) **2**:853–7.

Klein BEK, Klein R, Linton KLP, Intraocular pressure in an American community: the Beaver Dam Eye Study, *Invest Ophthalmol* (1992) **33**:2224–8.

Levene RZ, Low tension glaucoma: a critical review and new material, *Surv Ophthalmol* (1980) **19**:621–63.

Lewis RA, Hayreh SM, Phelps CD, Optic disk and visual field correlations in primary-open angle low-tension glaucoma, *Am J Ophthalmol* (1983) **6**:148–52.

Leydhecker W, Akiyama K, Neumann HG, Der intraokulare Druck gesunder menschlicher Augen, *Klin Monatsbl Augenheilkd* (1958) **133**:662–70.

Linner E, Stromberg U, The course of untreated ocular hypertension. A tonographic study, *Acta Ophthalmol* (1964) **42**:836–48.

Miller KM, Quigley HA, Comparison of optic disc features in low-tension and typical open-angle glaucoma, *Ophthalmic Surg* (1987) **13**:882–9.

Motolko M, Drance SM, Douglas GR, Visual field defects in low-tension glaucoma: comparison of defects in low-tension glaucoma and chronic open angle glaucoma, *Arch Ophthalmol* (1982) **100**:1074–7.

Motolko M, Drance SM, Douglas GR, The visual field defects of low-tension glaucoma: a comparison of the visual field defects in low-tension glaucoma with chronic open angle glaucoma, *Doc Ophthalmol Proc Series* (1983) **35**:107–11.

Nicolela MT, Drance SM, Various glaucomatous optic nerve appearances, *Ophthalmology* (1996) **103**:640–9.

Noureddin BN, Poinoosawmy D, Fietzke FW, Hitchings RA, Regression analysis of visual field progression in low tension glaucoma, *Br J Ophthalmol* (1991) **75**:493–5.

Perkins ES, The Bedford glaucoma survey. 1. Long term follow-up borderline cases, *Br J Ophthalmol* (1973) **57**:179 (abst).

Phelps CD, Hayreh SS, Montague PR, Comparison of visual field defects in the low-tension glaucomas with those in the high-tension glaucomas, *Am J Ophthalmol* (1984) **98**:823–5.

Samuelson TW, Spaeth GL, Focal and diffuse visual field defects: their relationship to intraocular pressure, *Ophthalmic Surg* (1993) **24**:519–25.

Schappert-Kimmijser J, A five-year follow-up of subjects with intraocular pressure of 22–30 mmHg without anomalies of the optic nerve and visual field typical for glaucoma at first investigation, *Ophthalmologica* (1971) **162**:289–95.

Schulzer M, Normal-tension Glaucoma Study Group. Errors in the diagnosis of visual field progression in normal-tension glaucoma, *Ophthalmology* (1994) **101**:1589–95.

Sjogren H, A study of pseudoglaucoma, *Acta Ophthalmol* (1946) **24**:239–94.

Spaeth GL, A new classification of glaucoma including focal glaucoma, *Surv Ophthalmol* (1994) **38 (suppl)**:S95–S15.

Tielsch JM, Sommer A, Witt K, Katz J, Royall RM, Blindness and visual impairment in an American urban population: the Baltimore Eye Survey, *Arch Ophthalmol* (1900) **108**:286–90.

Tuulonen A, Airaksinen PJ, Optic disc size in exfoliative, primary open angle and low tension glaucoma, *Arch Ophthalmol* (1992) **5**:211–13.

von Graefe A, Uber die glaucomatose Natur die Amaurosen mit Sehnervenexcavation und uber das Weses und die Classification des Glaucomas, *Archiv Ophthalmol* (1861) **8**:271–97.

von Graefe A, Amaurose mit Sehnervenexcavation, *Archiv Ophthalmol* (1857) **3**:484–7.

von Graefe A, Die Iridectomie bei Amaurose mit Sehnervenexcavation, *Archiv Ophthalmol* (1857) **3**:546–8.

Zeiter JH, Shin DH, Juzych MS, Jarvi TS, Spoor TC, Zwas F, Visual field defects in patients with normal-tension glaucoma and patients with high-tension glaucoma, *Am J Ophthalmol* (1992) **114**:758–63.

12 Ocular blood flow and glaucoma

Alon Harris and Larry Kagemann

Introduction

Over 100 years ago, Wagemann and Salzmann observed vascular sclerosis in many of their glaucoma patients. Through the years, numerous other researchers uncovered pieces of the blood flow puzzle: documenting reductions in the capillary beds, sclerosis of nutritional vessels, vascular lesions and degeneration, and other circulatory pathologies in glaucoma. Recently, in a study designed specifically to test vascular function of the vessels feeding the eye, the presence of a reversible vasospasm was documented in some normal-tension glaucoma patients. A century of observation and circumstantial evidence supporting a vascular component in the pathogenesis of glaucoma are now supported by direct experimental evidence. This transition from theory to fact took 100 years because the technology required to make such specialized measurements of hemodynamic function has only recently become available. Now that the link has been established, there has been a focus on ocular hemodynamics in glaucoma, and the effect of intraocular pressure-reducing medication on blood flow to the eye.

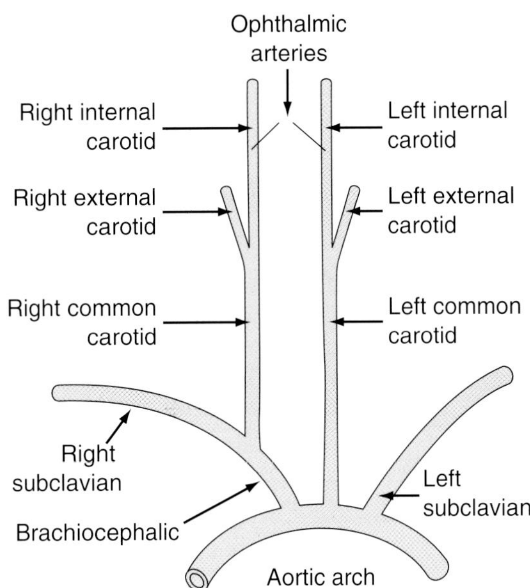

Figure 12.1 Anatomy of the gross circulation to the eye
The ophthalmic artery is the only branch of the internal carotid artery outside the cranium.

Ocular vasculature

The ophthalmic artery is the source for blood flow to the eye, but the left and right ophthalmic arteries drive blood from the heart through slightly different routes. The left carotid artery is one of three branches of the aortic arch. The right carotid artery is a branch of the brachiocephalic artery, itself one of the three branches of the aortic arch. Both left and right common carotids split to form the internal and external carotid arteries. The only branch of the internal carotid artery outside the cranium is the ophthalmic artery (Fig. 12.1).

The ophthalmic artery supplies two major ocular vascular beds: the retinal and uveal systems. The retinal vasculature is supplied by a single central retina artery (CRA). The CRA enters the globe through the center of the optic nerve and forms four branches: one for each quadrant of the retina. The uveal system supplies the iris, ciliary body, and choroidal vasculature through a number of anterior and posterior ciliary arteries. The posterior ciliary arteries (PCA) have been the focus of attention in glaucoma research. It is the PCAs which

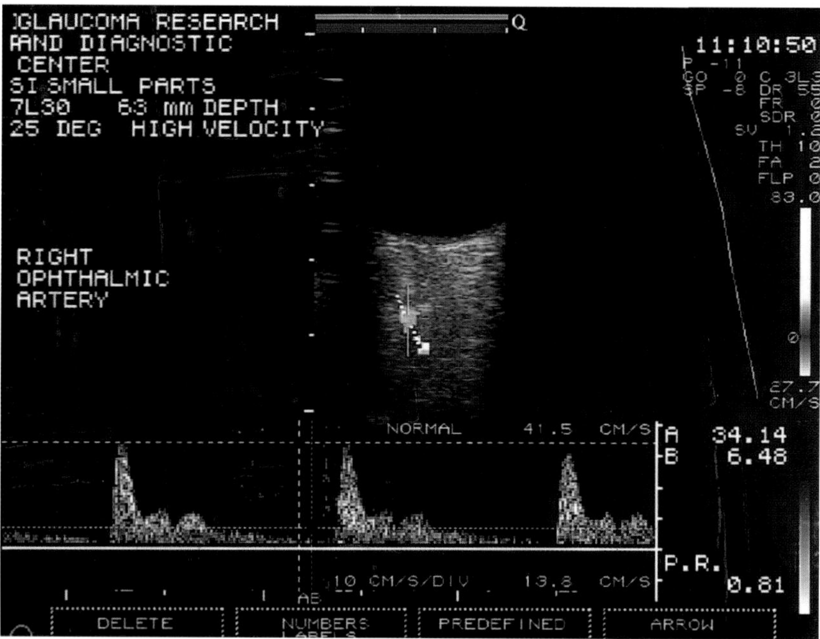

Figure 12.2 Imaging of the ophthalmic artery
Imaging of the ophthalmic artery requires a velocity setting of high, and a depth of 63 mm. Smaller vessels, measured in the vicinity of the nerve head, require settings for slow velocities and only 42 mm.

feed the various deep regions of the optic nerve head, with the exception of the superficial nerve fiber layer, which is supplied by branches of retinal arteries.

Techniques for examining ocular blood flow

Color Doppler imaging

Fundamentals

Ultrasound uses sound waves to locate structures in the body. By timing the delay between sound transmission and echo, ultrasound can measure the depth location of anatomic structure, e.g. A scan ultrasound measurements of axial length. The time between transmission of a sound wave into the eye and the returning echo from the back of the eye provides a precise measurement of axial length. This measurement does not require clear optical media and can be performed in the presence of many ophthalmic diseases. By sweeping the A scan in a line through the eye, a map of structural locations through a slice is obtained. This is commonly known as B scan ultrasound and has been used to produce gray-scale images of ophthalmic structures. Color Doppler imaging (CDI) is based on B scan technology, with an additional processing step. The frequencies of the returning B scan sound waves are analyzed. When a wave is reflected by a moving source, such as flowing blood cells, it is Doppler shifted to a different frequency. The amount of the shift is described by the Doppler equation:

$$\text{Doppler Shift} = \frac{2 \times V_{\text{blood}}}{\text{Wavelength}} \quad \text{Cos } \theta$$

where V_{blood} is the blood flow velocity, Wavelength is the wavelength of the incident sound wave, and Cos θ is the cosine of the angle between the blood velocity vector and the incident sound-wave vector. Doppler shifted sound is displayed using color-coded pixels within the gray-scale image. Red pixels represent movement toward the CDI probe, and blue represents movement away from the probe. Samples of Doppler shifts (or velocities as calculated using the equation above) may be collected from specified vessels within the image. Data are collected in real time during the cardiac cycle. A number of data may be obtained from the resulting velocity waveform. The peak systolic velocity (PSV) is located by the ultrasonographer and is equal to the greatest observable velocity obtained by the blood during systole. The end diastolic blood velocity (EDV) is also located by the ultrasonographer (Fig. 12.2). Using both these measurements, Porcelot's resistive index (RI) may be computed, which is described by:

$$\text{RI} = \frac{\text{PSV} - \text{EDV}}{\text{PSV}}$$

RI is an indication of the resistance to flow in the vasculature distal to the point of measurement.

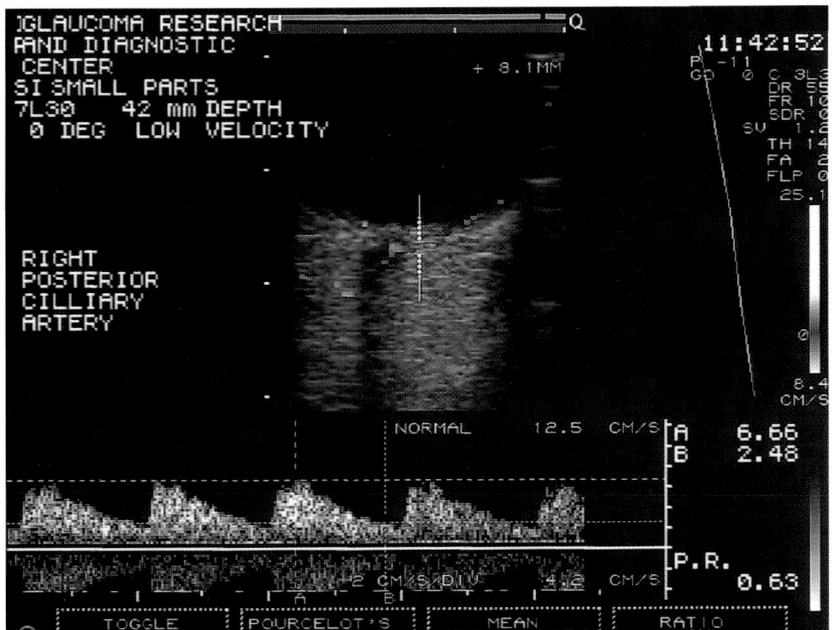

Figure 12.3 Color Doppler imaging waveforms
The waveform of the posterior ciliary artery lacks the dicrotic notch visible in the central retinal artery and well pronounced in the ophthalmic artery.

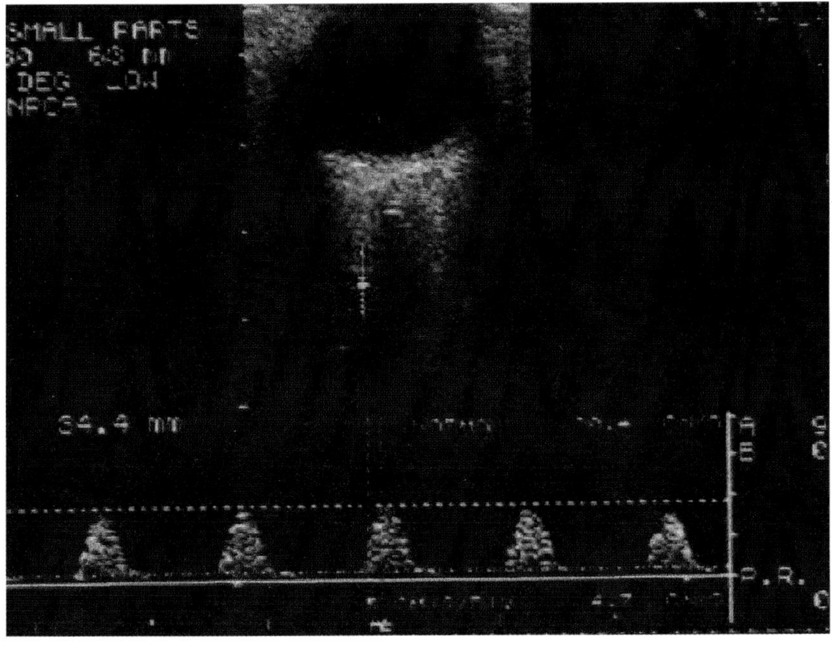

Figure 12.4 Color Doppler imaging waveforms
Waveforms of blood velocity in vasculature feeding high resistance areas take on a 'haystack' appearance.

Hemodynamic measurements

CDI is used to measure blood flow velocities in the ophthalmic, central retinal and posterior ciliary arteries. Due to the large difference between the ophthalmic and smaller CRA and PCAs, the system settings are changed to appropriate ranges of depth and velocity.

The waveforms of the various vessels provide additional information. The dicrotic notch is clearly evident in the ophthalmic artery (OA) waveform (Fig. 12.2), while still evident yet less pronounced in the CRA and missing from the PCA (Fig. 12.3). In glaucomatous eyes with high resistance to flow, PCA waveforms take on the appearance of a haystack with almost no end diastolic flow (Fig. 12.4). CDI thus allows quantification of flow velocities in the retrobulbar vasculature in research and clinical settings. The appearance of waveforms may also provide insight into the condition of the patients' ocular vascular health.

Angiography

Fundamentals

Ophthalmic angiography dates back to 1961 when, at the Indiana University School of Medicine, Novotny and Alvis first described a method for photographing fluorescein as it passed through the human retina. Their early technique was limited to one image every 12 seconds. Today fluorescein angiography can be performed with a scanning laser ophthalmoscope (SLO). Temporal resolution has increased to 30 images per second, and spatial resolution is maximized by using a scanning laser to illuminate the fundus one point at a time. Images obtained from the SLO are recorded on video tape, and not directly captured digitally, due to the large amount of image data. While the improvements in image collection are important, improvements in image interpretation and analysis continue to provide new insight into the physiology and pathophysiology of ocular hemodynamics.

Video images obtained from SLO angiography are analyzed using digital video analysis equipment. Each frame of a video segment of interest is digitized. This allows the brightness in specified areas to be quantified. As dye enters retinal vessels, the vessels become bright. By quantifying the brightness in two locations on a retinal vessel, the amount of time for fluorescein dye to move from a proximal to a distal location may be measured. Utilizing the image-processing capabilities of a video analysis system, the distance between the two brightness measurement locations may also be measured. Combining distance and time data yields the mean dye flow velocity (MDV) through retinal vessels (Fig. 12.5). If the same system is used to measure vessel diameter, volumetric flow through the retinal arteries may be calculated.

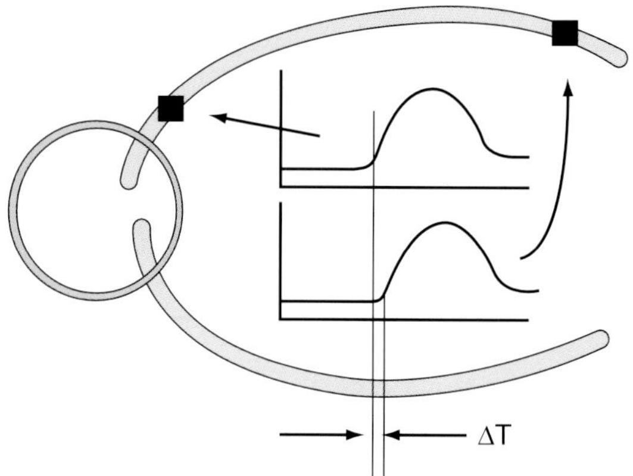

Figure 12.5 Dye transit time
The amount of time required for dye to travel through a retinal artery may be measured by plotting the brightness of two points in time. Here, some amount of time, ΔT, was required for dye to travel between the two black measurement squares.

Hemodynamic measurements at 40 degrees

The image series illustrated in Figure 12.6 displays frames from the early phase of a fluorescein angiogram. This series was obtained on the Rodenstock SLO 101 using the argon laser and a fluorescein angiography filter. The image is a 40-degree image of the retina. In order to obtain an accurate measurement, sample areas on retinal arteries are located on a length of vessel void of branches. A plot of the brightness of a vein in time may be used with the arterial plots in order to measure the arteriovenous passage (AVP) time. The AVP time is an indication of the overall status of retinal microcirculation, requiring passage of dye from retinal arteries to retinal veins.

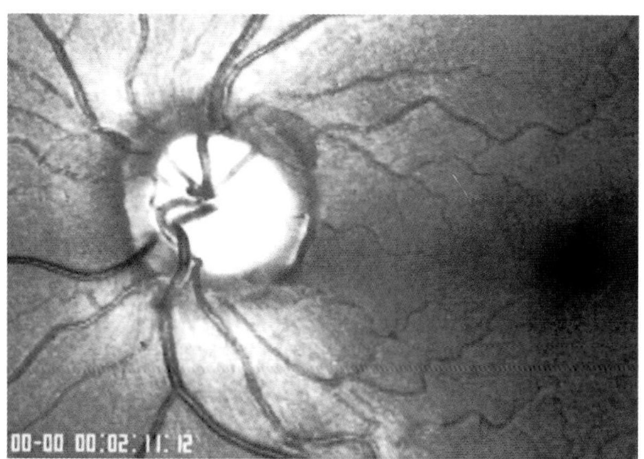

(a)

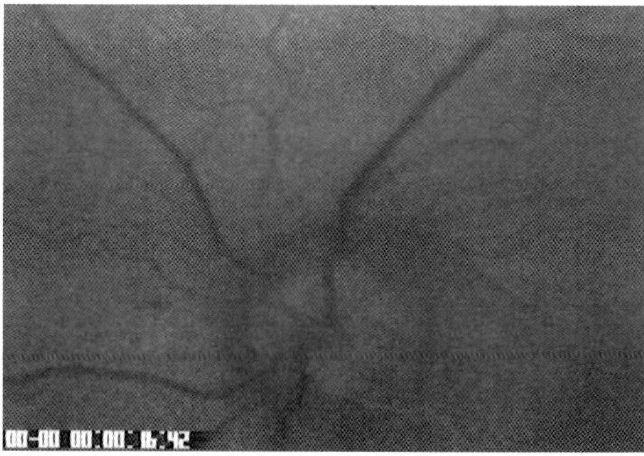

(b)

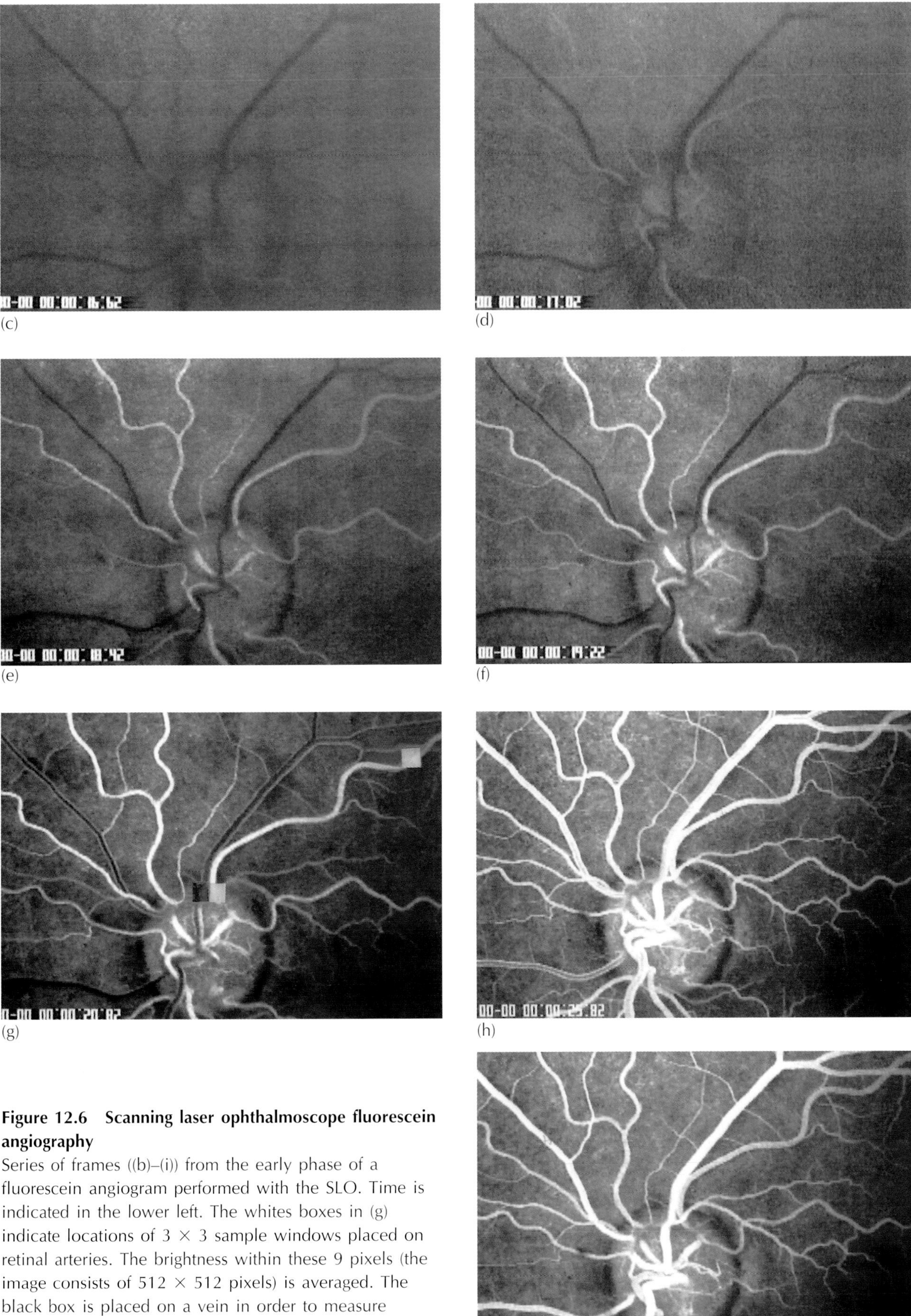

(c) (d) (e) (f) (g) (h) (i)

Figure 12.6 Scanning laser ophthalmoscope fluorescein angiography

Series of frames ((b)–(i)) from the early phase of a fluorescein angiogram performed with the SLO. Time is indicated in the lower left. The whites boxes in (g) indicate locations of 3 × 3 sample windows placed on retinal arteries. The brightness within these 9 pixels (the image consists of 512 × 512 pixels) is averaged. The black box is placed on a vein in order to measure arteriovenous passage time. Frame (a) displays a red free image obtained before angiography begins.

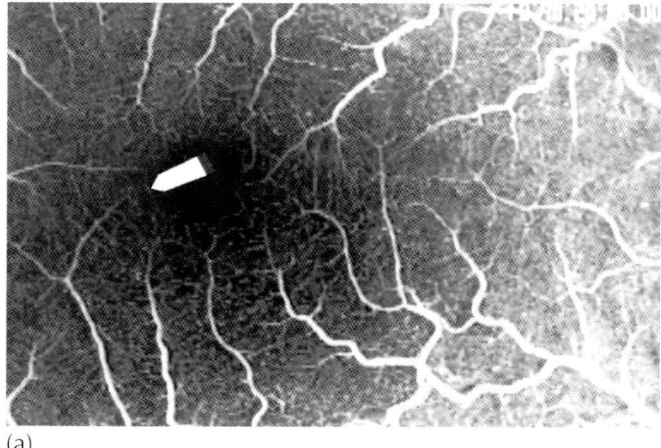
(a)

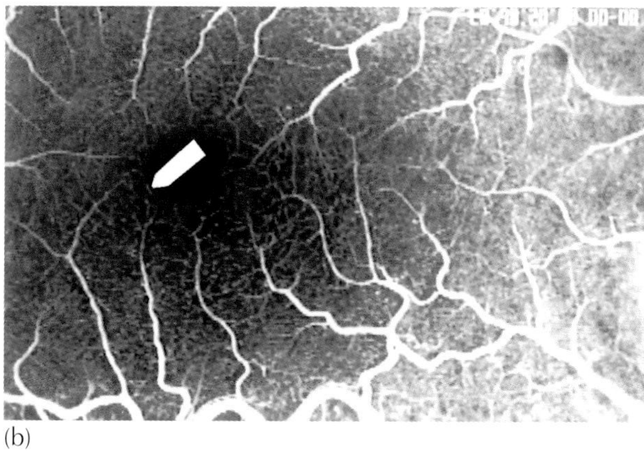
(b)

Figure 12.7 20-degree SLO angiography
Twenty-degree SLO angiography is used to measure capillary blood velocity in the perifoveal retina. This method can also be used to measure capillary velocities on the optic disc. Two successive frames ((a) and (b)) of a 20-degree image of the macula show the movement of fluorescein through the superficial nerve-fiber layer capillaries.

Hemodynamic measurements at 20 degrees

Measurements of blood velocity in the perifoveal retina were first estimated using the blue field entoptic phenomenon. Illuminated by a light blue light, the leukocytes cast a shadow on retinal receptors. In the perifoveal region, where the retinal capillaries thin to a single layer, these moving shadows are visible; the average subject describes their appearance as that of spermatozoa in a microscope. Using the blue field effect, Riva constructed a blue field entoptic simulator. The simulator allows a subject to adjust the density, speed, and pulsatility of simulated leukocyte shadows on a computer screen to match his own. Besides the subjectivity of this process, the problem with estimating blood velocity based on the movement of leukocytes is that leukocytes are much bigger than the retinal capillaries. Forcing their way through the capillaries, they must fold up by rubbing on the endothelial wall. Outnumbering the leukocytes by 600 to 1, the erythrocytes move more readily through the capillaries, making the forced movement of leukocytes an unrepresentative description of retinal capillary hemodynamics.

The SLO's high spatial and temporal resolution makes it possible to record microdroplets of fluorescein dye passing through the perifoveal capillaries. Dark areas between the bright droplets are thought to be rouleaux formations of erythrocytes. These droplets therefore represent the movement of red blood cells through the capillaries. If the intent of blood flow measurement is better understanding of the delivery of oxygen to tissue, this method, which concentrates on the movement of erythrocytes, is preferred for description of the velocity through retinal capillaries. Quantification is accomplished using the same system as the one used for measurement of the mean dye velocity in 40-degree angiograms. The number of frames required for bolus transit across the capillary is used to determine time, and the digital video analysis system is used to measure the length of the capillary. Combined, a precise measurement of capillary transit velocity (CTV) is obtained. In Figure 12.7, two successive frames of a 20 degree video segment are shown.

Thus, retinal blood velocities can be measured in the large retinal arteries using 40-degree fluorescein angiography, and capillary velocities in both the perifoveal and optic disc areas can be measured using a 20-degree field. Either measurement requires both an SLO and a video analysis system. Currently, the software required for this analysis is not commercially available.

Indocyanine green angiography: a new quantification method

Indocyanine green (ICG) dye is excited by near infrared light with maximum excitation at 805 nanometers, and maximum emission at 835 nanometers. These wavelengths of light are able to penetrate the retinal pigment epithelial layer and produce excellent images of choroidal structure. These structures are not visible using a 488 nanometer argon laser during fluorescein angiography. A technique has been developed which allows quantification of choroidal hemodynamics using ICG angiograms.

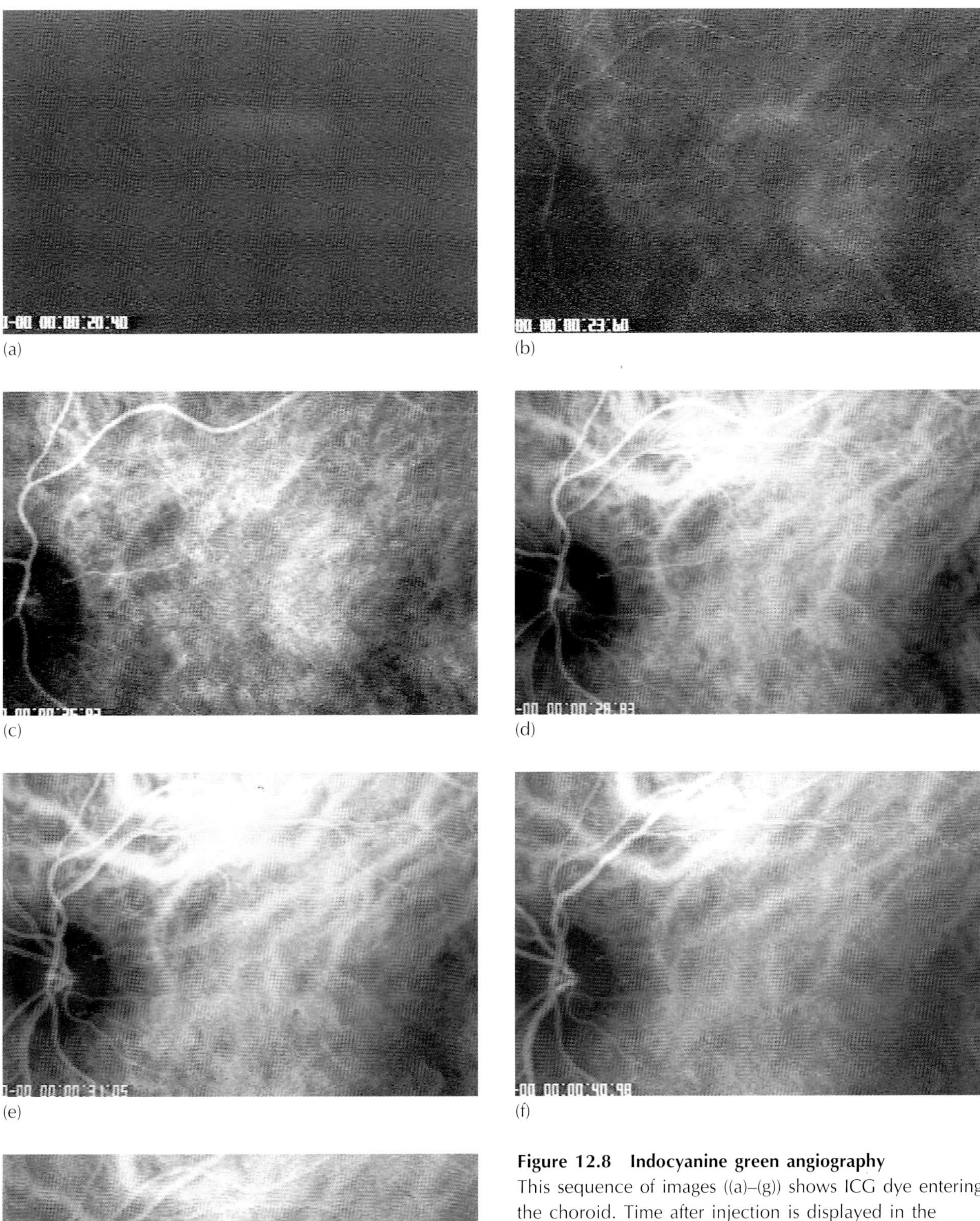

Figure 12.8 Indocyanine green angiography
This sequence of images ((a)–(g)) shows ICG dye entering the choroid. Time after injection is displayed in the lower left.

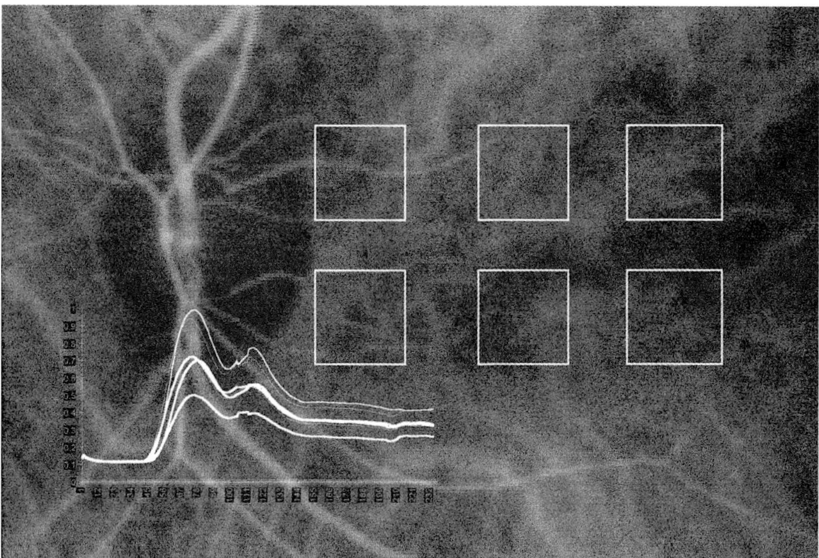

Figure 12.9 Indocyanine green angiography
Six large areas of choroidal hemodynamics are analyzed using ICG angiography. The average brightness of each area is graphed against time.

A modified injection technique is used. Twenty-five milligrams of ICG is dissolved into 2cc of dilute. One cubic centimeter of the solution is injected per examination. The small volume of dye allows a rapid injection time of less than one second. The injection is immediately followed by a 2cc saline flush. Like fluorescein angiography, verbal commands are used to guide subject fixation. Figure 12.8 demonstrates the appearance of dye in the choroid following intravenous injection. For ICG angiography, the nasal edge of the disc is situated at the edge of the 40-degree field of view. Examinations are recorded on S-VHS video tape and processed off-line. A digital image processor with customized software is used to perform the analysis. Six locations on the image are identified; two are near the optic disc located superiorly and inferiorly on the temporal side and four around the macula (Fig. 12.9). The average brightness in each of the six areas is computed for each frame of the angiogram. Area brightness is graphed with time on the x axis and brightness on the y axis. The analysis identifies three parameters from the brightness maps: slope, time to achieve 10% of total brightness, and curve width. The slope provides information concerning the average speed of dye entry into each area. The 10% time provides a more precise but noisier look at dye velocity into each area. The width of the curve provides information on the amount of time required for dye to enter and then leave the choroid. The mean value and range of all six areas are also computed.

Laser Doppler techniques

Laser Doppler technology has been employed to quantify ophthalmic blood flow in research. Until recently, the prevalent ophthalmic laser Doppler device was that of Riva's Occlux 5000, whose instrument consists of a modified fundus camera with the addition of a fiber-optic system. The operator must position an illuminating laser onto a location of interest, and a detector over the illumination point. The complexity and difficulty of operation have kept the Riva Laser Doppler Flowmeter (LDF) from gaining popularity clinically or in research.

Heidelberg Engineering GmbH of Heidelberg, Germany, has produced a scanning version of the LDF. The Heidelberg Retinal Flowmeter (HRF) scans the fundus, creating a map of retinal blood flow (Fig. 12.10). Three flow parameters are displayed: volume, flow, and velocity. Values are in arbitrary units, absolute values depending on the optical scattering characteristics of individual eyes.

As technology improves, the temporal and spatial resolution of hemodynamic measurements improves. When resolution surpasses the dimensions of capillaries new problems in data interpretation occur. Previous technologies, including Riva's LDF, measure flow per volume of tissue to describe local hemodynamics. When capillaries and the areas between them can be resolved, a quantitative method is required to describe this new information. Utilizing the high spatial resolution of the HRF, an analysis technique has been developed which quantifies capillary density in concert with quantification of blood flow within those same capillaries. Using the HRF, flow measurements of living tissue are obtained at a resolution sufficient to discern capillaries and the tissue between them (Fig. 12.11). The percentage of tissue between capillaries is calculated as a percentage of total tissue volume.

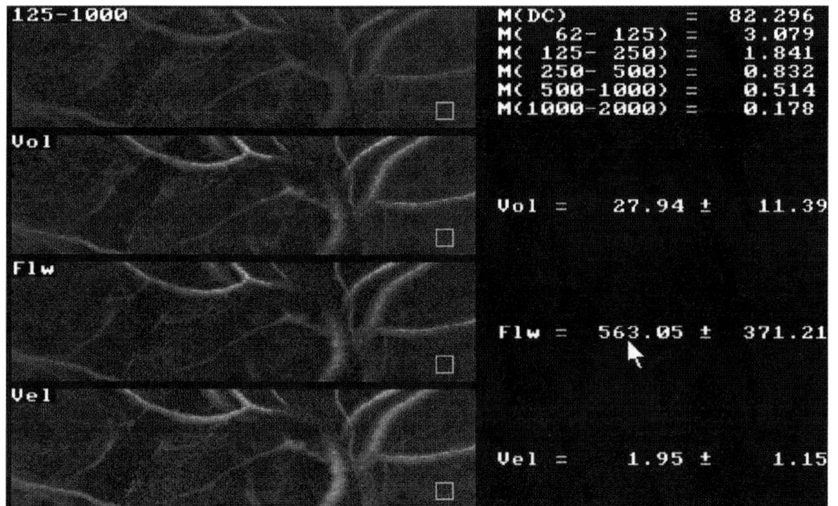

Figure 12.10 Heidelberg Retinal Flowmeter
The HRF produces a map of blood volume, flow, and velocity.

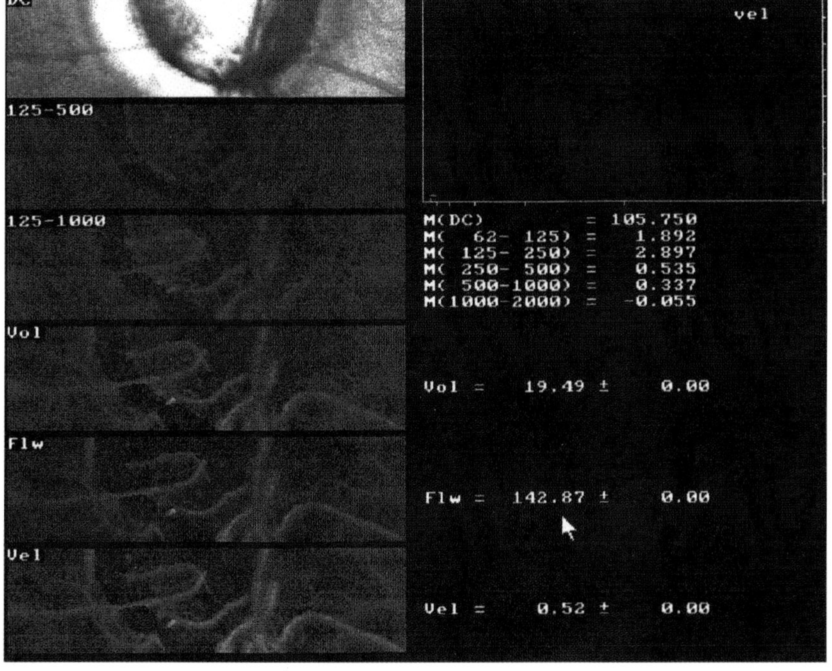

Figure 12.11 Heidelberg Retinal Flowmeter
A single pixel is used to probe the image and obtain all valid flow points.

Individual flow measurements within those same capillaries are described in a histogram (Fig. 12.12). Cumulative percentage landmarks are then used to describe the distribution of capillary flow. This provides a complete assessment of the hemodynamics in a given tissue.

Conclusions

Reporting use of these techniques, the literature contains numerous examples of altered blood flow in ophthalmic disease. What do the differences between normals and various glaucoma groups mean? Current technologies cannot be used to determine if altered blood flow is primary or secondary to nerve damage. Longitudinal studies may provide better insight into the role of ocular blood flow deficits in disease progression, but at a great cost in time and materials. As technology improves, more direct measurements may provide the answers to some basic questions:

- How great a blood flow deficit is necessary to cause glaucomatous damage?
- What is the threshold of perfusion deficit before nerve cell damage occurs?
- How can we identify this threshold?

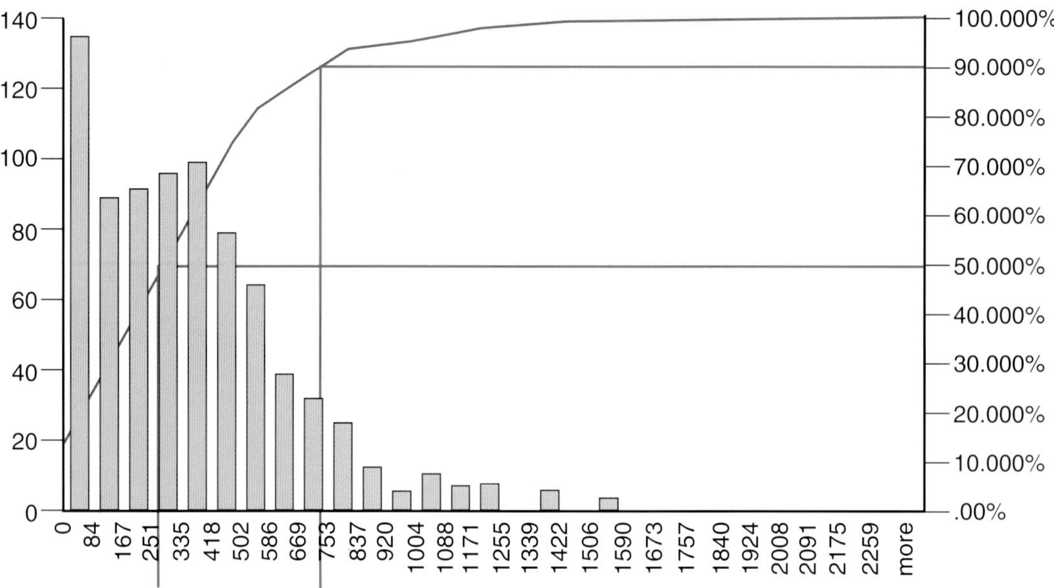

Figure 12.12 Heidelberg Retinal Flowmeter
Flow values are displayed on a histogram.

Measurement of metabolism may provide the answer. Several types of measurements would be of interest. Desired measurements include retinal oxymetry, quantification of metabolites, reduction/oxidation potentials, or perhaps ATP/NADH+ levels. Using spectral analysis of reflected light, work is underway in the development of retinal oxymetry, but a system suitable for clinical use is still years in the future. These measurements will allow us to fine tune glaucoma medications as we gain understanding of how various drugs affect the environment in which neurons must survive.

FURTHER READING

Anderson DR, Vascular supply to the optic nerve of primates, *Am J Ophthalmol* (1970) **70**:341.

Araki M, Anatomical study of vascularization of optic nerve, *Acta Soc Ophthalmol Jpn* (1975) **79**:101.

Duke-Elder WS, Text-book of ophthalmology. In: Vol 3 (St Louis, MO: CV Mosby, 1940), 3354.

Elschnig, *Hendbuch der speziellen pathologiseher Anatomie und Histologie. Volume 1* (Berlin: Julius Springs, 1928).

Gabel VP, Birngruber R, Nasemann J, Fluorescein angiography with the scanning laser ophthalmoscope, *Lasers and Light in Ophthalmol* (1988) **2**:35–40.

Harris A, Kagemann L, Cioffi GA. Assessment of human ocular hemodynamics: major review, *Surg Ophthalmol* (1998) **42**:509–33.

Harris A, Sergott RC, Spaeth GL, Katz JL, Shoemaker JA, Martin BJ, Color Doppler analysis of ocular vessel blood velocity in normal-tension glaucoma, *Am J Ophthalmol* (1994) **118**:642–9.

Hayreh SS, Structure and blood supply of the optic nerve. In: Heilmann K, Richardson KT, eds. *Glaucoma: conceptions of a disease: pathogenesis, diagnosis, therapy* (Stuttgart: George Theime, 1978), 78–96.

Kagemann L, Harris A, Cantor LB, Chung HS, Kristinsson JK, A new method for evaluating choroidal blood flow in glaucoma: area dilution analysis (ARVO), *Invest Ophthalmol Vis Sci* (1997) **38/4 (suppl)**:4892 (abst).

Lauber H, Treatment of atrophy of the optic nerve, *Arch Ophthalmol* (1936) **16**:555–68.

Loewenstein A, Cavernous degeneration, necrosis and other regressive processes in optic nerve with vascular disease of the eye, *Arch Ophthalmol* (1945) **34**:220–5.

Novotny HR, Alvis DL, A method of photographing fluorescence in circulating blood in the human retina, *Circulation* (1961) **24**:82–6.

Onda E, Cioffi GA, Bacon DB, Van Buskirk EM, Microvasculature of the anterior human optic nerve, *Am J Ophthalmol* (1995) **120**:92–102.

Pourcelot L, Indications de l'ultrasonographie Doppler dans l'etude des vaisseaux peripheriques, *Revue du Praticien* (1975) **25**:4671–80.

Powis RL, Color flow imaging: understanding its science and technology, *J Diag Med Ultrasound* (1988) **4**:236–45.

Reese AB, McGavic JS, Relation of field contraction to blood pressure in chronic primary glaucoma, *Arch Ophthalmol* (1942) **27**:845–50.

Riva CE, Grunwald JE, Sinclair SH, Laser Doppler measurement of relative blood velocity in the human optic nerve head, *Invest Ophthalmol Vis Sci* (1982) **22**:241–8.

Riva CE, Petrig B, Blue field entoptic phenomenon and blood velocities in the retinal capillaries, *J Opt Soc Am* (1980) **70**:1234–8.

Sinclair SH, Azar-Cavanagh M, Soper KA, et al. Investigations of the source of the blue field entoptic phenomenon, *Invest Ophthalmol Vis Sci* (1989) **30**:668–73.

Taylor KJW, Holland S, Doppler US part I. Basic principles, instrumentation, and pitfalls, *Radiology* (1990) **174**:297–307.

Wagemann A, Salzmann P, Anatomische Untersuchungen uber einseitige Retinitis Haemorrhagica mit Secondar–Glaucom nebst Mittheilungen uber dabei beobachtete Hypopyoian-Keratitis, *Arch fur Ophthalmologie* (1892) **38**:213.

Webb RH, Hughes GW, Delori FC, Confocal scanning laser ophthalmoscope, *Appl Opt* (1987) **26**:1492–9.

Williamson TH, Harris A, Color Doppler ultrasound of the eye and orbit, *Surv Ophthalmol* (1996) **40**:225–67.

Wolf S, Toonen H, Koyama T, Meyer-Ebrecht D, Reim M, Scanning laser ophthalmoscopy for the quantification of retinal blood-flow parameters: a new imaging technique. In: Nasemann JE, Burk ROW, eds. *Scanning laser ophthalmoscopy and tomography* (Munich: Quintessenz, 1990), 91–6.

13 The developmental glaucomas

Carlo E Traverso and Diane C Lundy

Introduction

The congenital glaucomas are a broad group of entities defined as glaucoma associated with a developmental anomaly which is present at birth. Included in this group are primary congenital glaucoma as well as glaucoma associated with other developmental anomalies, both ocular and systemic. The term developmental glaucoma is synonymous with congenital glaucoma.

Primary congenital glaucoma

Primary congenital glaucoma is characterized by an isolated trabeculodysgenesis in the absence of visible iris or corneal abnormalities. On examination, two major types of peripheral iris profiles may be seen: a flat iris insertion and a 'wrap around' configuration (Figs 13.1 and 13.2). A more severe variant of the disease exhibits peripheral iris stromal atrophy and anomalous iris vessels (Figs 13.3–13.6). Figure 13.5

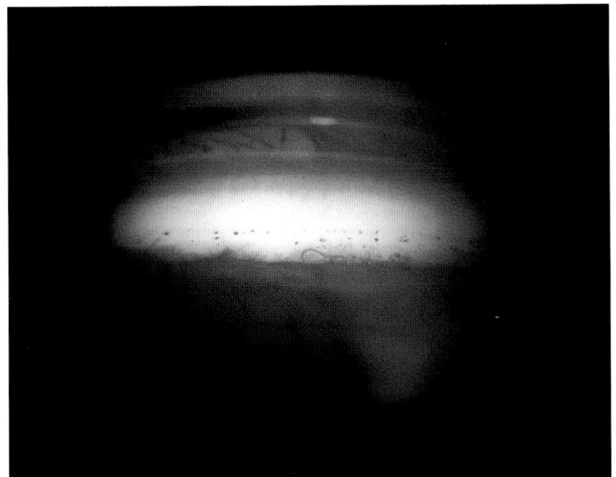

Figure 13.1 Developmental glaucoma, gonioscopic view
Note flat iris profile with anterior insertion. The iris processes extend irregularly over the ciliary band and pigment granules are scattered up to Schwalbe's line. One anomalous vascular loop is visible over the trabecular meshwork.

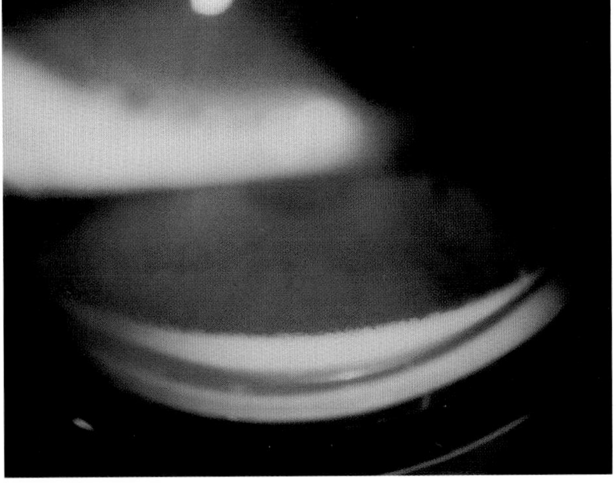

Figure 13.2 Developmental glaucoma, gonioscopic view
Note concave peripheral iris profile with 'wrap around' configuration.

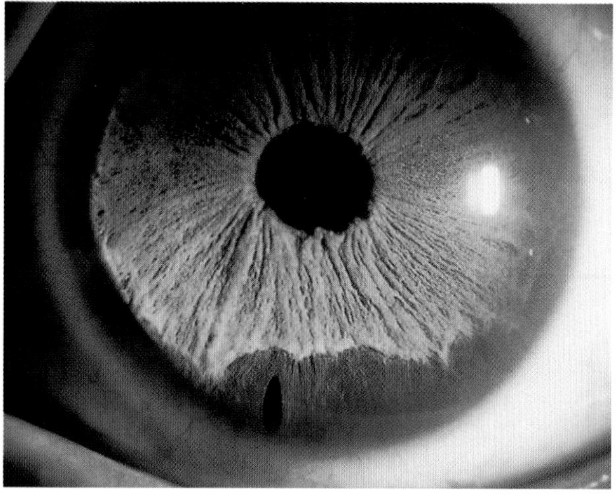

Figure 13.3 Iris hypoplasia
The superficial stroma is thin, especially in the inferior periphery and there is hypoplasia of the sphincter muscle.

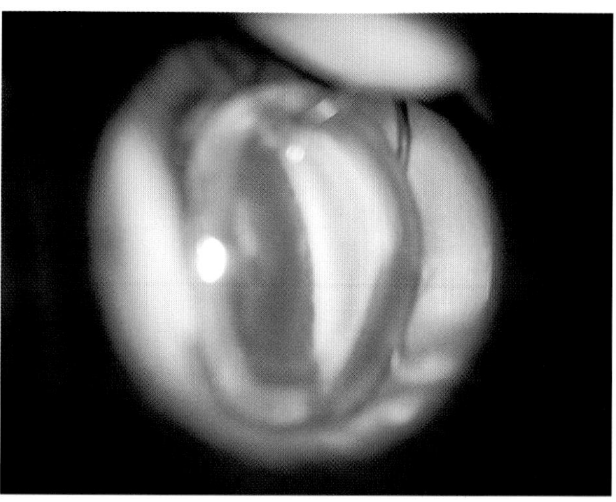

Figure 13.4 Gonioscopic view of anomalous vessels on iris surface

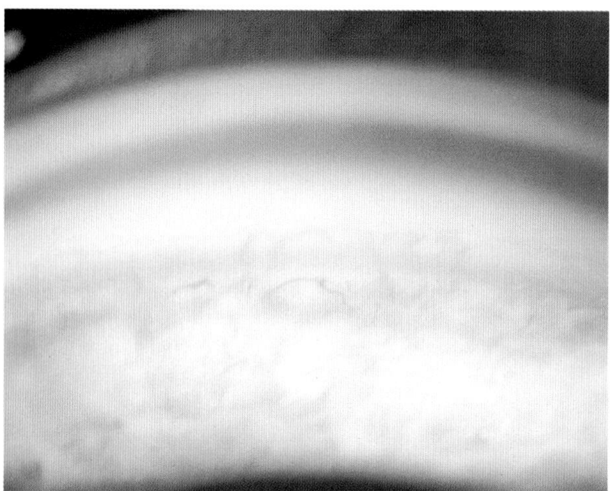

Figure 13.5 Gonioscopic view of normal iris surface vessels for comparison
Note exposed greater iris circle vessels which are commonly seen in patients with light-colored irides.

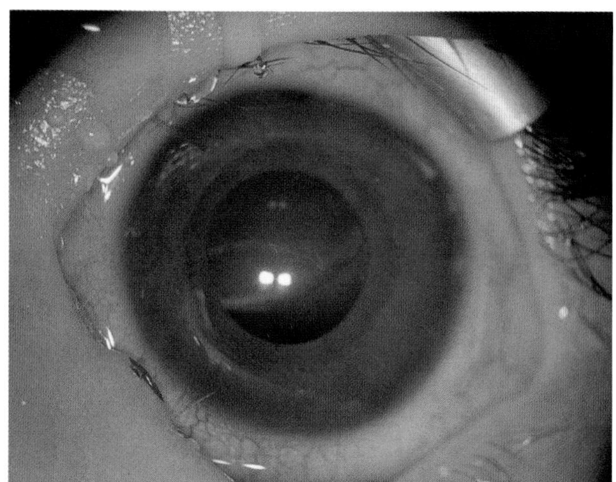

Figure 13.6 Spontaneous lens subluxation in a 12-month old infant with primary congenital glaucoma and buphthalmos

illustrtates normal iris vessels for comparison. The inheritance is sporadic with glaucoma occurring in approximately 1/12 500 live births, although a higher incidence is seen in the setting of consanguinity. Two-thirds of the patients are male with bilateral disease in approximately 75% of cases. Some clinicians further classify congenital glaucoma by age of onset: congenital (at birth), infantile (after birth, up to age 2 years), and juvenile (after age 2 years).

The treatment of primary congenital glaucoma is largely surgical (see Chapter 19), although medications may be used acutely to gain control of intraocular pressure and minimize corneal edema while awaiting surgery. Prognosis is related to the age of disease onset with a poorer prognosis associated with onset at birth. Even with successful IOP control, visual outcome may be limited by associated ocular problems such as myopia, retinal detachment, and lens subluxation from pressure-induced buphthalmos (Fig. 13.6), as well as corneal decompensation and amblyopia.

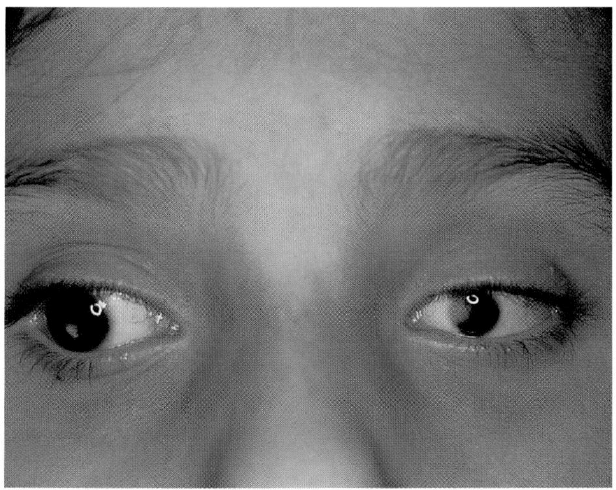

Figure 13.7 Microcornea OS in patient with Rieger's anomaly and bilateral glaucoma

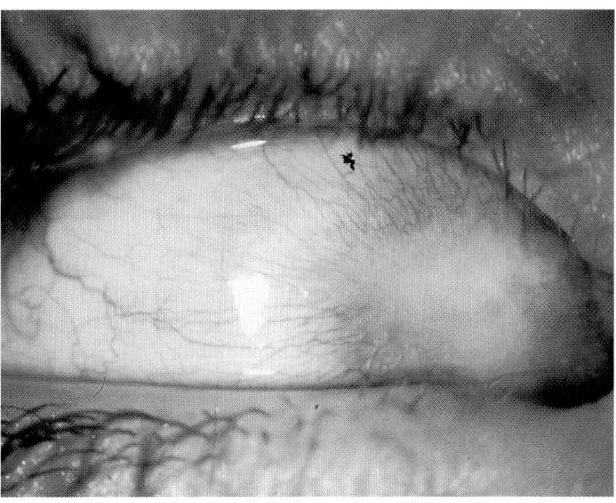

Figure 13.8 Sclerocornea

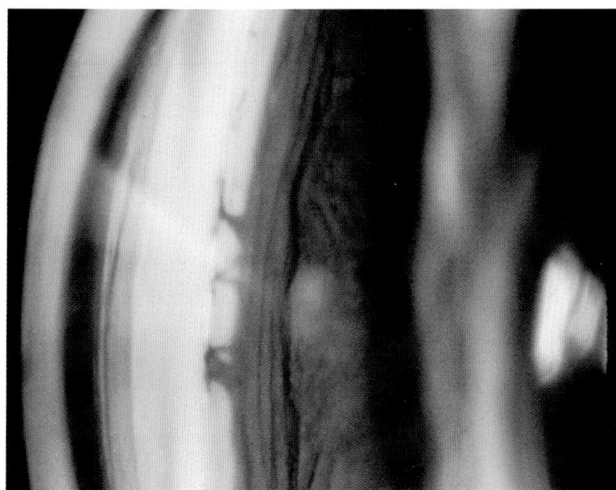

Figure 13.9 Axenfeld's anomaly, gonioscopic view
T-shaped strands of iris tissue bridge over the angle recess up to Schwalbe's line.

Congenital glaucoma associated with inherited anomalies

Ocular anomalies

Corneal anomalies

Microcornea, defined as a corneal diameter of less than 10 mm, is not a specific disease but rather associated with other ocular conditions such as persistent hyperplastic primary vitreous, nanophthalmos, micro-ophthalmos, rubella, and Rieger's syndrome (Fig. 13.7). Glaucoma may result from angle closure secondary to anterior segment crowding. Similarly, cornea plana and sclerocornea can be associated with angle anomalies and glaucoma (Fig. 13.8).

Iris/corneal anomalies

Axenfeld/Rieger/Peter's comprise a group of conditions known as anterior segment dysgenesis syndrome to reflect their proposed etiology. Recalling that corneal endothelium, trabecular meshwork, Schlemm's canal, and the iris stroma all develop from neural crest tissue, it is hypothesized that altered embryologic development of neural crest tissue leads to the spectrum of clinical findings in this group of diseases.

Axenfeld's anomaly is characterized by T-shaped iris strands drawn up to a prominent Schwalbe's line as well as anterior iris stromal atrophy (Figs 13.9 and 13.10). It is bilateral with an autosomal-dominant inheritance pattern. Up to 50% of patients may develop glaucoma which presents in infancy or later.

Rieger's anomaly is further along this clinical spectrum and shares many of the findings of Axenfeld's with a greater degree of anterior iris stromal atrophy. Findings include polycoria, corectopia, and pupillary distortion (Figs 13.11–13.13). Like Axenfeld's anomaly (and unlike iridocorneal endothelial syndrome), it is bilateral with an autosomal-dominant inheritance pattern. Glaucoma is present in roughly 50% of patients with onset in infancy or later. Nonocular anomalies may also be present and include dental (hypo- and microdentia), facial (hypotelorism, malar hypoplasia), and

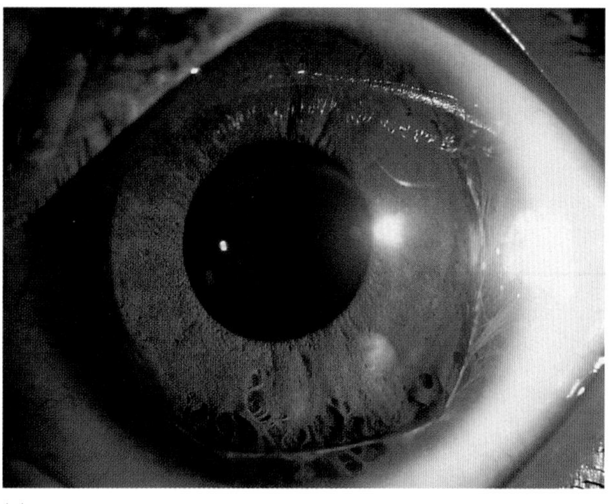

(a)

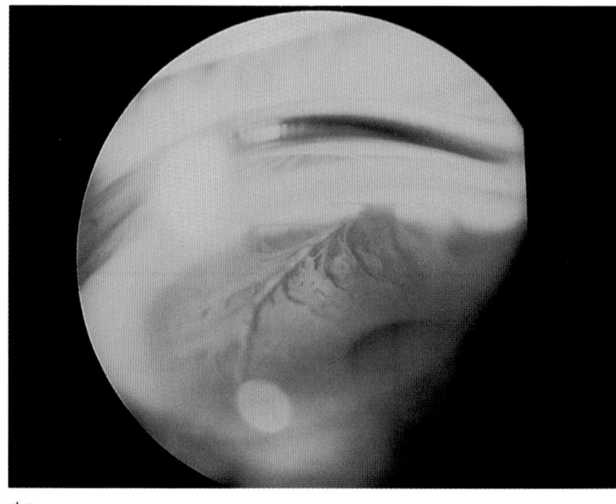

(b)

Figure 13.10 Axenfeld's anomaly with posterior embryotoxon
(a) The posterior embryotoxon seems to have been pulled from the angle wall so that it lies over the iris surface like a clothes-line.

(b) Gonioscopic view shows the suspended embryotoxon as a refractile rope with multiple strands of iris attached to it.

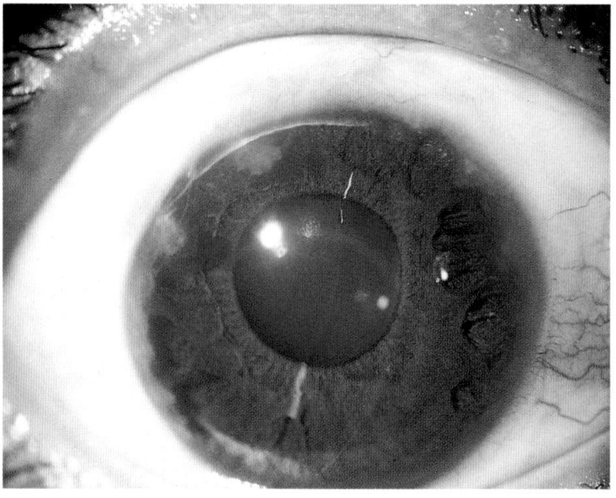

Figure 13.11 Rieger's anomaly
Note adhesions extending to the midperiphery of the cornea. A posterior embryotoxon is prominent in the superior quadrant.

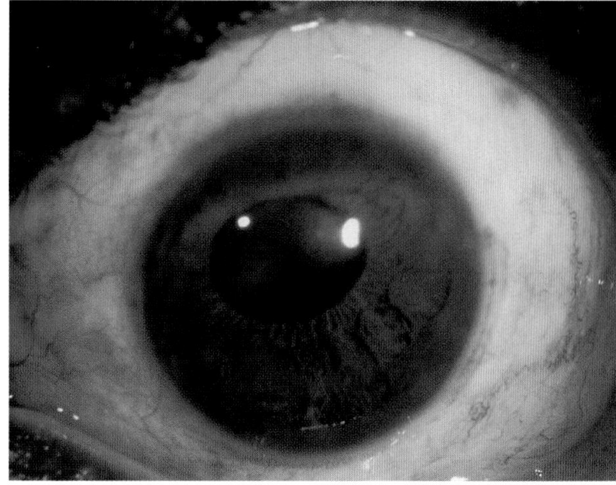

Figure 13.12 Rieger's anomaly
There are wide adhesions and the cornea is hazy in the affected areas.

systemic findings (short stature, cardiac defects, empty sella, deafness, and mental deficiency). The term Rieger's syndrome is used when nonocular and systemic findings are present.

Peter's anomaly is characterized by a central cornea opacity and adhesions between the iris collarette and corneal endothelium. Often there is absence of corneal endothelium and Descemet's membrane as well as stroma thinning underlying the central corneal opacity. Lenticular opacity may be present as well (Fig. 13.14). Of patients, 50% will develop open-angle glaucoma, even in the presence of normal-appearing angle structures. Glaucoma may present in infancy or later.

Iris anomalies
Aniridia is a bilateral inherited ocular abnormality which may occur sporadically or with an autosomal-dominant pattern. The sporadic form is associated with

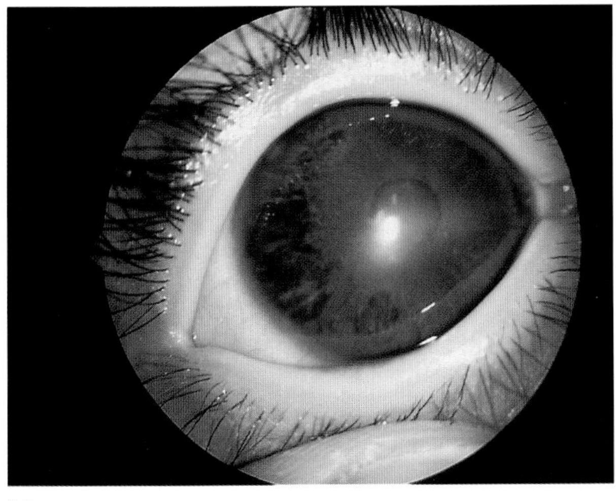

(a)

(b)

Figure 13.13 Rieger's anomaly
(a) Note marked iris hypoplasia with thinning of the peripheral anterior iris stroma allowing view of the posterior pigmented epithelium. (b) Transillumination defect of iris at 6 o'clock position.

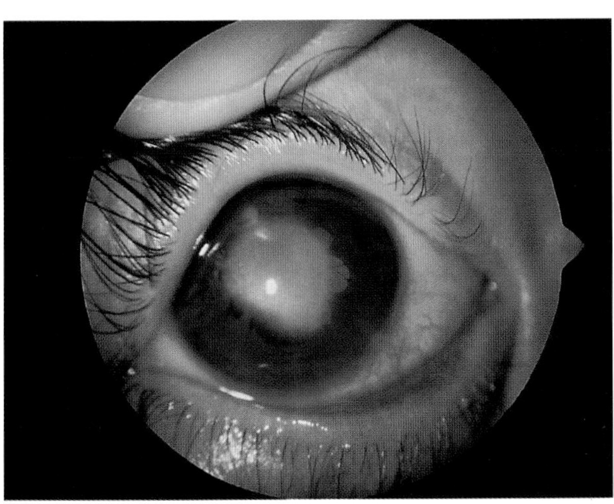

Figure 13.14 Peter's anomaly
Note central corneal opacity and iridocorneal adhesions.

a 20% prevalence of Wilm's tumor. In addition to glaucoma, ocular findings include: rudimentary stump of iris, corneal pannus, cataract, ectopia lentis, optic nerve and foveal hypoplasia, and nystagmus (Figs 13.15–13.17). The mechanism for intraocular pressure elevation may be adhesion of the iris stump to trabecular meshwork with progressive angle closure (late), or a primary trabeculodysgenesis (early). Glaucoma usually presents in the first three decades of life.

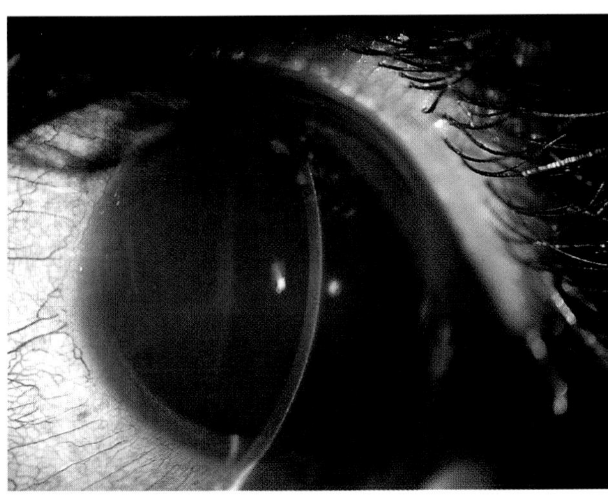

(a)

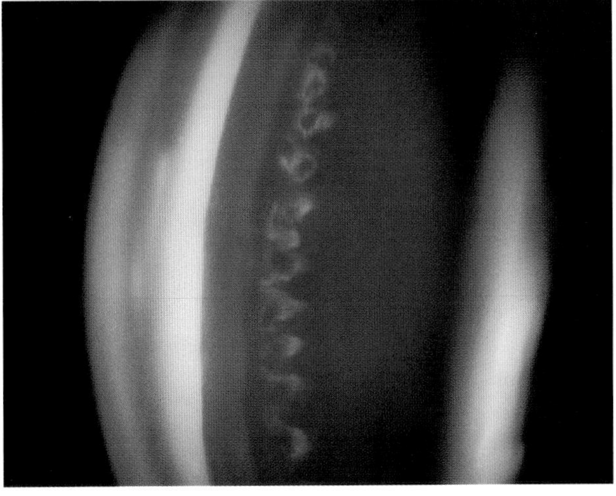

(b)

Figure 13.15 Aniridia
(a) Slit-lamp view. (b) Gonioscopic view. The angle is open.

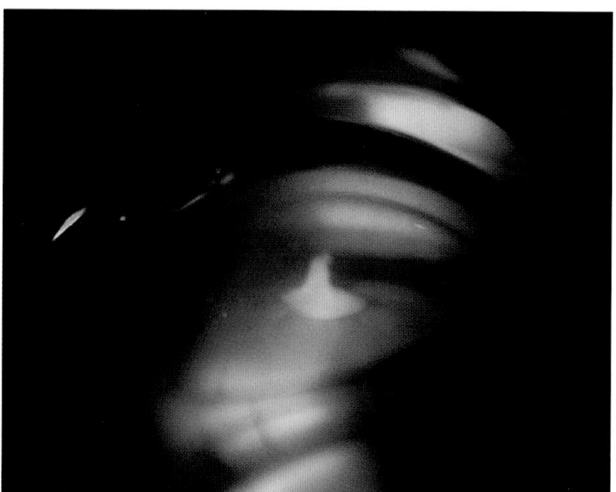

Figure 13.16 Aniridia, gonioscopic view
There is a peripheral iris stump only. Note lens opacity with anterior pyramidal cataract.

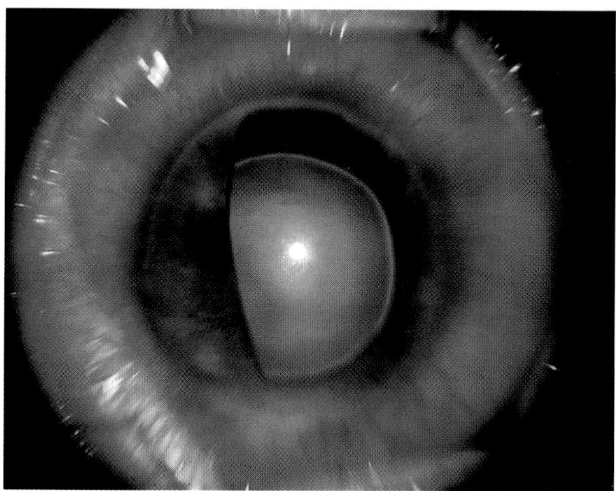

Figure 13.17 Aniridia, partial, slit-lamp view

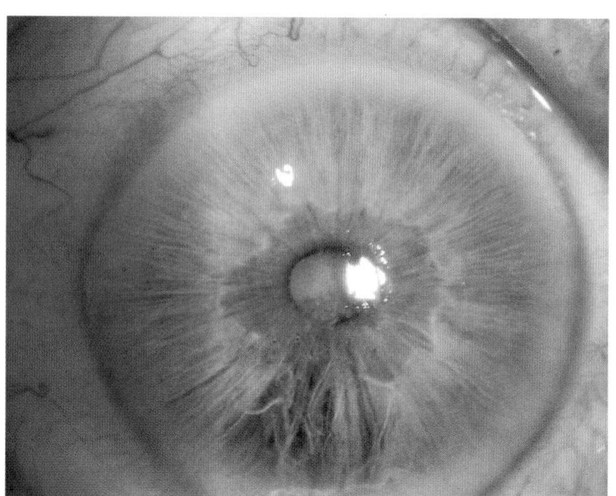

Figure 13.18 Iridoschisis in a 70-year-old patient with senile cataract

Iridoschisis usually occurs after the sixth decade of life but occasionally is seen in children. There is bilateral patchy iris dissolution in which the anterior stroma separates from the posterior stroma, most often in the inferior quadrants (Fig. 13.18). Iris strands from the anterior iris stroma may project into the angle causing peripheral anterior synechiae, leading to pressure elevation. Alternatively, pupillary block can occur with release of pigment and debris which further compromises outflow. Glaucoma occurs in about 50% of patients and is managed medically. Patients in whom pupillary block plays a significant role may benefit from laser peripheral iridotomy.

Lens

Microspherophakia may occur as an isolated finding or in association with systemic syndromes (see below). Clinically, the edges of the small spheric lens can be seen through the mid-dilated pupil. Other typical findings are high myopia and a shallow anterior chamber in a young person. Zonular laxity can lead to pupillary block with acute or chronic angle closure. Miotics make the pupillary block worse since they result in further anterior lens displacement.

Vitreous

Persistent hypertrophic primary vitreous—see micro-ophthalmia.

Globe

Nanophthalmos

The nanophthalmic eye is small but normally shaped. Small corneal diameter and short anterior-posterior length combined with a normal-sized lens leads to anterior segment crowding and angle-closure glaucoma in the fourth to sixth decades (Fig. 13.19). Increased scleral thickness may lead to choroidal effusions, which can occur spontaneously or following filtering surgery.

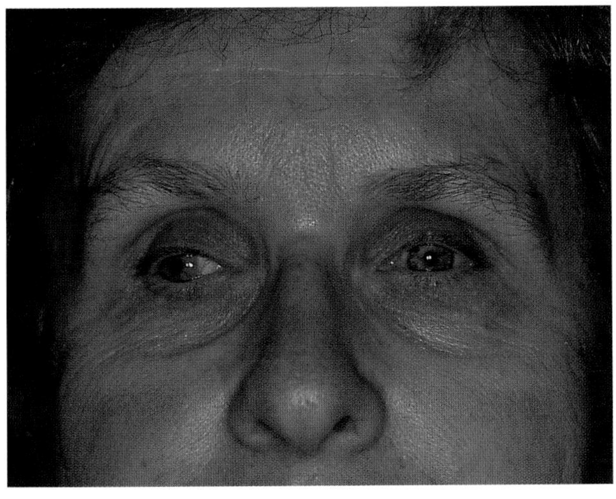

(a)

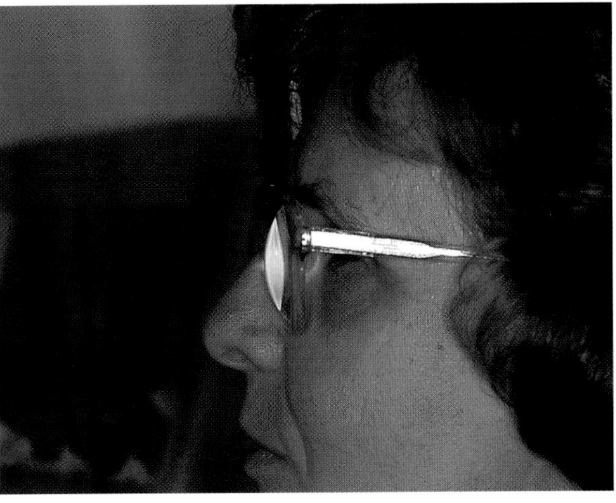

(b)

Figure 13.19 Nanophthalmos
(a) Note small-appearing eyes.

(b) The patient wearing her spectacles (the patient is phakic).

Systemic anomalies

Lowe's syndrome

Lowe's syndrome is an X-linked recessive condition with findings of aminoaciduria and mental retardation in affected males. Characteristic ocular findings are cataracts and open-angle glaucoma in infancy.

Sturge–Weber syndrome

The hallmark of the Sturge–Weber syndrome is the hemangioma. Facial hemangiomas are most common and occur in the distribution of cranial nerve V. When cranial hemangiomas are present, there may be an associated seizure disorder. Ocular findings include lid, choroidal, and episcleral hemangiomas (Fig. 13.20). Glaucoma may occur due to a primary angle dysgenesis (early) or increased episcleral venous pressure (late). Filtering surgery, which carries an increased risk of suprachoroidal hemorrhage, should be undertaken with great caution in patients with evidence of increased episcleral venous pressure such as blood in Schlemm's canal or dilated episcleral vessels.

Neurofibromatosis (von Recklinghausen's disease)

Neurofibromatosis is an autosomally inherited condition characterized by multiple neurofibromas, pigmented skin lesions (café au lait spots), osseous malformations, and associated tumors of the brain, spinal cord, and optic nerves. The skin neurofibromas may involve the eyelids and glaucoma occurs most commonly in this setting. The glaucoma may be due to a primary angle dysgenesis, synechial angle closure from neurofibroma tissue on the iris, or from direct infiltration of the angle by iris neurofibroma tissue.

Lens malposition syndromes

Several systemic conditions are associated with lens malposition and resulting pupillary block. Attenuated and broken zonules can lead to bilateral lens subluxation or complete dislocation into the anterior chamber (Fig. 13.21). Lens subluxation is typically superiorly in Marfan's syndrome and inferiorly in homocystinuria.

Marfan's syndrome has an autosomal-dominant inheritance and is characterized by arachnodactyly and tall stature. In addition to lens malposition and glaucoma, other ocular findings include microphakia, myopia, and retinal detachment. Systemic abnormalities include cardiac valve defects and congenital weakness of the aorta which may lead to the development of dissecting thoracic aortic aneurysms.

Homocystinuria is a rare autosomal recessively inherited defect of the enzyme cystathione synthetase. Patients are characteristically lightly pigmented and may have osteoporosis, mental retardation, and seizures as well as tall stature. General anesthesia carries a significant risk of thrombotic vascular occlusions and should be avoided in these patients.

Patients with Weill–Marchesani syndrome exhibit short stature with short fingers and microspherophakia.

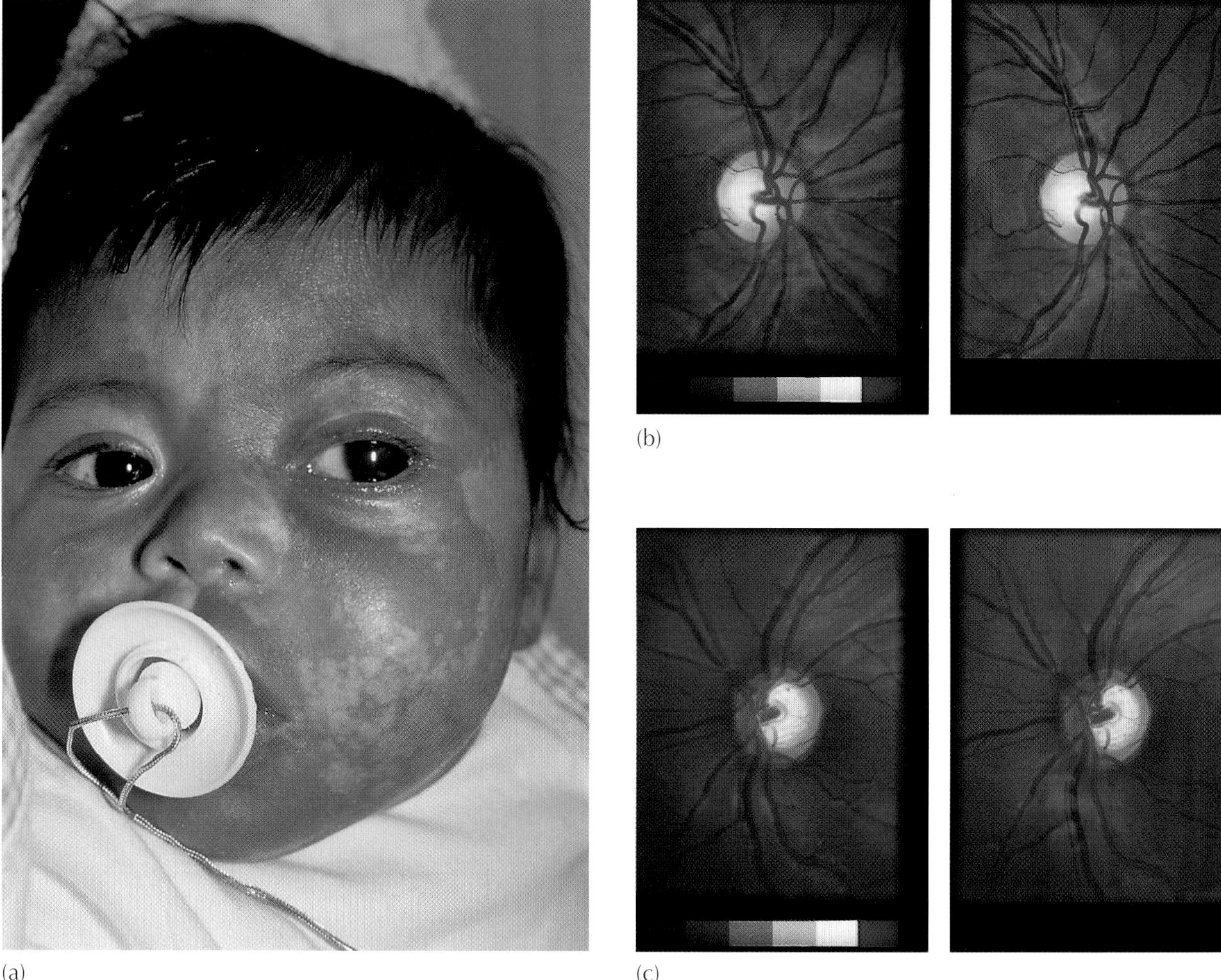

(a) (b) (c)

Figure 13.20 Sturge–Weber syndrome
(a) External examination. There is extensive facial hemangioma involving the trigeminal nerve. Note left hemifacial hypertrophy and buphthalmos in the left eye secondary to elevated intraocular pressure. (b) Normal fundoscopic examination of right eye. (c) Fundoscopic examination of left eye with cupping of optic nerve and 'tomato catsup' choroidal hemangioma.

Patient history and examination

Historical information which should be obtained includes: time of symptom onset, previous medical or surgical treatment, family history of glaucoma, family history of ocular or systemic congenital abnormality, perinatal history (gestation, maternal infections, drug use, delivery), and consanguinity.

The examination of the patient is crucial for diagnosis and management, since most decisions and treatment options will be formulated solely on the basis of measured objective findings. The collection of objective findings can be performed at three levels: office evaluation, examination under sedation, and examination under anesthesia. The choice of examination level is made according to the patient's age and degree of co-operation, the ability and habits of the examining ophthalmologist as well as the anticipated amount of ocular manipulation. Below six months of age, a reasonably detailed examination can be carried out by pacifying the infant with feeding.

After the crying triggered by administration of topical anesthetics has subsided, intraocular pressure measurement and gonioscopy are often possible without sedation. More complete examination (axial length, fundus photography, etc.) may warrant sedation or anesthesia with its attendant effects on intraocular measurement (see below).

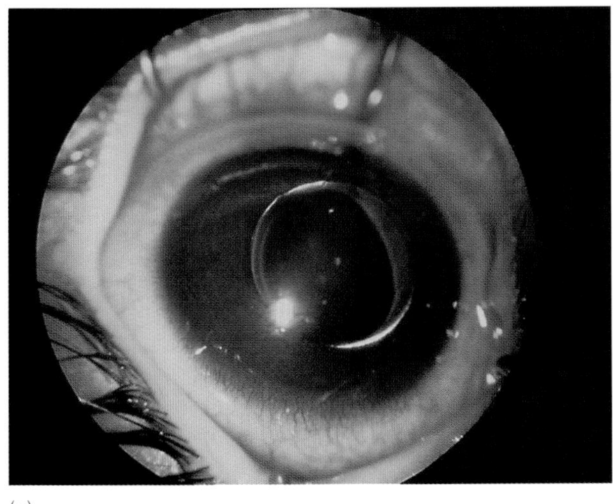
(a)

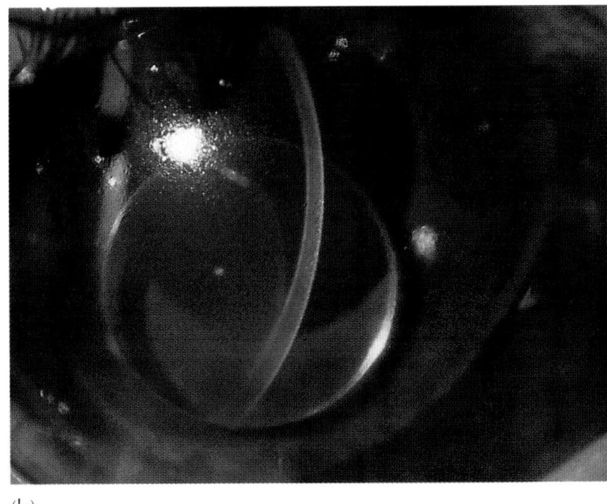
(b)

Figure 13.21 Homocystinuria with dislocation of the lens into the anterior chamber ((a) and (b))

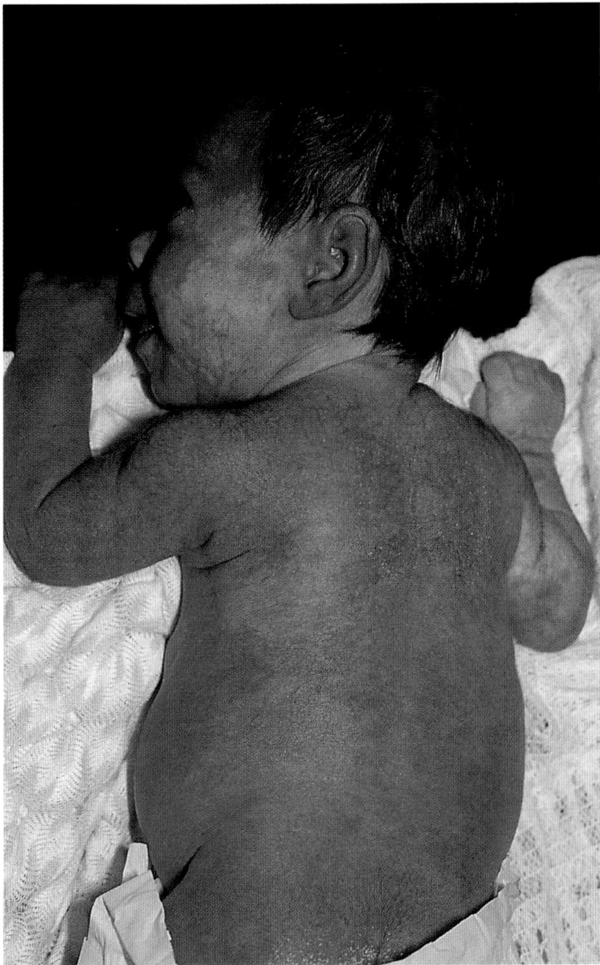

Figure 13.22 External examination of infant with Klippel–Trenaunay–Weber syndrome and bilateral developmental glaucoma
Note hemangiomas of trunk and limbs.

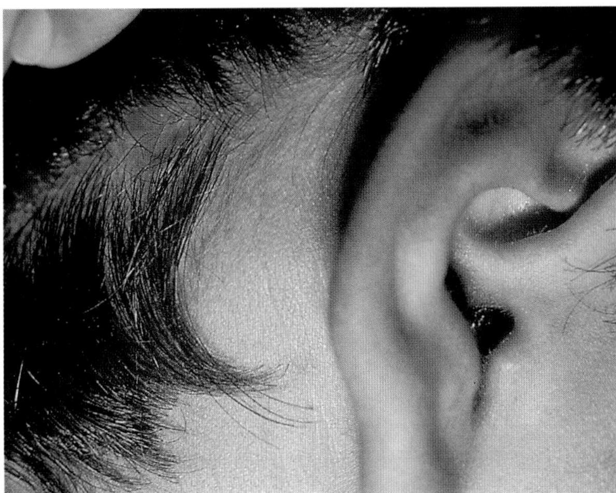

Figure 13.23 Head and neck examination of patient with developmental glaucoma
Note ear-lobe malformation and scalp fibroma.

Examination should commence with the nonocular structures to include the body, head, face, and extremities (Figs 13.22–13.26). Nonocular findings may help make the diagnosis of a systemic syndrome associated with developmental glaucoma. Attention is next directed to the ocular examination beginning with assessment of visual function (acuity, nystagmus, and amblyopia) as well as determination of gross visual field defects, if possible.

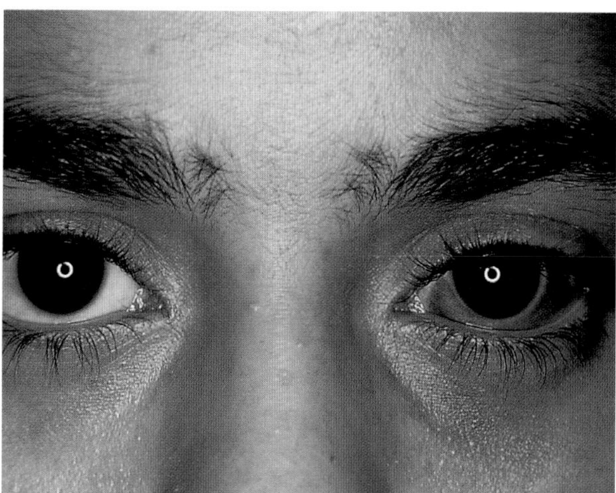

Figure 13.24 External examination in patient with oculodermal melanocytosis involving the second branch of the trigeminal nerve and elevated intraocular pressure left eye
Note pigmentation of left lower lid and left sclera/episclera.

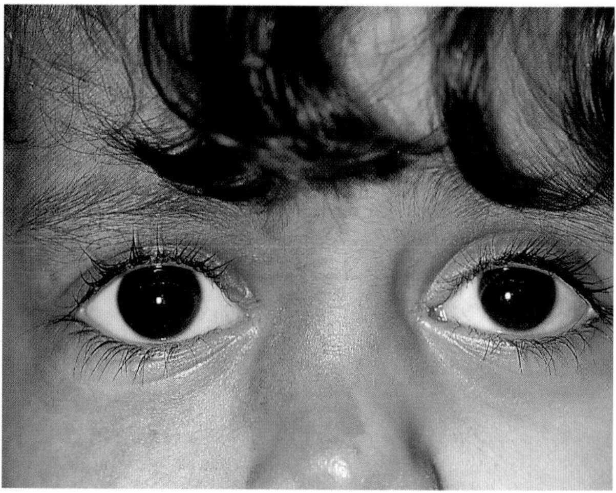

Figure 13.25 External examination of patient with Sturge–Weber syndrome
Note right facial hemangioma involving the second branch of the trigeminal nerve.

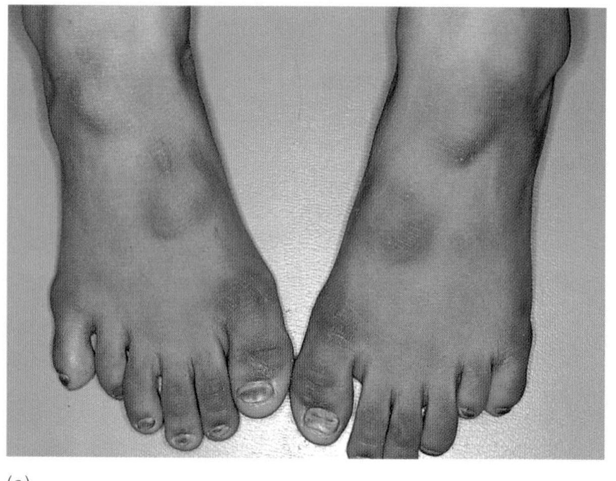

(a)

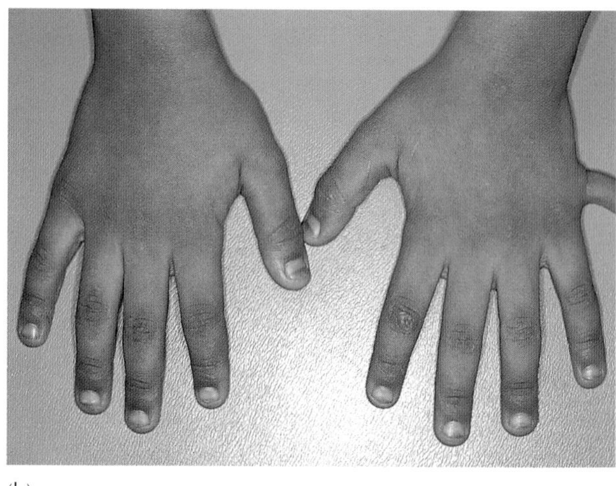

(b)

Figure 13.26 External examination of patient with developmental glaucoma and polydactyly
(a) Of feet.

(b) Of hands.

Intraocular pressure may be measured in a number of settings and by a variety of methods. In the office, the young (less than 6 months old) infant can usually undergo accurate measurement with topical anesthetic while nursing. The Tonopen or Schiotz tonometer are most commonly used in this setting. For infants under sedation or general anesthesia, the pneumotometer or Perkins type are additional methods (Figs 13.27 and 13.28). Since most sedatives do not have a corneal anesthetic effect, use of topical anesthetic should be considered. During examination under general anesthesia, the best time for tonometry is right after induction. There are numerous factors which affect tonometry measurements regardless of the method used, including sedation and anesthesia, corneal abnormalities, and positive pressure on the periocular tissues (Figs 13.29 and 13.30).

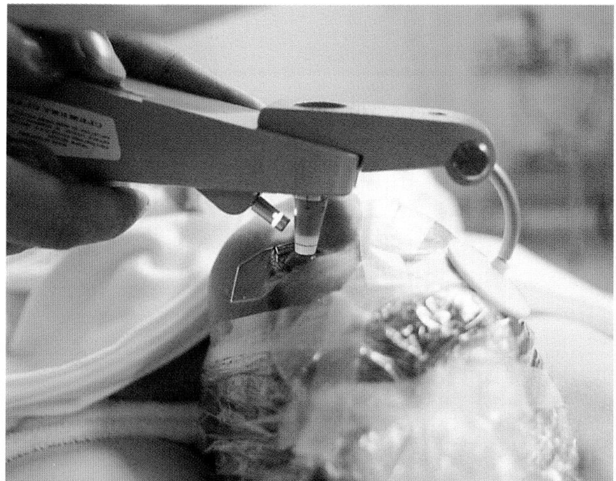

Figure 13.27 Perkins applanation tonometer
The counterbalance modification to the Goldmann applanation tonometer allows measurement of intraocular pressure in the supine position during examination under anesthesia.

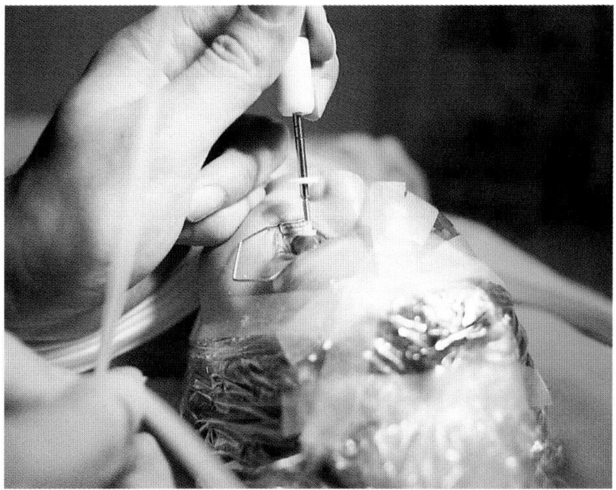

Figure 13.28 Pneumotonometer in use to measure intraocular pressure during examination under anesthesia

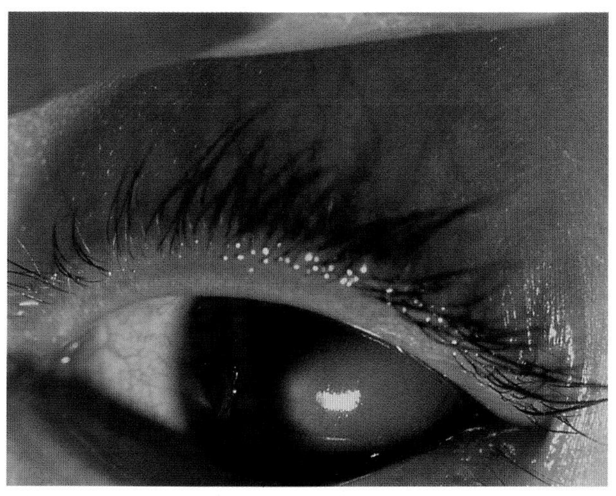

(a)

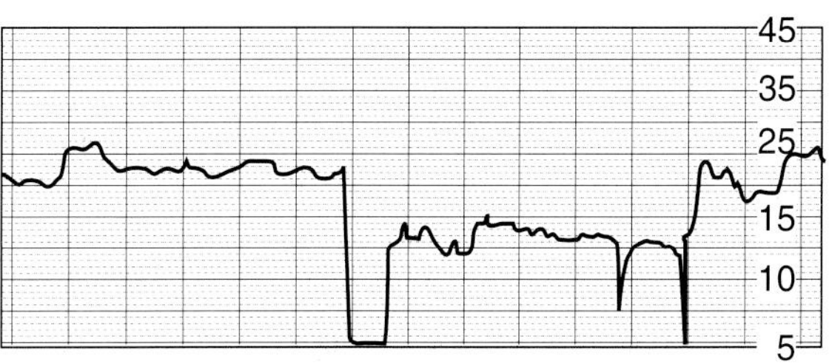

(b)

Figure 13.29 Tonometry artifacts, corneal abnormalities
In this eye, differing tonometry tracings were obtained over normal and abnormal cornea. (a) External corneal examination.

(b) Tonometry tracings (photographs courtesy of M Jaafar, MD, Washington, DC).

The external examination often reveals the characteristic triad of photophobia, buphthalmos, and epiphora secondary to elevated intraocular pressure-induced globe and corneal enlargement (Figs 13.31 and 13.32). Corneal enlargement and decompensation with edema may be reversible with effective lowering of intraocular pressure (Fig. 13.33). Corneal diameter is measured and monitored as an indication of long-term intraocular pressure control in young children (Fig. 13.34). Beyond the age of 3–4 years, there is limited enlargement because the sclera and cornea are less distensible. Dramatic changes may be seen in patients with advanced disease resulting in corneal ectasia or scleral thinning (Fig 13.35). Often, a less obvious degree of scleral thinning is present in these children which poses a risk of inadvertent perforation with scleral incisions and suture passes during glaucoma filtering and shunt surgery (Fig. 13.36).

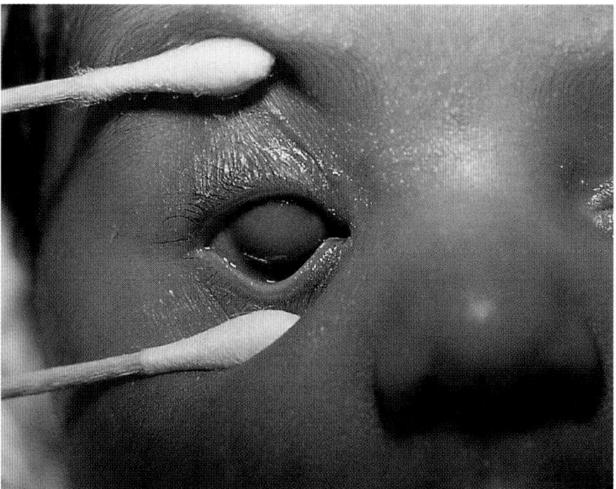

Figure 13.30 Tonometry artifacts, tight lids
When the lid fissure is very small, one might artificially increase intraocular pressure by applying pressure through the lids. This illustrates a method of opening the fissures by placing cotton-tipped applicators over the bony orbits to minimize this artifact.

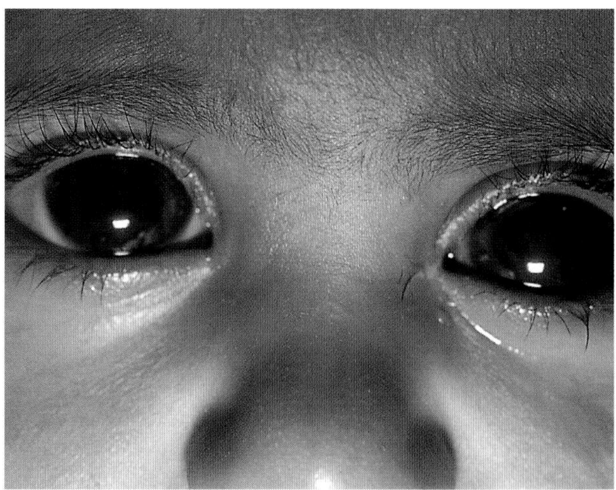

Figure 13.31 Epiphora and corneal diameter enlargement in child with congenital glaucoma

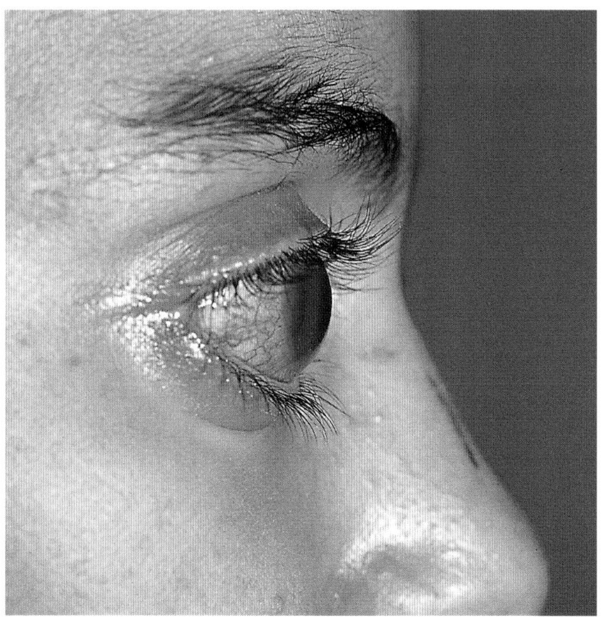

(a)

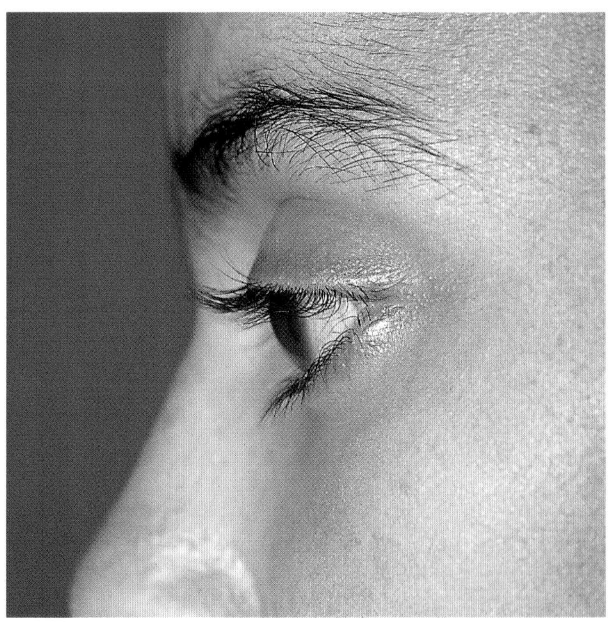

(b)

Figure 13.32 Buphthalmos in right eye of child with congenital glaucoma
(a) Right eye.
(b) Normal left eye.

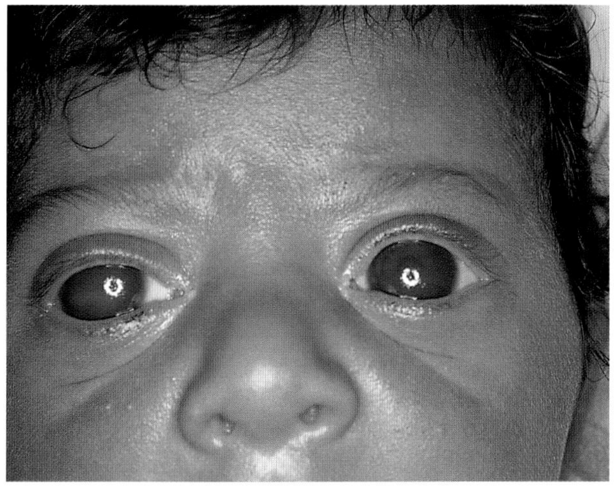

(a)

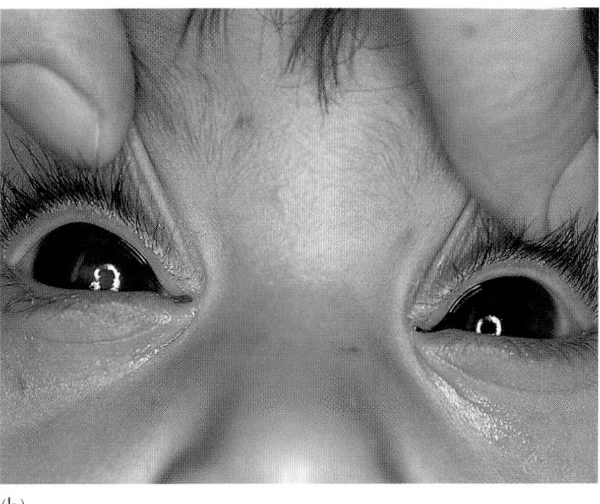

(b)

Figure 13.33 Reversible corneal edema in congenital glaucoma
(a) Bilateral corneal edema at pressures of 40 mmHg.
(b) Resolution of edema following trabeculotomy (pressure less than 20 mmHg).

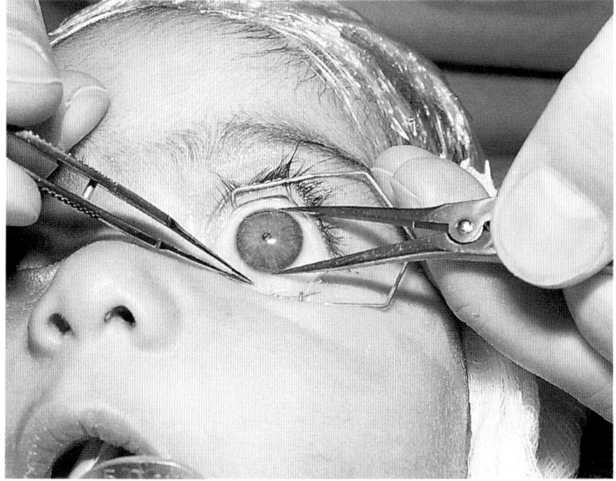

Figure 13.34 Measurement of corneal diameter during examination under anesthesia
Diameters are measured in the vertical and horizontal meridians with calipers.

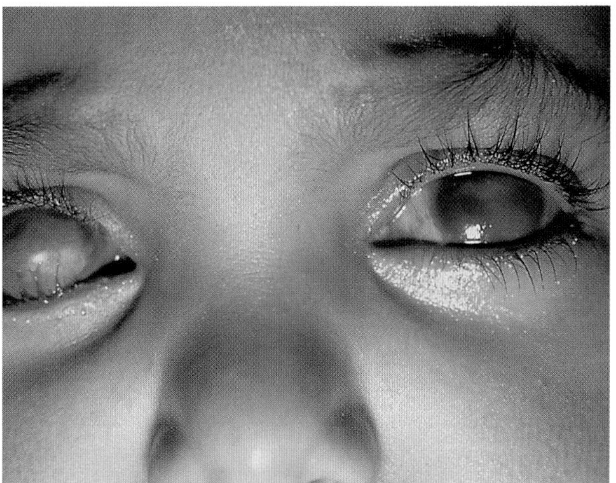

Figure 13.35 Corneal ectasia

Penlight examination of the cornea may reveal gross abnormalities such as an opacity or an irregular light reflex indicative of corneal edema. Slit-lamp examination (Fig. 13.37) permits a more detailed examination of the cornea and other anterior segment structures. Corneal findings include epithelial and stromal edema and breaks in Descemet's membrane. When Descemet's membrane is overstretched by pressure-induced corneal enlargement, linear breaks may occur. These breaks can result in acute stromal edema with accompanying photophobia (Fig. 13.38). Both edges of the ruptured membrane roll up, and when the cornea eventually clears, a typical pattern of rail-like defect is evident at the level of Descemet's membrane. Breaks occurring in congenital glaucoma are known as Haab's striae and are characterized by a horizontal orientation or a location parallel to the limbus (Fig. 13.39). They are

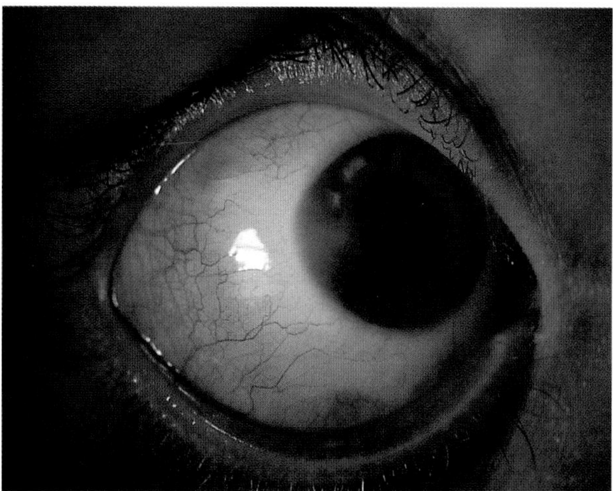

Figure 13.36 Scleral thinning with bluish appearance of underlying choroid

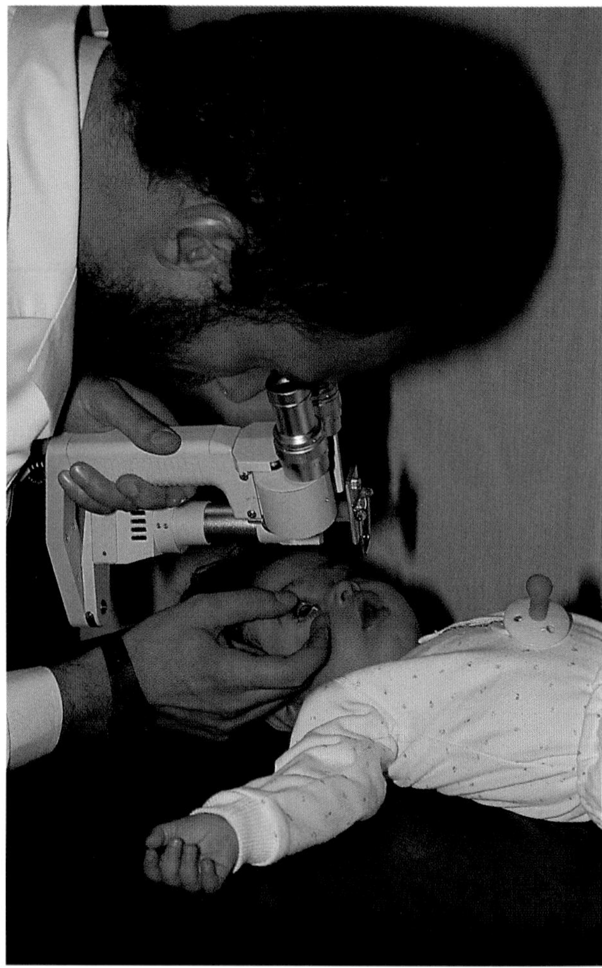

Figure 13.37 Examination under sedation; portable slit-lamp examination of anterior segment

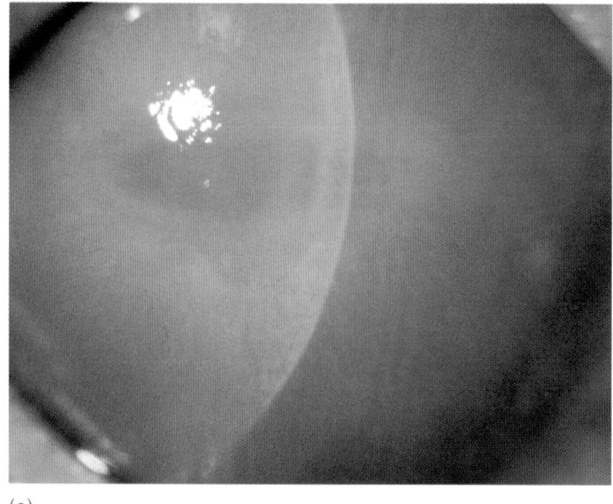

(a)

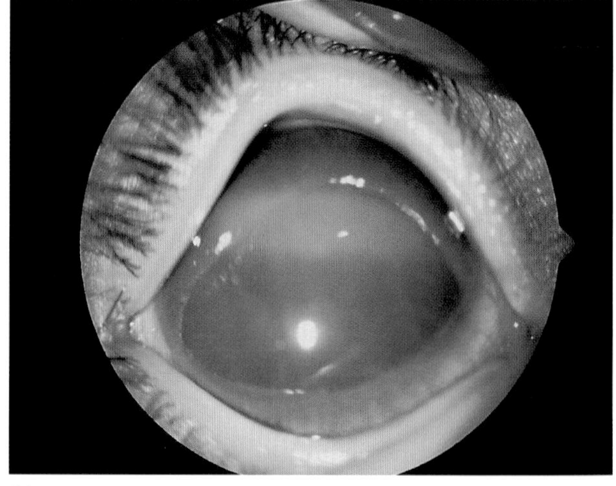

(b)

Figure 13.38 Acute corneal stromal edema secondary to breaks in Descemet's membrane
(a) Diffuse stromal edema.
(b) Clearing with scar over site of rupture.

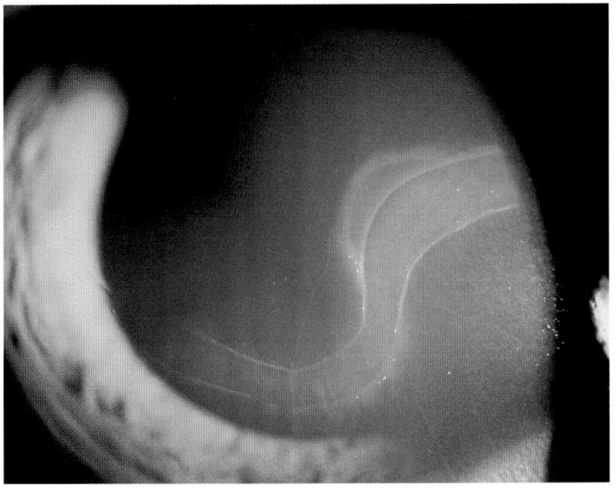

Figure 13.39 Haab's striae in congenital glaucoma
Note typical pattern of rail-like refractile material at the level of Descemet's membrane.

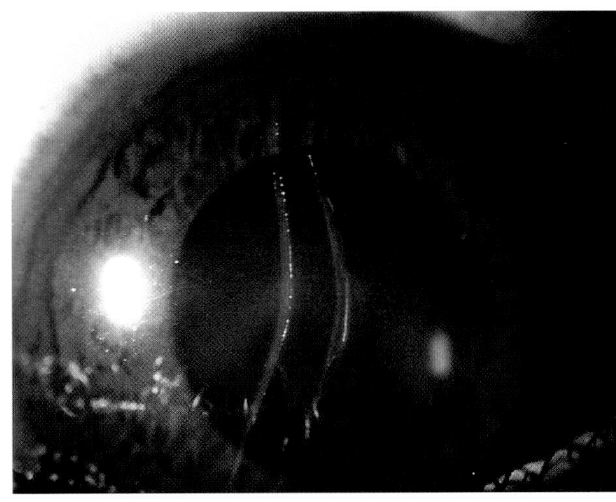

Figure 13.40 Birth trauma and breaks in Descemet's membrane
This child underwent a difficult forceps delivery. Note the vertical orientation of the corneal defect,

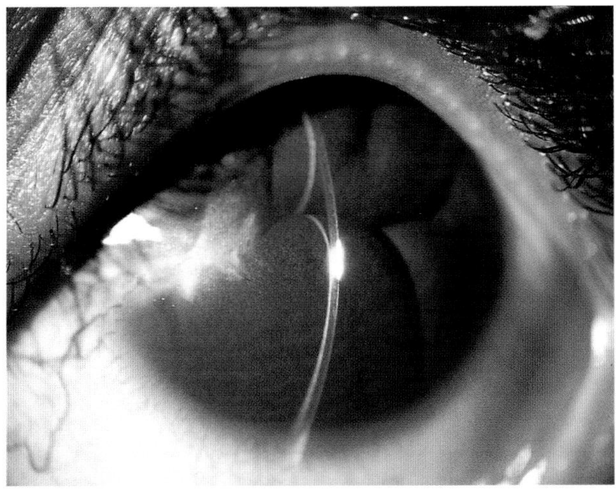

Figure 13.41 Shallow anterior chamber secondary to occluded pupil with complete pupillary block
This child had suffered a perforating injury in the past.

usually seen in the setting of elevated intraocular pressure and enlarged corneal diameter (greater than 10.5 mm in the horizontal meridian in the newborn infant). On the other hand, breaks due to birth trauma tend to run in any direction and are accompanied by normal intraocular pressure and normal corneal diameters (Fig. 13.40). Iris abnormalities such as atrophy and abnormal vessels are noted and the anterior chamber depth is assessed (Fig. 13.41). Lens clarity and position are noted as well as any evidence of phakodonesis.

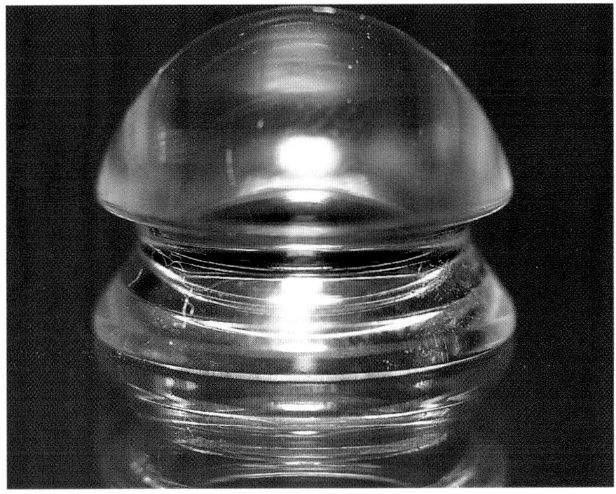

(a)

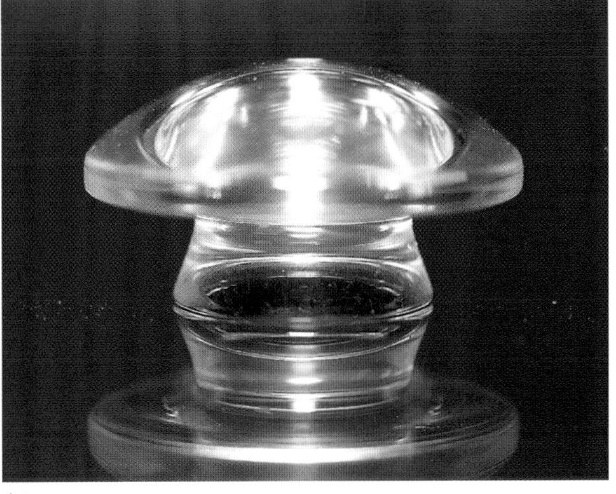

(b)

Figure 13.42 Direct goniolenses
(a) Koeppe lens. (b) Layden lens.

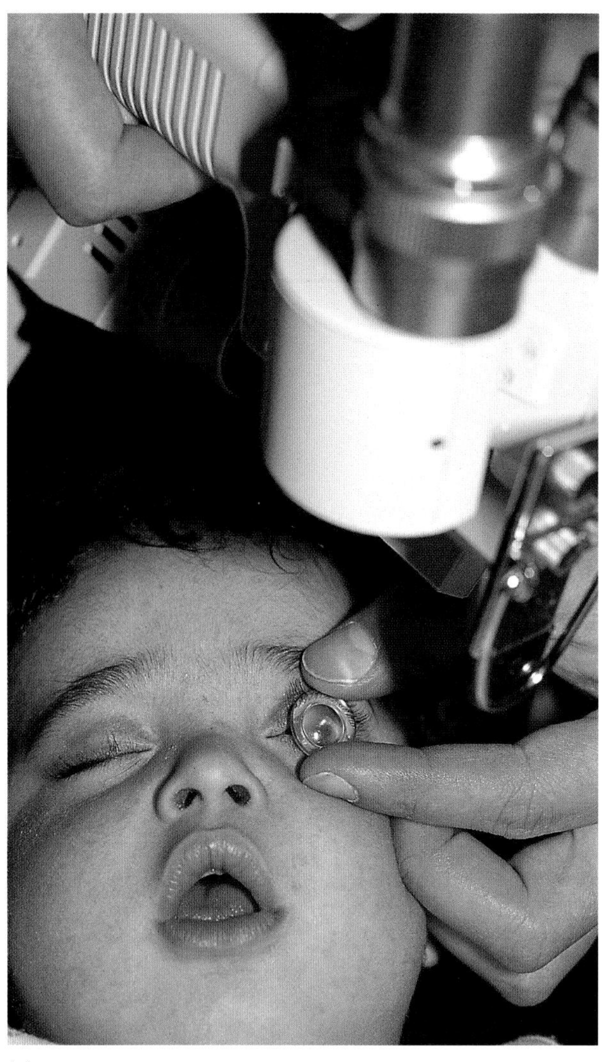

(a)

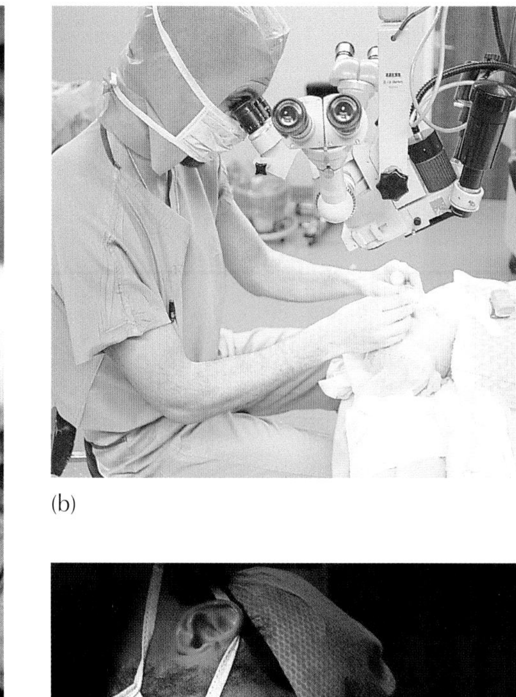

(b)

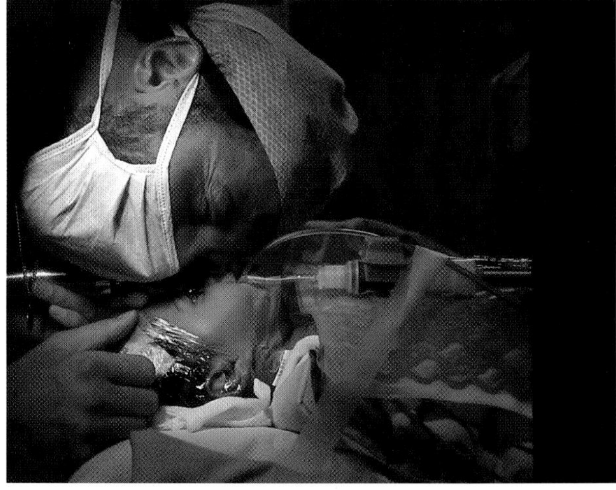

(c)

Figure 13.43 Gonioscopy with a direct goniolens and various light/magnification systems

(a) Portable slit lamp. (b) Tilted surgical microscope. (c) Direct ophthalmoscope with high plus lens dialed in.

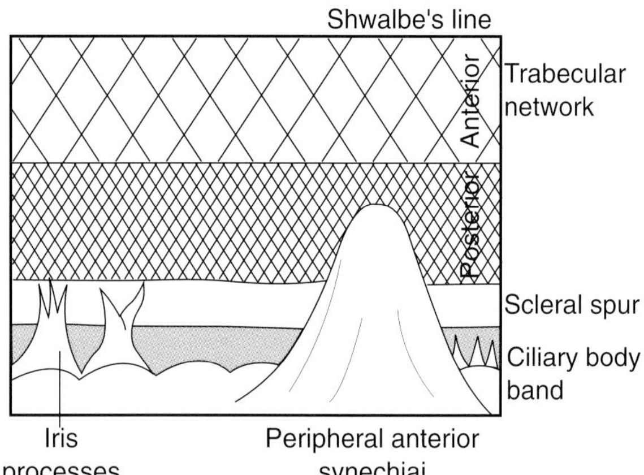

Figure 13.44 Anatomic landmarks on gonioscopy

Note the difference between peripheral iris processes and peripheral anterior synechiae.

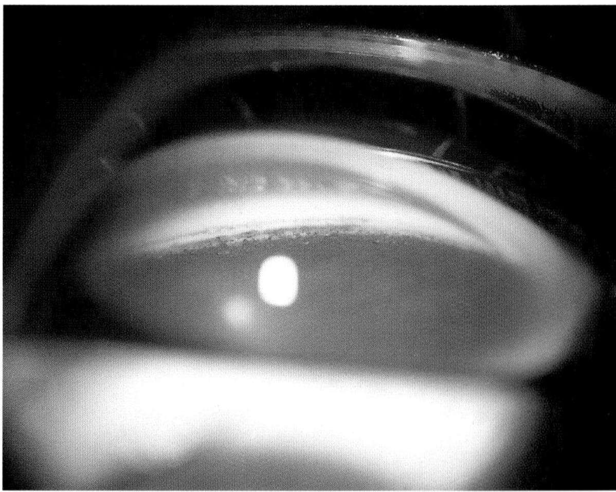

Figure 13.45 Primary congenital glaucoma, gonioscopic view

The iris insertion is posterior and flat. The ciliary body band is covered by iris processes and is barely visible. Grayish pigment is visible just anterior to Schwalbe's line.

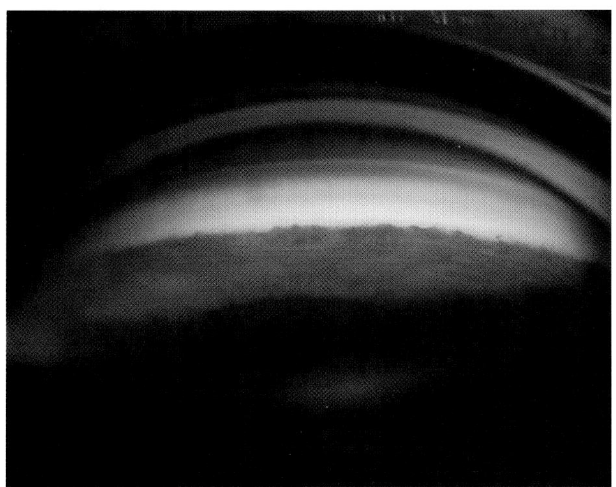

Figure 13.46 Primary congenital glaucoma, gonioscopic view
The iris insertion is anterior and flat. The tissue of the iris base extends to cover the scleral spur and most of the trabecular meshwork.

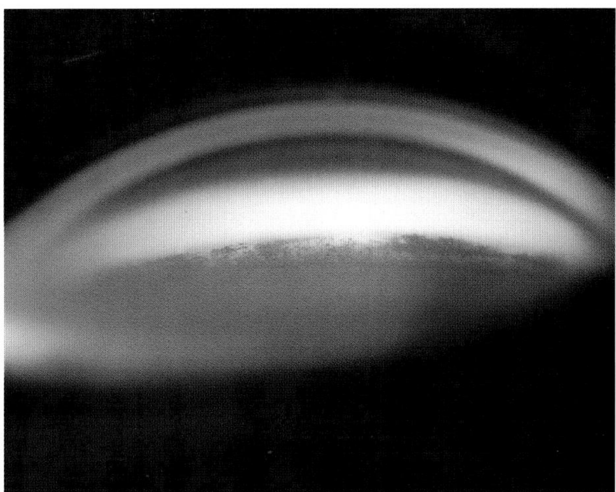

Figure 13.47 Primary congenital glaucoma, gonioscopic view
Pigmented granules of iris-like tissue appear to be enmeshed in a grayish membrane covering the trabecular meshwork.

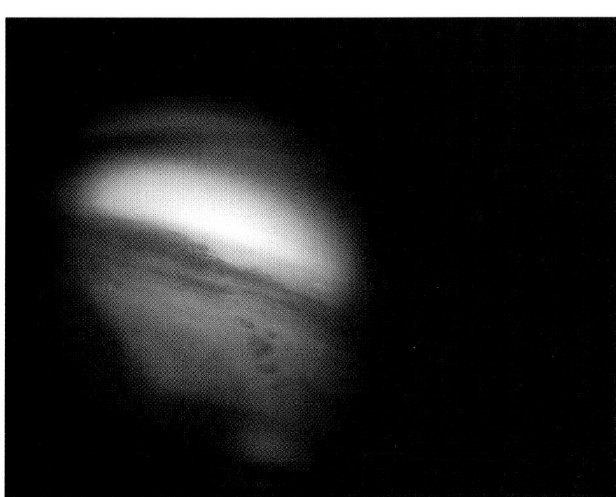

Figure 13.48 Primary congenital glaucoma, gonioscopic view
A grayish membrane covers the angle from the iris root to Schwalbe's line. Strands of irregular uveal meshwork extend forward on the left side of the picture.

Gonioscopy can be performed with an indirect gonioprism or a direct goniolens (see Chapter 5). The Zeiss four-mirror gonioprism or a direct goniolens (Koeppe or Layden) is preferred over the Goldmann lens since no contact gel is required (Fig. 13.42). Impaired visibility from contact gel may hinder posterior pole examination or anterior segment trabecular incisional surgery. Advantages of the direct goniolens include a magnified, 360 degree, distortion-free view of the angle in addition to a view of the posterior pole through the undilated pupil. The lens also stabilizes the globe in the awake (co-operative) patient with nystagmus or acts as a lid speculum in the sedate/anesthetized infant (Fig. 13.42). Light and magnification are obtained by means of either a portable slit lamp, the operating microscope, or a light source coupled with binoculars (Fig. 13.43). In normal infants, the trabecular meshwork has a pinkish, moist, transparent appearance. In trabeculodysgenesis, the color is more white/gray. However, since the normal infant angle features are often indistinguishable from primary trabeculodysgenesis, the diagnosis of developmental glaucoma cannot be ruled out solely on the basis of a 'normal' angle (Fig. 13.44). Noteworthy angle features include the profile of the peripheral iris, the true level of the iris insertion (Figs 13.45 and 13.46), visibility of the scleral spur and ciliary body band, presence of a prominent Swalbe's line (posterior embryotoxon), presence of a membrane over the angle (Figs 13.47 and 13.48), iris strands or adhesions, and angle vessels (Figs 13.49–13.51).

A dilated fundus examination is recommended unless goniotomy/trabeculotomy is planned during the same anesthesia. In eyes with small pupils, hazy cornea, or nystagmus, a reasonable view of the posterior pole may be obtained by using a direct goniolens such as the Koeppe lens with magnification and a light source (see Fig. 13.43c). A direct ophthalmoscope may be used but three-dimensional anatomy is not appreciated with this method and is especially important when evaluating the optic nerve head. Examination and documentation of the disc are of paramount importance for the diagnosis

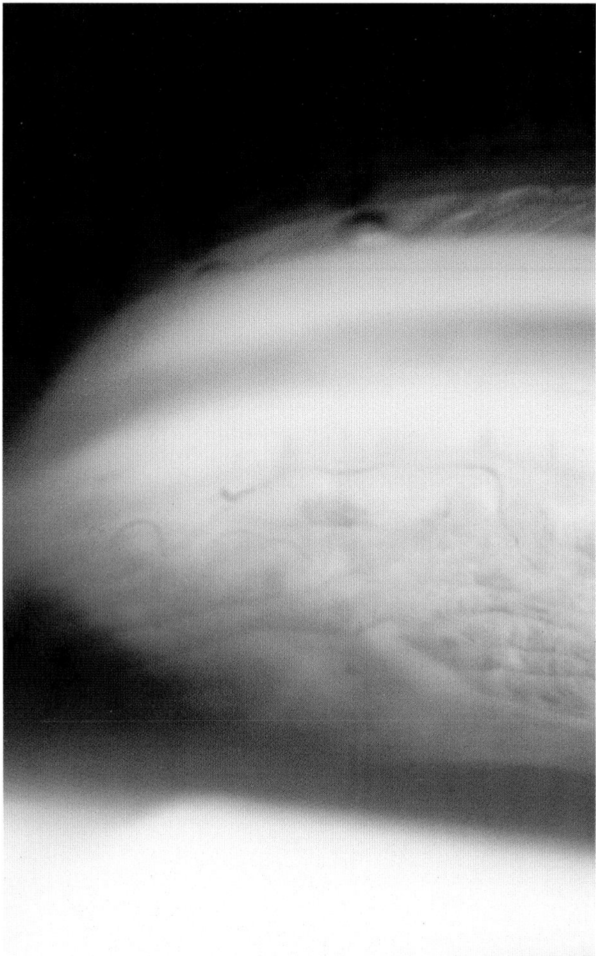

Figure 13.49 Juvenile glaucoma, gonioscopic view Anomalous iris vessels loop in the periphery of the iris bridging over Schwalbe's line.

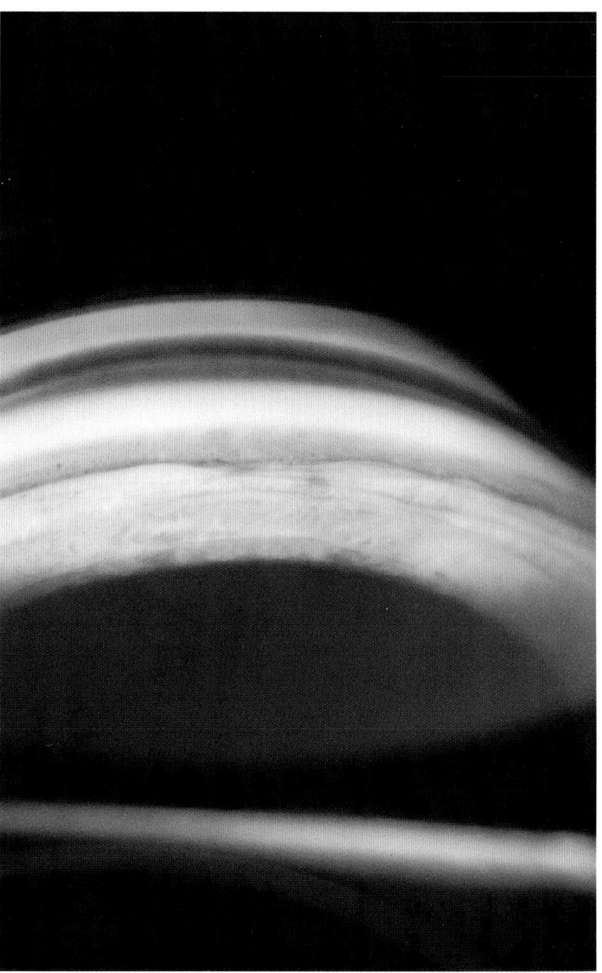

Figure 13.50 Sturge–Weber syndrome, gonioscopic view In this patient the uveal meshwork is covering the angle structures up to Schwalbe's line.

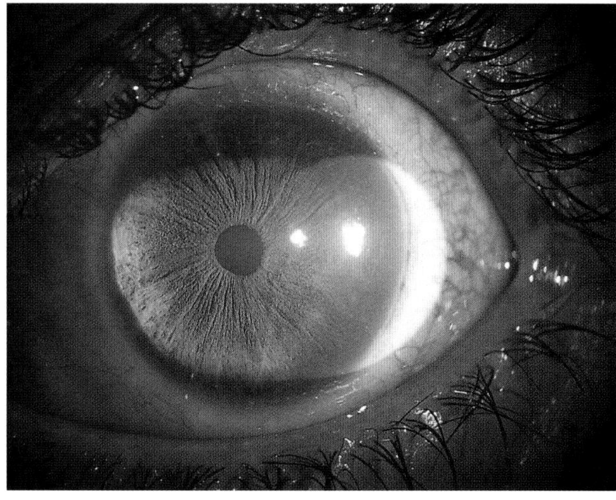

(a)

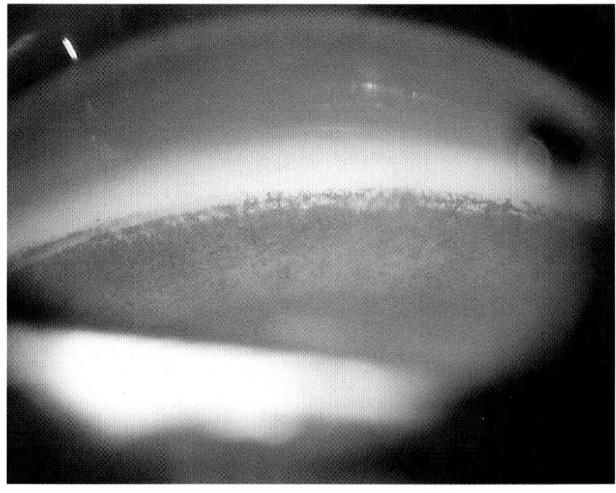

(b)

Figure 13.51 Primary congenital glaucoma with iris hypoplasia
(a) Slit-lamp view. The sphincter is not visible. Radial spokes are the only iris feature.

(b) Gonioscopic view. There is concavity of the peripheral iris. Strands of iris tissue extend to form a band over the trabecular meshwork. In the bottom part of the picture, darker pigment outlines Schwalbe's line.

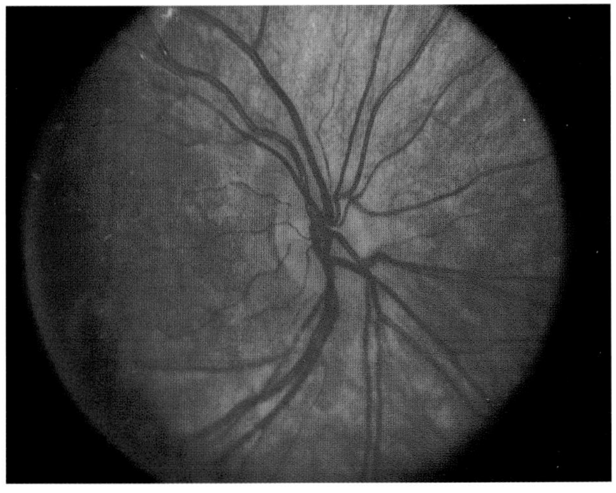

(a)

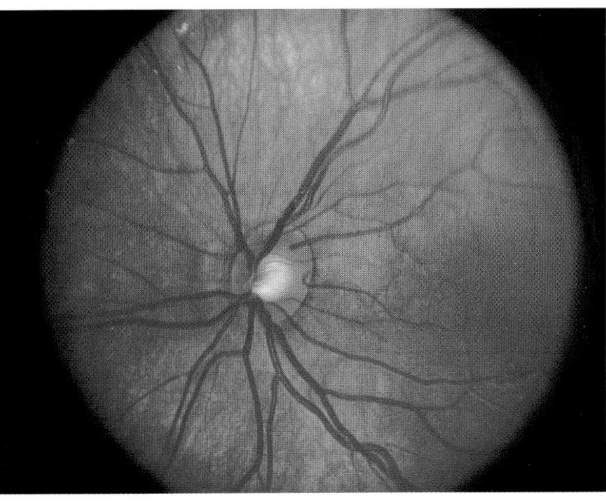

(b)

Figure 13.52 Disc rim asymmetry
In this 11-month-old infant, the difference between (a) OD and (b) OS is striking, indicating more severe glaucomatous damage in OS.

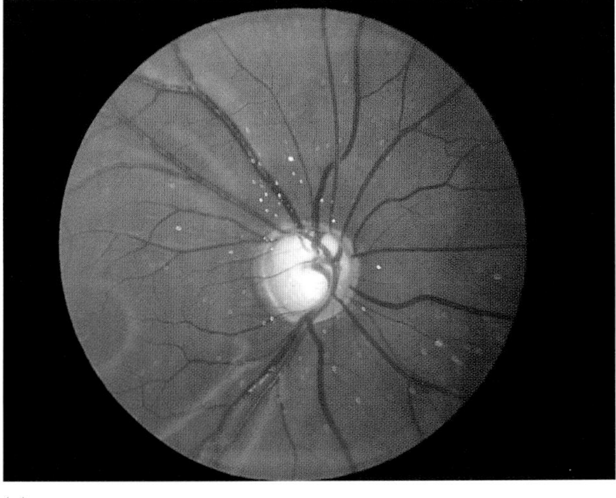

(a)

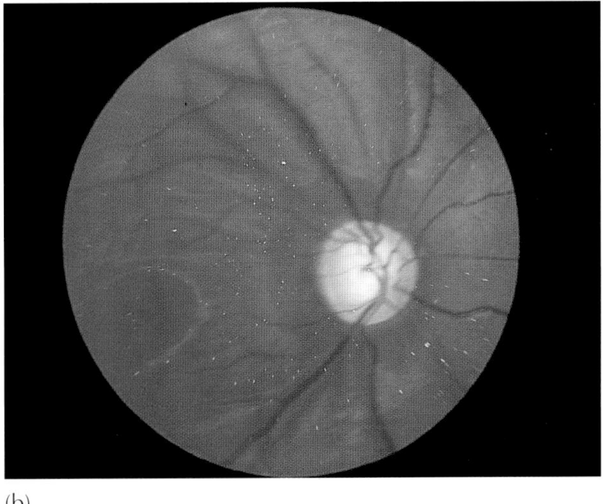

(b)

Figure 13.53 Change in optic nerve cupping with IOP changes
(a) Before surgery with IOP levels approximately 40 mmHg. (b) After surgery with IOP of 14 mmHg.

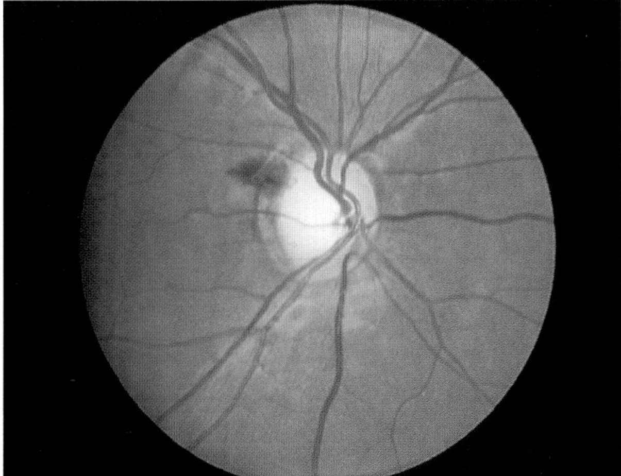

Figure 13.54 Disc hemorrhage in a case of childhood glaucoma

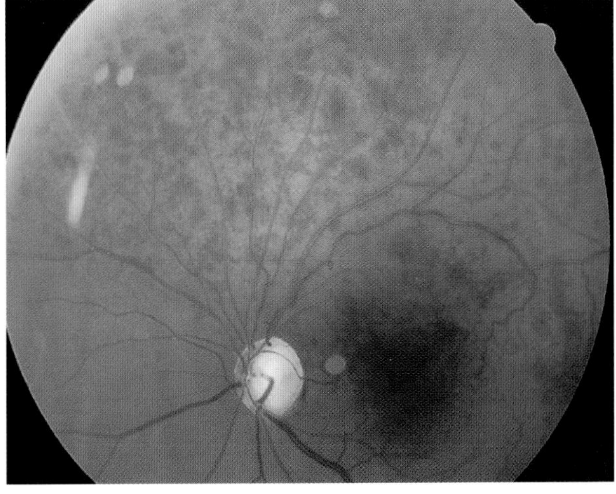

Figure 13.55 Branch retinal vein occlusion in a case of advanced juvenile glaucoma

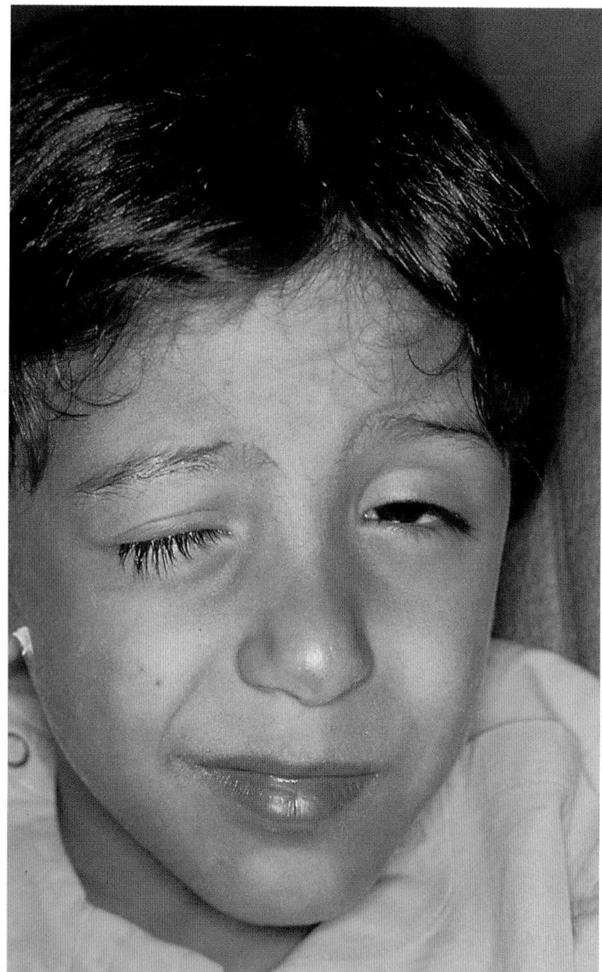

(a)

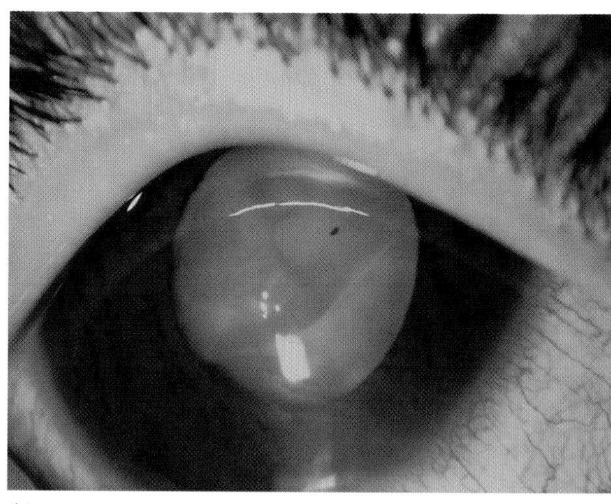

(b)

Figure 13.56 Differential diagnosis of epiphora and photophobia: trauma
This patient complained of epiphora and photophobia (a) but had a history of penetrating trauma (b) with corneal laceration and perforation of the lens.

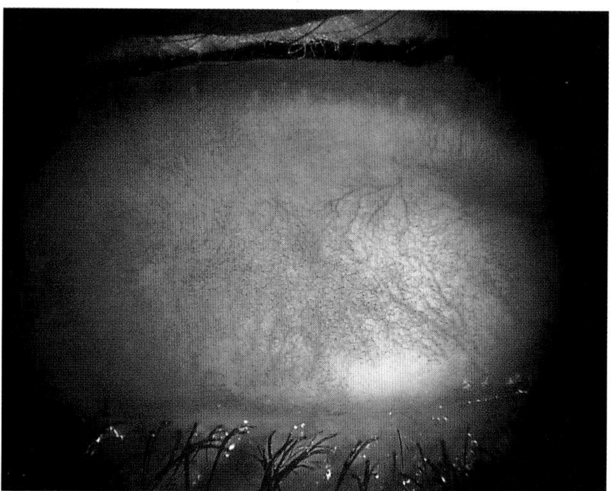

Figure 13.57 Conjunctivitis is a cause of epiphora and photophobia

and management of developmental glaucomas. Disc asymmetry and enlarged (greater than 0.3) cup are rare in normal infants and children (Fig. 13.52). Reversal of cupping with normalization of intraocular pressure is typically seen in infants and young children due to the distensibility of the scleral canal and lamina cribrosa (Fig. 13.53). On the other hand, disc hemorrhage and venous occlusion with elevated pressure are unusual in this age group (Figs 13.54 and 13.55).

Differential diagnosis

Epiphora, blepharospasm, and photophobia in the infant or young child comprise the classical triad of congenital glaucoma. Together or isolated, they are a sign of irritation due to the corneal edema secondary to elevated intraocular pressure and rupture of Descemet's membrane. However, they are not pathognomonic and other causes must be considered, as summarized in Table 13.1.

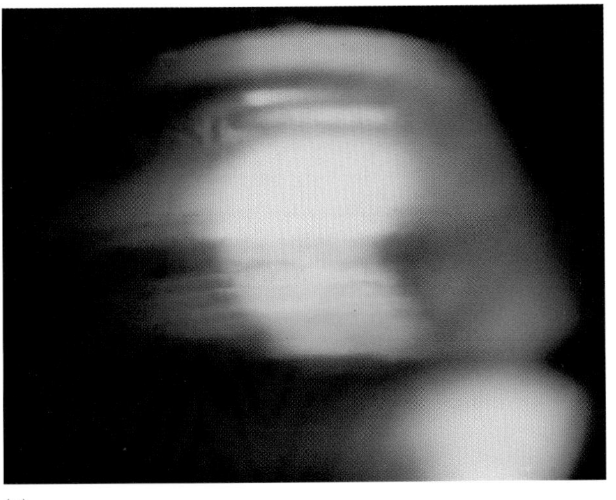

(a)

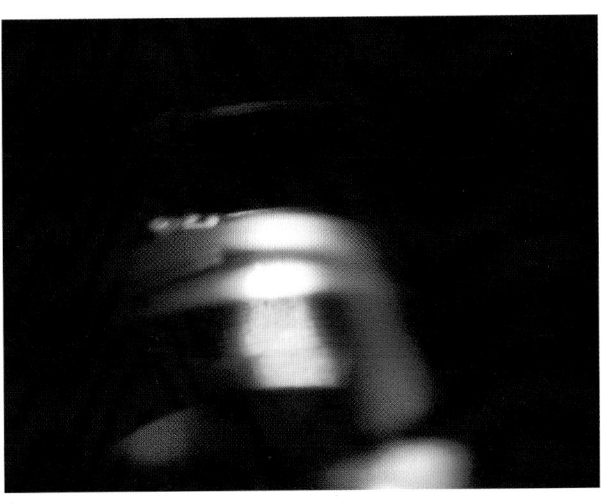

(b)

Figure 13.58 Traumatic angle recession
(a) This can be differentiated from a naturally occurring posterior iris insertion by examining the fellow eye (b).

Figure 13.59 Optic nerve atrophy in a patient who suffered child abuse.

Table 13.1 **Differential diagnosis of the signs of developmental glaucoma.**

Epiphora	Blepharospasm	Photophobia
Lacrimal duct obstruction	Corneal abrasion	Corneal abrasion
Acute dacryocystitis	Keratitis	Keratitis
Conjunctivitis	Trauma	Trauma
Trauma		Aniridia
		Albinism

Elevated intraocular pressure can be due to topical steroid use, traumatic angle recession (Fig. 13.58), or traumatic globe perforation with pupillary block (Figs 13.56–13.59). Acquired optic atrophy can be seen in retinitis pigmentosa or post-trauma as in the battered child syndrome (Fig. 13.59).

FURTHER READING

Cross HE, Maumanee AE, Progressive dissolution of the iris, *Surv Ophthalmol* (1973) **18**:186–92.

De Luise VP, Anderson DR, Primary infantile glaucoma, *Surv Ophthalmol* (1983) **28**:1–19.

Hoskins HD, Jr, Shaffer RN, Heterington J, Jr, Anatomical classification of the developmental glaucomas, *Arch Ophthalmol* (1984) **102**:1331–8.

Mintz-Hittner HA, Aniridia. In: Ritch R, Shields MB, Krupin T, eds. *The glaucomas* (St Louis, MO: CV Mosby 1996), 859–71.

Progressive changes in the angle in congenital aniridia, with development of glaucoma, *Am J Ophthalmol* (1974) **78**:842–6.

Quigley HA, Childhood glaucoma: results with trabeculotomy and study of reversible cupping, *Ophthalmology* (1982) **89**:219–23.

Richardson KT, Optic cup symmetry in normal newborn infants, *Invest Ophthalmol* (1968) **7**:137–41.

Shaffer RN, Weiss DI, *Congenital and pediatric glaucomas* (St Louis, MO: CV Mosby 1970).

Steinle NI, Tomey KF, Senft S, Bergqvist G, Traverso CE, Nutritional status and development of congenital glaucoma patients. Prelimary observations. In: Moyal MF, ed. *Dietetics in the 90s. Role of the dietitian/nutritionist* (London: John Libbey Eurotext, 1988), 87–90.

Weatherill JR, Hart CT, Familial hypoplasia of the iris stroma associated with glaucoma, *Br J Ophthalmol* (1969) **53**:433–7.

14 Medical therapy for glaucoma

Alan L Robin, Gary D Novack and Neil T Choplin

Introduction

At present, therapy for glaucoma consists of lowering the intraocular pressure. There is good correlation between the level of intraocular pressure and the risk of the presence or progression of visual field loss. Many believe (with little evidence that this is the case) that lowering intraocular pressure in patients without visual field damage (i.e. ocular hypertensives or glaucoma suspects) will decrease their risk of developing visual field damage. There are however, ongoing studies to address this question, such as the Ocular Hypertension Treatment Trial.

In deciding to treat (or not treat) a particular patient, an assessment must be made of that patient's risk and possible mode of visual loss. Therapy is instituted if it is concluded that the risk of not lowering the intraocular pressure outweighs the risks and costs of therapy. Having made a decision to treat, the physician is obligated to make therapeutic decisions that maximize patient benefit while minimizing risks of adverse reactions, cost, and inconvenience. The choices, therefore, are driven by safety concerns (*primum non nocere*) as well as efficacy.

Target pressure

Regardless of the mode of treatment, one must decide on a 'target pressure' when treating the glaucoma patient. The concept of a target pressure presumes that by attaining an adequately low intraocular pressure the optic nerve will be protected from further damage and the patient from further visual field loss. How low is 'adequately low'? The answer is part science and part empiric. Generally, the target pressure should be at least 20% lower than the mean pretreatment pressure. In addition, the target is dictated by the course of the disease in the eye being treated and that of the fellow eye, and by the degree of optic nerve damage already present—the greater the damage, the lower the target, as it is felt that the more damaged nerve is vulnerable to additional damage at lower pressures than a less damaged nerve. Once a target pressure is determined, it should be pursued, taking whatever therapeutic steps necessary (including surgery) to achieve it. On the other hand, one must be flexible in assigning a target pressure. If, on attaining the target, the patient continues to lose visual field, one must be willing to revise the target downward (after ruling out noncompliance and nonglaucomatous etiologies for progressive cupping and visual field loss). Table 14.1 lists different goals that have been used for initial therapy.

Table 14.1 **Potential goals in the lowering of intraocular pressure (IOP).**

Lower IOP:

- by 50%
- by 33%
- by 25%

Keep IOP:

- below 23 mmHg
- below 21 mmHg
- below 16 mmHg
- as low as you safely can

Considerable debate has taken place regarding medical versus laser versus surgical therapy for lowering intraocular pressure in glaucoma, particularly early in the course of the disease. In the UK, trabeculectomy is the preferred initial treatment for primary open-angle glaucoma. Arguments for early surgical treatment include the efficacy of trabeculectomy for reducing pressure and the lower cost of surgery compared to life-long medical therapy. On the other hand, surgery has associated risks and complications not present with medical therapy (such as endophthalmitis and expulsive choroidal hemorrhage). Initial reports from the UK indicated that surgery was more effective than laser or medical therapy for preserving visual function. However, re-analysis of the same data indicated that achieving a pressure below 16 mmHg, by whatever means, was associated with better stabilization of the disease. The long-term efficacy of medical versus surgical treatment, in terms of preservation of visual field, awaits the conclusion of additional studies such as the Collaborative Initial Treatment of Glaucoma Study, currently underway at multiple centers in the USA. At present, a rationale still exists for initiating glaucoma treatment with medications, with an individualized therapeutic goal in mind, adjusting the medication according to the patient's responses and disease progression, with surgery as an option should it be necessary. Most patients in the USA diagnosed with glaucoma, or felt to be at risk for the development of glaucomatous optic neuropathy, are presently treated initially with medical therapy.

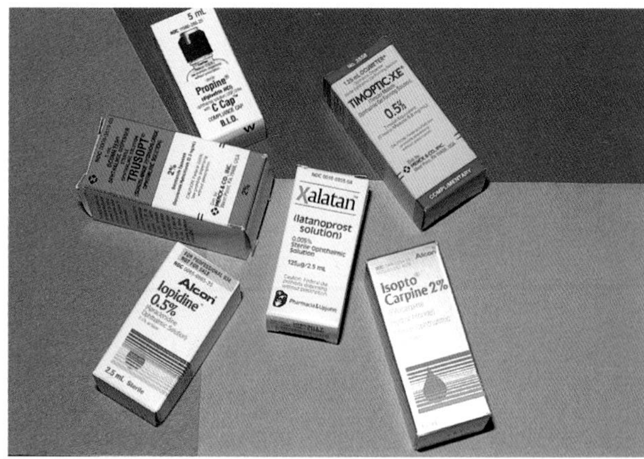

Figure 14.1 Glaucoma medication classes
There are currently six different classes of glaucoma medications on the market. These are (clockwise from upper left): adrenergic agonists (epinephrine, divivalyl-epinephrine), beta adrenergic blockers (timolol, levobunolol, metipranolol, carteolol, betaxolol), cholinergics or miotics (pilocarpine, carbachol, cholinesterase inhibitors), $alpha_2$ adrenergic agonists (apraclonidine, brimonidine), carbonic anhydrase inhibitors (oral: acetazolamide, methazolamide; topical: dorzolamide, brinzolamide), and (center) prostaglandin analogues (latanoprost).

Principles of medical therapy for glaucoma

Once the decision to treat has been made, and a target pressure chosen, there is a multitude of medications (in various formulations) from six different classes to choose from (Fig. 14.1). The field may be narrowed by taking into consideration various patient factors which have a direct bearing on the risk versus benefit ratio, as well as increasing the likelihood that the patient will even take the medication. These are summarized in Table 14.2.

The patient's general medical history is one of the most important considerations in formulating a plan of medical therapy. Many of the more serious (even life-threatening) side-effects of therapy can be avoided by carefully screening out patients who are poor candidates for a particular medication. For example, a patient with severe asthma has a contraindication for nonselective topical beta-adrenoreceptor antagonists, as the use of such medication may induce bronchospasm. Coexisting ophthalmic conditions may also dictate therapeutic choices. In the aphakic or pseudophakic patient, one might hesitate to use epinephrine due to the risk of cystoid macular edema. Similarly, miotics should be avoided in patients with cataracts (the miosis may further compromise vision) or uveitis (miotics may exacerbate the breakdown of the blood–aqueous barrier).

Table 14.2 **Social, medical, and physical factors affecting medication choices.**

- patient's financial status
- patient's ability to instill drop into eye
- patient's social schedule
- patient's reliability
- patient's perception of the disease as being blinding
- patient's social status (i.e. red or discolored eyes are acceptable)
- presence of cataract
- presence of intraocular inflammation
- phakic status
- medical problems
- systemic allergies
- topical allergies

Compliance

Since glaucoma is usually an asymptomatic disease, patients may have difficulty accepting the diagnosis and the need for life-long medication, particularly when vision is good and they have no pain or discomfort. They may believe that all is well and the

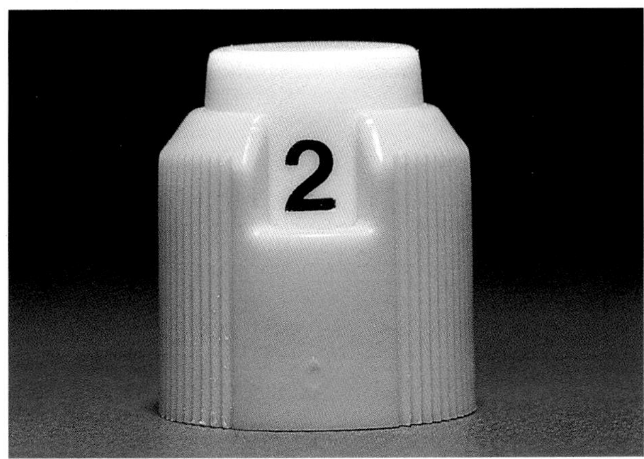

Figure 14.2 Compliance cap
One manufacturer of glaucoma medications designed this 'compliance cap' as an aid to patients in remembering to take their eye drops. This cap is for a twice-daily medication—it has positions for '1' and '2', corresponding to the *next* dose due. As the cap is replaced on the bottle after administration of a dose, the patient continues to turn it until the next number appears. After taking the morning dose, the cap would then be turned to '2', indicating that the evening dose is next. Another cap is available for once-daily dosing and this displays the days of the week (see Fig. 14.6a).

Table 14.3 **Factors which might affect a patient's decision to take an eye drop.**
• patient's co-ordination and ability to administer the drop • user-friendliness of the drop bottle • comfort of the drop • cost of the medication • topical side-effects of the medication • systemic side-effects of the medication

diagnosis must be wrong. This perception decreases compliance since the patient does not realize the potential gravity of the situation, and the medications may burn or sting and may be expensive. It is important to take the time to explain the disease process, demonstrate the potential for (or the presence of) visual field loss, and how following the prescribed treatment plan may reduce the risk of visual loss.

Even 'convinced and committed' patients have limits on what they can successfully manage, especially when multiple medications are prescribed. Compliance studies show a strong correlation between increasing numbers of medications and declining compliance. Increased frequency of installation also correlates with lower compliance. Even once or twice a day medications, such as the beta-adrenoreceptor antagonists, may be taken incorrectly, with patients taking them more often than needed and thereby increasing the risk for systemic side-effects. Devices such as the 'compliance cap' (Fig. 14.2) may help minimize such problems in some patients. However, considering that the average glaucoma patient is over 70 years of age and may be taking one or more nonglaucoma medications, it is not surprising that many patients are often not taking their medications as directed. Some of the many factors that influence compliance are listed in Table 14.3.

Gauging efficacy

Having tailored a medical regimen that the patient can manage, how do we know it is working? Since intraocular pressure has a diurnal variation that may be exaggerated in the glaucoma patient, how can we be sure that any pressure reduction is due to the therapy? The one eye trial addresses this important question. Generally, medications are added one at a time in a stepwise fashion (exceptions to this might be the patient with advanced disease and very high pressures who needs an expeditious trial of medical therapy prior to surgery). In the one-eye trial, the medication being added (or used initially) is instilled in one-eye while the untreated eye serves as a 'control'. After a suitable interval, intraocular pressure is again measured. Any reduction in the 'control' eye is due to diurnal variation. Reduction in the treated eye is due to diurnal variation *plus* medication effect. The difference between the treated and untreated eyes (pre- and post-treatment) is the therapeutic effect of the medication. A difference of at least 15–20% Hg or more might be considered to be a therapeutic response to the trial medication. Even though medications such as the beta-adrenoreceptor antagonists and alpha agonists exhibit some 'consensual' or contralateral effect (medication effect is seen in the nontreated eye), this is still a valuable method to determine whether a particular medication works in a given patient. Some medications are simply ineffective in a given patient (not all medications work in all individuals). More commonly, a medication may have some pressure-lowering effect but not attain the 'target'. Therefore, many patients will require more than one medication to attain their target. By using the one-eye trial with each therapeutic addition, one can have confidence that the medications being taken are actually effective, avoiding the risk and expense of medications which may not be contributing to the treatment. Stopping a medication in one eye as a trial may also be used periodically to assess ongoing efficacy, especially when a patient has been on a multiple drug regimen for a long time and there has been no progression of the disease. Additionally, it is wise to simplify rather than add. If one class of medications does not work, trying another class of medications, rather than adding to an ineffective class, is important.

Reducing systemic absorption

All topically applied medications leave the eye via the nasal lacrimal drainage system and are systemically absorbed when they come into contact with the mucosa in the oral and nasal pharynx. This results in decreased ocular contact time (with less ocular absorption and possibly lowered efficacy) and increased chance for systemic side-effects. Two fairly simple techniques may be used to decrease passage of topically applied medication down the nasolacrimal duct. The first technique is simply to close the eyelids for two minutes after instillation of the eye drop. This inhibits action of the 'lacrimal pump' associated with blinking that is responsible for the movement of tears across the cornea from the temporal side (where the lacrimal gland is) to the nasal side (where the drain is located). The second technique is punctal occlusion, in which pressure is applied to the area of the puncta and nasolacrimal sac (again, for two minutes following drop instillation) as illustrated in Figure 14.3. Both techniques, especially in combination, prolong ocular contact time to the drug, enhancing absorption, while minimizing its systemic absorption via transit down the nasolacrimal duct. Decreased serum levels of topically applied medications have been demonstrated following the use of these techniques.

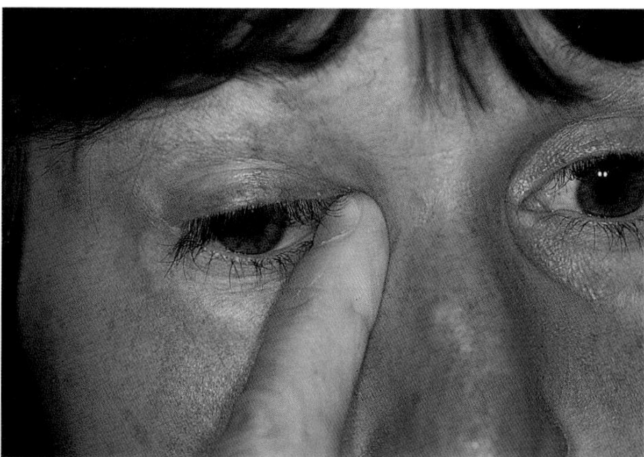

Figure 14.3 Nasolacrimal occlusion
If digital pressure is placed over the area of the puncta and nasolacrimal duct after instilling a topical medication, passage of nonabsorbed medication down the duct and into the nose will be reduced, thus decreasing systemic levels and the potential for systemic side-effects. This maneuver should be combined with simple eyelid closure for a period of one to two minutes, which decreases the movement of tears (and medication dissolved in them) towards the puncta.

Additional factors

There may be more to preserving vision in glaucoma patients than simply lowering the intraocular pressure. This is an area of active research at present. There is some evidence that some of the medications used to lower intraocular pressure may have an idiosyncratic ability to increase optic nerve vascular perfusion, perhaps by mechanisms such as calcium channel blockade. Although this remains to be proven in humans, such additional therapeutic effects may be important in certain patients.

Available agents

During the past two decades, since the introduction of topical beta-adrenoreceptor antagonists, the choices for intraocular pressure-lowering therapy have more than doubled. At present in the USA there are six different classes of medications used to lower intraocular pressure in the treatment of glaucoma and ocular hypertension. These are beta-adrenoreceptor antagonists; epinephrine compounds; carbonic anhydrase inhibitors; miotics; alpha-adrenergic agonists; and prostaglandin analogues.

Different considerations are involved in the decisions over initial therapy (i.e. the first drug to be used) and additive therapy (i.e. what drug to add next if the initial drug doesn't lower the pressure to the target or if the target has been lowered). The decision as to which drug to use as primary therapy should be based on efficacy but with the least number of adverse effects, lowest cost, and ease of use, i.e. a favorable risk/benefit ratio. Additionally, the likelihood of the medication to retard the progression of visual field loss (in addition to lowering the pressure) must be considered (see below). The two classes of medications which have the best pressure-lowering ability are the beta-adrenoreceptor antagonists and the prostaglandins. However, at present in the USA, the available topical prostaglandin analogue, latanoprost, is not approved as primary therapy. Therefore, when safe to do so, most patients are treated initially with a beta-adrenoreceptor antagonist.

If initial therapy fails to achieve the target pressure, or additional pressure lowering is desired, additional medication must be considered. Second and third-line drugs are almost always from different classes

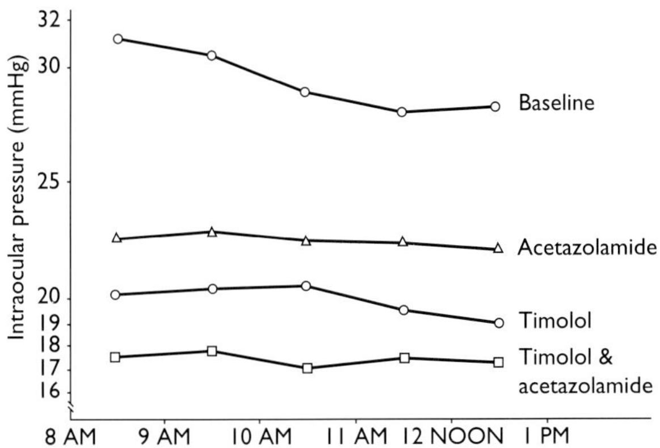

Figure 14.4 Additivity of glaucoma medications
The graph illustrates a modified diurnal curve of intraocular pressure in a glaucoma patient at baseline (top), following administration of acetazolamide alone (second from top), timolol alone (third from top), and the combination of acetazolamide and timolol (bottom). Note how the intraocular pressure after the administration of the combination of drugs (bottom curve) is lower than after administration of either drug alone, demonstrating the additive nature of the two drugs. In this case, both medications have similar mechanisms of action, i.e. suppression of aqueous humor production, although each drug accomplishes this by different means.

from medications already being used, as medications within the same class rarely add to each other. Best additivity will most likely occur if the drugs have different mechanisms of action, although sometimes agents with the same mechanism of action will work well together. Figure 14.4 illustrates the additivity of a topical beta-adrenoreceptor antagonist and an oral carbonic anhydrase inhibitor, both of which decrease pressure through aqueous humor production suppression. In choosing from the various medications currently on the market, it remains important to consider simplicity in administration and the overall daily medication administration schedule; if it becomes too complex the patient will miss doses, leading to decreased compliance.

Beta-adrenoreceptor antagonists

Beta-adrenergic receptors are found in many different cells in the body, primarily in vascular smooth muscle, the heart, bronchial smooth muscle, kidneys, and the ciliary body. There are two subclasses of beta receptors, $beta_1$ and $beta_2$. Stimulation of the receptor causes relaxation of smooth muscle while blockade will cause contraction. The receptors in the heart and blood vessels are primarily $beta_1$, while those in the lung are primarily $beta_2$. The beta receptors within the eye are involved with the regulation of aqueous humor production, showing a marked decrease (with concomitant lowering of intraocular pressure) when blocked. Thus, beta-adrenoreceptor antagonists are very effective intraocular pressure-lowering agents. Agents which exhibit the ability to block both $beta_1$ and $beta_2$ receptors are known as 'nonselective', while agents which primarily block $beta_1$ are known as 'cardioselective' or simply as 'selective'. Such agents have the theoretical advantage of causing less bronchospasm by not binding to beta receptors in the lung.

Timolol maleate (Fig. 14.5a), available in 0.25% and 0.5% concentrations, was the first commercially available nonselective beta-adrenoreceptor antagonist in the USA. It has become the 'gold standard' in beta-adrenoreceptor antagonist therapy. Both concentrations of timolol maleate lower intraocular pressure by decreasing aqueous flow approximately 30–35% (6–8 mmHg). Initial studies to determine the appropriate dosing were based upon short-term dose response studies. Even the 0.001% solution significantly lowers intraocular pressure. Used chronically, timolol maleate solution is effective when used once daily. More recently, a gel-forming suspension formulation has been developed (Timoptic-XE). Chronically, the gel once daily is at least as effective as the solution twice daily (Fig. 14.5c). The gel formulation may have less systemic effects due to less passage down the nasolacrimal duct, attributed to its ability to remain within the conjunctival fornices. However, the gel used once daily has not been compared to conventional timolol used once daily. Allergic reactions to the XE vehicle have been reported, as illustrated in Figure 14.5d. Also, the gel can cause blurred vision. Another formulation of timolol, timolol hemihydrate (Betimol, not illustrated), has been introduced as a twice-daily drug, with similar efficacy to timolol maleate.

Three other nonselective beta-adrenoreceptor antagonists, all with similar efficacy to timolol, are available in the USA (Fig. 14.6). Levobunolol hydrochloride is also marketed in 0.25% and 0.5% concentrations. The primary metabolite of levobunolol (Fig. 14.6a), dihydrolevobunolol, is also an active beta-adrenoreceptor antagonist which lowers intraocular pressure. The drug has been shown to be effective administered once daily in both concentrations. However, no study has shown levobunolol to be more effective than timolol. The drug is off patent and is available generically.

Carteolol (Ocupress, (Fig. 14.6b)) is relatively new in the USA but is one of the largest-selling beta-adrenoreceptor antagonists globally. It is available in a 1.0% concentration which is comparable in efficacy to 0.5% of timolol maleate. Carteolol possesses a quality known as 'intrinsic sympathomimetic activity' (ISA), which produces an early transient adrenergic

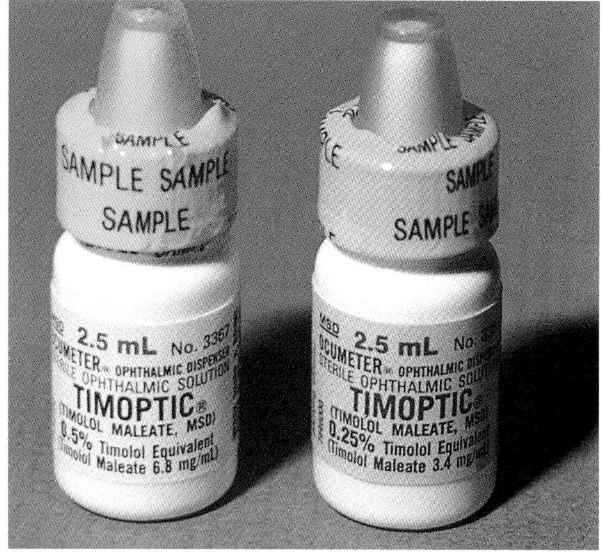

(a)

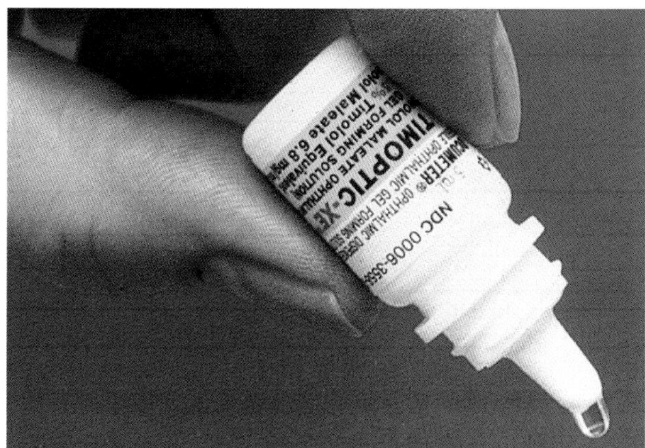

(b)

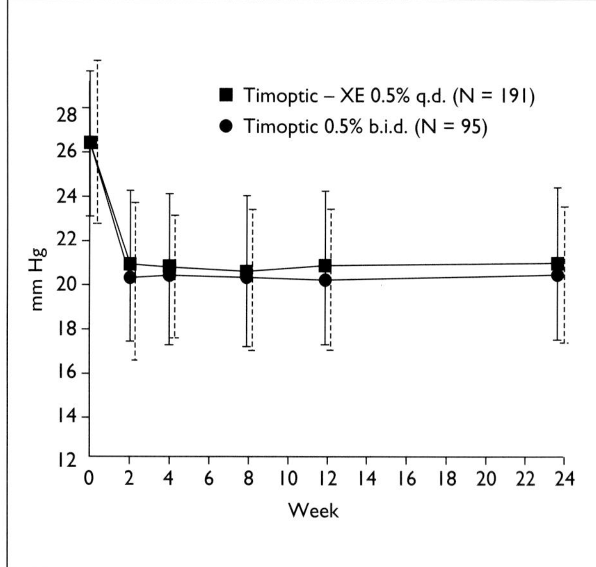

(c)

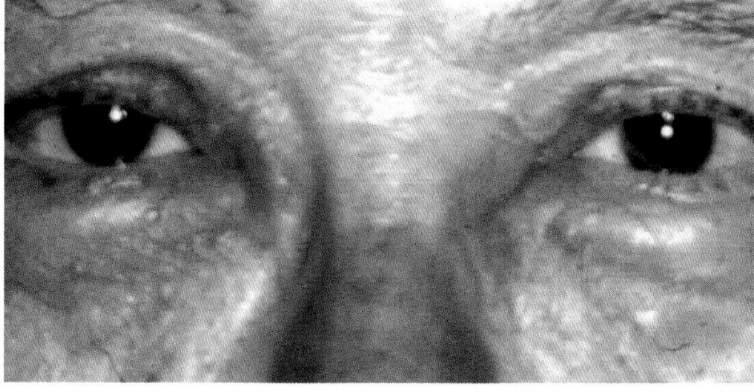

(d)

Figure 14.5 Timolol

(a) The first nonspecific beta-adrenoreceptor antagonist, timolol maleate is available in 0.25% and 0.5% solutions. By convention, the label and cap color for most 0.25% beta-adrenoreceptor antagonists is blue, while the 0.5% uses yellow. Pictured is Timoptic from Merck, Inc. Not shown is timolol hemihydrate, marketed as Betimol from Ciba, Inc. in the same concentrations. (b) Timoptic-XE from Merck is a reformulation of timolol maleate in a gel-forming liquid vehicle. The vehicle is a heteropolysaccharide derived from gellan gum, originally developed as a food additive. This vehicle contains a 'thixotropic' property which allows it to liquify upon mild agitation (i.e. turning the bottle over and shaking once) and turning back to a gel upon contact with cations in the precorneal tear film. The gel then takes up residence in the conjunctival fornices and releases medication slowly over time as the gel is removed by tear flow. This allows for decreased frequency of administration, and the XE products are marketed for once-daily administration. Because a slight blur can occur from the gel, the medication may best be administered at bedtime. (c) Timoptic-XE administered once daily is therapeutically equivalent to Timoptic solution administered twice daily. (d) Allergic reactions may occur to the XE vehicle. This photograph, showing an acute allergic reaction to Timoptic-XE, was taken the day after the patient administered his first drop of the drug into each eye. He had been on Timoptic solution for years and was switched to the XE for 'convenience'.

agonist effect not found in other marketed ophthalmic beta-adrenoreceptor antagonists, and is thought to reduce some of the potential side effects. One theoretical advantage of carteolol to other nonselective beta-adrenoceptor antagonists is its demonstrated ability to cause less lowering of serum HDL-C compared to timolol, which in turn theoretically reduces the increased risk of myocardial infarction associated with reduced serum HDL-C. No clinical study has ever demonstrated an increased risk of myocardial infarction from topical beta-adrenoreceptor antagonist therapy.

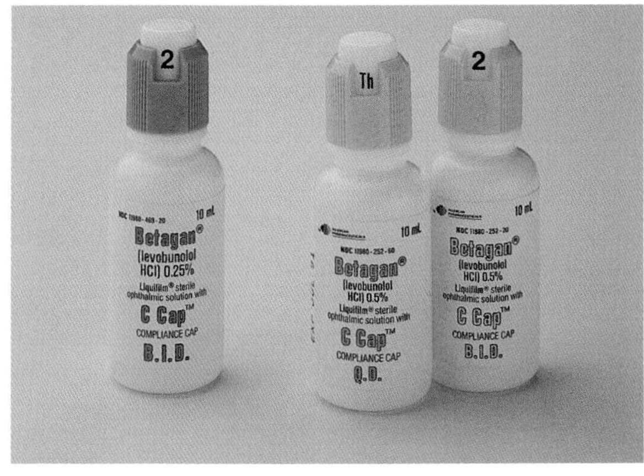

(a)

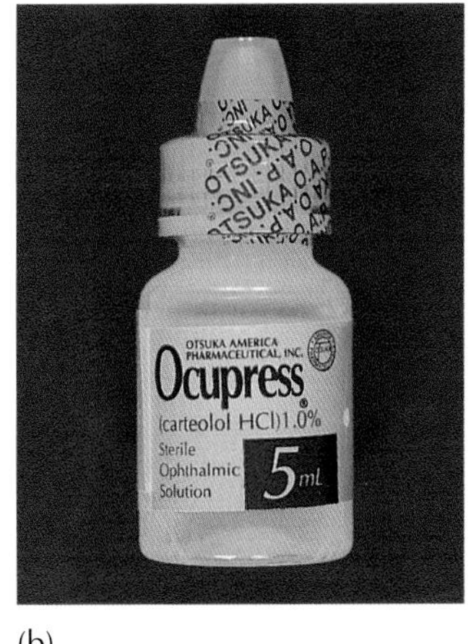

(b)

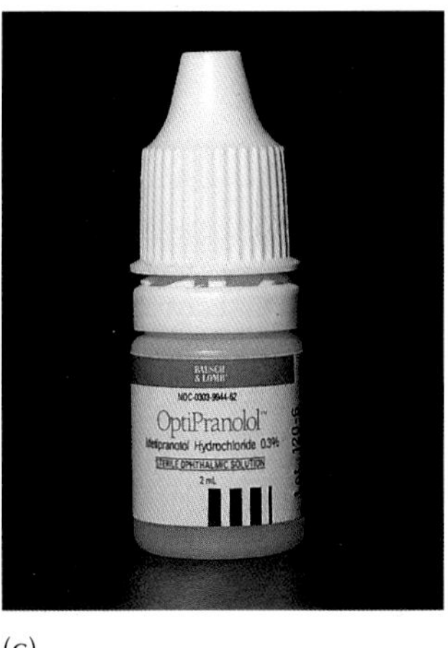

(c)

Figure 14.6 Other nonspecific beta-adrenoreceptor antagonists
All the nonspecific beta-adrenoreceptor antagonists are essentially therapeutically equivalent. They each have their own marketing claims (see text). (a) Levobunolol hydrochloride, marketed by Allergan, Inc. as Betagan. The blue top is 0.25% and the yellow is 0.5%. Note the 'compliance cap' (see Fig. 14.2). The outside bottles have the twice-daily 'C' cap while the center bottle is the once daily. Levobunolol is also available generically. (b) Carteolol, marketed as Occupress by Otsuka Pharmaceuticals. (c) Metipranolol, marketed as Optipranolol by Bausch & Lomb, Inc.

Finally, metipranolol (Optipranolol, Fig. 14.6c) is marketed in a 0.3% strength in the USA. It offers some cost savings over the other available agents, at least as originally marketed. The drug has caused granulomatous uveitis in some formulations, particularly those marketed outside the USA.

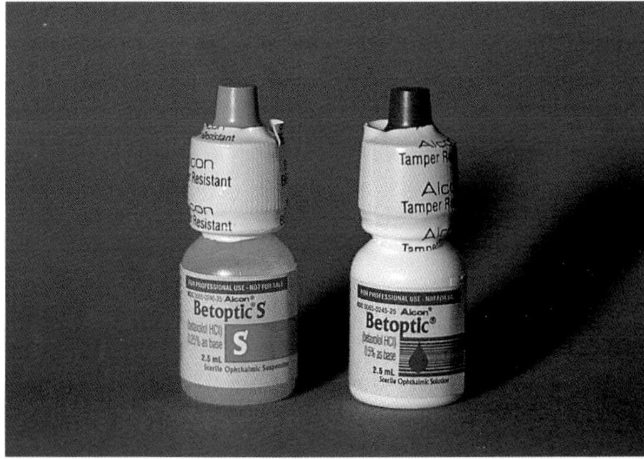

Figure 14.7 Betaxolol
Betaxolol is the only $beta_1$ specific beta-adrenoreceptor antagonist available. It is marketed by Alcon, Inc. in two formulations, Betoptic-S 0.25% suspension (left) and Betoptic 0.5% solution (right). The 0.25% suspension is more comfortable and causes less stinging and burning than the 0.5% solution; they are both administered twice daily and are therapeutically equivalent.

Betaxolol (Fig. 14.7) is the only commercially available topical relatively $beta_1$ selective intraocular pressure-lowering medication. It is available as both a 0.25% suspension (Betoptic-S) and a 0.5% solution (Betoptic). The suspension is more comfortable than the solution in most individuals, but the two are equally efficacious. Both formulations lower intraocular pressure approximately 20% from baseline, which is approximately 2 mmHg less than any of the nonselective beta-adrenoreceptor antagonists. One of the main advantages of betaxolol is its reduced affinity for $beta_2$ receptors (hence its label as a selective $beta_1$ blocker) and thus it is less likely to produce bronchospasm in susceptible individuals (Fig. 14.8). It must be noted, however, that $beta_1$ selectivity is relative, and betaxolol may still cause bronchospasm in susceptible individuals. All beta-adrenoreceptor antagonists must be used with caution in any patient with a history of reactive airway disease.

Even though the intraocular pressure-lowering of betaxolol may be less than that of the nonselective beta-adrenoreceptor antagonists, some authorities have advocated betaxolol as first-line therapy. Betaxolol has minimal effects on both resting pulse rate and exercise-induced tachycardia. It is safer in patients with mild reactive airway disease. Some feel that betaxolol is the beta-adrenoreceptor antagonist of choice in individuals who have diabetes. Systemic administration of betaxolol has no effect on serum lipids. There is also a suggestion that betaxolol causes less central nervous side-effects (i.e. depression) than nonselective beta-adrenoreceptor antagonists due to

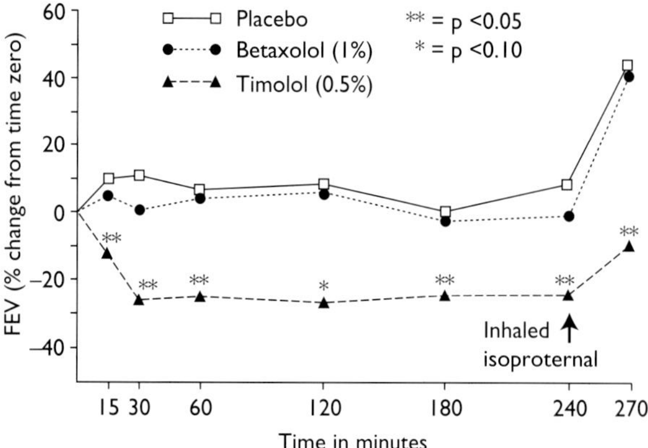

Figure 14.8 Pulmonary effects of beta-adrenoreceptor antagonists

Blockade of $beta_2$ receptors allows contraction of smooth muscle in the bronchial tree, and may result in bronchospasm, especially in patients with pre-existing reactive airway disease (asthma, emphysema, chronic bronchitis). Airway resistance may be measured by determining the amount of air forcibly expelled within one second, known as forced expiratory volume, or FEV_1. The graph illustrates the effect of different beta-adrenoreceptor antagonists on FEV_1. The lower curve demonstrates decreased FEV_1 following administration of timolol, a nonspecific beta-adrenoreceptor antagonist which blocks both $beta_1$ and $beta_2$ receptors. The upper curve illustrates that the effect of betaxolol is similar to placebo in causing minimal to no change in FEV_1 since it does not affect $beta_2$ receptors. Also note how FEV_1 returns to and surpasses baseline following administration of isoproterenol, a beta agonist which causes relaxation of the bronchial smooth muscle and relieves the bronchospasm.

less penetration of the blood–brain barrier. Additionally, betaxolol appears to reach a lower concentration in both the anterior chamber and blood stream than do nonselective beta blockers. Part of this could also be related to noncorneal penetration differences between betaxolol and other beta-adrenoreceptor antagonists. When administered chronically, it has a shorter cumulative effect. Betaxolol's effect on aqueous flow lasts only days, while the effect of non selective beta-adrenoreceptor antagonists may last for weeks. Betaxolol is therefore more likely to be better tolerated and less likely to cause systemic side-effects than other beta-adrenoreceptor antagonists. If untoward side-effects occur, they may disappear more quickly than with a nonselective beta blocker. Additionally, betaxolol may have the ability to increase blood flow to the optic nerve. This may be due to an intrinsic calcium channel blocking activity. This may be advantageous in the appropriate patient.

Both ocular and systemic side-effects occur with topical beta-adrenoreceptor antagonists. Common ocular side-effects include decreased corneal sensation, punctate keratitis, dry eye, allergic blepharoconjunctivitis, lid dermatitis, blurred vision, and decreased accommodation. Systemic side-effects include exacerbation of reactive airway disease (emphysema, asthma, chronic bronchitis), congestive heart failure, heart block, hypotension, hallucinations, confusion, erectile dysfunction, depression, and fatigue. A number of deaths have been reported from status asthmaticus and idiosyncratic cardiac events.

Adrenergic agents

Epinephrine and dipivalyl-epinephrine

Topical epinephrine applied to the glaucomatous eye lowers the intraocular pressure between 10 and 30%. Acceptable (in terms of comfort and stability) formulations of epinephrine have been in use since the early 1950s, as either bitartrate, hydrochloride, or borate salt solutions. Maximum pressure lowering occurs within 2–4 hours of administration, with a duration of action between 12 and 24 hours; hence administration is usually twice daily. Because epinephrine can dilate the pupil, it should be used with caution (if at all) in angle closure glaucoma or in patients with narrow angles. There is some controversy over the mechanism of action of topically applied epinephrine. It is believed to cause a short-lived increase in aqueous production, with sustained increased outflow, believed to be mostly through nonconventional, i.e. uveoscleral, pathways.

Although largely replaced by some of the newer classes of medications available nowadays, epinephrine may still have some indications. It may be a useful drug in younger patients with open-angle glaucoma or those with early cataract (because it does not cause miosis), in additive therapy to miotics and carbonic anhydrase inhibitors (particularly in patients with contraindications to beta-adrenoreceptor antagonist therapy), and in patients with inflammatory glaucoma. Additivity to beta-adrenoreceptor antagonists is variable. One study comparing the additivity of epinephrine to a nonselective beta-adrenoreceptor antagonist (timolol) or a selective beta-adrenoreceptor antagonist (betaxolol) suggested better additivity to the selective beta-adrenoreceptor antagonist. This suggests that the action of epinephrine may be mediated through $beta_2$ receptors (the ones not blocked by betaxolol but blocked by timolol).

Topical epinephrine therapy is associated with systemic, local, and intraocular side-effects, causing intolerance to the drug in about 20% of patients trying it. Systemic side-effects include headaches,

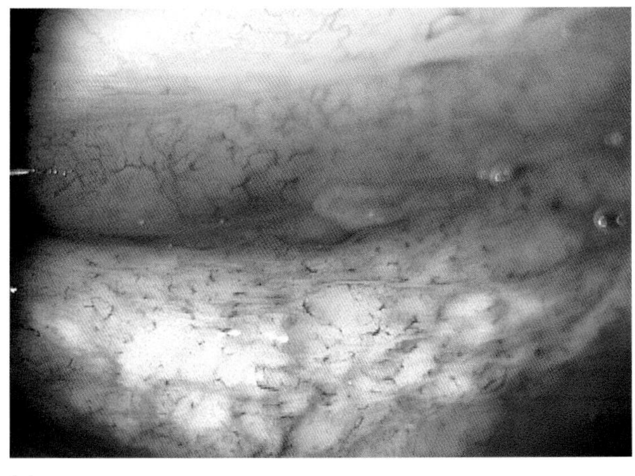

(a)

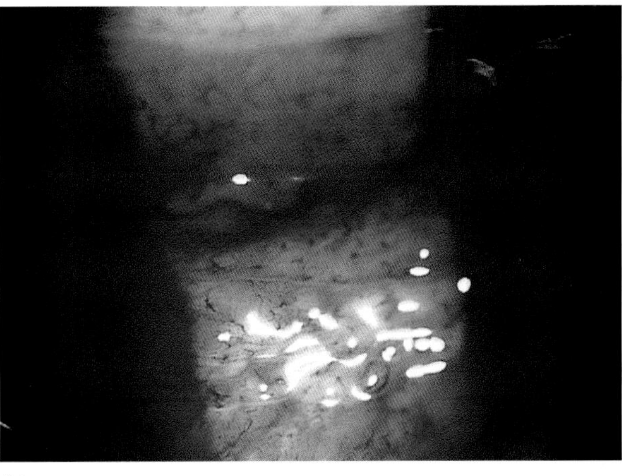

(b)

Figure 14.9 Follicular conjunctivitis
This allergic reaction is typical of that commonly seen to such drugs as epinephrine, dipivalyl-epinephrine, apraclonidine, brimonidine, and dorzolamide. (a) Note redness, mucoid discharge, and follicles. (b) Close-up of the follicles in the inferior conjunctival fornix. This reaction will subside within a few weeks of stopping the offending medication.

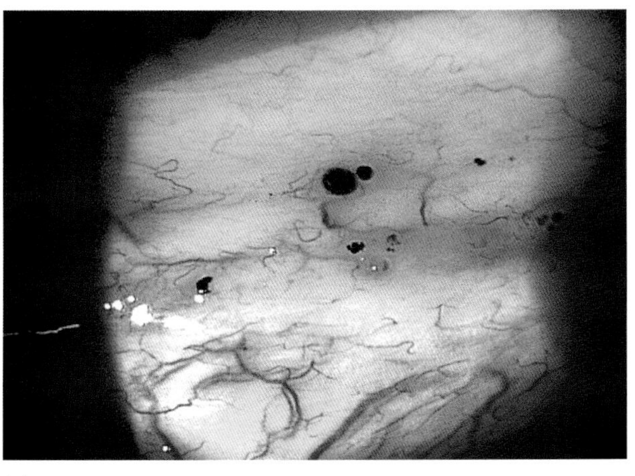

(a)

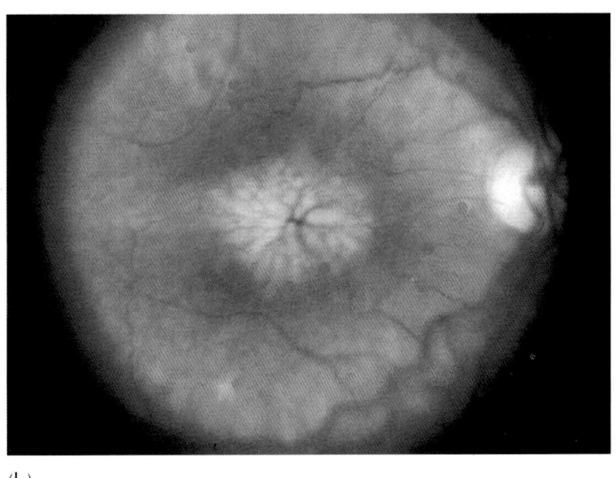

(b)

Figure 14.10 Complications of epinephrine therapy
(a) Chronic administration of epinephrine may result in the deposition of black particles in the conjunctiva. Known as adrenochrome deposits, they represent black oxidation products of the drug. They are usually asymptomatic, but occasionally cause irritation by rubbing on the cornea. (b) Late-phase fluorescein angiogram demonstrating the typical 'petaloid' appearance of cystoid macular edema in an aphakic patient with blurred vision, being treated with epinephrine for elevated intraocular pressure. The cause of the edema is not fully understood, but may be related to vasoconstriction in the macula due to diffusion of epinephrine to the retina, more likely to occur in eyes that have lost the barrier effect of the posterior lens capsule. The edema will most likely resolve upon cessation of the drug.

elevated blood pressure, tachyarrythmias, and strokes. Local side-effects include conjunctival hyperemia, adrenochrome deposits, and, commonly, allergic blepharoconjunctivitis (Fig. 14.9). Intraocular side-effects include pupillary dilatation, corneal endothelial effects, reduction in ocular blood flow due to vasospasm, rebound hyperemia, and, in aphakic and some pseudophakic patients, cystoid macular edema (Fig. 14.10).

Attempts to reduce the side-effects of epinephrine therapy while increasing absorption into the eye resulted in the development of an epinephrine 'prodrug', dipivalyl-epinephrine, also known as dipivefrin or DPE. The substitution of pivalyl acid for each of the hydroxyl groups on the epinephrine molecule results in 1) a compound that is inactive as it comes out of the bottle, thus having a lower potential for systemic side-effects; and 2) a compound with

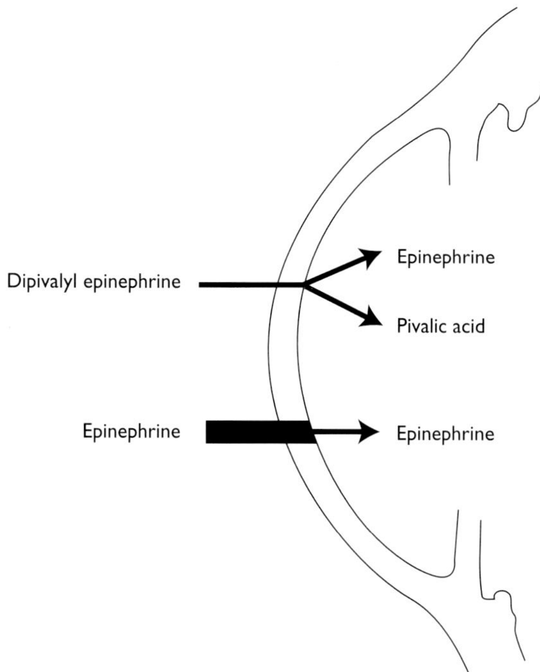

Figure 14.11 Dipivalyl-epinephrine
The substitution of pivalyl acid for the hydroxyl groups on the epinephrine molecule results in a drug that 1) is more highly lipid soluble than the parent compound, allowing for approximately 17 times greater penetration across the cornea into the eye; 2) is clinically inactive outside the eye, virtually eliminating systemic side-effects; 3) may be administered in much lower dosing (0.1% versus 1–2%), contributing to increased safety; and 4) that may be tolerated if the parent compound is not. As shown in the top of the diagram, dipivalyl-epinephrine is 'activated' to epinephrine as it crosses the cornea, where an esterase cleaves off the pivalyl acid from each site. A much higher concentration of epinephrine must be applied to achieve the same intraocular level as dipivalyl-epinephrine, as illustrated in the bottom of the diagram. It is estimated that 0.1% dipivalyl-epinephrine is the therapeutic equivalent of 1.5% ephinephrine.

markedly increased lipid solubility over the epinephrine molecule with greater penetrability into the eye, allowing for a lower concentration of the drug presented to the eye. As the drug penetrates the cornea, esterases cleave the pivalyl moieties, thus activating the drug to epinephrine (Fig. 14.11). DPE has approximately 17 times more penetrability into the eye than epinephrine, and a 0.1% concentration has the pressure-lowering ability equivalent to about 1.5% epinephrine. Although the systemic side-effects have been reduced with DPE, local reactions, particularly allergy, remain a problem.

Alpha$_2$ adrenergic agonists

Clonidine is a potent centrally acting alpha$_2$ adrenergic agonist used to treat systemic hypertension. Applied topically in concentrations of 0.25% and 0.5%, clonidine will lower intraocular pressure but also elicits severe systemic hypotension. Modification of the molecule led to the development of para-aminoclonidine, also known as apraclonidine, marketed as Iopidine. The 1% solution of apraclonidine has been shown to be effective in blunting postoperative pressure rises following ophthalmic laser procedures and cataract surgery. The 0.5% solution has been approved for 'short-term' adjunctive therapy for lowering intraocular pressure pending surgery. The alpha$_2$ agonists lower intraocular pressure by decreasing aqueous flow. Chronic use of apraclonidine has been limited by a high allergy rate of approximately 25%. The allergic reaction is similar to that seen in epinephrine, as illustrated in Figure 14.9a and b. Other side-effects include conjunctival blanching and lid retraction, attributed to alpha$_1$ effects.

Brimonidine tartrate has been introduced into the USA for chronic use in the treatment of ocular hypertension and glaucoma. Marketed as Alphagan, the drug is thought to have greater selectivity for the alpha$_2$ receptor than apraclonidine. In addition to decreasing aqueous flow, brimonidine may also lower pressure by increasing uveoscleral outflow. In a one-year study, the drug has been demonstrated to be equally effective for lowering intraocular pressure as 0.5% timolol when both were administered twice daily, with no difference in pressure at peak (2 hours after administration) but statistically significantly less efficacious as timolol at trough (12 hours after administration). The drug has been approved for use three times daily. The allergy rate to brimonidine is about 12%. In the one-year study, only about 8% of patients were discontinued due to inadequate response. Side-effects include dry mouth, fatigue and drowsiness, systemic hypotension, and allergy.

Carbonic anhydrase inhibitors

Carbonic anhydrase is an enzyme found predominantly in the ciliary epithelium, the kidney, the central nervous system, and red blood cells. It catalyzes the combination of water and carbon dioxide to form bicarbonate and hydrogen ions. Within the ciliary epithelium hydrogen ions are exchanged for sodium ions, some bicarbonate is exchanged for chloride, and bicarbonate and/or chloride are actively transported into the aqueous with sodium and water passively following. Inhibition of the carbonic anhydrase enzyme can result in marked reduction in aqueous humor formation (approximately 40%), and lowering of the intraocular pressure.

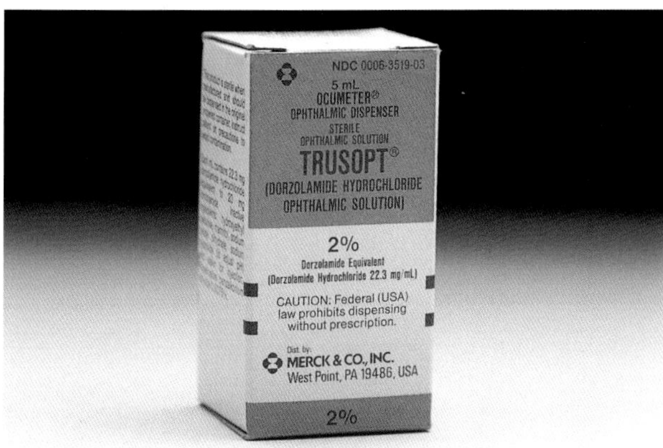

Figure 14.12 Dorzolamide
The first topically active carbonic anhydrase inhibitor, dorzolamide, is marketed as Trusopt by Merck, Inc. It is effective as monotherapy when administered three times daily, and lowers intraocular pressure approximately 20% from baseline. It is also effective as additive therapy, where twice-daily administration may be sufficient.

The first clinically active orally administered carbonic anhydrase inhibitor, acetazolamide, was introduced in the mid-1950s. It is currently available in 125 and 250 mg tablets for four time daily administration and as 500 mg time-release capsules (Diamox Sequals) for twice-daily use. A number of other agents have been marketed, notably methazolamide and ethoxzolamide. Methazolamide has a theoretical advantage over acetazolamide in that it is much less bound to plasma protein, and hence may be administered in lower doses (usually 25–50 mg two to four times daily) and may thus elicit less systemic toxicity than acetazolamide.

Clinical use of the carbonic anhydrase inhibitors, especially long term, is limited by the potential for systemic side-effects. Since all carbonic anhydrase inhibitors are sulfa derivatives, they must be used with caution, if at all, in patients with sulfa allergies. More common reactions include anorexia, weight loss, fatigue and drowsiness, general malaise, tingling and numbness in the hands and feet, metallic taste in the mouth after ingestion of carbonated beverages, gastrointestinal upset (including diarrhea and nausea), potassium loss with the attendant complications of hypokalemia (which could be fatal in patients taking digitalis), kidney stones (less common with methazolamide), systemic acidosis, and shortness of breath. Idiosyncratic reactions may result in a fatal aplastic anemia, estimated to occur in 1 in 18 000 patients. The indications for oral carbonic anhydrase inhibitors include short-term adjunctive therapy, particularly for acute pressure rises, and perhaps long-term use in patients who are unwilling or unable to administer an eye drop, particularly if argon laser trabeculoplasty has failed.

The limitations of oral carbonic anhydrase inhibitors and decades of continued research culminated in the development and release of the first topically active carbonic anhydrase inhibitor, dorzolamide (Trusopt, Fig. 14.12). Used three times daily, the drug is approximately equal in efficacy to betaxolol, and slightly less effective than timolol. It is an excellent additive drug to topical beta-adrenoreceptor antagonists, resulting in reductions in intraocular pressure reaching 35% from baseline. Many glaucoma specialists are of the opinion that twice-daily dosing of dorzolamide is sufficient when the drug is used as additive therapy, although the effectiveness of twice-daily dosing when used in combination with other drugs for 24-hour pressure control is unproven. The drug is fairly well tolerated with minimal or no systemic side-effects, with the exception of a bitter taste in the mouth in some individuals. Stinging and burning (occurring approximately three times more frequently than with timolol), punctate keratopathy, corneal edema, and follicular conjunctivitis (Fig. 14.9) have also been commonly seen. Since dorzolamide is a sulfa derivative, it should not be used in patients with known sulfa allergy.

Brinzolamide (Azopt, Alcon, Inc.) is a new topical carbonic anhydrase inhibitor recently approved for use in the USA. Administered two or three times daily, it is similar in efficacy to dorzolamide. Of greatest potential utility is that brinzolamide is rated as more comfortable than dorzolamide. Since comfort is an important contributor to compliance, the main advantage of brinzolamide is that patients may be more likely to take it.

Cholinergic agonists (miotics)

Stimulation of the longitudinal muscle of the ciliary body (via the parasympathetic pathways mediated by acetylcholine) increases traction on the scleral spur, which in turn increases the tension on the trabecular meshwork, resulting in increased outflow facility. Effective lowering of intraocular pressure may be achieved by direct stimulation of the cholinergic receptors by drugs which mimic naturally occurring acetylcholine (directly applied acetylcholine is ineffective because it is broken down by esterases in the cornea). Indirect stimulation may be achieved by use of drugs which inhibit the enzymatic breakdown of naturally occurring acetylcholine. Direct-acting cholinergics include pilocarpine (Fig. 14.13) and carbachol, while the indirect-acting cholinesterase inhibitors include phospholine iodide and eserine. Use of cholinergics

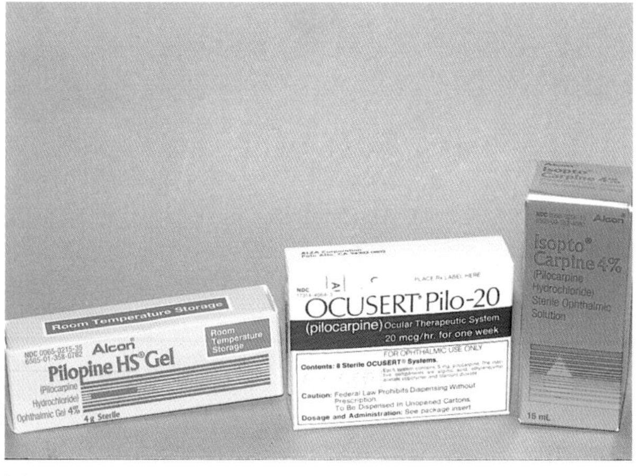

(a)

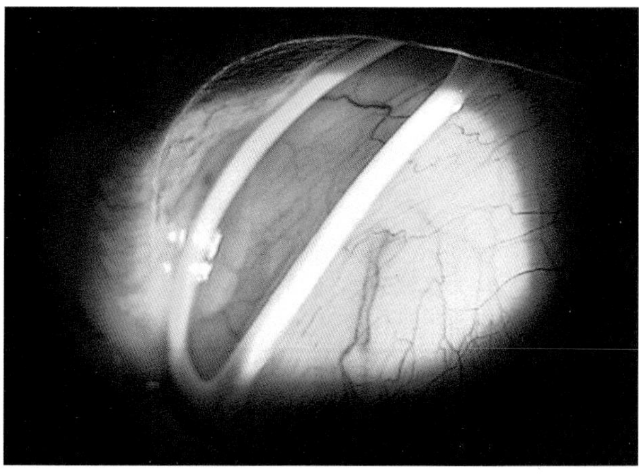

(b)

Figure 14.13 Pilocarpine
(a) Various formulations of pilocarpine, from left to right: 1) Pilopine HS Gel, a 4% formulation which provides effective pressure control over a 24-hour period following bedtime administration; 2) Ocusert, a semi-permeable membrane system which slowly releases pilocarpine over a one-week period when left in place in the conjunctival fornix; and 3) pilocarpine solution. (b) Close-up of an Ocusert in the upper fornix.

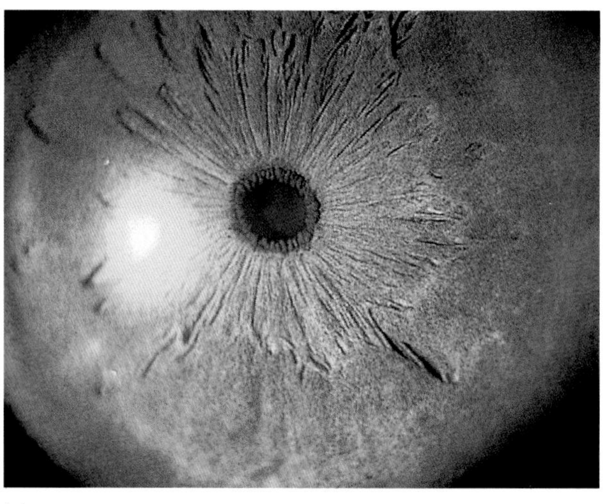

(a)

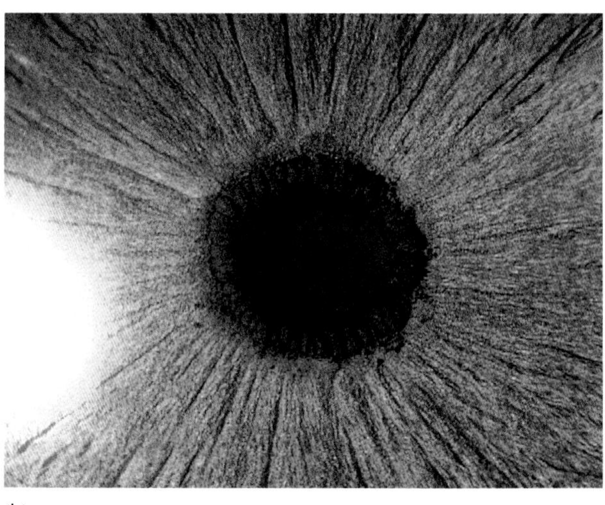

(b)

Figure 14.14 Ocular side-effects of cholinergics
(a) Miosis, which may cause blurred vision and dimness, especially in patients with cataract. (b) Pigment epithelial cysts at the pupillary margin, related to chronic use of cholinergics.

is limited by the side-effects which occur through stimulation of other cholinergic receptors in the eye, i.e. accommodative spasm with induced myopia due to stimulation of the circular muscle of the ciliary body, and miosis (Fig. 14.14a) with decreased vision (especially in patients with early cataracts) due to stimulation of the iris sphincter. Prolonged use of miotics may result in conjunctival hyperemia, pigment epithelial cysts of the iris sphincter (Fig. 14.14b), inability to dilate the pupil due to fibrosis, uveitis due to breakdown of the blood–aqueous barrier (miotics are relatively contraindicated in inflammatory glaucoma and neovascular glaucoma), and systemic symptoms from cholinergic stimulation (salivation, tearing, urinary frequency, diarrhea, excessive sweating). Strong miotics such as carbachol or phospholine iodide may cause cataract formation (phospholine should best be used in aphakic or pseudophakic patients, where it is generally well tolerated and highly effective), and may cause retinal detachment through traction on the vitreous base. Additionally, anesthesiologists must be told when patients are using phospholine iodide, since inhibition of systemic cholinesterase may prolong the action of succinylcholine (used for paralysis during induction of general anesthesia), resulting in difficulty taking the patient off the ventilator. Headache is very common when starting patients on miotic therapy due to ciliary spasm. Treatment should start with very low concentrations, increasing the concentration based upon the response observed. The patients should be advised that the headache will ease up over an 'adjustment' period lasting a few days.

Pilocarpine in various formulations (Fig. 14.13a) is the most commonly used cholinergic and one of the least expensive glaucoma medications. It has been available for over 100 years, and is the only agent derived from naturally occurring substances. In drop form, pilocarpine must be administered four times daily due to its limited duration of action. More darkly pigmented eyes usually require higher concentrations of the drug. Alternative delivery systems have been developed in an attempt to decrease the required frequency of application. These include a 4% gel preparation for use once daily at bedtime (theoretically the miotic effect will 'wear off' during sleep while the pressure-lowering effect lasts for 24 hours), and time-release discs (Ocuserts, available in the equivalent of 2% and 4%, Fig. 14.13b) which reside in the conjunctival fornix and release the drug over a one-week period. Carbachol and phospholine iodide, being stronger agents, usually are administered twice daily, although carbachol may be administered three or four times daily if necessary.

Prostaglandin analogues

The prostaglandin analogues represent the newest class of medications to be introduced for the lowering of intraocular pressure. Topically applied prostaglandins, although highly effective, had been plagued by marked hyperemia and miosis. The search for a tolerable, effective agent yielded latanoprost, the analogue of prostaglandin$F2_{alpha}$. Marketed as Xalatan, the drug is highly effective as a once-daily medication, shown to lower intraocular pressure 25–35% when administered at bedtime. It is the first drug to be shown to be more effective than twice-daily timolol for lowering intraocular pressure in clinical trials. Its unique mechanism of action is through increased uveoscleral outflow. Latanoprost is generally well tolerated, although hyperemia and irritation prompt a small percentage of patients to discontinue therapy. Some systemic side-effects have been reported, including whitening and elongation of the eyelashes, postmenopausal spotting, and a self-limited flu-like upper respiratory syndrome. Cases of cystoid macular edema have been seen in both pseudophakic and phakic patients. An unusual complication of chronic therapy with latanoprost, observed in 7–10% of patients, is a darkening of the iris (Fig. 14.15). Thought to be due to an increase of pigment within the pigmented cells of the iris, this complication has been seen in hazel or blue-green eyes. Since latanoprost has been shown to be capable of lowering intraocular pressure in eyes with already low pressures, and has not been shown to be vasoactive, it may be the ideal drug to use in patients with glaucoma requiring very low pressures.

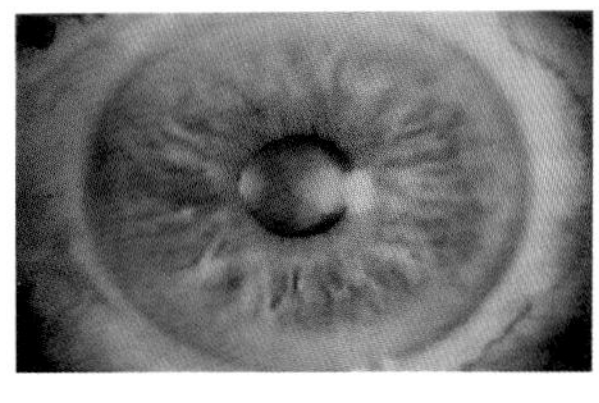
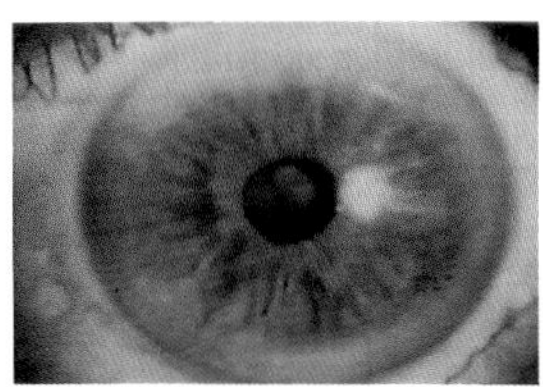
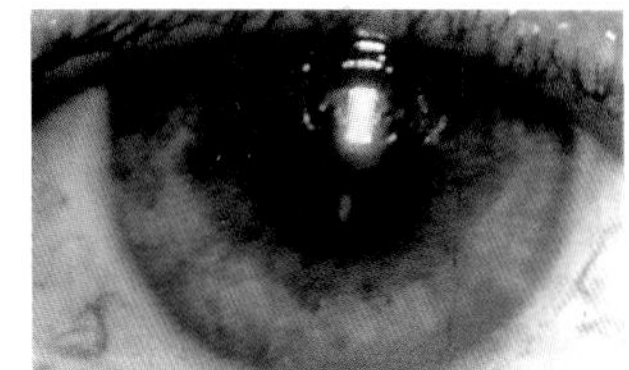
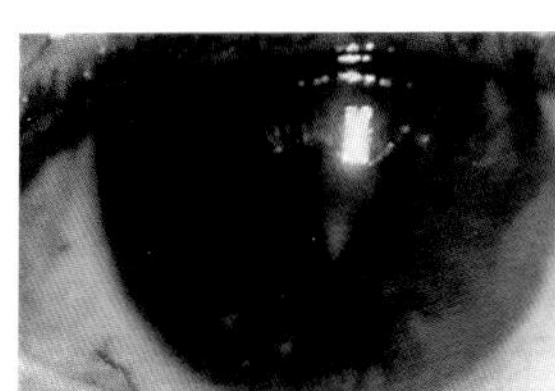

Figure 14.15 Iris color change from latanoprost
Chronic administration of latanoprost (Xalatan, Pharmacia-Upjohn) may result in darkening of the iris in approximately 7% of patients, particularly in those with hazel, blue-green, or multicolored irides. These photographs are from two different patients, with the earlier photograph on the left. The color change is due to the accumulation of pigment within existing melanosomes.

The future of medical therapy for glaucoma

New drugs

The search for the ideal glaucoma medication continues. Perhaps in the future we will have a medication that is highly effective, easy to administer, and free of side-effects. Within the past few years we have seen the introduction of the topical carbonic anhydrase inhibitor (dorzolamide), two $alpha_2$ adrenergic agonists proven safe and effective for chronic use (apraclonidine and brimonidine), and a highly effective prostaglandin analogue (latanoprost). Medications under investigation include new prostaglandins and topical carbonic anhydrase inhibitors. New drug-delivery vehicles are also under investigation designed to decrease frequency of administration or lower the required concentration of currently available drugs, all designed to increase the safety and efficacy of the drugs. Additionally, intense research is now ongoing by many companies to find medications that protect the optic nerve, rather than simply lower intraocular pressure (see below).

Combination therapy

Obviously, there is value in keeping medical therapy as simple as possible in order to maximize compliance and minimize patient confusion and inconvenience. This is part of the rationale for combining two agents into a single container. One of the oldest combinations is that of epinephrine and pilocarpine, which has generally fallen from favor since the requirement for four-times daily dosing of the pilocarpine meant an overdose of epinephrine. Newer combinations include timolol/pilocarpine (Fig. 14.16) and betaxolol/ pilocarpine. Additional products of this type are in development and may be available in the near future. A combination of timolol and dorzolamide (Cosopt) may also soon be available.

Neuroprotection

The ultimate goal of glaucoma therapy is to prevent or halt optic nerve damage. In the vast majority of patients, it would seem that lowering the intraocular pressure accomplishes that. However, it may be incorrect to look at intraocular pressure and set 'targets' for treatment, since other mechanisms, such as blood flow or genetics, may be more important in certain patients. The mechanisms leading to optic nerve damage are not well known, nor is the relationship between intraocular pressure and nerve damage. As the mechanisms become elucidated, new therapies may be developed to protect the optic nerve from damage, independent of pressure lowering.

One mechanism that may play a role is ocular blood flow, and drugs that improve blood flow (or don't decrease it as a side-effect) may prove beneficial in neuroprotection. Calcium channel blockers, for example, represent a class of medications which may improve systemic blood flow through vasodilatation. In patients with normal blood pressure, however, the use of calcium channel blockers may cause intolerable systemic hypotension. Certain topical pressure-lowering drugs already in clinical use, such as betaxolol, may have some intrinsic calcium channel blocking ability, which may contribute to their ability to stabilize the disease.

The topical beta-adrenoreceptor antagonists have also been investigated as to their effect on blood

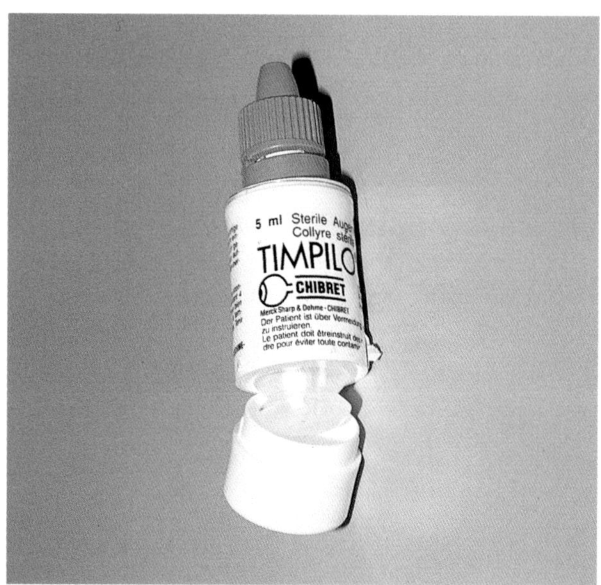

Figure 14.16 Combination therapy
Combining two medications within the same bottle has the theoretical advantage of decreasing the frequency with which the patient must administer doses, which may in turn result in better compliance. With the exception of pilocarpine/epinephrine, combination drugs are not currently available in the USA. Illustrated is the combination of timolol and pilocarpine ('Timpilo').

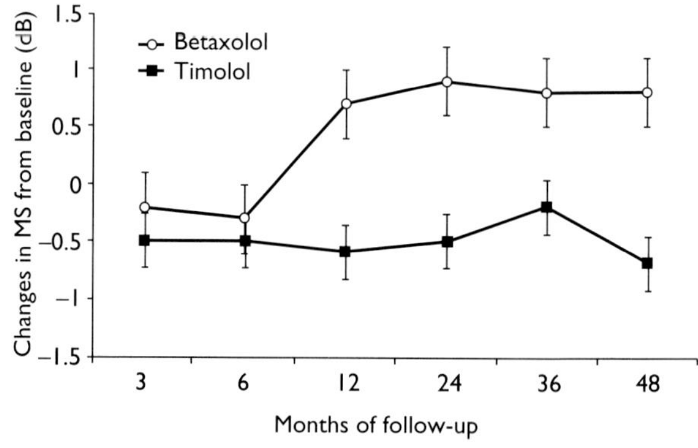

Figure 14.17 Preservation of visual field
The goal of glaucoma therapy is to prevent visual field loss from occurring or progressing. The graph illustrates the long-term change in mean retinal sensitivity as determined by visual field testing, comparing patients treated with timolol with those treated with betaxolol. The group treated with timolol show minimal change over the 4-year period, while there is a suggestion of improvement in sensitivity in the group treated with betaxolol. These findings may be interpreted as a 'neuroprotective' effect of betaxolol. Despite the fact that betaxolol does not lower intraocular pressure as well as timolol, this effect may be mediated through effects (or lack of effect) on ocular blood flow. This is an area of active research.

flow. In one study, betaxolol was shown to have less detrimental effect on end-diastolic blood velocity in the ocular circulation than the nonspecific beta-adrenoreceptor antagonists. A long-term study comparing visual fields in patients treated with timolol with those in patients treated with betaxolol showed a slight increase in mean sensitivity in the betaxolol patients (Fig. 14.17), despite the fact that betaxolol does not lower intraocular pressure as well as timolol. Could this mean that betaxolol has some as yet undefined neuroprotective effect? Further investigation is needed.

Mechanisms of cell death as they apply to the optic nerve are also under investigation. It is known that when an axon dies, it releases substances, such as glutamate, into the extracellular environment that may trigger the death of neighboring cells by a mechanism known as apoptosis. Agents are being sought to prevent triggering apoptosis in otherwise undamaged neurons. One drug under investigation for this is brimonidine. One study, involving a focal crush injury to the optic nerve in the rat, has shown that brimonidine is capable of reducing the spread of injury. Whether or not this has any applicability to glaucoma management remains to be seen. Other drugs under investigation include oral neuroexcitatory drugs currently being used outside the USA for the treatment of senile dementias. It may be that some day the treatment of glaucoma will place less emphasis on intraocular pressure control and will involve topical or oral agents that prevent or retard neuronal death.

FURTHER READING

Airaksinen PJ, Valkonen R, Stenborg T et al., A double-masked study of timolol and pilocarpine combined, *Am J Ophthalmol* (1987) **104**:587–90.

Airaksinen PJ, Valkonen R, Stenborg T et al., A double-masked study of timolol and pilocarpine combined, *Am J Ophthalmol* (1988) **105**:437.

Akingbehin AO, Granulomatous uveitis and metipranolol, *Br J Ophthalmol* (1993) **77**:536–7 (letter).

Akingbehin T, Villada JR, Metipranolol-associated granulomatous anterior uveitis, *Br J Ophthalmol* (1991) **75**:519–23.

Akingbehin T, Villada JR, Metipranolol-induced adverse reactions. II. Loss of intraocular pressure control, *Eye* (1992) **6**:280–3.

Akingbehin T, Villada JR, Walley T. Metipranolol-induced adverse reactions. I. The rechallenge study, *Eye* (1992) **6**:277–9.

Allen RC, Cagle GD, Bruce LA, Controlled clinical evaluation of betaxolol (0.5%) ophthalmic solution intraocular pressure and adjunctive therapy, *Program and Abstracts, Glaucoma Soc Meeting, Turin (XXV Int Congress Ophthalmology)* (1986) **1**:20.

Ashton P, Podder SK, Lee VH, Formulation influence on conjunctival penetration of four beta blockers in the pigmented rabbit: a comparison with corneal penetration, *Pharm Res* (1991) **8**:1166–74.

Bacon PJ, Brazier DJ, Smith R, Smith SE, Cardiovascular responses to metipranolol and timolol eyedrops in healthy volunteers, *Br J Clin.Pharmacol* (1989) **27**:1–5.

Ball SF, Schneider E, Cost of beta-adrenergic receptor blocking agents for ocular hypertension, *Arch Ophthalmol* (1992) **110**:654–7.

Barnebey HS, Robin AL, Zimmerman TJ et al., The efficacy of brimonidine in decreasing elevations in intraocular pressure after laser trabeculoplasty, *Ophthalmology* (1993) **100**:1083–99.

Beck RW, Moke P, Blair RC, Nissenbaum R, Uveitis associated with topical beta-blockers, *Arch Ophthalmol* (1996) **114**:1181–82.

Becker B, Use of methazolamide (Neptazane) in the therapy of glaucoma, *Am J Ophthalmol* (1960) **49**:1307–11.

Becker B, Middleton W, Long-term acetazolamide (Diamox) administration in the therapy of glaucomas, *Arch Ophthalmol* (1955) **54**:187–92.

Blackwell B, Treatment adherence, *Br J Psychiatry* (1976) **129**:513–31.

Boger WP, Steinert RF, Puliafito CA, Pavan-Langston D, Clinical trial comparing timolol ophthalmic solution to pilocarpine in open-angle glaucoma, *Am J Ophthalmol* (1978) **86**:8–18.

Calissendorff B, Maren N, Wettrell K, Ostberg A, Timolol versus pilocarpine separately or combined with acetazolamide—effects on intraocular pressure, *Acta Ophthalmol* (1980) **58**:624–31.

Camras CB, the Brinzolamide Primary Therapy Study Group I, A triple-masked, primary therapy study of the efficacy and safety of b.i.d and t.i.d.-dosed brinzolamide 1% compared to t.i.d.-dosed dorzolamide 2% and b.i.d.-dosed timolol 0.5%, *Invest Ophthalmol Vis Sci* (1997) **38**:S560–S560 (abst).

Charap AD, Shin DH, Petursson G et al., The effect of varying drop size on the efficacy and safety of a topical beta-blocker, *Ann Ophthalmol* (1988) **21**:351–7.

Christ T, Kessler C, (Are metipranolol eyedrops responsible for intraocular side effects?) Verursachen Metipranololhaltige

Augentropfen intraokulare Nebenwirkungen? *Ophthalmologe* (1992) **89**:455–61.

Coakes RL, Brubaker RF, The mechanism of timolol in lowering intraocular pressure, *Arch Ophthalmol* (1978) **96**:2045–8.

Coleman AL, Diehl D, Jampel HD, Bachorik PS, Quigley HA, Topical timolol decreases plasma high-density lipoprotein cholesterol level, *Arch Ophthalmol* (1990) **108**:1260–3.

Collignon-Brach J, Long-term effect of ophthalmic beta-adrenoreceptor antagonists on intraocular pressure and retinal sensitivity in primary open-angle glaucoma, *Curr Eye Res* (1992) **11**:1–3.

David R, Spaeth GL, Clevenger CE et al., Brimonidine in the prevention of intraocular pressure elevation following argon laser trabeculoplasty, *Arch Ophthalmol* (1993) **111**:1387–90.

David R, Zangwill L, Stone D, Yassur Y, Epidemiology of intraocular pressure in a population screened for glaucoma, *Br J Ophthalmol* (1987) **71**:766–71.

Dean T, May J, Chen HH, Kyba E, McLaughlin M, DeSantis L, Brinzolamide (AL-4862) suspension is a new topically active carbonic anhydrase inhibiter in the Dutch belted rabbit and cynomolgus monkey, *Invest Ophthalmol Vis Sci* (1997) **38**:S813–S813 (abst).

Dickstein K, Aarsland T, Comparison of the effects of aqueous and gellan ophthalmic timolol on peak exercise performance in middle-aged men, *Am J Ophthalmol* (1996) **121**:367–71.

DuBiner HB, Hill R, Kaufman H et al., Timolol hemihydrate vs timolol maleate to treat ocular hypertension and open-angle glaucoma, *Am J Ophthalmol* (1996) **121**:522–8.

Fraunfelder FT, Shell JW, Herbst SF, Effect of pilocarpine ocular therapeutic systems on diurnal control of intraocular pressure, *Ann Ophthalmol* (1976) **8**:1031–9.

Freedman SF, Freedman NJ, Shields MB et al., Effects of ocular carteolol and timolol on plasma high-density lipoprotein cholesterol level, *Am J Ophthalmol* (1993) **116**:600–11.

Freedman SF, Shields MB, Freedman NJ et al., Topical beta blockers and plasma lipids: carteolol vs. timolol, *Invest Ophthalmol Vis Sci* (1993) **34**(Suppl):927.

Gaul GR, Will NJ, Brubaker RF, Comparison of a non-cardioselective beta adrenoreceptor blocker and a cardioselective blocker in reducing aqueous flow in humans, *Arch Ophthalmol* (1989) **107**:1308–11.

Gordon RN, Ritch R, Liebmann JM, Greenfield DS, Lama P, Alpha-agonist allergy: is there a cross-reactivity between apraclonidine and brimonidine? *Invest Ophthalmol Vis Sci* (1997) **38**:S559–S559 (abst).

Hass I, Drance SM, Comparison between pilocarpine and timolol on diurnal pressures in open-angle glaucoma, *Arch Ophthalmol* (1980) **98**:480–1.

Hayashi M, Yablonski ME, Novack GD, Cook DJ, True outflow facility determined by fluorophotometry in human subjects, *Exp Eye Res* (1989) **48**:621–5.

Hommer A, Nowak A, Huber-Spitzy V, Multicenter double-blind study with 0.25% timolol in Gelrite (TG) once daily vs. 0.25% timolol solution (TS) twice daily. German Study Group, *Ophthalmologe* (1995) **92**:546–9.

Kaiser HJ, Flammer J, Messmer C, Stumpfig D, Hendrickson P, Thirty-month visual field follow-up of glaucoma patients treated with ?-blockers, *J Glaucoma* (1992) **1**:153–5.

Kass MA, Gordon M, Meltzer DW, Can ophthalmologists correctly identify patients defaulting from pilocarpine therapy? *Am J Ophthalmol* (1986) **101**:524–30.

Kass MA, Gordon M, Morley RE, Meltzer DW, Goldberg JJ, Compliance with topical timolol treatment, *Am J Ophthalmol* (1987) **103**:188–93.

Kass MA, Meltzer DW, Gordon M, Cooper D, Goldberg J, Compliance with topical pilocarpine treatment, *Am J Ophthalmol* (1986) **101**:515–23.

Katz IM, Berger ET, Effects of iris pigmentation on response of ocular pressure to timolol, *Survey Ophthalmol* (1979) **23**:395–8.

Kaufman PL, Prostaglandins and cholinomimetics, *Arch Ophthalmol* (1997) **115**:911–12.

Kessler C, Possible bilateral anterior uveitis secondary to metipranolol (OptiPranolol) therapy, *Arch Ophthalmol* (1994) **112**:1277 (letter).

Kessler C, Christ T, The incidence of uveitis in glaucoma patients using metipranolol, *J Glaucoma* (1993) **2**:166–70.

Kitazawa Y, Multicenter double-blind comparison of carteolol and timolol in primary open-angle glaucoma and ocular hypertension, *Adv Ther* (1993) **10**:95–131.

Kolker AE, Visual prognosis in advanced glaucoma: a comparison of medical and surgical therapy for retention of vision in 101 eyes with advanced glaucoma, *Trans Am Ophthalmol Soc* (1977) **75**:539–55.

Krieglstein GK, Novack GD, Voepel E et al., Levobunolol and metipranolol: comparative ocular hypotensive efficacy, safety and comfort, *Br J Ophthalmol* (1987) **71**:250–3.

Laurence J, Holder D, Vogel R et al., A double-masked, placebo-controlled evaluation of timolol in gel vehicle, *J Glaucoma* (1993) 177–82.

Levobunolol Study Group, Levobunolol: a four-year study of efficacy and safety in glaucoma treatment, *Ophthalmology* (1989) **96**:642–5.

Leydhecker W, Akiyama K, Neumann HG, Der intraokulare druck gesunder menshlicher augen, *Klin Mbl Augenheilk* (1958) **133**:662–70.

Linden C, Alm A, Latanoprost and physostigmine have mostly additive ocular hypotensive effects in human eyes, *Arch Ophthalmol* (1997) **115**:857–61.

Lofors KT, Hovding G, Viksmoen L, Aasved H, Bergaust B, Bulie T, Twelve-hour IOP control obtained by a single dose of timolol/pilocarpine combination eye drops, *Acta Ophthalmol* (1990) **68**:323–6.

Long DA, Johns GE, Mullen RS et al., Levobunolol and betaxolol: a double-masked controlled comparison of efficacy and safety in patients with elevated intraocular pressure, *Ophthalmology* (1988) **95**:735–41.

Lyden M, Applebaum HJ, Effect of ophthalmic metipranolol and timolol on exercise-induced tachycardia, *J Glaucoma* (1995) **4**:124–29.

Melles RB, Wong IG, Metipranolol-associated granulomatous iritis, *Am J Ophthalmol* (1994) **118**:712–15.

Merte HJ, Stryz JR, Mertz M, Comparative studies of initial pressure reduction using 0.3% metipranolol and 0.25% timolol in eyes with wide-angle glaucoma, *Klin Mbl Augenheilk* (1983) **182**:286–9.

Mertz M, Results of a 6 weeks' multicenter double-blind trial: metipranolol vs timolol. In: Merte H-J ed, *Metipranolol: pharmacology of beta-blocking agents and use of metipranolol in ophthalmology* (Springer-Verlag: Vienna and New York, 1984) 93–105.

Messmer C, Stumpfig D, Flammer J, Effect of betaxolol and timolol on visual fields in glaucoma patients, *Klin Mbl Augenheilk* (1991) **198**:330–1.

Migdal C, What is the appropriate treatment for patients with primary open-angle glaucoma: medicine, laser, or primary surgery? *Ophthalmic Surg* (1996) **26**:108–9.

Midgal C, Gregory W, Hitchings R, Long-term functional outcome after early surgery compared with laser and medicine in open-angle glaucoma, *Ophthalmology* (1994) **101**:1651–6.

Mottow-Lippa LS, Lippa EA, Naidoff MA, Clementi R, Bjornsson T, Jones K, .008% timolol ophthalmic solution. A minimal-effect dose in a normal volunteer model, *Arch Ophthalmol* (1990) **108**:61–4.

Novack GD, Ophthalmic beta-blockers since timolol, *Surv Ophthalmol* (1987) **31**:307–27.

Ober M, Scharrer A, Novack GD, Lue JC, Die lokale subjektive Vertraglich keit von Levobunolol und Metipranolol in einer Doppelblink-Vergliechsstudie bie Patienten mit erhohtem intraokularem druck, *Ophthalmologica* (1986) **192**:159–64.

O'Connor GR, Granulomatous uveitis and metipranolol, *Br J Ophthalmol* (1993) **77**:536–7 (letter).

Puustjarvi T, Aine E, Hakala T, The effect of two timolol and pilocarpine combinations versus timolol 0.5% in the treatment of open-angle glaucoma, *Chibret Intl J Ophthalmol* (1990) **7**:68–71.

Puustjarvi TJ, Repo LP, Aarnisalo E et al., Timolol-pilocarpine fixed-ratio combinations in the treatment of chronic open angle glaucoma: a controlled multicenter study of 48 weeks, *Arch Ophthalmol* (1992) **110**:1725–29.

Puustjarvi T, Aine E, Hakala T, Die wirkung von timolol/pilocarpin-kombinationen mit konstantem verhßltnis verglichen mit 0,5%igem timolol bei der behandlung des weitwinkel-glaukoms, *Fortschr Ophthalmol* (1988) **85**:76–8.

Reiss GR, Brubaker RF, The mechanism of betaxolol, a new hypotensive agent, *Ophthalmology* (1983) **90**:1369–72.

Robin AL, Ocular hypotensive efficacy and safety of a combined formulation of betaxolol and pilocarpine, *Trans Am Ophthalmol Soc* (1996) **94**:89–101.

Rosenlund EF, The intraocular pressure lowering effect of timolol in gel-forming solution, *Acta Ophthalmol Scand* (1996) **74**:160–2.

Schultz JS, Hoenig JA, Charles H, Possible bilateral anterior uveitis secondary to metipranolol (Optipranolol) therapy, *Arch Ophthalmol* (1993) **111**:1606–7.

Schuman JS, Clinical experience with brimonidine 0.2% and timolol 0.5% in glaucoma and ocular hypertension, *Surv Ophthalmol* (1996) **41**(Suppl 1):S27–37.

Schuman JS, Horwitz B, Choplin NT, David R, Albracht D, Chen K, Chronic Brimonidine Study Group, A 1-year study of brimonidine twice daily in glaucoma and ocular hypertension, *Arch Ophthalmol* (1997) **115**:847–52.

Serle JB, A comparison of the safety and efficacy of twice daily brimonidine 0.2% versus betaxolol 0.25% in subjects with elevated intraocular pressure. The Brimonidine Study Group III, *Surv Ophthalmol* (1996) **41** (Suppl 1):S39–47.

Shedden AH, Long-term, double-masked evaluation of the efficacy and safety of a timolol maleate ophthalmic gel forming solution, *Ophthalmology* (1993) **100**:111 (abst).

Shedden AH, Timolol maleate in gel-forming solution: a novel formulation of timolol maleate, *Chibret Intl J Ophthalmol* (1994) **10**:32–6.

Sherwood MB, Migdal CS, Hitchings RA et al., Initial treatment of glaucoma: surgery or medications, *Surv Ophthalmol* (1993) **37**:293–305.

Soderstrom MB, Wallin O, Granstrom P-A, Thorburn W, Timolol-pilocarpine combined vs. timolol and pilocarpine given separately, *Am J Ophthalmol* (1989) **107**:465–70.

Soll DB, Evaluation of timolol in chronic open-angle glaucoma: once-a-day vs twice-a-day, *Arch Ophthalmol* (1980) **98**:2178–81.

Sommer A, Intraocular pressure and glaucoma, *Am J Ophthalmol* (1989) **107**:186–8.

Sommer A, Enger C, Witt K, Screening for glaucomatous visual field loss with automated threshold perimetry, *Am J Ophthalmol* (1987) **103**:681–4.

Stewart R, the Brinzolamide Comfort Study Group I, The ocular comfort of t.i.d.-dosed brinzolamide 1% compared to t.i.d.-dosed dorzolamide 2% in patients with primary open-angle glaucoma or ocular hypertension, *Invest Ophthalmol Vis Sci* (1997) **38**:S559–S559 (abst).

Stewart WC, Carteolol, an ophthalmic adrenergic blocker with intrinsic sympathomimetic activity, *J Glaucoma* (1994) **3**:339–45.

Stewart WC, Shields MB, Allen RC et al, A 3-month comparison of 1% and 2% carteolol and 0.5% timolol in open-angle glaucoma, *Graefes Arch Clin Exp Ophthalmol* (1991) **229**:258–61.

Stewart WC, Sine C, Cate E, Minno GE, Hunt HH, Daily cost of adrenergic blocker therapy, *Arch Ophthalmol* (1997) **115**:853–6 (abst).

Strahlman ER, Deasy D, Panebianco D, Timolol/Dorzolamide Combination Study Group, A two-week pilot activity study of a fixed combination of timolol and dorzolamide hydrochloride, *Invest Ophthalmol Vis Sci* (1993) **34**(Suppl):1148 (abst).

Strahlman E, Tipping R, Vogel R, A double-masked, randomized 1-year study comparing dorzolamide (Trusopt), timolol, and betaxolol. International Dorzolamide Study Group, *Arch Ophthalmol* (1995) **113**:1009–16.

Strahlman E, Tipping R, Vogel R, Dorzolamide Dose-Response Study Group, A six-week dose-response study of the ocular hypotensive effect of dorzolamide with a one-year extension *Am J Ophthalmol* (1996) **122**:183–94.

Strahlman ER, Vogel R, Tipping R, Clineschmidt CM, The use of dorzolamide and pilocarpine as adjunctive therapy to timolol in patients with elevated intraocular pressure. The Dorzolamide Additivity Study Group, *Ophthalmology* (1996) **103**:1283–93.

Sturm A, Vogel R, Binkowitz B, Timolol-Pilocarpine Clinical Study Groups, A fixed combination of timolol and pilocarpine: double-masked comparisons with timolol and pilocarpine, *J Glaucoma* (1992) **1**:7–13.

Sugiyama K, Enya T, Kitazawa Y, Ocular hypotensive effect of 8-hydroxycarteolol, a metabolite of carteolol, *Int Ophthalmol Clinics* (1989) **13**:85–9.

Uusitalo RJ, Palkama A, Efficacy and safety of timolol/pilocarpine combination drops in glaucoma patients, *Acta Ophthalmol (Copenh)* (1994) **72**:496–504.

Watanabe TM, Hodes BL, Bilateral anterior uveitis associated with a brand of metipranolol, *Arch Ophthalmol* (1997) **115**:422 (letter).

Weinreb RN, Caldwell DR, Goode SM et al., A double-masked three-month comparison between 0.25% betaxolol suspension and 0.5% betaxolol ophthalmic solution, *Am J Ophthalmol* (1990) **110**:189–92.

Yablonski ME, Zimmerman TJ, Waltman SR, Becker B, A fluorophotometric study of the effect of topical timolol on aqueous humor dynamics, *Exp Eye Res* (1978) **27**:135–42.

Yalon M, Urinowsky E, Rothkoff L, Frequency of timolol administration, *Am J Ophthalmol* (1981) **92**:526–9.

Zimmerman TJ, Cost of ?-blocker therapy, *Arch Ophthalmol* (1997) **115**:914.

15 Laser surgery in the treatment of glaucoma

Richard A Hill

Introduction

The development of the laser and its application in clinical medicine have been particularly important in ophthalmology. This chapter discusses the use of the laser in the treatment of glaucoma. Conditions for which lasers have proven to be useful include angle-closure glaucoma (iridectomy), plateau iris (iridoplasty), open-angle glaucoma (trabeculoplasty, laser sclerostomy), postoperative regulation of intraocular pressure following trabeculectomy (suture lysis), 'refractory' glaucomas (ciliodestructive procedures) and other miscellaneous conditions.

In 1960 Maiman first demonstrated stimulated emission of radiation using a ruby crystal and a flash-lamp. The device used light amplification for the stimulated emission of radiation and is now known by the acronym 'laser'. Light produced by a laser is monochromatic (one wave length, determined by the

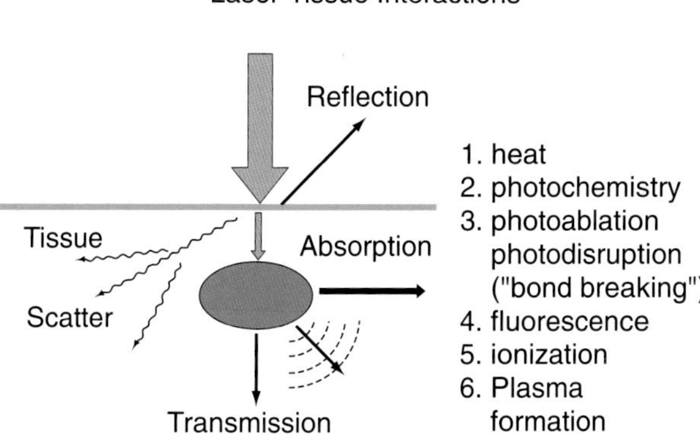

Figure 15.1 Laser–tissue interactions
Laser light may be reflected, scattered, absorbed, transmitted or create plasma. (Courtesy M Berns, Beckman Laser Institute and Medical Clinic, University of California, Irvine.)

'lasing' medium), spatially coherent (phase correlation across beam) and temporally coherent (wavelength is stable). When laser light interacts with ocular tissue, it is either reflected, scattered, transmitted or absorbed (Fig. 15.1). Clinically useful laser–tissue interactions can be classified as photochemical, thermal (photocoagulation and photothermoablation) or ionizing (Fig. 15.2). Light in the range of 400–1100 nanometers (nm) will easily pass through cornea, aqueous, lens and vitreous.

In current glaucoma therapy, intraocular laser effects are achieved by two main mechanisms. In the first mechanism, spatial confinement of photons occurs by absorption of photons by the ocular chromophores melanin, hemoglobin, and xanthophyll or water (Figs 15.3 and 15.4). The deposition of energy at first causes denaturation of proteins as the tissue temperature rises. This is clinically useful for iridoplasty or coagulation of bleeding vessels. If irradiance is greatly increased (continuous wave power/area) thermally induced focal destruction of the target tissue occurs (photocoagulation). If the temperature rises above the boiling point of water, a steam bubble is seen to form which contains water vapor and gaseous byproducts of the tissue destroyed. This produces a typical laser ablation (Fig. 15.5) in which both the surrounding edema zone of thermally altered tissues decreases and energy needed decreases (Fig. 15.6) as spatial confinement of energy increases. In addition to chromophore selection, thermal damage may be limited or extended by altering the exposure time relative to the thermal relaxation time (approximately 1 microsecond) for biologic tissues (Fig. 15.7). In glaucoma therapy by continuous wave lasers (trabeculoplasty, iridectomy, cyclophotocoagulation and iridoplasty), melanin is the major chromophore. Its absorption decreases over the 400–1000 nm range. This decreases spatial confinement of laser energy for longer wavelength lasers. In addition, longer

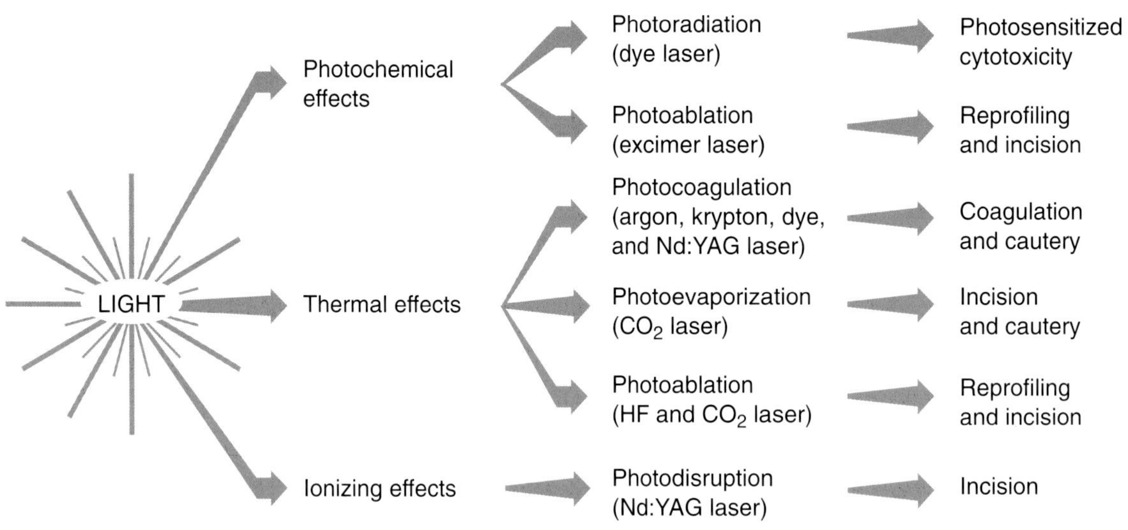

Figure 15.2 Clinically useful laser–tissue interactions
(Adapted from L'Esperance FA Jr, *Ophthalmic lasers* (St Louis, MO: Mosby, 1989: 65) and Nelson JS, Berns MW, Basic laser physics and tissue interactions, *Contemp Dermatol* (1988) **2**:2.)

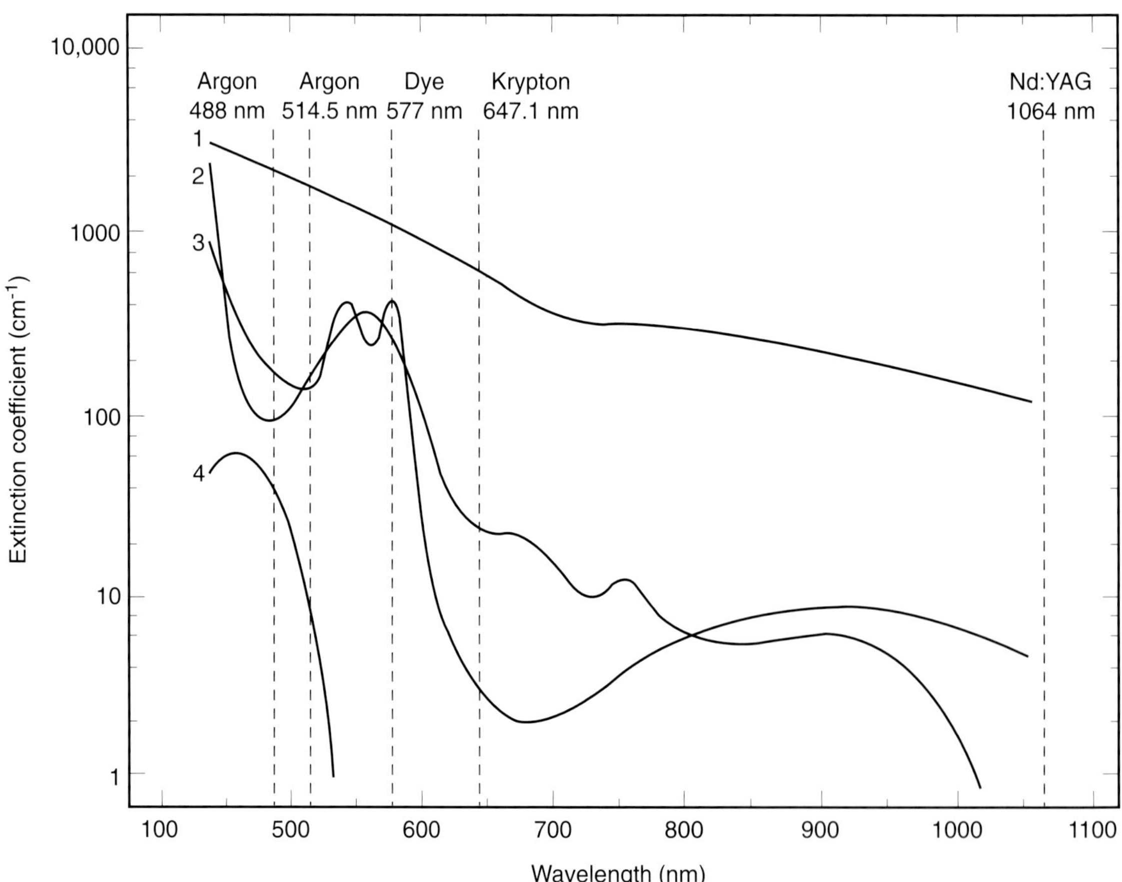

Figure 15.3 Extinction coefficient versus wavelength for ocular chromophores
Curve 1 = melanin; curve 2 = reduced hemoglobin; curve 3 = oxygenated hemoglobin; curve 4 = macular xanthophyll (Adapted from L'Esperance, FA Jr, *Ophthalmic lasers* (St Louis, MO: Mosby, 1989: 68).)

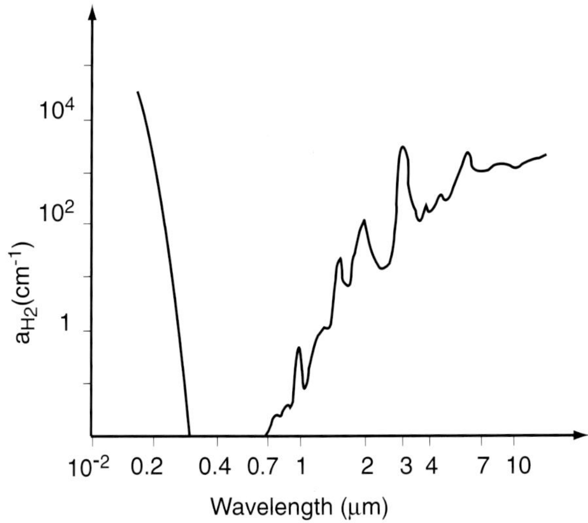

Figure 15.4 Absorption of photons by water
Water, as a chromophore, has intense absorption in the ultraviolet and usable peaks in the infrared at 2.1 μm (holmium lasers) and 2.94 μm (erbium lasers).

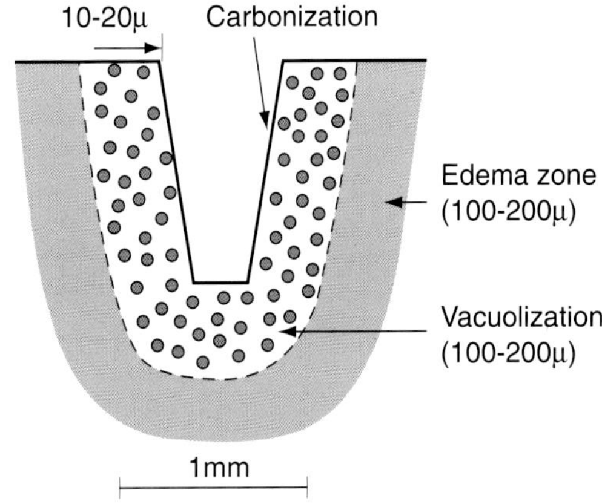

Figure 15.5 Typical effects of a pulsed laser on biologic tissues
The edema zone represents tissue thermally denatured and is of variable thickness depending on spatial confinement of the laser light and laser pulse duration. (Adapted from Nelson JS, Berns MW, Basic laser physics and tissue interactions, *Contemp Dermatol* (1988) **2**:2.)

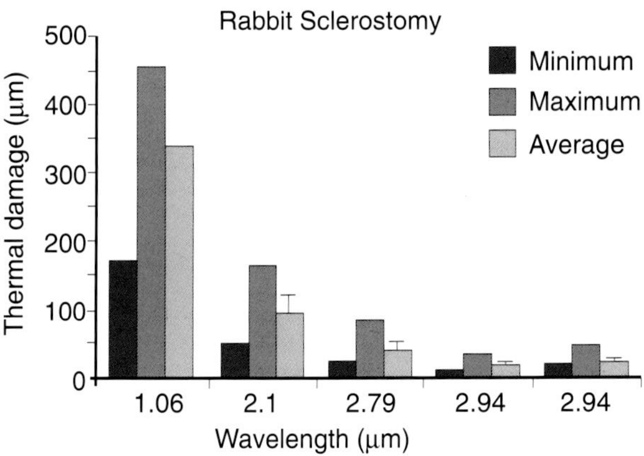

Figure 15.6 Energy required for tissue ablation decreases as spatial confinement increases
This results in maximum efficiency for lasers operating near water absorption peaks (Fig. 14.4). (Reprinted with permission, *Investigative Ophthalmology and Visual Science* (1991) **32(9)**:58–63.)

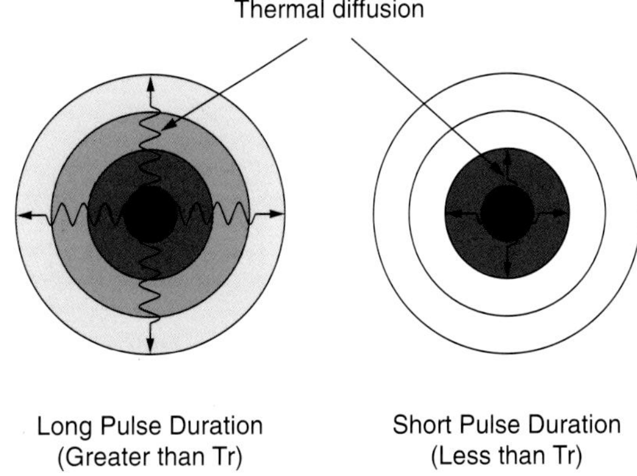

Figure 15.7 Tissue thermal damage
Tissue thermal damage increases by diffusion when laser pulses are longer than the thermal relaxation time (Tr) for biologic tissues. (Courtesy S Nelson, Beckman Laser Institute and Medical Clinic, University of California, Irvine.)

wavelength will exhibit less scatter, further increasing penetration into tissues. Although this facilitates some procedures such as trans-scleral Nd:YAG cyclophotocoagulation, it tends to create less of a surface effect (which provides clinical feedback) in other procedures such as trabeculoplasty.

The second major mechanism by which laser affects ocular tissue occurs at the focal point of short pulse, high-power lasers (Nd:YAG, Nd:YLF), which create optical breakdown or plasma formation. The individual laser pulses are delivered over extremely short intervals which results in an extraordinarily high irradiance at the focal point of the laser. This irradiance is sufficient to strip electrons from atoms of molecules creating a cloud of ions and electrons (plasma). This plasma cloud can initially absorb photons and later scatter them providing some protection for underlying tissues. After the initial plasma cloud forms, it expands rapidly creating

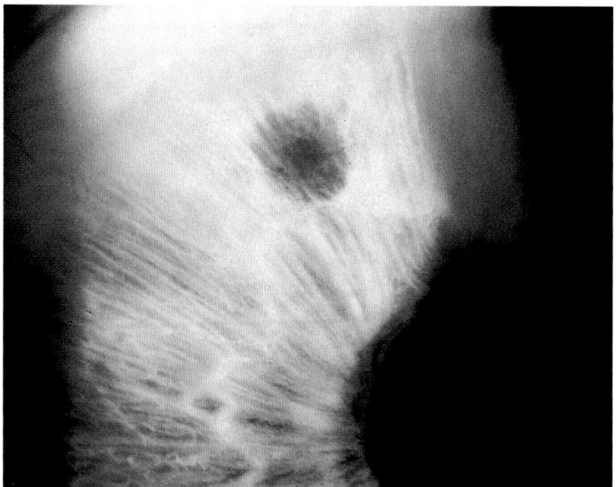

Figure 15.8 Argon laser iridectomies
Argon laser iridectomies are typically rounded with zones of thermal damage extending beyond the opening (see also Fig. 14.5).

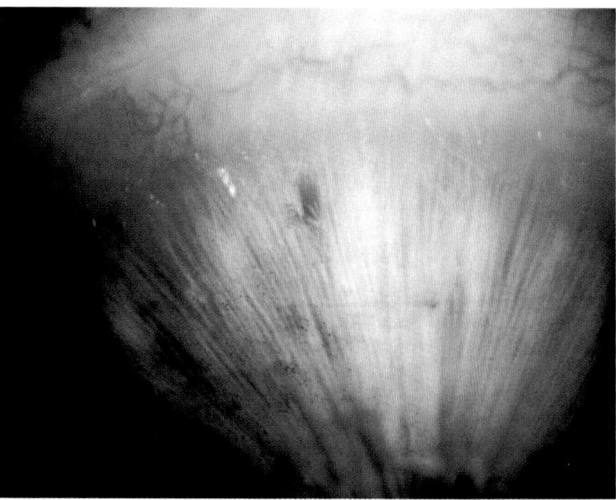

Figure 15.9 Neodymium: YAG laser iridectomies
Typical slit-like iridectomy produced by short pulse Nd:YAG laser.

stresses that exceed the structural limits of the target tissue. This ablation mechanism is chromophore independent, and useful for iridectomy formation in light-colored irides.

Laser peripheral iridectomy

Early attempts at iridectomy formation with coherent light sources were not successful because of poor spatial confinement of the laser energy. The longer wavelength photons traveled deeper into the iris and were less well absorbed by melanin. The application of lasers with shorter wavelengths and better spatial confinement of applied energy (such as ruby and argon) led to the reproducible creation of laser iridectomies. The argon laser was widely embraced and strategies for dealing with situations of excessive chromophore (dark irides) or insufficient chromophore (light irides) were developed by Ritch (contraction burn) and Hoskins/Migliazzo (bubble formation). In the early 1980s the argon laser iridectomy (Fig. 15.8) largely replaced incisional iridectomy as initial therapy for angle closure with pupillary block. In the mid-1980s short-pulsed neodymium:YAG lasers became widely available for iridectomies. Its mechanism of action is chromophore independent and works well in all iris colors. The radial orientation of iris fibers yields slit-like iridectomies (Fig. 15.9). The simplicity of the procedure and lower iridectomy closure rates have led to rapid and widespread acceptance. In addition, the use of apraclonidine prophylaxis decreased the incidence and severity of postlaser intraocular

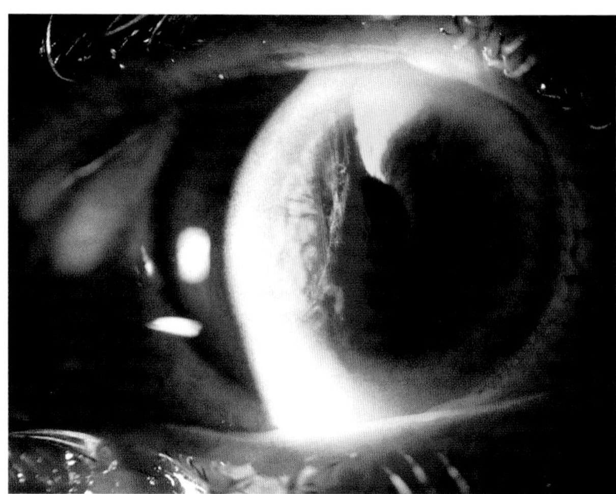

Figure 15.10 Bleeding in a patient after Nd:YAG iridectomy
Bleeding in a patient after Nd:YAG iridectomy requiring argon laser coagulation to stop. On questioning the patient, NSAIDs were being taken for arthritis but not declared as a current medication.

pressure elevations. There are, however, a number of situations where the argon laser has retained utility. For example, in the angle-closure patient on anticoagulants or in an eye with chronic inflammation, the argon laser creates a zone of thermally induced tissue coagulation (Fig. 15.5) which can also be used to prevent bleeding or stop bleeding resistant to contact lens pressure (Fig. 15.10). Other uses of the argon laser include pretreating a spongy,

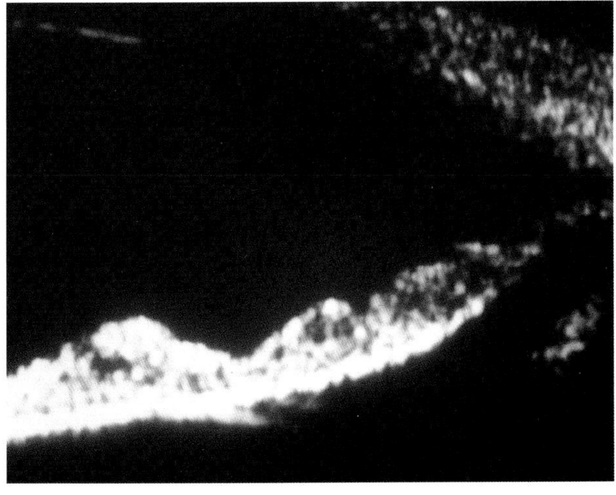

(a)

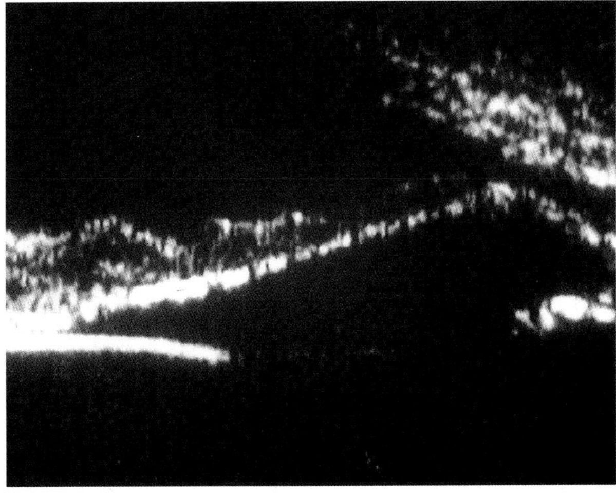

(b)

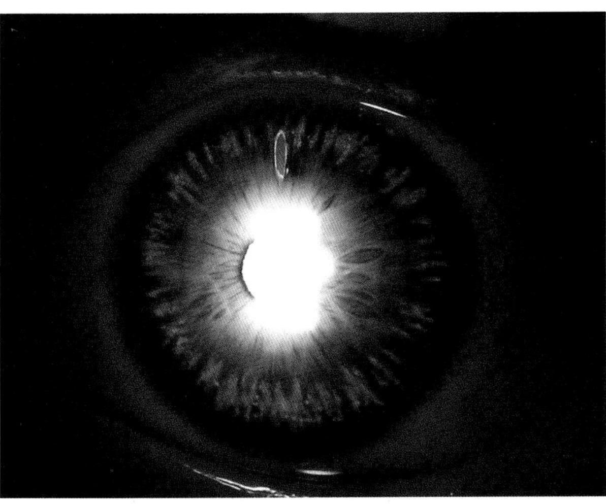

(c)

Figure 15.11 Ultrasound biomicroscopy in a patient with pigment dispersion glaucoma
(a) Before and (b) after Nd:YAG laser iridectomy. (c) Demonstrates transillumination defects and iridectomy. Intraocular pressures have normalized without medications two years' posttreatment. (Figures (a) and (b) courtesy of Dr Robert Ritch.)

thick, brown iris to minimize shredding with subsequent application of Nd:YAG energy, and in iridoplasty to break an attack of angle closure when the surgeon is unable initially to create a laser iridectomy or the angle remains occluded or occludable after laser peripheral iridectomy.

Patient evaluation

The patient examination with a Zeiss 4-mirror or similar-shaped gonioscope should show occludable or occluded angles which open with compression. In patients with pigment dispersion, laser iridectomy reverses iris concavity and iridozonular contact (Fig. 15.11a, b and c), although additional pilocarpine therapy may be necessary for residual irido-ciliary contact. Lastly, an iridectomy may be useful in treating postoperative complications such as iris bombè caused by posterior synechiae formed in eyes with chronic inflammation (Fig. 15.12).

Contact lens selection

An Abraham or Wise iridectomy lens (Fig. 15.13) will increase safety and facilitate the laser iridectomy. The use of a viscous artificial tear solution to place the contact lens (such as Celluvisc™) increases patient comfort postoperatively.

Patient preparation

Apraclonidine (Iopidine™) preoperatively and postoperatively will limit pressure spikes and bleeding with iridectomies. The use of pilocarpine will thin the iris and allow for more peripheral placement of the iridectomy which will decrease the possibility of postoperative glare symptoms. The operation should be performed in an area of iris normally covered by eyelid. Thin areas of iris such as crypts or transillumination defects in pigment dispersion (after pilocarpine use) are preferable locations.

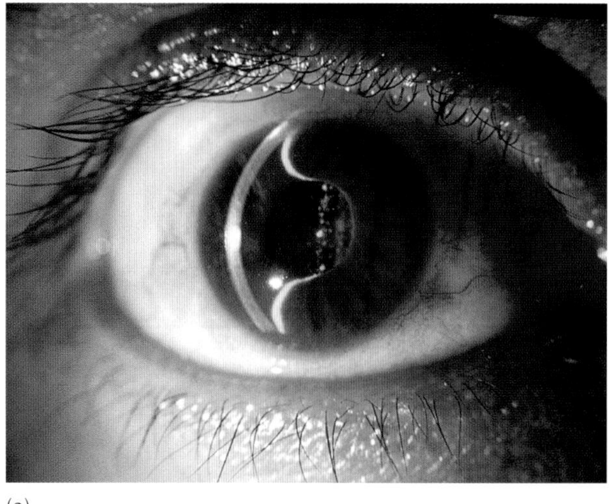

(a)

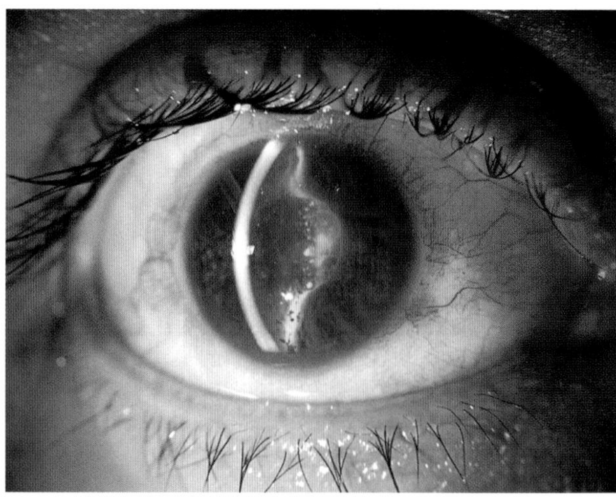

(b)

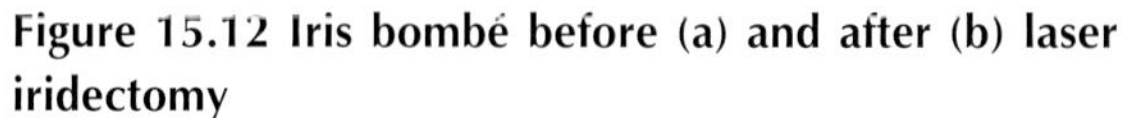

Figure 15.12 Iris bombé before (a) and after (b) laser iridectomy

Technique

Continuous or quasi-continuous wave laser iridectomy

Continuous wave lasers include argon, krypton, ruby, frequency doubled Nd:YAG and diode. Historically, the 'hump', 'drumhead' and 'chipping away' techniques have been described for argon laser iridectomy. The chipping-away technique is most commonly used. This technique is simple and straightforward. The patient must be instructed not to look at the laser light; a slight upward or inward orientation of the eye will further decrease the chances of a posterior pole laser burn. A high power (+) lens will minimize fundus irradiance should an errant laser pulse go through a patent iridectomy. Laser spots of 50 μm size are placed at exactly the same site until the anterior lens capsule can be visualized. The surgeon adjusts the continuous wave power and exposure times based on observed laser–tissue interactions. Darker irides that absorb laser energy well may char at 0.1 second exposure time and consideration should be given to shorter exposures. Conversely, lighter irides with poorer absorption must first be heated to denature tissue, decreasing transmission which increases focal scatter and heating. In practical applications, the argon laser is useful for medium-brown irises. It is also useful for pretreating thick spongy irides to minimize shredding with the application of Nd:YAG energy, coagulating vessels in patients on anticoagulants and stopping hemorrhage unresponsive to contact lens pressure (Fig. 15.10). If continuous wave power needs to be above 1.0 W or exposure times above 0.1 second, consideration should be given to the use of a Nd:YAG laser. In most situations this is the laser of choice for this procedure.

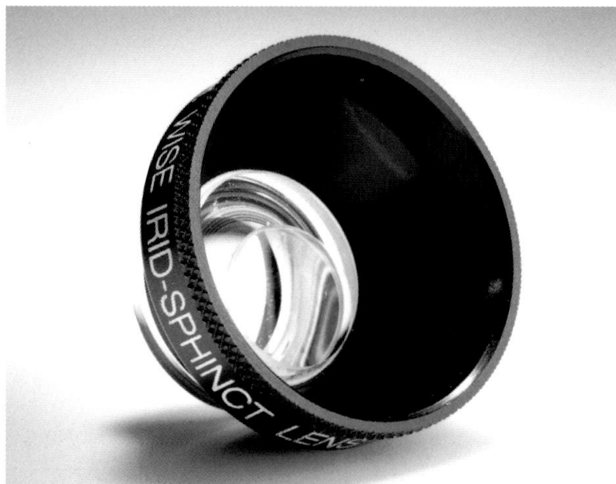

Figure 15.13 The Wise iridectomy lens
Using the Wise iridectomy lens as an example, corneal irradiance is decreased 91%, spot size on the iris is decreased 62% (increasing irradiance 7×) and potential fundus irradiance minimized by causing a 230% increase in beam diameter. (Courtesy Ocular Instruments.)

Nd:YAG laser iridectomy

The Nd:YAG laser is the laser of choice for the creation of laser iridectomies. In general,

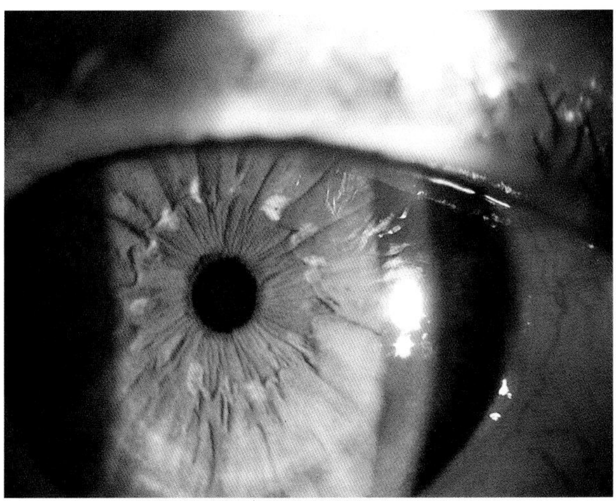

Figure 15.14 Pupilloplasty
Pupilloplasty incorrectly performed at a continuous wave power too high and a duration too short. There has been pigment release and a partial, superficial effect.

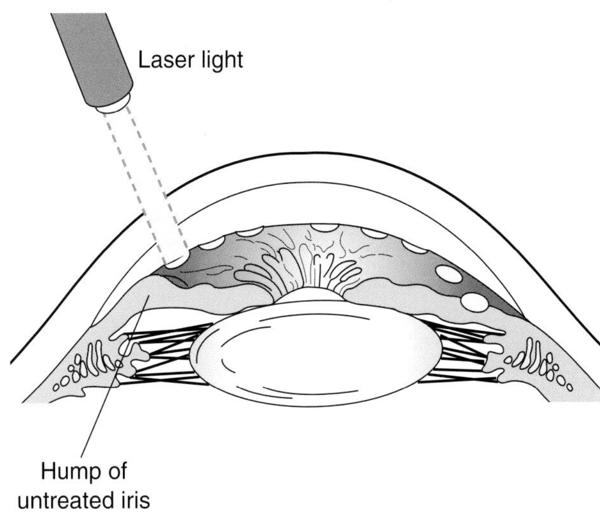

Figure 15.15 The mechanical effect of low continuous wave power, long exposure laser treatments on peripheral iris contour

2.5–4.0 mJ/pulse at 1–2 pulses per burst are usually sufficient to create Nd:YAG laser iridectomies. The use of a high plus power lens also helps create a shallow cutting effect. A coated, high-power Abraham or Wise lens (Fig. 15.13) is placed with the aid of topical anesthesia. The patient is asked to look slightly down and a thinner area of superior iris is sought out. The aiming beam is placed directly on the surface of the iris. Lighter-colored, thinner irides will yield to a few laser pulses, while darker, thicker irides may require multiple pulses. As the stroma thins, pulses per burst and energy per burst may be decreased to minimize danger to the crystalline lens. The risk to the lens may further be reduced by iridectomy placement in the far periphery, adjusting the oculars of the slit lamp delivery system to make the operator's retina conjugate with the focal point of the laser and careful focusing. Regardless of the laser used, the anterior lens capsule must be visualized; transillumination defects are not adequate to establish patency of an iridectomy. Neodymium: YAG laser iridectomies tend to be slit-like because of the radial orientation of iris fibers (Fig. 15.9). A small amount of bleeding is common with this technique. It may be stopped by increasing pressure on the contact lens. Rarely this is not sufficient and an argon laser may be used with a large spot (200–500 μm), longer duration 0.2 second) and low power burn (200–350 mW) (Fig. 15.10). The postlaser pressure check should be at slightly over an hour in order to detect the majority of postlaser pressure spikes. Corticosteroids are used at q.i.d. frequency and the patient seen at one day postoperatively (if a pressure spike has occurred or if the clinical situation dictates) and at one week for gonioscopy and to confirm discontinuation of steroids.

Central and peripheral iridoplasty

Central iridoplasty, or photomydriasis, is useful on rare occasions. Typically, a glaucoma patient who is controlled on medical therapy which includes miotics, who has a pupillary diameter less than 2 mm, may complain of poor vision and dimness, especially if an early cataract is present. Such a patient may experience an improved quality of vision if the pupil can be enlarged to greater than 2 mm by laser pupilloplasty. Long (0.2 second), large (200 μm) and low continuous wave power are used to shrink iris tissue. Spots are placed in a circular fashion every 30 degrees around the pupil and only the minimum number of spots needed to increase pupillary size over 2 mm are used. Lenticular opacities can occur. These tend to be more common in lighter-colored irides with poorer spatial confinement of the laser energy. The operator should be vigilant for eye motion as the laser energy is applied close to the pupil. If the duration of the burn is shortened and continuous wave power increased, pigment release and a superficial partial effect will result (Fig. 15.14).

Selected narrow angles may be widened by peripheral iridoplasty, particularly if the configuration is one of plateau iris and the narrowing is not due to pupillary block. In current practice, iridoplasty is performed by inducing a deep thermal contraction burn in iris stroma causing mechanical retraction from the filtering angle by flattening of the iris contour (Fig. 15.15). The laser parameters chosen to facilitate this type of laser tissue interaction are long (0.5 second), large (500 μm) and low power (200–350 mW). If bubble formation occurs, the operator should stop energy application in midpulse and decrease continuous wave power. The laser energy can be delivered through an Abraham contact lens to the most peripheral portion of the iris accessible. Five to six spots are usually placed per quadrant with 1000 μm (two laser spot) spacing. In cases of plateau iris or nanophthalmos, the laser light may need to be delivered even more peripherally and a gonio lens will facilitate this. In this case the spot size should be reduced to 200 μm. In general, eyes with more chromophore (dark irides) will require less continuous wave power, and lighter irides, more. Iridoplasty is also a useful adjunct for cases that retain an appositional closure of the filtering angle after iridectomy or in cases where an iridectomy cannot be initially created. Iridoplasty may also be useful to facilitate the performance of laser trabeculoplasty in eyes with a plateau iris configuration.

Laser trabeculoplasty

Introduced originally by Wise and Witter, laser trabeculoplasty (LTP) is a frequently performed glaucoma procedure with good long-term follow-up. A variety of lasers have been used to perform trabeculoplasty. The most commonly used is the argon laser. In using this laser, operator macular photic stress may be reduced by using the argon green only rather than both the blue and green. In addition, the use of a contact lens with a metal halide coating will reduce the hazards of reflected light. The Ritch trabeculoplasty lens (Fig. 15.16) has two different angles on its mirrors; 64 degrees for the superior angle and 59 degrees for the inferior angle. In addition a plano-convex button is positioned over each mirror which provides 1.4× magnification. This reduces a 50 μm spot to 35 μm and doubles irradiance. A standard 1 or 2-mirror lens (Fig. 15.17) without a plano-convex condensing lens has an angle of 62 degrees and produces a 54 μm spot from the original 50 μm beam which also slightly decreases irradiance. If a 1-mirror lens is used, the patient is asked to move the eye in the direction of the treating mirror to accommodate the slight variance in filtering angle anatomy. Tilting the lens will introduce astigmatic error, creating an oval beam and altered irradiance (energy per surface area).

LTP is generally indicated for the reduction of intraocular pressure in patients with primary open-angle glaucoma, although it is generally successful in patients with glaucoma associated with the pigment dispersion syndrome and the exfoliation syndrome. It may also work in patients with steroid-induced glaucoma. It is usually used when the patient has reached maximum tolerated medical therapy, and in such cases usually does not allow the discontinuation of any of the medications being used. The procedure carries an initial success rate between 70 and 80%, but patients should be advised that the effect may wear off over time; approximately 10% per year of eyes will return to pretreatment pressures. Retreatment (after 360 degrees of the angle has already been treated) carries only about a 30% chance of success, and consideration should be given to filtering surgery once LTP has failed.

Preparation

Preoperatively and postoperatively, the patient is given apraclonidine (Iopidine™), unless an allergy dictates the use of another ocular hypotensive agent. Anesthesia is achieved with topical proparicaine. Viscous artificial tear solution such as Celluvisc™ may be used with the laser lens to maximize patient comfort postoperatively.

Procedure

Standard parameters of a 50 μm spot size and an exposure time of 0.1 second are usually employed. The suggested application site is the junction of the pigmented and nonpigmented trabecular meshwork. Application of laser energy at this position, easily found except in nonpigmented filtering angles, will further reduce the incidence of pressure spikes and peripheral anterior synechiae formation. This site can be found immediately below the termination of the parallelepipid of light in a long thin slit beam under high magnification (Fig. 15.18). The degree of pigmentation found in the trabecular meshwork and whether or not the treating lens increases irradiance will suggest to the operator what continuous wave power to select initially. In most filtering angles, 700 mW is sufficient. A general rule of thumb is to subtract 100 mW of power for each stepwise increase in trabecular pigmentation. Continuous wave power should be sufficient to produce blanching or small bubble formation at 0.1 second exposure time (Fig. 15.19). Laser power meters may not be accurate and the surgeon should always believe the observed laser–tissue interaction over the power meter. An operator should also vary the power output for variations in angle pigmentation encountered intraoperatively. Treatment at too high

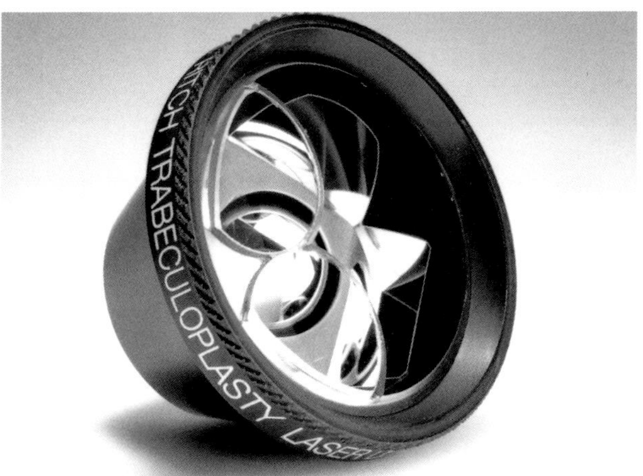

Figure 15.16 The Ritch lens
The Ritch lens has two different angles on its mirrors: 64 degrees for the superior angle and 59 degrees for the inferior angle. In addition a plano-convex button is positioned over each mirror which provides 1.4× magnification. This reduces a 50 μm spot to 35 μm and doubles irradiance. (Courtesy Ocular Instruments.)

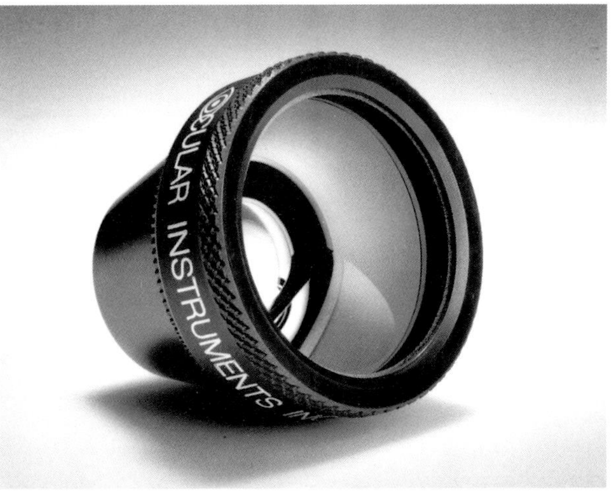

Figure 15.17 A standard 1 or 2-mirror lens
A standard 1 or 2-mirror lens without a plano-convex condensing lens has an angle of 62 degrees and produces a 54 μm spot from the original 50 μm beam (magnification = 0.93) which also slightly decreases irradiance. (Courtesy Ocular Instruments.)

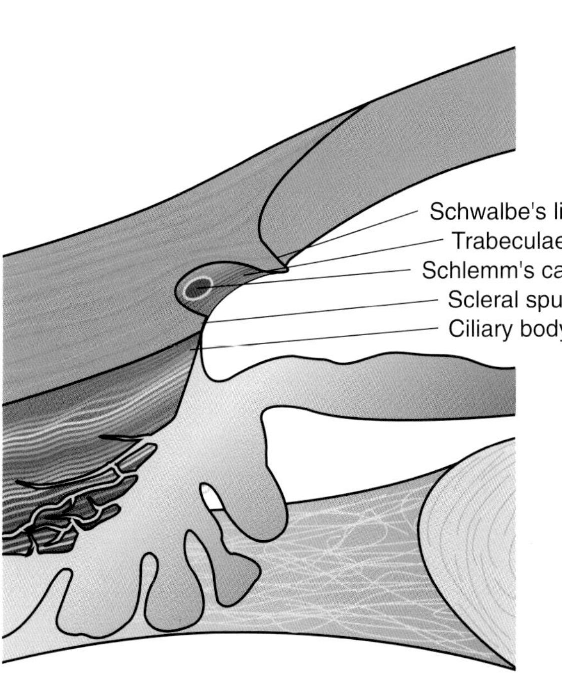

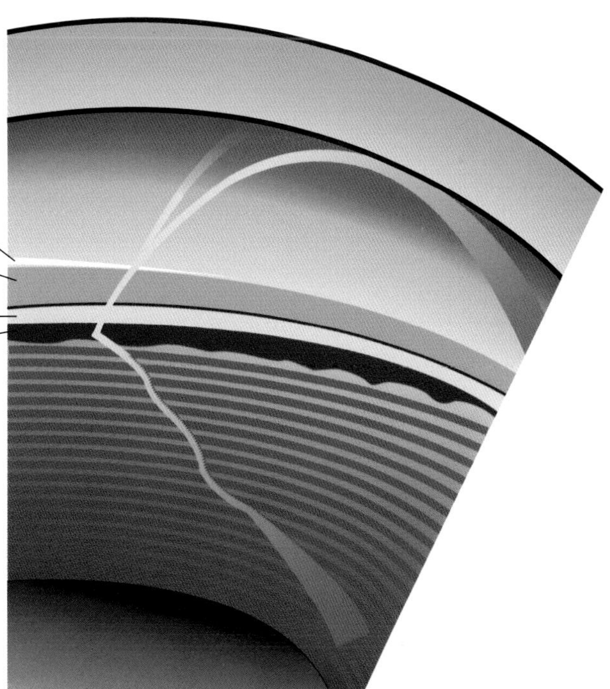

Figure 15.18 The junction of the filtering and nonfiltering trabecular meshwork
This is located posterior to Schwalbe's line, located at the terminus of the two focal lines representing the anterior and posterior surfaces of the cornea. (Adapted from Gorin and Posner *Slit Lamp Gonioscopy*, Williams and Williams Co, 1957.)

an irradiance or posterior placement may lead to small focal peripheral anterior synechiae formation (Fig. 15.20). Both standard 1 and 2-mirror lens as well as specialty lens have been used for this procedure. Before the treating lens is rotated, the operator should note angle landmarks to avoid overlapping a treated area. Finally, careful focusing is important for a uniform treatment. Focusing starts with adjusting the oculars of the laser to make the operator's retina conjugate with the focal point of the laser. If the lens is tilted, irradiance is decreased and a larger area irradiated. Also, if the spot size is

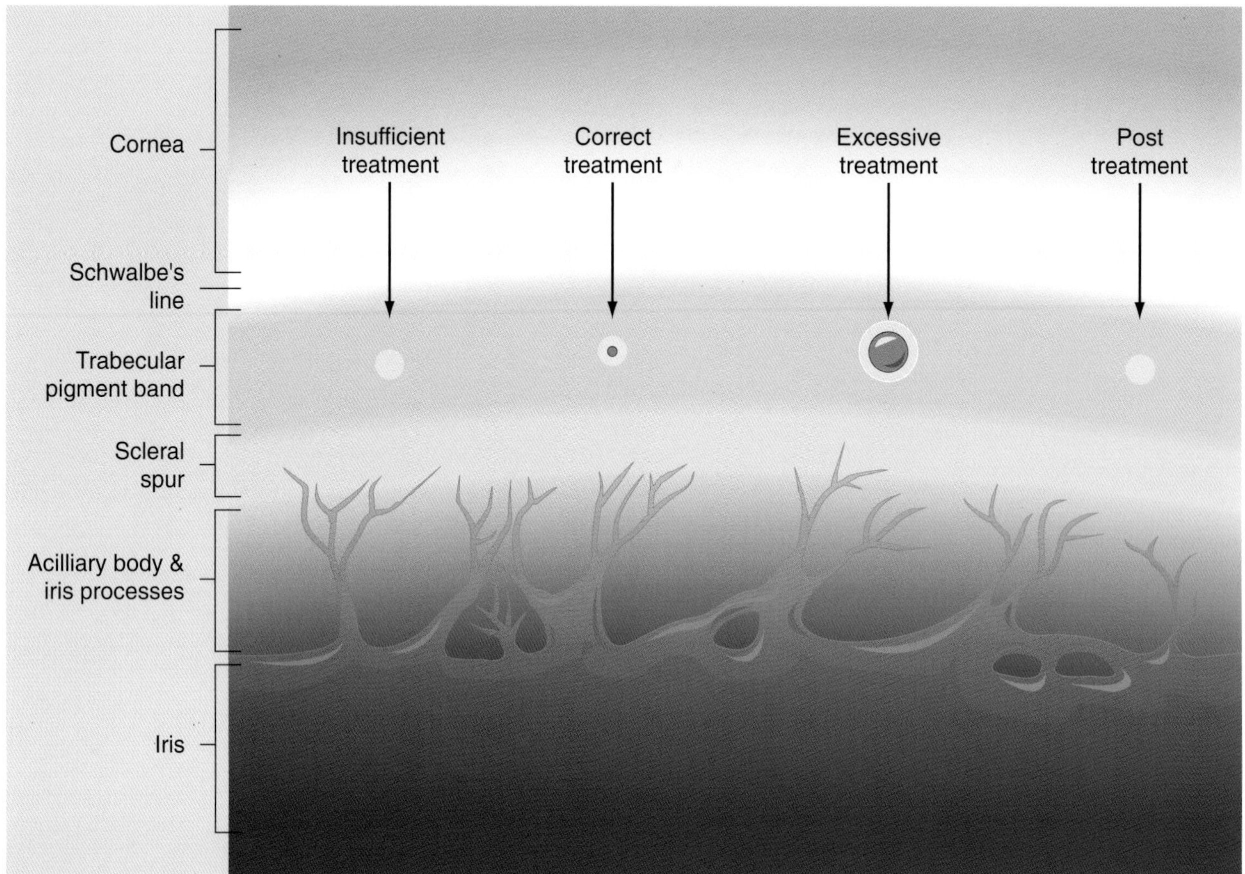

Figure 15.19 Correct level of energy delivered during argon laser trabeculoplasty results in a small, transient vapor bubble

The correct treatment site is at the terminus of the arrow under the text—Correct treatment.

increased by poor focusing the irradiance decreases by the square of the difference.

Treating the eye in divided sessions or limiting laser treatment spots to 50–60 will minimize chances of a postoperative laser-induced pressure spike. The operator should be consistent in the order of treatment, treating a total of 360 degrees in two sessions (inferior then superior, nasal then temporal, right side then left side, etc.) or 360 degrees with fewer laser spots in one session. Historically the former treatment technique affords a better treatment effect. In eyes with small central islands of remaining visual field, the operator may wish to subdivide the sessions further to minimize the chances of a laser-induced intraocular pressure spike.

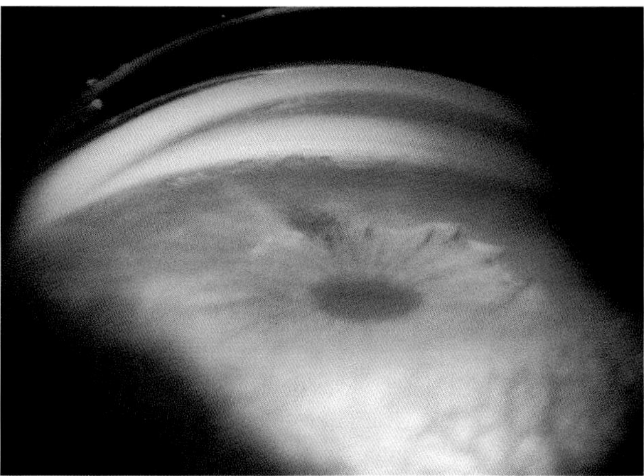

Figure 15.20 Peripheral anterior synechiae formation after argon laser trabeculoplasty

Two lasers also used in trabeculoplasty differ in their laser–tissue interactions from those of argon. The frequency-doubled quasi-continuous wave (high-frequency repetition) Nd:YAG (532 nm) laser's micropulses that make up each macropulse are at the thermal relaxation time of sclera. This probably decreases surface tissue denaturing and scatter, resulting in slightly deeper photon penetration. In addition, the slightly longer wavelength is less well absorbed by melanin allowing deeper penetration. This will decrease observed surface effects. The second type of laser in use is the diode laser. These lasers, currently operating around 810 nm, have increased scleral transmission over 488/514 nm (argon) or 532 nm (frequency-doubled Nd:YAG) and

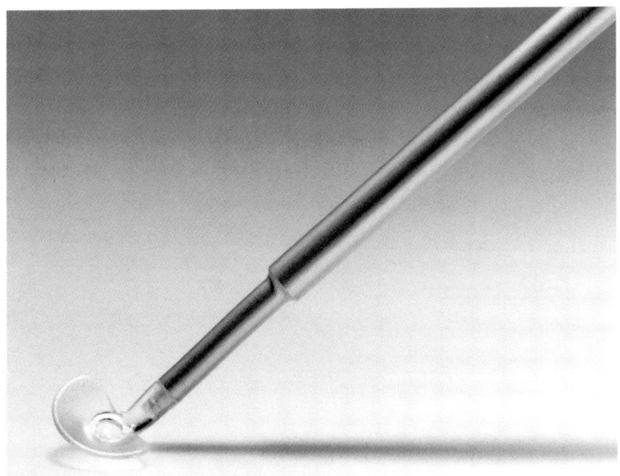

Figure 15.21 The Hoskins laser suture lysis lens
The Hoskins laser suture lysis lens has a 120 diopter lens providing 1.2× magnification. This decreases a 50 μm spot to about 42 μm in use. (Courtesy Ocular Instruments.)

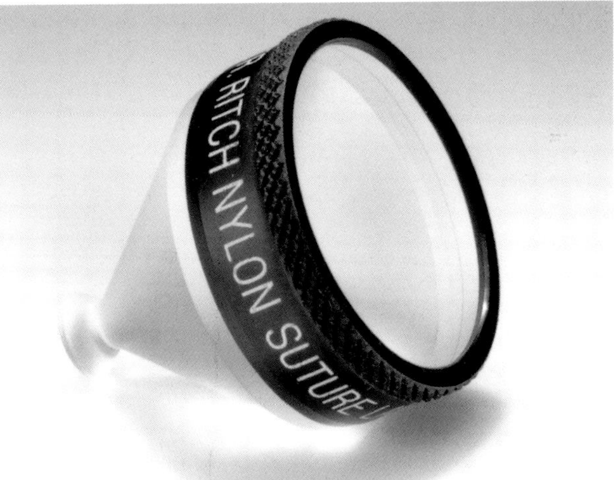

Figure 15.22 The Ritch laser suture lysis lens
The Ritch laser suture lysis lens does not provide magnification. The notch is useful for holding the eye lid but slightly cuts down the viewing field. (Courtesy Ocular Instruments.)

decreased melanin absorption. This results in deeper penetration which may explain the relative lack of visible surface effect.

Postoperative care

On completion of trabeculoplasty, a final drop of apraclonidine is given to the patient. The intraocular pressure is checked at 1–2 hours post-treatment. Corticosteroids are started at q.i.d. frequency and if a pressure spike did not occur, the patient is asked to return in one week to ensure discontinuation of topical steroids. Nonsteroidal anti-inflammatory agents are an alternative for known steroid responders. The risk of an IOP elevation > 10 mmHg after ALT with apraclonidine prophylaxis is small. The final procedure related visit is at 4–6 weeks postoperatively to assess the effects of treatment unless the clinical situation dictates differently.

Laser suture lysis

One of the most significant advancements in filtration surgery, the selective cutting of sutures after trabeculectomy, has had a profound effect on decreasing immediate postoperative hypotony and its sequelae while maintaining the benefits of full-thickness surgery. The effective window for melting of sutures without antimetabolites is 0–21 days, with effectivity falling rapidly after 14 days. The use of antimetabolites such as 5-fluorouracil extends this greatly and sutures can be melted with good effect up to 30 days postoperatively. The use of mitomicin-C deserves special mention. This potent agent also suppresses aqueous production and suture lysis should be undertaken with caution. In general, an increased interval to suture lysis will decrease the chances of hypotony and also decrease the effect. Suture lysis after the use of mitomicin-C may even be attempted in the face of a failed filter with good results; the length of time that this may be effective to is not known. There are some limits in that nylon sutures will depigment over time and will heat more slowly. Great care should be taken to avoid buttonhole formation during suture lysis after the use of mitomicin-C. The technique requires the use of a continuous wave argon or quasi-continuous wave laser (frequency-doubled Nd:YAG; 532 nm), argon dye (610 nm), krypton (647.1 nm) or diode (810 nm) laser. In a postoperative eye with any blood or hemoglobin present in the subconjunctival space, the most useful lasers are those that can emit 610 nm laser light. This wavelength is poorly absorbed by hemoglobin and decreases the possibility of a conjunctival buttonhole. If hemoglobin is absent, there is some evidence that yellow (585 nm) or orange (610 nm) may limit conjunctival damage.

Patient evaluation and preparation

The number and the effect each scleral flap suture had at the time of surgery should be reviewed. Phenylephrine (2.5%) may be given to reduce congestion of the tissues before treatment. Three laser suture lysis lenses are available (Figs 15.21–15.23). All three lenses thin and blanch overlying tissues allowing

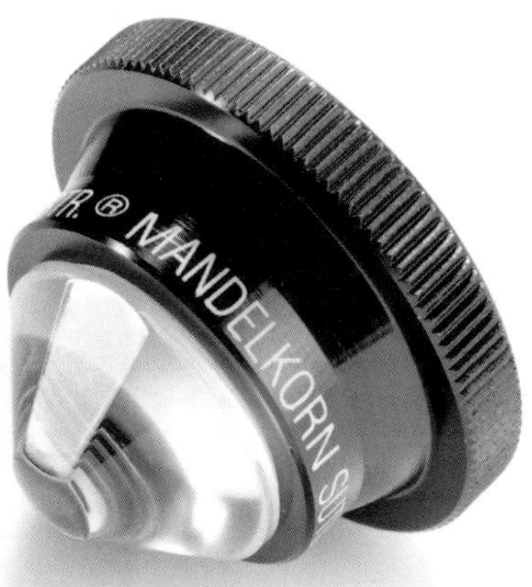

Figure 15.23 The Mandelkorn laser suture lysis lens
The Mandelkorn laser suture lysis lens provides 1.32× magnification decreasing a 50 μm spot to 38 μm and increasing irradiance at the level of the suture 1.7×. (Courtesy Ocular Instruments.)

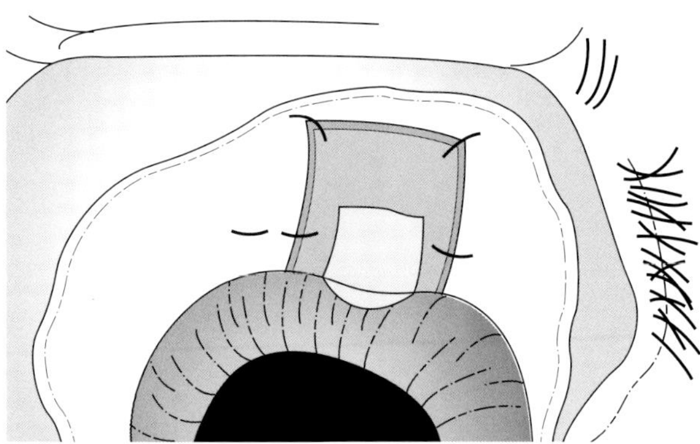

Figure 15.24 Laser suture lysis
The limbal sutures should be cut first. Premature lysis of the posterior corner sutures may cause profound hypotony.

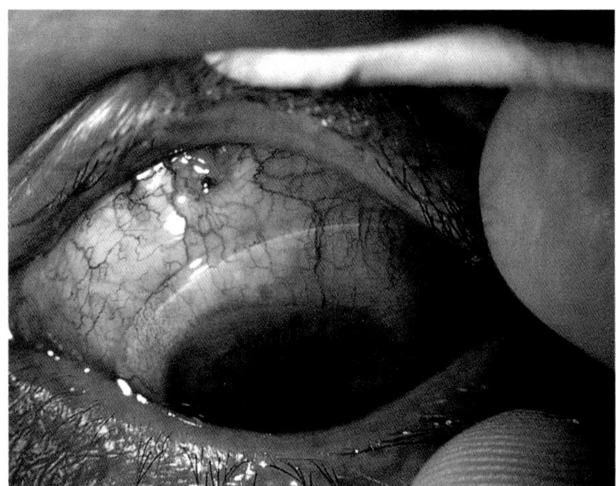

Figure 15.25 The McCalister contact lens
The McCalister contact lens providing tamponade after a full-thickness erbium:YAG laser sclerostomy. Both the laser sclerostomy and suture closing the conjunctival entry wound are visible.

visualization of the sutures. All three lenses help hold the eyelid; the Hoskins and Ritch lenses have flanges for this purpose. The Hoskins and Mandelkorn laser suture lysis lenses provide magnification and smaller spot sizes which effectively increase irradiance. This should be taken into account when selecting continuous wave power and exposure duration. Care should be taken in handling the Hoskins lens as the neck is somewhat fragile.

Procedure

Topical anesthetic agents are used. The patient is asked to look down and the iridectomy is used to locate the approximate area of the scleral flap. The continuous wave power should start low (50 μm; 0.1 second, 400 mW) with caution directly proportional to the relative potency of antimetabolite employed and amount of blood in the subconjunctival space. The laser spot should be focused on the suture to produce one long cut end which will lay flat. After successful lysis the melted suture ends will retract (Fig. 15.24); occasionally the suture blanches but does not retract. This indicates that sufficient tension in the suture to cause retraction does not exist and that no extra filtration can be gained by pursuing this suture. The one suture per session rule should be observed, especially when mitomicin-C has been used. Additional sutures may be cut after careful evaluation a few hours after the initial attempt. In emergent situations aqueous may be released from the paracentesis created at surgery to temporize. Complications are mainly limited to small conjunctival buttonholes from the laser and hypotony with or without buttonhole formation. These may be treated with patching and with or without aqueous suppressants as the clinical situation dictates. If antimetabolites have been used, a McCalister contact lens without patching may be used to help close the conjunctival defect (Fig. 15.25). This lens provides tamponade and may be tolerated for 1–2 weeks if needed. The use of aqueous suppressants is also an option with this lens.

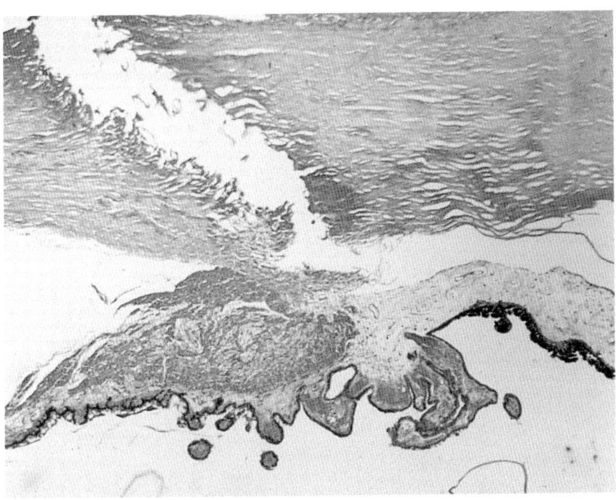

Figure 15.26 Lateral thermal damage
Lateral thermal damage after Ho:YAG laser sclerostomy is in the range of 100–150 μm.

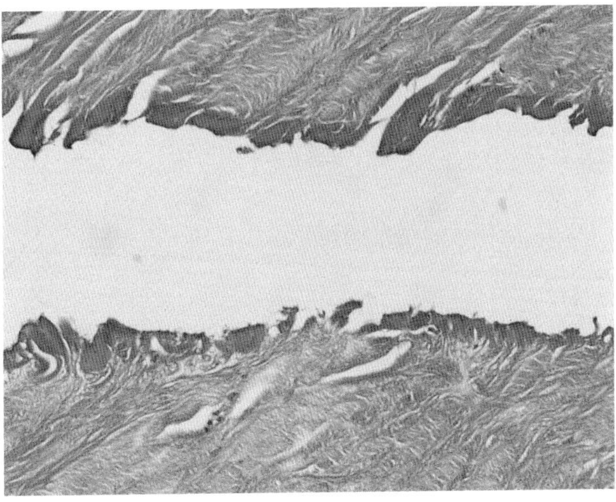

Figure 15.27 Lateral thermal damage
Lateral thermal damage after Er:YAG laser sclerostomy is in the range of 10–20 μm.

Laser sclerostomy

Laser sclerostomy formation has generated an intense, transient, interest. The promise of a procedure which rapidly creates a sclerostomy with minimal or no conjunctival dissection has great appeal to the glaucoma surgeon. Approaches which have been investigated include Q-switched and continuous wave infrared lasers, excimer lasers, pulsed dye lasers using exogenous chromophores delivered by iontophoresis and pulsed infrared lasers. The pulsed infrared lasers (Holmium (Ho, 2.1 μm) and Erbium (Er, 2.94 μm)) have had the most extensive clinical evaluations and have received FDA premarket approval. Both of these lasers emit in the infrared, near water absorption peaks. The intense water absorption of light at these wavelengths (Er >> Ho) creates a spatial confinement of energy allowing vaporization and ejection of material out of the ablation crater. The ablation efficiency and thermal damage are proportional to the intensity of water absorption at the wavelength emitted, with Er having a higher efficiency and requiring less total energy than Ho (Figs 15.6, 15.26 and 15.27). Early experience with both lasers showed that the average diameters of sclerostomies needed to be in the 300 μm range for acceptable success rates. In addition, 5-fluorouracil was also needed to produce surgical success rates that compared to trabeculectomy. The intense water absorption found at these wavelengths (Fig. 15.4) precluded slit lamp delivery requiring a minimally invasive ab externo fiberoptic delivery. The Ho unit (Fig. 15.28) utilized a fiberoptic delivery system with a side-firing probe which was advanced in a tangential manner to the limbus for delivery of laser energy

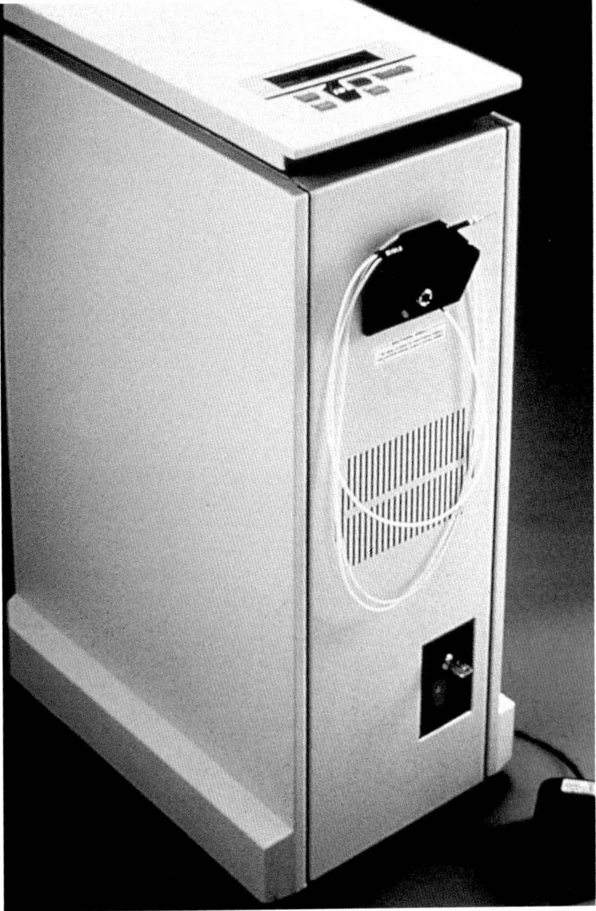

Figure 15.28 The Sunrise Technologies Ho:Th:YAG laser
The Sunrise Technologies Ho:Th:YAG laser for glaucoma filtration surgery is a pulsed solid-state device using a fiberoptic delivery and side-firing handpiece. (Courtesy Andrew Iwach.)

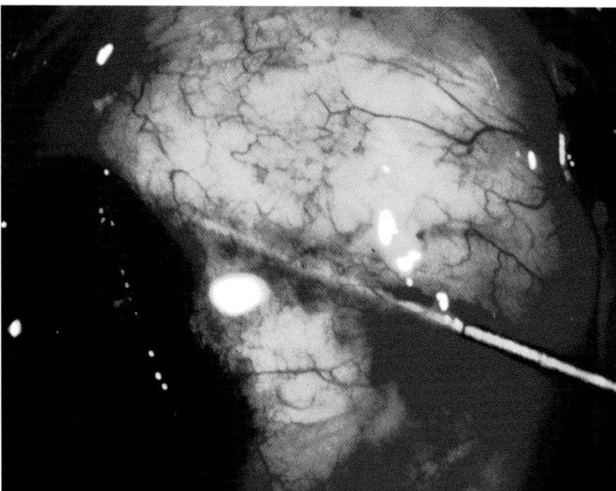

Figure 15.29 The delivery system for the Sunrise Technologies Ho:Th:YAG laser
This used a side-firing probe requiring careful angulation and a tangential approach to the limbus. (Courtesy Andrew Iwach.)

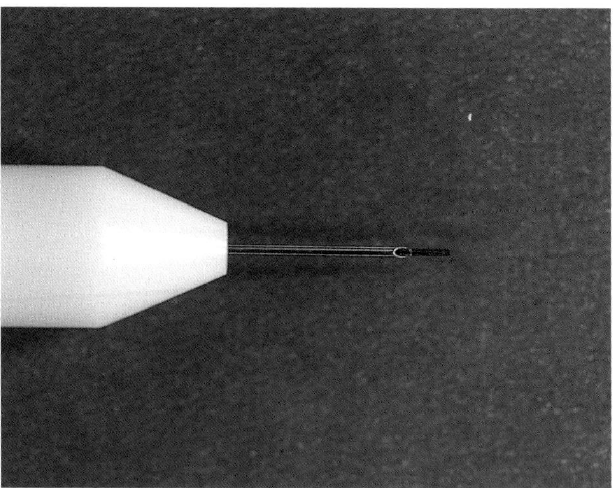

Figure 15.31 The delivery system for the Candela Er:YAG laser
This used a compound fiber delivery system to deliver laser energy to a condensing lens where it was focused into a short low hydroxyl-fused silica fiber for delivery to the eye. The end-firing fiberoptic requires a perpendicular approach to the limbus.

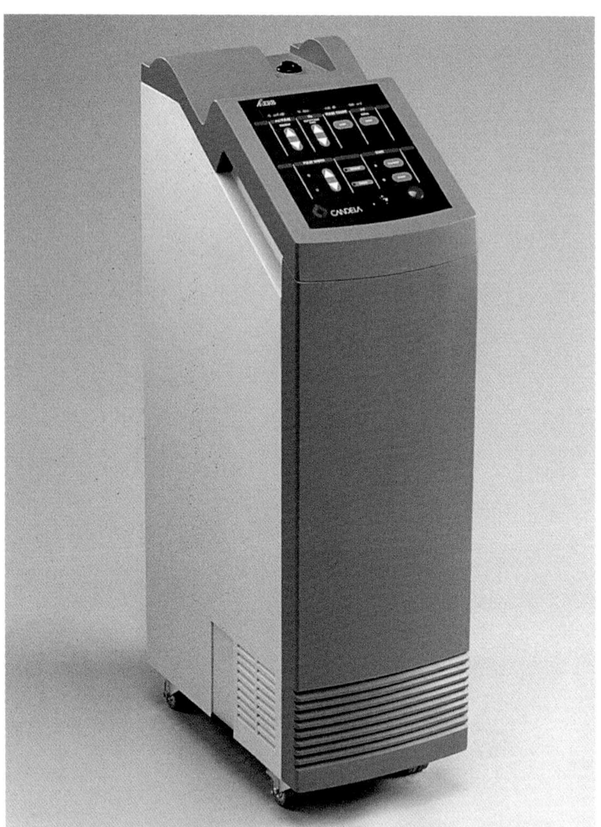

Figure 15.30 The Candela Er:YAG laser
The Candela Er:YAG laser for glaucoma filtration surgery is a solid-state variable pulse-width device. A compound fiber using ZrF2 carries energy to a lens in the handpiece where it is focused into a short low hydroxyl-fused silica fiberoptic for treatment. (Courtesy Candela Laser Corp.)

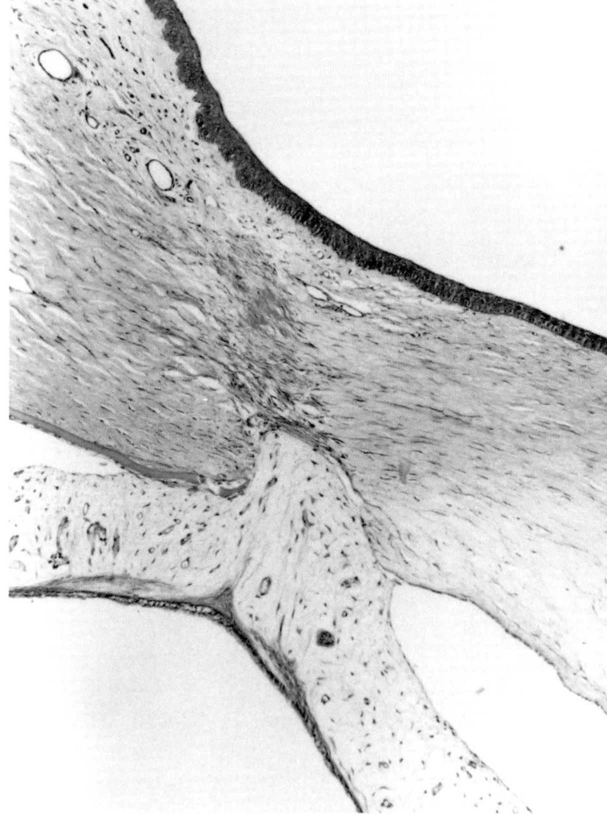

Figure 15.32 Iris incarceration
Iris incarceration occurs at a high frequency with an ab externo approach to filtering surgery.

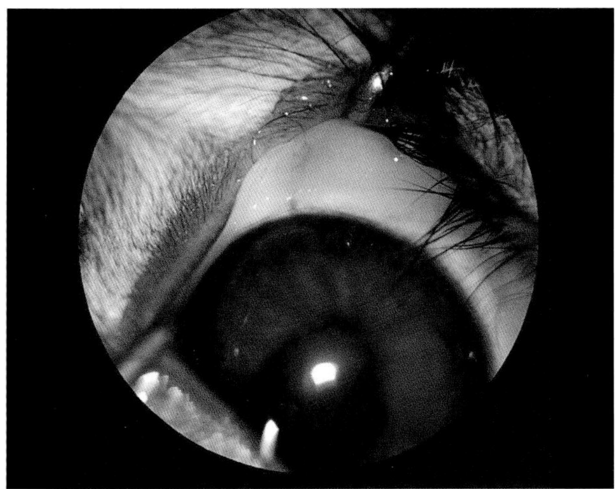

Figure 15.33 Early postoperative appearance of an Er:YAG laser sclerostomy in a rabbit model

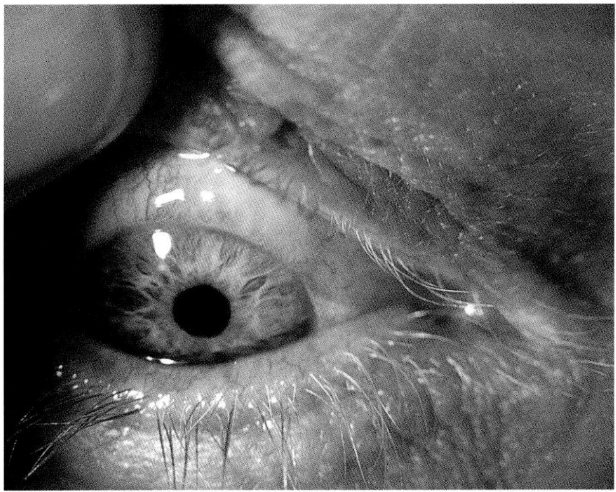

Figure 15.34 A small localized avascular bleb typical of those created by laser sclerostomy
Although this patient was a success, postoperative complications included kissing choroidal effusions following by iris incarceration and acute pressure rise to 45 mmHg requiring treatment with an argon laser to retract iris out of the sclerostomy. Final visual acuity was reduced by four lines.

(Fig. 15.29). The laser energy was delivered in the range of 80–120 mJ/pulse until the operator could hear a difference in the ablation report or see gas bubbles in the anterior chamber. The Er unit (Fig. 15.30) utilized an end-firing compound fiber which was advanced through a stainless-steel sheath once the limbus was reached (Fig. 15.31). Laser energy was delivered in the range of 4–8 mJ/pulse until the fiberoptic tip was seen to advance into the anterior chamber, gas bubbles were seen to form or the helium:neon aiming beam was seen in the anterior chamber. Both techniques produce a full-thickness sclerostomy and postoperative tamponade techniques such as the McCalister contact lens (Fig. 15.25) are utilized to minimize the sequelae of hypotony. New complications such as iris incarceration also frequently occurred (Fig. 15.32). The filtering blebs created tended to be localized and avascular (Figs 15.33 and 15.34). Although these lasers were FDA approved, when compared to trabeculectomy, they had lower success rates, higher rates of complication and required the large initial expense of a laser. They do however retain some utility in revision of failing/failed filters as an alternative to needling.

Cyclodestructive procedures

Introduction

It has been over 60 years since Weve and Voght introduced diathermy and penetrating diathermy respectively as cyclodestructive techniques. In this time electrolysis, beta irradiation, cryotherapy, xenon arc, ultrasound, surgical excision and various visible and infrared lasers have been tried in an attempt to improve on this type of glaucoma surgery. In current practice, laser-based cyclodestructive procedures are useful in the treatment of glaucomas with poor surgical prognosis in which trabeculectomy with antimetabolites or aqueous drainage devices have failed. In addition, these procedures may also be used to decrease pain and to lower pressure in cases with limited visual potential. The most frequently used techniques are laser-based contact and noncontact cyclophotocoagulation using neodymium:YAG or diode-based laser systems. The use of these techniques causes considerable pain, inflammation and visual loss; they should therefore be treatments of last recourse (Fig. 15.35). Initial reports of sympathetic ophthalmia were in eyes with previous ocular surgery, creating controversy. Subsequently, there have been reports of sympathetic ophthalmia occurring in eyes after cyclophotocoagulation, not previously operated. Laser–tissue interactions vary somewhat depending on the wavelength and the peak power delivered. High-power, pulsed lasers (20 microseconds), such as the Microrupter series, cause more tissue disruption. Continuous wave lasers require a longer exposure time to deliver sufficient energy to cause cyclophotocoagulation; the effects are more of a coagulative nature. Distinctive pops that are heard are steam bubbles disrupting uveal tissue. The reported rates of phthisis are in excess of

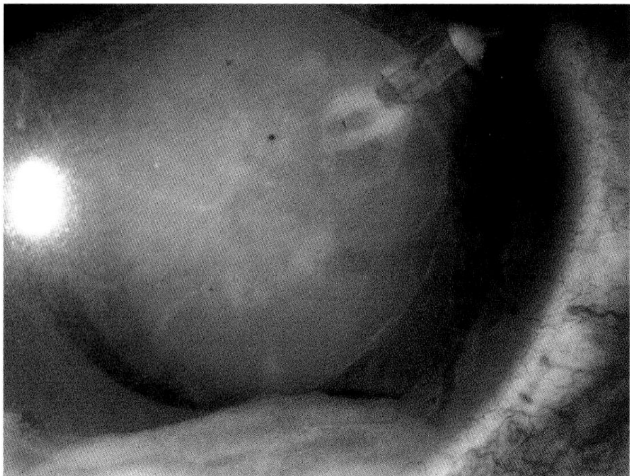

Figure 15.35 Tremendous inflammatory responses are possible after cyclophotocoagulation
(Courtesy James Martone, MD.)

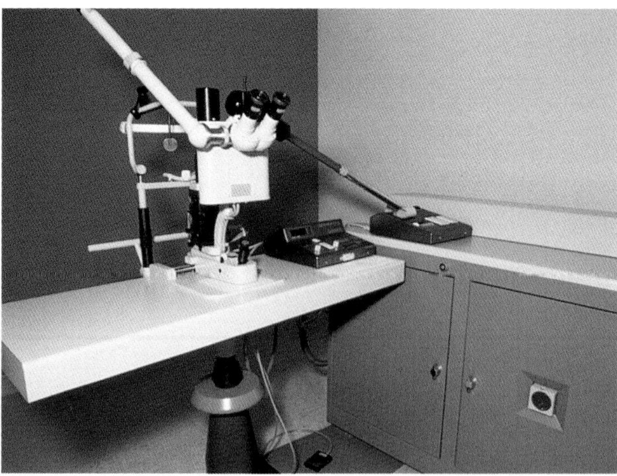

Figure 15.36 The Microrupter III Nd:YAG laser used for noncontact cyclophotocoagulation

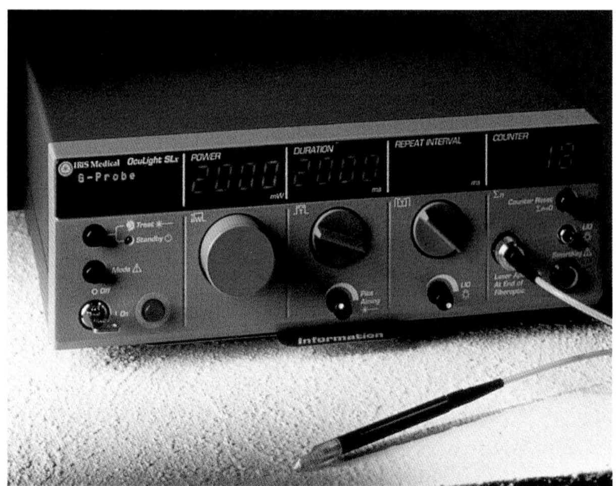

Figure 15.37 The Oculight SLX (Iris Medical, Mountain View, CA) diode photocoagulator

the occurrence of choroidal hemorrhage or loss of fixation in eyes with advanced glaucoma undergoing trabeculectomy. This argument in favor of cyclophotocoagulation should perhaps be revisited by surgeons. Although laser-based treatments produce less pain than cyclocryotherapy, they should be performed under retrobulbar anesthesia and the patients given a 3–4 day supply of moderate-strength analgesic such as Vicodin™.

Patient preparation

All cyclodestructive procedures are performed under retrobulbar anesthesia using a mixture of short-acting (2% lidocaine) and long-acting (0.75% bupivacaine) local anesthetics. In the event that general anesthesia is used the operator should remember to administer a retrobulbar block for postoperative comfort. Apraclonidine may also be given preoperatively if not currently used by the patient to blanch conjunctiva and minimize the chances of an IOP spike.

Contact trans-scleral cyclophotocoagulation

A variety of continuous wave lasers based on either Nd:YAG or diode laser technology are available for this technique. The Surgical Laser Technologies, Oaks, PA and Lasag Microrupter III (Fig. 15.36) are representative of the Nd:YAG group. Diode-based units include the Oculight SLX (Iris Medical, Mountain View, CA) (Fig. 15.37) and the DC-3000 (Nidek Inc., Palo Alto, CA). These contact delivery systems use exposures much longer than the pulsed high peak power Nd:YAG systems; the tissue effects therefore tend to be somewhat less explosive and more coagulative. The use of a contact fiberoptic probe also creates a focal relative desiccation of sclera, increasing scleral transmission of laser light. The use of operator and assistant eye protection is mandatory and great care should be used when pointing the muzzle end of the fiberoptic. The patient is placed in the supine position and given retrobulbar anesthesia. An eye lid speculum is placed and the nonoperative eye patched shut. If the globe is either

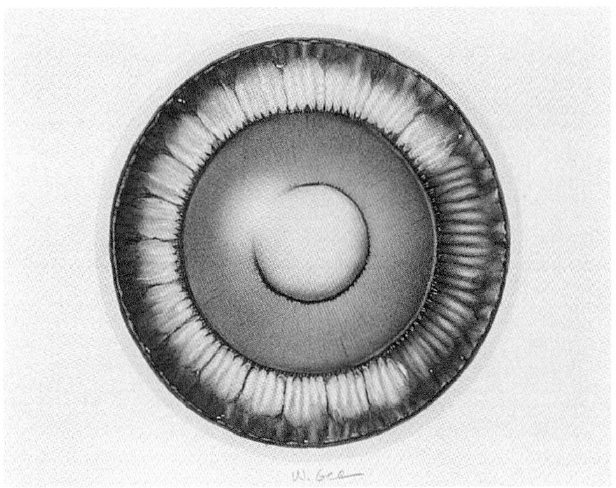

Figure 15.38 An alternative to 360 degree placement with sparing in the 3 and 9:00 positions suggested for diode laser cyclophotocoagulation

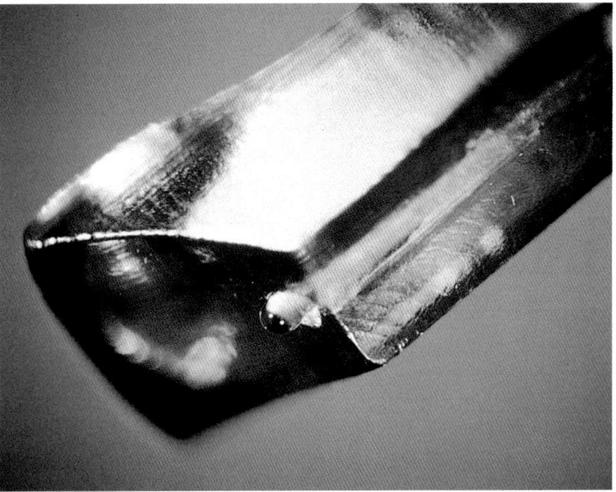

Figure 15.39 The G-probe for use with the Oculight SLX (Iris Medical, Mountain View, CA) diode photocoagulator

The probe is adapted to the contour of the limbus providing the correct orientation of the fiberoptic delivery system.

very long or short, transillumination should be used to localize the ciliary body. The Nd:YAG technique differs slightly from the diode technique. In using the SLT unit the anterior edge of the probe is held 0.5–1 mm posterior to the limbus and 8–10 applications of 5–6 J are placed for 360 degrees, sparing the 3:00 and 9:00 positions. In non-Caucasian patients with increased melanin (chromophore) or in eyes with neovascular glaucoma, continuous wave power is decreased to 5–6 mW. When using a diode laser such as the Oculight SLX, suggested settings are 2.5 seconds at 1750 mW. A popping sound considered desirable in Nd:YAG techniques is not desirable with this laser as this is more of a coagulating technique. The proposed treatment area differs slightly; the region spared is 45 degrees above and below the temporal horizontal midline (Fig. 15.38). Energy is delivered to the eye through the G-Probe (Fig. 15.39) which is a handpiece containing the fiberoptic for laser delivery. It is contoured to fit the limbus providing the correct spacing to deliver the laser energy to the ciliary body.

Noncontact trans-scleral cyclophotocoagulation

Currently, the noncontact technique uses the Microrupter series lasers (Lasag, Thun, Switzerland). The Microrupter II is used in the free-running mode which delivers multiple joule, 20 microsecond pulses. To separate the focal points of the He:Ne aiming laser (ocular surface) and the Nd:YAG laser (ciliary body), the focusing offset is set to 9 (Fig. 15.40). A lid speculum or the Shields contact lens may be used to facilitate treatment. Most commonly, 8–10 spots per quadrant are placed at a distance of 1–1.5 mm posterior to the limbus. The 3:00 and 9:00 positions are spared to avoid injury to the long posterior ciliary arteries. The operator may wish to consider transillumination of the globe for a more accurate location of the ciliary body in very long or short eyes. The energies used in most studies are in the 4–8 J range; 4–6 J are usually suggested at present.

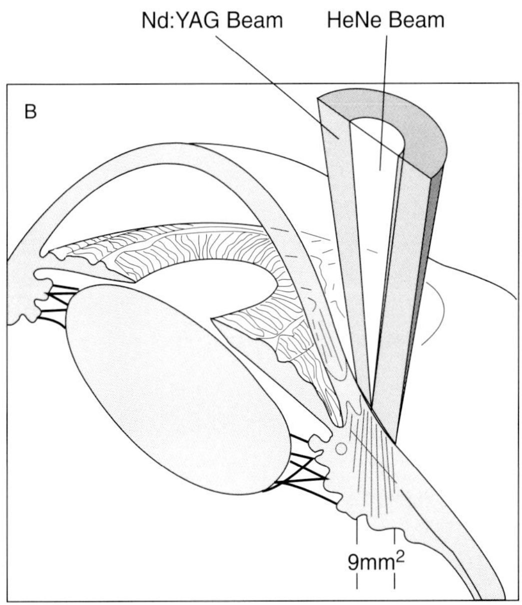

Figure 15.40 Microrupter series lasers

To separate the focal points of the He:Ne aiming laser (ocular surface) and the Nd:YAG laser (ciliary body), the focusing offset is set to 9 on the Microrupter series lasers.

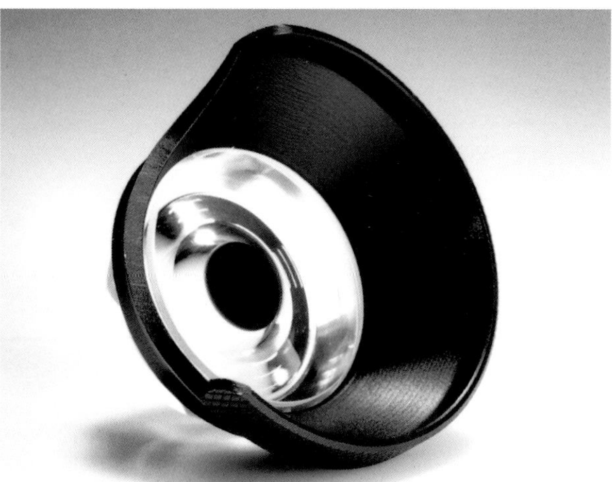

Figure 15.41 The Shields contact lens for trans-scleral cyclophotocoagulation
This lens compresses overlying tissues facilitating transfer of laser energy. A central opaque shields the eye, and etch marks at 1 mm interval increments allow accurate placement of laser energy. (Courtesy Ocular Instruments.)

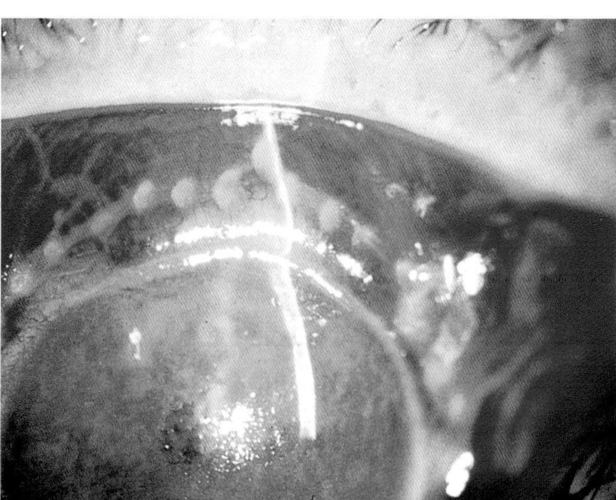

Figure 15.42 Conjunctival burns
Conjunctival burns produced by the noncontact method of cyclophotocoagulation without the use of the Shields contact lens. (Courtesy Anne Coleman.)

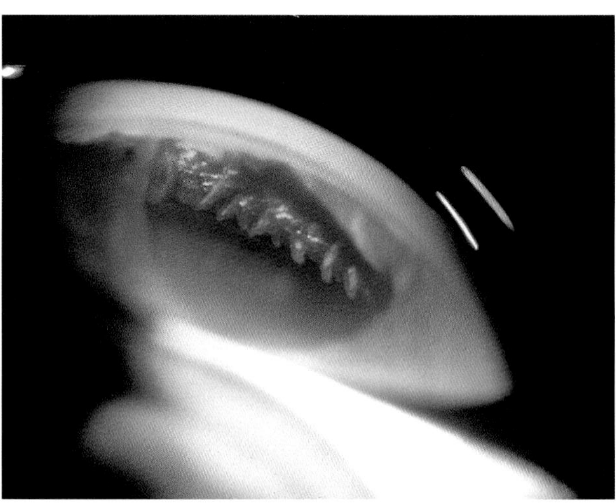

Figure 15.43 The effects of noncontact cyclophotocoagulation laser treatment
Visible through a sector iridectomy. (Courtesy James Martone, MD.)

The use of the Shields lens (Fig. 15.41) facilitates transfer of laser energy (eliminating conjunctival burns) (Fig. 15.42) and therefore the lower end of this energy range should be used to avoid overtreatment. The Shields lens also acts as a lid speculum, visual axis occluder and has marks at 1 mm increments for reproducible placement of laser spots.

Postoperative care

The eye is patched shut until the postoperative day-one examination. At this time prednisolone acetate 1% is started at 4–8 times per day based on induced inflammation. Atropine 1% is used twice daily for cycloplegia. The ocular hypotensive medications are adjusted based on clinical response and the patient asked to return in one week and one month post-operatively. Eyes may be retreated with decreased numbers of spots if the pressure is not adequate 4–6 weeks postoperatively.

Future directions for cyclodestructive surgery

Photodynamic therapy

The observation that photochemicals localize to the ciliary body has led to the study of photodynamic therapy for possible selective injury to the ciliary body. The principle of selective retention of photochemical by tumors or the ciliary body allows this tissue to be injured with little damage to nonlocalizing tissue as long as thermal damage thresholds are not exceeded. Among compounds being investigated, tin-ethyl-etiopurpurin has been shown to localize to the nonpigmented ciliary body in a rabbit model. Subsequent irradiation with low-level (nonthermal) laser light generates reactive oxidative species which cause localized damage in the tissue retaining the photochemical.

Aqueous misdirection

In cases of aqueous misdirection, the aqueous collects posterior to the anterior hyaloid face,

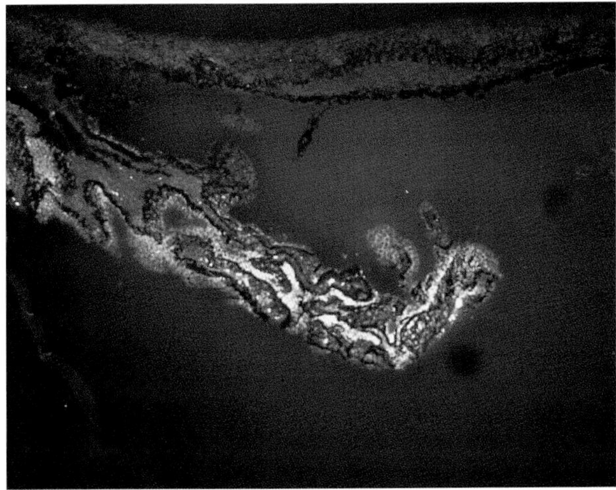

Figure 15.44 Photochemicals localize well to the ciliary body (silicon naphthalocyanine, 24 hours after IV infusion)
Newer photochemicals such as tin-ethyl-etiopurpurin can exhibit subselectivity, localizing to the nonpigmented ciliary body epithelium in rabbit models. (Reprinted with permission, Lasers in Surgery and Medicine.)

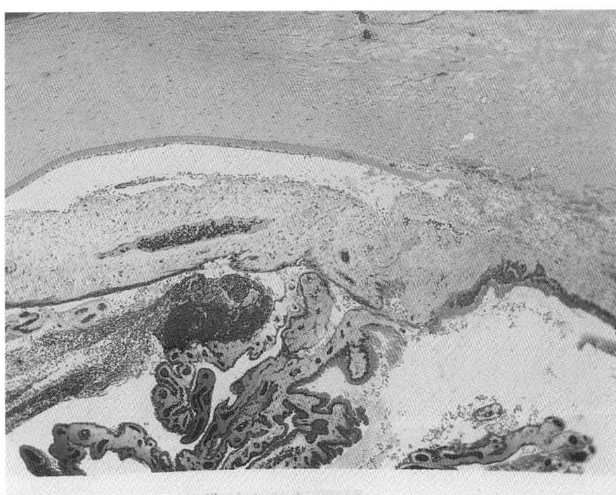

Figure 15.45 Injury by photodynamic therapy
When photochemicals selectively localize, a very specific injury can be created by photodynamic therapy—the local generation of reactive oxidative species by the interaction of photochemicals, light and oxygen. (Reprinted with permission, Lasers in Surgery and Medicine.)

pushing the lens (natural or pseudophakos) and iris forward, closing the angle. Surgical disruption of the hyaloid face may allow the trapped aqueous to resume its normal pathway and relieve the anteriorly directed forces. The anterior hyaloid face may be disrupted using a Q-switched Nd:YAG laser set at 4–11 mJ and a capsulotomy lens (Fig. 15.46). This energy may be delivered through the pupil or a large iridectomy in both phakic and pseudophakic patients. In addition, if the posterior capsule is intact, a capsulotomy should also be performed. Argon laser shrinkage of swollen ciliary processes through a large iridectomy has also been reported. The treatment should use a long, low, continuous wave-power burn. The effects of successful treatment are dramatic with rapid restoration of normal anterior chamber depth.

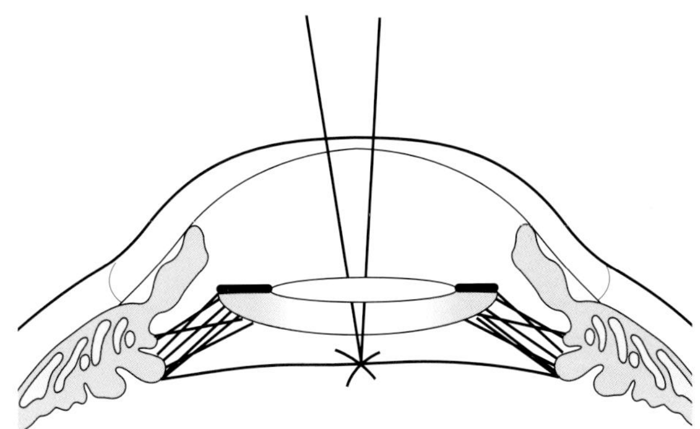

Figure 15.46 Aqueous misdirection
Aqueous misdirection may be stopped by disruption of the anterior hyaloid face. In pseudophakic patients with this problem, a capsulotomy should also be created.

Aqueous drainage implant tube occlusions

Occlusions and malpositions are common complications of aqueous drainage implants. The majority of these will require operative intervention. In some cases they may be treated by laser therapy. In situations where the drainage tube has been occluded by blood, fibrin or vitreous pushed forward by choroidal effusions, treatment should wait until the transient hypotony has resolved (Fig. 15.47). If the clinical situation can wait for this then the strands of vitreous may be cut where they enter the drainage tube with a Q-switched Nd:YAG laser using 1–2 mJ pulses and an iridectomy lens. This will leave a plug of vitreous in the drainage tube. This plug may be dislodged by focusing and releasing a 3–5 mJ pulse focused in the sealed portion of the tube just opposite the plug. This will dislodge the vitreous or

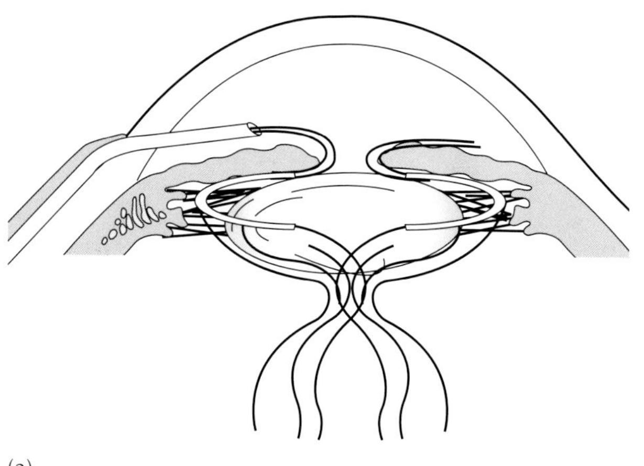

(a)

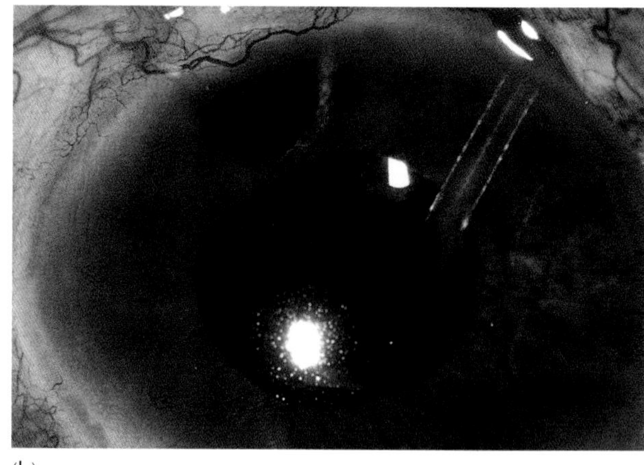

(b)

Figure 15.47 Drainage tubes occluded secondary to volume shifts
If drainage tubes have become occluded with vitreous secondary to volume shifts from choroidal effusions pushing the vitreous forward, waiting until the hypotony resolves will place the vitreous on traction, allowing it to be cut with a Nd:YAG laser. A second application will dislodge it into the anterior chamber or allow it to escape up the drainage tube into the filtering capsule. (a) schematic (b) clinical photograph showing vitreous plug one week after placement of an Ahmed Glaucoma Valve. (see also Fig. 17.23) (Photograph courtesy of Neil T. Choplin, MD)

fibrin into the anterior chamber or allow it to travel into the filtering capsule of the implant. If this fails, then operative intervention is warranted. Iris may also occlude the drainage tube. Evidence for iris bombè should be sought out and an iridectomy performed if needed. Iris may also be retracted by focal application of low, continuous wave-power, long-exposure argon laser energy.

Revision of the failing filter

The use of the laser to lyse flap sutures as intraocular pressure rises following filtering surgery has previously been discussed. In cases where a pigmented membrane may be visualized, an argon laser may be used to revise the filtering site. Argon lasers are also useful for performing a focal iridoplasty to treat iris incarceration complicating laser sclerostomy procedures. In most cases, the internal ostium will be patent, pigmented tissues absent and a Q-switched Nd:YAG laser will be required.

Procedure

After topical anesthesia, an Abraham or Wise lens is placed on the eye. If mitomicin-C was used, the scleral flap should be inspected for remaining sutures to cut even if many months have passed since surgery. The main risk of revision is creating a conjunctival buttonhole. Therefore, energy is increased until optical breakdown is observed and the focus used is slightly deep to the episcleral surface. At the conclusion of the procedure a modified Seidel test with a fluorescein strip is performed. Buttonholes created may be most comfortably treated with a McCalister contact lens, with or without aqueous suppressants. The use of a Simmons shell with a disposable contact lens, symblepharon ring (medium size) or patching have also been described. Although good success has been reported when a filter has worked on an extended basis, it is the experience of the author and others that this type of revision has low success. However, the cost and morbidity of these procedures are also low and selected patients may benefit. Ab externo pulsed infrared lasers (Er:YAG and Ho:Th:YAG) are also useful for revision of a failed filter as an alternative to bleb needling.

Treatment of hypotonous cyclodialysis clefts

Cyclodialysis clefts can be caused by blunt ocular trauma and surgical procedures involving the manipulation of iris. They seldom close spontaneously and a trial of cycloplegia with cessation of steroids will have even less success after the cleft has been present for six or more weeks. These clefts may be closed by the use of an argon laser.

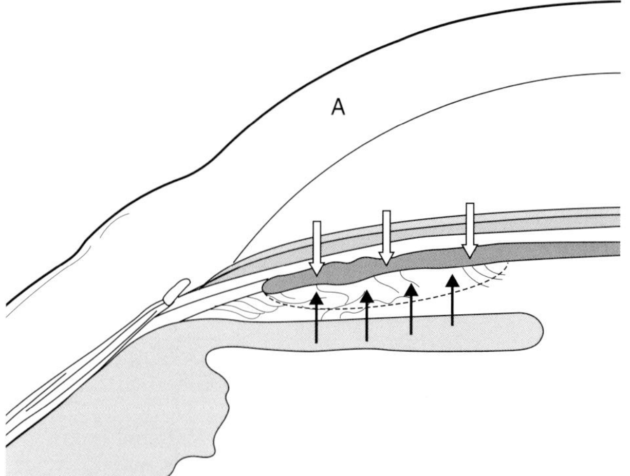

Figure 15.48 Cyclodialysis cleft
The scleral side (larger arrows) is treated first with high-power argon laser burns. The uveal side (smaller arrows) follows at power and exposure settings that create a marked surface effect.

Patient evaluation

The patient is given pilocarpine to open the cyclodialysis cleft maximally. Compression gonioscopy may also be helpful in diagnosis. If the anterior chamber has shallowed and the filtering angle is not visible the patient is given retrobulbar anesthesia and the chamber deepened by intracameral sodium hyaluronate (Healon), an agent that will irrigate easily from the eye. The number, extent and location of the clefts can now be established.

Procedure

If retrobulbar therapy was not necessary, anesthesia should be obtained with topical proparicaine. Topical anesthesia may be adequate but this depends on the individual's discomfort threshold and the continuous wave power required. Treatment is first by the placement of overlapping laser spots on the sclera surface. The spot size should be 100 μm and the exposure time 0.1 second. A continuous wave power is selected that will generate a small gas bubble on the scleral surface. This will require a high power (>1.5 W) and may cause discomfort requiring retrobulbar anesthesia. Secondly, the uveal side of the cleft is treated starting in the depths of the cleft as this tissue will contract, narrowing the cleft. The power delivered should be varied according to iris color, with lighter color receiving up to one watt and brown irises receiving slightly less (800–900 mW range initially). A marked surface effect should be seen on the uveal side of the cleft. Multiple treatments may be necessary.

Postoperative care

If viscoelastic was used to facilitate diagnosis and treatment it should be removed by irrigation from the paracentesis port using gentle downward pressure allowing wound gape. The patient is given atropine 1% three times daily and an antibiotic four times daily (if a paracentesis was made) for three days. The patient should also be instructed on the symptoms of an acute pressure rise and provided with an after-hours contact mechanism.

FURTHER READING

Abraham RK, Protocol for single-session argon laser iridectomy for angle-closure glaucoma, *Int Ophthalmol Clin* (1981) **21**:145.

Abraham RK, Miller GL, Outpatient argon iridectomy for angle-closure glaucoma: a 3-1/2 year study, *Adv Ophthalmol* (1977) **34**:186.

Adachi M, et al., Internal sclerostomy with a high-powered argon laser, *Acta Soc Ophthalmol Jpn* (1991) **95**:657.

Allingham RR, et al., Probe placement and power levels in contact transscleral neodymium:YAG cyclophotocoagulation, *Arch Ophthalmol* (1990) **108**:738.

Alward WLM, et al., Argon laser endophotocoagulation closure of cyclodialysis clefts, *Am J Ophthalmol* (1988) **106**:748.

Arden GB, et al., A survey of color discrimination in German ophthalmologists. Changes associated with the use of lasers and operating microscopes, *Ophthalmology* (1991) **98**:567.

Beckman H, Sugar HS, Neodymium laser cyclocoagulation, *Arch Ophthalmol* (1973) **90**:27.

Beckman H, Sugar HS, Laser iridectomy therapy of glaucoma, *Arch Ophthalmol* (1973) **90**:453.

Beckman H, et al., Limbectomies, keratectomies, and keratostomies performed with a rapid pulsed carbon dioxide laser, *Am J Ophthalmol* (1971) **71**:1277.

Beckman RL, et al., Erbium-YAG laser sclerostomy in humans—an update, *Invest Ophthalmol Vis Sci* (1993) **34**:1071.

Berlin MS, et al., Excimer laser photoablation in glaucoma filtering surgery, *Am J Ophthalmol* (1984) **103**:713.

Berringer TA, et al., Using argon laser blue light reduces ophthalmologists color contrast sensitivity. Argon blue and surgeons vision, *Arch Ophthalmol* (1989) **107**:1453.

Blok MDW, et al., Scleral flap sutures and the development of shallow or flat anterior chamber after trabeculectomy, *Ophthalmic Surg* (1993) **24**:309.

Boettner EA, Wolter JR, Transmission of the ocular media, *Ophthalmic Res* (1962) **1**:776.

Brancato R, Carassa R, Trabucchi G, Diode laser compared with argon laser for trabeculoplasty, *Am J Ophthalmol* (1991) **112**:50.

Brancato R, et al., Probe placement and energy levels in continuous wave neodymium-YAG contact transscleral cyclophotocoagulation, *Arch Ophthalmol* (1990) **108**:679.

Brown RH, et al., Neodymium:YAG vitreous surgery for phakic and pseudophakic malignant glaucoma, *Arch Ophthalmol* (1986) **104**:1464.

Brown RH, et al., ALO 2145 reduces the IOP elevation after anterior segment laser surgery, *Ophthalmology* (1988) **95**:378.

Brown SVL, Higginbotham E, Tessler H, Sympathetic ophthalmia following Nd:YAG cyclotherapy, *Ophthalmic Surg* (1965) **21**:736 (letter).

Cohen EJ, et al., Neodymium:YAG laser transscleral cyclophotocoagulation for glaucoma after penetrating keratoplasty, *Ophthalmic Surg* (1989) **20**:713.

Cohen JS, et al., Revision of filtration surgery, *Arch Ophthalmol* (1977) **95**:1612.

Cohn HC, Whalen WR, Aron-Rosa D, YAG laser treatment in a series of failed trabeculectomy, *Am J Ophthalmol* (1989) **108**:395.

Dailey RA, Samples JR, Van Buskirk EM, Reopening filtration fistulas with neodymium:YAG laser, *Am J Ophthalmol* (1986) **102**:491.

De Alwis TV, The long-term follow-up of patients treated with YAG laser to reopen closed or closing fistulae following glaucoma surgery, *Eye* (1993) **7**:444.

Del Priore LV, Robin AL, Pollack IP, Long-term follow-up of neodymium:YAG laser angle surgery for open-angle glaucoma, *Ophthalmology* (1988) **95**:277.

Del Priore LV, Robin AL, Pollack IP, Neodymium:YAG and argon laser iridectomy. Long-term follow-up in a prospective, randomized clinical trial, *Ophthalmology* (1988) **95**:1207.

Drake MV, Neodymium:YAG laser iridectomy, *Surv Ophthalmol* (1987) **32**:171.

Edward DP, et al., Sympathetic ophthalmia following neodymium:YAG cyclotherapy, *Ophthalmic Surg* (1989) **20**:544.

Emoto I, Okisaka S, Nakajima A, Diode laser iridectomy in rabbit and human eyes, *Am J Ophthalmol* (1992) **113**:321.

Epstein DL, Steinert RF, Puliafito CA, Neodymium:YAG laser therapy to the anterior hyaloid in aphakic malignant glaucoma, *Am J Ophthalmol* (1984) **98**:137.

Fankhauser F, et al., Optical principles related to optimizing sclerostomy procedures, *Ophthalmic Surg* (1992) **23**:752.

Fankhauser F, et al., Transscleral cyclophotocoagulation using a neodymium:YAG laser, *Ophthalmic Surg* (1986) **17**:94.

Farnath D, Margolis TI, Puliafito CA, Mid-infrared laser sclerostomy, *Laser Light Ophthalmol* (1988) **2**:196.

Federman JL, et al., Contact laser for transscleral photocoagulation, *Ophthalmic Surg* (1987) **18**:183.

Federman JL, et al., Contact laser thermal sclerostomy ab interno, *Ophthalmic Surg* (1987) **18**:726.

The Glaucoma Laser Trial Research Group, The Glaucoma Laser Trial (GLT). 2. Results of argon laser trabeculoplasty versus topical medicines, *Ophthalmology* (1990) **97**:1403.

Halkias A, Magauran DM, Joyce M, Ciliary block (malignant) glaucoma after cataract extraction with lens implanted treated with YAG laser capsulotomy and anterior hyaloidectomy, *Br J Ophthalmol* (1992) **76**:569.

Hampton C, et al., Evaluation of a protocol for transscleral neodymium:YAG cyclophotocoagulation in one hundred patients, *Ophthalmology* (1990) **97**:910.

Harbin TS Jr, Treatment of cyclodialysis clefts with argon laser photocoagulation, *Ophthalmology* (1982) **89**:1082.

Haut J, et al., Study of the first hundred phakic eyes treated by peripheral iridectomy using the Nd:YAG laser, *Int Ophthalmol* (1986) **9**:227.

Hawkins TA, Stewart WC, One year results of semiconductor transscleral cyclophotocoagulation in glaucoma patients, *Arch Ophthalmol* (1993) **111**:488.

Herbort CP, et al., Anti-inflammatory effect of diclofenac drops after argon laser trabeculoplasty, *Arch Ophthalmol* (1993) **111**:481.

Herschler J, Laser shrinkage of the ciliary processes: a treatment for malignant (ciliary block) glaucoma, *Ophthalmology* (1980) **87**:1155.

Higginbotham EJ, Kao G, Peyman G, Internal sclerostomy with the Nd:YAG contact laser versus thermal sclerostomy in rabbits, *Ophthalmology* (1988) **95**:385.

Hill RA, Ghosheh F, Kim JJ, et al., Photodynamic cyclodestruction in pigmented rabbits using tin ethyl etiopurpurin (SnET2), *Invest Ophthalmol Vis Sci* (1996) **37**:S408.

Hill RA, et al., Ab-interno neodymium:YAG versus erbium:YAG laser sclerostomies in rabbits, *Ophthalmic Surg* (1992) **23**:192–7.

Hill RA, et al., Apraclonidine prophylaxis for postcycloplegic IOP spikes, *Ophthalmology* (1991) **98**:1083.

Hillenkamp F, Interaction between laser radiation and biological systems. In: Hillenkamp F, Pratesi R, Sacchi CA, eds. *Lasers in biology and medicine* (New York: Plenum, 1980).

Ho T, Fan R, Sequential argon-YAG laser iridotomies in dark irides, *Br J Ophthalmol* (1992) **76**:329.

Hoskins HD, et al., Subconjunctival THC:YAG laser thermal sclerostomy, *Ophthalmology* (1991) **98**:1394.

Hosking HD, Migliazzo CV, Laser iridectomy—a technique for blue irides, *Ophthalmic Surg* (1984) **15**:448.

Hoskins HD Jr, Migliazzo C, Management of failing filtering blebs with the argon laser, *Ophthalmic Surg* (1984) **15**:731.

Hotchkiss ML, et al., Non-steroidal anti-inflammatory agents after argon laser trabeculoplasty: a trial with flurbiprofen and indomethacin, *Ophthalmology* (1984) **91**:969.

Iwach AG, Hoskins HD Jr, Laser sclerostomy for the management of glaucoma, *Curr Opin Ophthalmol* (1993) **4**:85.

Iwach AG, et al., Subconjunctival THC:YAG (holmium) laser thermal sclerostomy ab externo. A one-year report, *Ophthalmology* (1993) **100**:356.

Jaffe GJ, et al., Ab-interno sclerostomy with a high-powered argon endolaser, *Am J Ophthalmol* (1988) **106**:391.

Jaffe GJ, et al., Ab-interno sclerostomy with a high powered argon endolaser: clinicopathologic correlation, *Arch Ophthalmol* (1989) **107**:1183.

James WA Jr et al., Argon laser photomydriasis, *Am J Ophthalmol* (1976) **81**:62.

Joondeph HC, Management of postoperative and post-traumatic cyclodialysis clefts with argon laser photocoagulation, *Ophthalmic Surg* (1980) **11**:186.

Kalenak JW, et al., Transscleral neodymium:YAG laser cyclocoagulation for uncontrolled glaucoma, *Ophthalmic Surg* (1990) **21**:346.

Khuri CH, Argon laser iridectomies, *Am J Ophthalmol* (1973) **76**:490.

Kimbrough RL, et al., Angle-closure in nanophthalmos, *Am J Ophthalmol* (1979) **88**:572.

Kitazawa Y, Tanigucchi T, Sugiyama K, Use of apraclonidine to reduce acute IOP rise following Q-switched Nd:YAG laser iridectomy, *Ophthalmic Surg* (1989) **20**:49.

Klapper RM, Q-switched neodymium:YAG laser iridectomy, *Ophthalmology* (1984) **91**:1017.

Klapper RM, et al., Transscleral neodymium:YAG thermal cyclophotocoagulation in refractory glaucoma. A preliminary report, *Ophthalmology* (1988) **95**:719.

Klein HZ, Shields MB, Ernest JT, Two-stage argon laser trabeculoplasty in open angle glaucoma, *Am J Ophthalmol* (1985) **99**:392.

Krasnov MM, Naumidi LP, Contact transscleral laser cyclocoagulation in glaucoma, *Ann Ophthalmol* (1990) **22**:354.

Krasnov MM, Q-switched laser iridectomy and Q-switched laser goniopuncture, *Adv Ophthalmol* (1977) **34**:192.

Kurata F, Krupin T, Kolker AE, Reopening filtration fistulas with transconjunctival argon laser photocoagulation, *Am J Ophthalmol* (1984) **98**:340.

Latina MA, et al., Laser sclerostomy by pulsed dye laser and goniolens, *Arch Ophthalmol* (1990) **108**:1745.

Latina MA, et al., Gonioscopic ab interno laser sclerostomy: a pilot study in glaucoma patients, *Ophthalmology* (1992) **99**:1736.

Latina MA, Rankin GA, Internal and transconjunctival neodymium:YAG revision of late-failing filters, *Ophthalmology* (1991) **98**:215.

Lerman S, *Radiant energy and the eye* (New York: Macmillan, 1980).

L'Esperance FA Jr, *Ophthalmic lasers: photocoagulation, photoradiation, and surgery*, 3rd edn. (St Louis, MO: Mosby, 1989).

Lieberman MF, Suture lysis by laser and goniolens, *Am J Ophthalmol* (1983) **95**:257.

Lim AS, et al., Laser iridoplasty in the treatment of severe acute angle closure glaucoma, *Int Ophthalmol* (1993) **17**:33.

Little BC, Hitchings RA, Pseudophakic malignant glaucoma: Nd:YAG capsulotomy as a primary treatment, *Eye* (1993) **7**:102.

March WF, et al., Experimental YAG laser sclerostomy, *Arch Ophthalmol* (1984) **102**:1834.

McMillan TA, et al., The effect of varying wavelength on subconjunctival scleral laser suture lysis in rabbits, *Acta Ophthalmol (Copenh)* (1992) **70**:758.

Melamed S, Ashkenazi I, Blumenthal M, Nd:YAG laser hyaloidotomy for malignant glaucoma following one-piece 7mm intraocular lens implantation, *Br J Ophthalmol* (1991) **75**:501.

Melamed S, et al., Tight scleral flap trabeculectomy with postoperative laser suture lysis, *Am J Ophthalmol* (1990) **109**:303.

Minckler DS, Does Nd:YAG cyclotherapy cause sympathetic ophthalmia? *Ophthalmic Surg* (1989) **20**:543 (editorial).

Mittra RA, Allingham RR, Shields MB, Follow-up of argon laser trabeculoplasty: is a day-one postoperative IOP check necessary? *Ophthalmic Surg Lasers* (1995) **26**:410–13.

Morinelli EN, et al., Laser suture lysis after mitomycin C trabeculectomy, *Ophthalmology* (1996) **103**:306.

Nelson JS, Berns MW, Basic laser physics and tissue interactions. *Contemp Dermatol* (1988) **2**:2.

Noureddin BN, et al., Advanced uncontrolled glaucoma. Nd:YAG cyclophotocoagulation or tube surgery, *Ophthalmology* (1992) **99**:430.

Oh Y, Katz LJ, Indications and technique for reopening closed filtering blebs using the Nd:YAG laser: a review and case series, *Ophthalmic Surg* (1993) **24**:617.

Onda E, et al., Determination of an appropriate laser setting for THC:YAG laser sclerostomy ab-externo in rabbits, *Ophthalmic Surg* (1992) **23**:198.

Oram O, et al., Opening an occluded Molteno tube with the picosecond neodymium-yttrium-lithium fluoride laser, *Arch Ophthalmol* (1994) **112**:1023.

Ormerod LD, et al., Management of the hypotonous cyclodialysis cleft, *Ophthalmology* (1991) **98**:1384.

Ozler SA, et al., Infrared laser sclerostomies, *Invest Ophthalmol Vis Sci* (1991) **32**:2498.

Pappa KS, et al., Late argon suture lysis after mitomycin-C trabeculectomy. *Ophthalmology* (1993) **100**:1268.

Partamiam LG, Treatment of a cyclodialysis cleft with argon laser photocoagulation in a patient with a shallow anterior chamber, *Am J Ophthalmol* (1985) **99**:5.

Pavlin C J, Ritch R, Foster FS, Ultrasound biomicroscopy in plateau iris syndrome, *Am J Ophthalmol* (1992) **113**:390.

Perkins ES, Brown NA, Iridectomy with a ruby laser, *Br J Ophthalmol* (1973) **57**:487.

Pollack IP, Patz A, Argon laser iridectomy: an experimental and clinical study, *Ophthalmic Surg* (1976) **7**:22.

Potash SD, et al., Ultrasound biomicroscopy in pigment dispersion syndrome, *Ophthalmology* (1994) **101**:332.

Praeger DL, The reopening of closed filtering blebs using the neodymium:YAG laser, *Ophthalmology* (1984) **91**:373.

Quigley HA, Long-term follow-up of laser iridectomy, *Ophthalmology* (1981) **88**:218.

Rankin GA, Latina MA, Transconjunctival Nd:YAG laser revision of failing trabeculectomy, *Ophthalmic Surg* (1990) **21**:365.

Ritch R, Argon laser treatment for medically unresponsive attacks of angle-closure glaucoma, *Am J Ophthalmol* (1982) **94**:197.

Ritch R, *Techniques of argon laser iridectomy and iridoplasty* (Palo Alto, CA: Coherent Medical Press, 1983).

Ritch R, A new lens for argon laser trabeculoplasty, *Ophthalmic Surg* (1985) **16**:331.

Ritch R, Plateau iris is caused by abnormally positioned ciliary processes, *J Glaucoma* (1992) **1**:23.

Ritch R, Argon laser peripheral iridoplasty: an overview, *J Glaucoma* (1992) **1**:206.

Ritch R, Palmberg P, Argon laser iridectomy in densely pigmented irides, *Am J Ophthalmol* (1982) **94**:800.

Ritch R, Potash SD, Liebmann JM, A new lens for argon laser suture lysis, *Ophthalmic Surg* (1994) **25**:126.

Robin AL, Pollack IP, DeFaller JM, Effects of topical ALO 2145 (p-aminoclonidine hydrochloride) on intraocular pressure rise following argon laser iridectomy, *Arch Ophthalmol* (1987) **105**:1208.

Robin AL, Pollack IP, Argon laser peripheral iridotomies in the treatment of primary angle closure glaucoma: long-term follow-up, *Arch Ophthalmol* (1982) **100**:919.

Robin AL, et al., Effect of ALO 2145 on intraocular pressure following argon laser trabeculoplasty, *Arch Ophthalmol* (1987) **105**:656.

Robin AL, Pollack IP, A comparison of neodymium:YAG and argon laser iridotomies, *Ophthalmology* (1984) **91**:1011.

Savage JA, Simmons RJ, Staged glaucoma filtration surgery with planned early conversion from scleral flap to full-thickness operation using argon laser, *Ophthalmic Laser Ther* (1986) **1**:201.

Schrems W, Belcher CDI, Tomlinson CP, Neodymium:YAG laser iridectomy: a report of 200 cases, *Ophthalmic Laser Ther* (1987) **2**:33.

Schuman JS, et al., Contact transscleral Nd:YAG laser cyclophotocoagulation: midterm results, *Ophthalmology* (1992) **99**:1089.

Schuman JS, et al., Energy levels and probe placement in contact transscleral semiconductor diode laser cyclophotocoagulation in human cadaver eyes, *Arch Ophthalmol* (1991) **109**:1534.

Schuman JS, et al., Contact transscleral continuous wave neodymium:YAG laser cyclophotocoagulation, *Ophthalmology* (1990) **97**:571.

Schuman JS, et al., Experimental use of semiconductor diode laser in contact transscleral cyclophotocoagulation in rabbits, *Arch Ophthalmol* (1990) **108**:1152.

Schuman JS, Puliafito CA, Laser cyclophotocoagulation, *Int Ophthalmol Clin* (1990) **30**:111.

Schuman JS, et al., Holmium laser sclerectomy. Success and complications, *Ophthalmology* (1993) **100**:1060.

Schwartz AL, Love DC, Schwartz MA, Longterm follow-up of argon laser trabeculoplasty for uncontrolled open angle glaucoma, *Arch Ophthalmol* (1985) **103**:1482.

Schwartz AL, Weiss H, Bleb leak with hypotony after laser suture lysis and trabeculectomy with mitomycin-C, *Arch Ophthalmol* (1992) **110**:1049.

Shahinian LJ, Egbert PR, Williams AS, Histologic study of healing after ab interno laser sclerostomy, *Am J Ophthalmol* (1992) **114**:216.

Shields MB, Wilkerson MH, Echelman DA, A comparison of two energy levels for noncontact transscleral neodymium-YAG cyclophotocoagulation, *Arch Ophthalmol* (1993) **111**:484.

Shingleton BJ, et al., Long-term efficacy of argon laser trabeculoplasty, a ten-year follow-up study, *Ophthalmology* (1993) **100**:1324.

Simmons RJ, Discussion of Herschler J: Laser shrinkage of ciliary processes: a treatment for malignant glaucoma, *Ophthalmology* (1980) **87**:1158.

Simmons RB, et al., Comparison of transscleral neodymium:YAG cyclophotocoagulation with and without a contact lens in human autopsy eyes, *Am J Ophthalmol* (1990) **109**:174.

Simmons RB, et al., Transscleral Nd:YAG laser cyclophotocoagulation with a contact lens, *Am J Ophthalmol* (1991) **112**:671.

Sliney DH, Mainster MA, Potential laser hazards to the clinician during photocoagulation, *Am J Ophthalmol* (1987) **103**:758.

Smith J, Argon laser trabeculoplasty: comparison of bichromatic and monochromatic wavelengths, *Ophthalmology* (1984) **91**:355.

Spaeth GL, Baez K, Argon laser trabeculoplasty controls one third of cases of progressive, uncontrolled, open angle glaucoma for 5 years, *Arch Ophthalmol* (1992) **110**:491.

Spurny RC, Lederer CM Jr, Krypton laser trabeculoplasty, *Arch Ophthalmol* (1984) **102**:1626.

Starita RJ, Klapper RM, Neodymium:YAG photodisruption of the anterior hyaloid face in aphakic flat chamber: a diagnostic and therapeutic tool, *Int Ophthalmol Clin* (1985) **25**:119.

Stetz D, Smith HJ, Ritch R, A simplified technique for laser iridectomy in blue irides, *Am J Ophthalmol* (1983) **96**:249.

Tello C, et al., Ultrasound biomicroscopy in pseudophakic malignant glaucoma, *Ophthalmology* (1993) **100**:1330.

Thomas JV, Pupilloplasty and photomydriasis. In: Belcher CD, Thomas JV, Simmons RJ, eds. *Photocoagulation in glaucoma and anterior segment disease* (Baltimore, MD: Williams & Wilkins, 1984).

Ticho U, Ivry M, Reopening of occluded filtering blebs by argon laser photocoagulation, *Am J Ophthalmol* (1977) **84**:413.

Tomey KF, Traverso CE, Shammas IV, Neodymium:YAG laser iridectomy in the treatment and prevention of angle closure glaucoma: a review of 373 eyes, *Arch Ophthalmol* (1987) **105**:476.

Tomlinson CP, Brigham M, Belcher CD III, Suture manipulation with the argon laser, *Ophthalmic Laser Ther* (1987) **2**:151.

Trope GE, Ma S, Mid-term effects of neodymium:YAG transscleral cyclocoagulation in glaucoma, *Ophthalmology* (1990) **97**:73.

Van Buskirk EM, Reopening filtration fistulas with the argon laser, *Am J Ophthalmol* (1982) **94**:1.

Van Rens GH, Transconjunctival reopening of an occluded filtration fistula with the Q-switched neodymium:YAG laser, *Doc Ophthalmol* (1988) **70**:205.

Vogel A, Dlugos C, Nuffer R, et al., Optical properties of human sclera and their consequences for transscleral laser applications, *Lasers Surg Med* (1991) **11**:331–40.

Walsh JT, Flotte TJ, Deutsch TF, Er:YAG laser ablation of tissue: effect of pulse duration and tissue type on thermal damage, *Lasers Surg Med* (1989) **9**:314.

Weber PA, et al., Argon laser treatment of the ciliary processes in aphakic glaucoma with flat anterior chamber, *Am J Ophthalmol* (1984) **97**:82.

Wetzel W, et al., Laser sclerostomy ab externo using the erbium:YAG laser. First results of a clinical study, *Ger J Ophthalmol* (1994) **3**:112.

Wilensky JT, Welch D, Mirolovich M, Transscleral cyclocoagulation using a neodymium:YAG laser, *Ophthalmic Surg* (1985) **16**:95.

Wilson RP, Javitt JC, Ab interno laser sclerostomy in aphakic patients with glaucoma and chronic inflammation, *Am J Ophthalmol* (1990) **110**:178.

Wise JB, Ten-year results of laser trabeculoplasty, *Eye* (1987) **1**:45.

Wise JB, Munnerlyn CR, Erickson PJ, A high-efficiency laser iridectomy-sphincterotomy lens, *Am J Ophthalmol* (1986) **101**:546.

Yassur Y, et al., Iridectomy with red krypton laser, *Br J Ophthalmol* (1986) **70**:295.

16 Filtering surgery

J Brent Bond and Richard P Wilson

Introduction

For roughly 100 years, surgical attempts have been made to lower intraocular pressure by establishing continual filtration of aqueous from the anterior chamber to the subconjunctival space. A wide variety of techniques were used until the early 1970s when 'trabeculectomy', as described by Cairns in 1968, became the preferred technique for glaucoma filtering surgery. The popularity of trabeculectomy has been due to a much lower postoperative complication rate compared to previous procedures. Its safety is due to the partial-thickness scleral flap overlying the filtration site, decreasing the incidence of early postoperative complications owing to overfiltration which had often been seen with the 'full thickness' procedures. Because of this decreased complication rate, trabeculectomy has become the filtering procedure of choice, and over the last 20 years much of the work done in glaucoma surgery has been directed towards modifications of the basic procedure, attempting to lower the complication rate further and increase the success rate. In this chapter, a basic trabeculectomy technique is presented with attention to details of its performance. Modifications of the technique are also presented, including various suture techniques and the use of antimetabolites.

General principles

Filtering surgery is usually indicated when the patient's glaucoma is observed to worsen at the present level of intraocular pressure, usually after establishing maximum tolerated medical therapy, and possibly following failure of argon laser trabeculoplasty. Surgery may also be indicated when the target intraocular pressure has not been achieved by other means and the disease is expected to worsen.

During filtering surgery, the conjunctiva should be handled as little as possible and as meticulously as possible. The conjunctiva overlying the area of the filtration site should never be touched. Nontoothed forceps, such as utility forceps or Pierce–Hoskins forceps, should be used when handling conjunctiva.

Bleeding conjunctival and scleral vessels must be painstakingly cauterized. Even slight oozing, which would be of little significance in other types of ocular surgery, can significantly decrease the chance of successful glaucoma filtering surgery. Any subconjunctival blood in the area of the filtration bleb can result in scarring, limiting the size and functional capacity of the filtration bleb. A 23 gauge needle tip cautery may be used for precise cauterization of small vessels, and may also be used within the anterior chamber to stop bleeding of iris or ciliary body vessels.

The surgeon must make certain prior to entering the anterior chamber that the scleral flap is dissected anteriorly enough so that the sclerostomy site will enter the anterior chamber and will not be over the ciliary body. Careful observation is required in patients with altered limbal anatomy from previous surgery. When a limbal-based conjunctival flap is being developed in such a patient, careful and patient dissection is often required to extend the dissection anteriorly enough for appropriate placement of the filtration site.

After initial suturing of the scleral flap, the surgeon should reform the anterior chamber to a normal depth and pressure and then always evaluate the amount of filtration obtained prior to closing the conjunctiva. As described below, further manipulation can be done to adjust filtration to a specific level of outflow, rather than simply placing a predetermined number of sutures in the scleral flap for every case. This intraoperative adjustment is crucial for obtaining a consistently successful result.

Techniques

Preparation

After sterile prepping and draping, the lid speculum should be inserted with care taken that the speculum does not cause pressure on the globe. A traction suture should be placed in such a way as to infraduct the globe maximally, exposing conjunctiva as far superiorly and posteriorly as possible, especially if a limbal-based conjunctival flap is being used. This is crucial for making the conjunctival incision as far posterior as possible, preferably 10 mm posterior to the limbus, so that the area of the postoperative filtering bleb will not be limited by scar tissue from the conjunctival incision. Either a corneal traction suture or a superior rectus bridle suture may be used. The corneal traction suture has the advantage of avoiding the rare instance of scleral perforation which may occur with the larger needle and less well visualized needle pass of the superior rectus bridle suture, and also avoids bleeding at the superior rectus and postoperative ptosis that may occur rarely with the superior rectus bridle suture. However, the corneal traction suture has the disadvantage that dissection through the Tenons is more laborious. Also, the other disadvantage of the corneal traction suture is the possibility, especially in myopes with pliable sclera, that when the eye is forcibly infraducted near the end of the surgery for closure of the limbal-based conjunctival flap, the traction at the superior limbus will distort the anatomy enough at the filtration site so that the wound cleft will gape with outflow of aqueous and inability to maintain a formed chamber during conjunctival wound closure.

Placement of a corneal traction suture is best done with a 6-0 Vicryl suture on an S-29 needle through superior peripheral clear cornea. Care should be taken not to enter the anterior chamber. If the filtration site is to be offset either superonasally or superotemporally, then the traction suture should be centered in the quadrant to be used. The globe needs minimal stabilization during passage of this suture, with a cellulose sponge being sufficient to hold the globe steady for needle passage. With this suture and also with the bridle suture placement, the surgeon should remember at all times to resist the tendency to grasp conjunctiva on the superior bulbar portion of the globe anywhere near the planned filtration site.

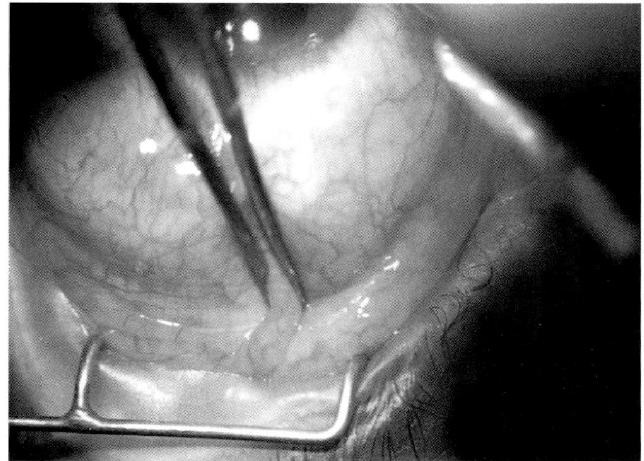

Figure 16.1 Traction suture
A muscle hook may be used to turn the eye inferiorly. The superior rectus muscle is then grasped with a forceps and lifted to allow placement of a bridle suture. This allows the suture line, with its foreign body reaction, to be as far as possible from the site of filtration.

A superior rectus bridle suture is best done with a 4-0 silk suture on a taper-point needle. The superior rectus muscle can be grasped with a forceps by either infraducting the globe with a muscle hook pressing into the inferior fornix and grasping the muscle posteriorly under direct visualization (Fig. 16.1), or by sliding the closed forceps into the superior fornix and then opening the forceps, rotating it perpendicularly to the globe, and with firm downward pressure grasping the superior rectus. The globe can then be infraducted and the bridle suture placed underneath the muscle. Since toothed forceps are necessary for grasping the superior rectus, a conjunctival buttonhole may occur, but it will be far posteriorly in the area of the conjunctival incision.

Conjunctival flap dissection

In the past, there has been no consensus among surgeons as to whether a limbal-based or fornix-based conjunctival flap is associated with a better surgical result. The surgeon who only occasionally performs filtering surgery may feel more comfortable with a fornix-based approach and perhaps have more assurance that the scleral flap dissection and anterior chamber entry is positioned appropriately anteriorly. A significant disadvantage of the fornix-based approach is the higher chance of a wound leak. Prior to usage of antimetabolites, a small leak was usually of no consequence except for perhaps resulting in a less extensive bleb. However, with the use of antimetabolites, such a leak may have much

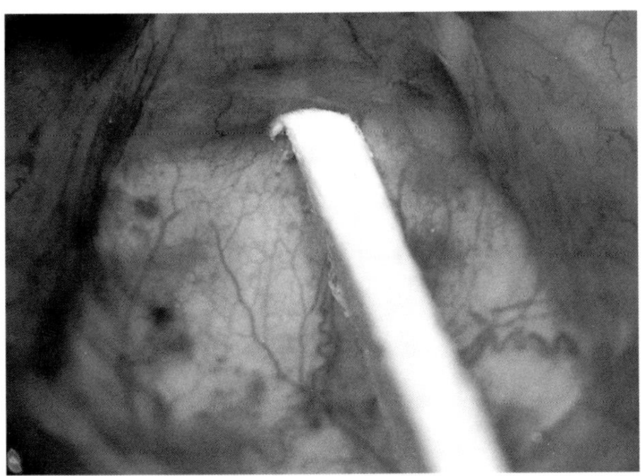

Figure 16.2 Blunt dissection
A cellulose sponge is used to dissect down to the limbus bluntly, minimizing the chance of a buttonhole.

more grave consequences. The leak may take much longer to seal or not seal at all, putting the patient at risk of blebitis, flat anterior chamber and hypotony with or without choroidal detachment. A further disadvantage of the fornix-based approach is that a wound leak may be induced if laser suture lysis or digital ocular compression is needed in the early postoperative period. The use of the limbal-based flap with its intact limbal conjunctival barrier reduces these concerns, perhaps making it the approach of choice at least when antimetabolites are to be used.

When using a limbal-based conjunctival flap, the conjunctiva is incised with Westcott scissors at least 10 mm posterior to the superior limbus. The incision is extended in either direction for a total of about 10–15 mm of length, taking care that the entire length of the incision remains at least 10 mm posterior to the limbus. If a corneal traction suture is used, then the Tenon's is grasped with a nontoothed forceps, such as the Pierce–Hoskins, by both the assistant and the surgeon in order to tent it upward, taking care not to include the superior rectus muscle. Tenon's is then incised with the Westcott scissors down to bare scleral and the Tenon's incision is extended for at least the entire length of the conjunctival incision and perhaps several millimeters further on either side to allow comfortable stretching of the tissue forward. The conjunctival–Tenon's flap complex can then be stretched forward and downward over the cornea with sharp dissection with Westcotts through episcleral attachments several millimeters posterior to the limbus. This dissection should always be done under direct visualization with the flap stretched anteriorly, thereby making inadvertent buttonhole incision much less likely. Once the episcleral attachments have been incised, then the remainder of the forward dissection can be done bluntly with a cellulose sponge, in order to decrease the likelihood of buttonhole formation (Fig. 16.2). However, it is important to make certain that the Tenon's fibers are dissected as far forward into the corneo-scleral sulcus as possible. In some patients, such as young patients or African-American patients, the Tenon's may be too thick for the dissection to be completed with the cellulose sponge and therefore the final remaining fibers must be dissected with a 67 blade tip oriented vertically to the scleral surface and scraped circumferentially along the base of the Tenon's attachments. The remaining tissue can then be pushed forward into the sulcus as desired. Patient and complete anterior dissection of the conjunctival flap is crucial to allow proper placement of the scleral flap dissection.

If a superior rectus bridle suture is used, the only difference from the technique just described is with the conjunctival and Tenon's incision. With the bridle suture, the surgeon should grasp conjunctiva only with the nontoothed forceps just anterior to the bridle suture and pull the conjunctiva forward on stretch and incise it with the blunt Westcott scissors. Tenon's is grasped in a like manner but without the need for an assistant to also grasp this tissue since it is in effect already tented by the bridle suture. As this Tenon's incision is done over the superior rectus, care should be taken not to cut into muscle. The incision is then extended as previously described.

If a fornix-based conjunctival flap approach is elected, a limbal conjunctival incision of about 8 mm is initiated at either end of what will be the extent of the peritomy. This is done by tenting the conjunctiva near the limbus with nontoothed forceps and beginning the incision with the Westcott scissors. This is carefully extended along the length of the peritomy. Then Tenon's is incised in a like manner. Blunt dissection with the blunt Westcott scissors should be done posteriorly underneath Tenon's along the length of the limbal incision to allow for good posterior exposure, to encourage larger posterior bleb development and to allow posterior placement of mitomycin if necessary.

Scleral flap dissection

The size and shape of the scleral flap is of no significance. However, most surgeons prefer either a

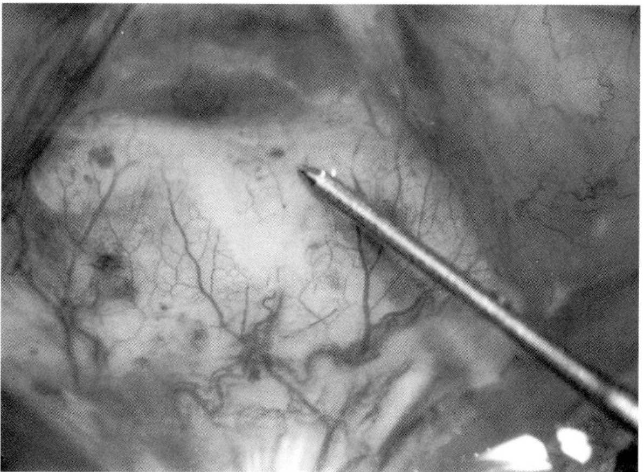

Figure 16.3 Scleral flap
Cautery may be used to outline the scleral flap.

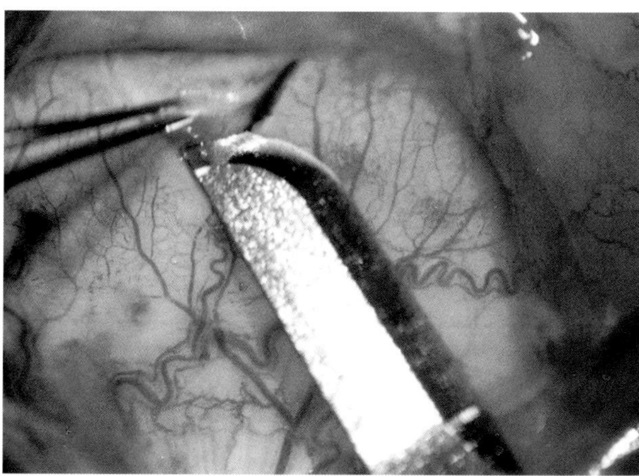

Figure 16.4 Dissecting the scleral flap
The posterior tip of the scleral flap is grasped firmly and lifted anteriorly towards the microscope. The best surgical plane will be found at the base of the flap where the scleral fibers pull apart.

square or a triangular flap with the anterior base of the flap being 2–4 mm with the length likewise ranging from 2 to 4 mm. Prior to dissection of the flap, the surgeon should confirm its appropriate placement anteriorly and then outline the desired dimensions with the needle-point cautery (Fig. 16.3). A 67 blade should then be used to outline the scleral flap with a scleral incision of one half to two thirds scleral thickness. The posterior-most aspect of the scleral flap is then grasped with forceps and the flap is dissected forward with the blade held almost flat against the sclera (Fig. 16.4). During this dissection, the scleral flap should be pulled continually anteriorly with the forceps so that the dissection is done with the tip of the blade under direct visualization. As the dissection continues anteriorly, the thickness of the flap can continually be assessed and modified as necessary. If a particularly low postoperative pressure is believed necessary, then the anterior portion of the flap can be made thinner. If it is especially important to avoid overfiltration in a particular patient, the surgeon can make certain that the scleral flap remains quite thick. The dissection should be continued anteriorly until the cornea is seen in the bed of the flap, and/or until the knife blade can be visualized in clear cornea (Fig. 16.5).

Paracentesis track

After completion of the scleral flap dissection, a clear cornea paracentesis track is made (Fig. 16.6). The globe is fixated by firmly grasping the sclera with a 0.12 mm forceps, taking care not to touch conjunctiva with this toothed forceps. A 25 gauge or 27 gauge, 5/8-inch sharp needle on a 1 or 3 cc syringe is then passed through clear cornea, attempting to make the track about 2 mm long so that it will be self-sealing. The track should be begun just on the clear corneal side of the limbus and is produced without ever pointing the needle posteriorly. The needle must always be oriented parallel to the plane of the iris with the bevel up. The correct technique involves rotating the globe superiorly with the fixating hand as much as pushing the needle forward. A 15 degree blade, such as a Beaver 75, may alternatively be used. The entry into the anterior chamber should be over iris, not lens, but the surgeon must

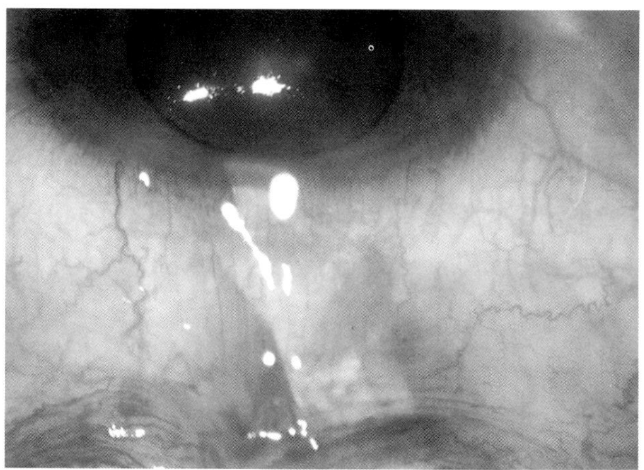

Figure 16.5 Dissecting the scleral flap
The dissection is carried forward until the knife blade can be seen in clear cornea anterior to the limbus.

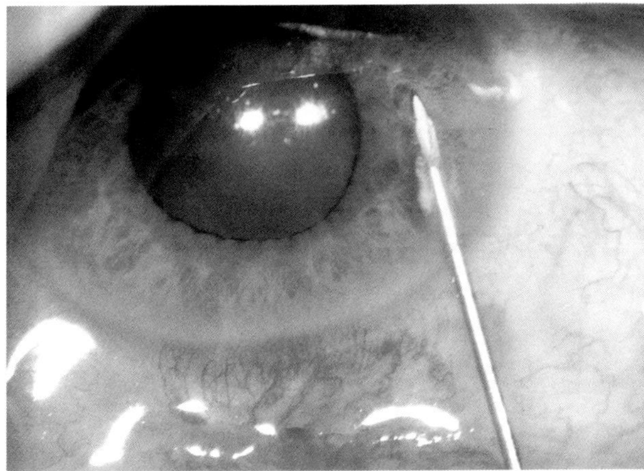

Figure 16.6 Making a paracentesis track
A paracentesis track is made with a 27 gauge needle before the eye is entered for the trabeculectomy block. Subsequent filling of the anterior chamber with balanced salt solution is done through a 30 gauge needle.

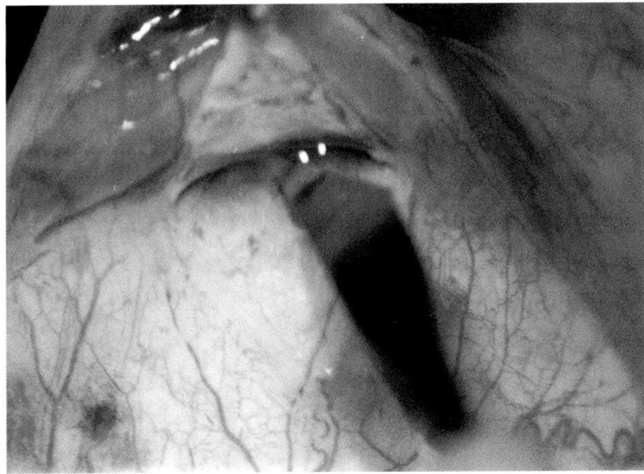

Figure 16.7 Trabeculectomy block
A blade such as the Beaver 75 or a 15 degree blade is used to make the anterior–posterior incisions for the trabeculectomy block.

make certain that the full bevel of the needle tip is within the anterior chamber before withdrawing the needle. In general, the location of the track is left to the preference of the surgeon. Some prefer always to make the track on the side of the dominant hand with the track being placed superiorly and oriented towards the inferior limbus. Others prefer always to place the track with a more horizontal orientation temporally, requiring use of either hand, depending on which eye is undergoing the surgery. This is for the purpose of allowing easier access to the track if the anterior chamber must be reformed in the early postoperative period.

Corneo-scleral block excision

Similar to the sizing of the scleral flap, the size of the opening into the anterior chamber is not in itself important. However, the proximity of the opening to the edge of the scleral flap is of crucial importance. In the patient who may need a particularly low pressure with a high-flow filter, the surgeon may wish to excise the corneo-scleral block up to the very edge of the scleral flap. Certainly this will then require tight suturing of the scleral flap over that area and will increase the risk of overfiltration, but may be necessary in selected patients. For a more conservative filter, the block excision may be positioned centrally underneath the flap with perhaps a millimeter of tissue remaining between the internal opening and the edge of the scleral flap. Also, the surgeon can preferentially orient the direction of the filtration by offsetting the block excision much closer to one side of the scleral flap than the other. Often for a right-hand dominant surgeon, this may mean offsetting the internal block excision to the left edge of the scleral flap, relative to the surgeon's view, so that placement of scleral flap sutures will be with a more easily controlled forehand pass of the suture. There are several different techniques of excising the corneo-scleral block of tissue. One technique involves excision of the block with a sharp-point blade and Vannas scissors and another uses a sharp-point blade and a punch, such as the Kelly Descemet punch or the Luntz– Dodick punch. If a limbal-based conjunctival flap has been used, the assistant will need to stretch it anteriorly over the cornea to maintain a clear view for the surgeon. The surgeon then grasps the posterior aspect of the scleral flap with the nondominant hand, reflects it anteriorly and, with the dominant hand, makes an incision into the anterior chamber through clear cornea parallel to the base of the scleral flap (Fig. 16.7). This incision should be 1–3 mm long depending upon how big an internal block of tissue the surgeon wishes to excise. Most surgeons excise a block of tissue from 1 to 3 mm in width. Care must be taken to make certain that this incision is full thickness into the anterior chamber. If a punch is to be used, it should be positioned through the incision so that a full-thickness block of corneo-scleral tissue will be excised. The punch should be positioned so that the tissue is excised from the posterior lip of the anteriorly placed incision. The punch should be positioned as close to the edge of the scleral flap as the surgeon desires, offsetting the excision towards the dominant hand as desired by the surgeon. Several punches may be required to obtain the desired size of opening. Care should be taken that a thin lip of Descemet

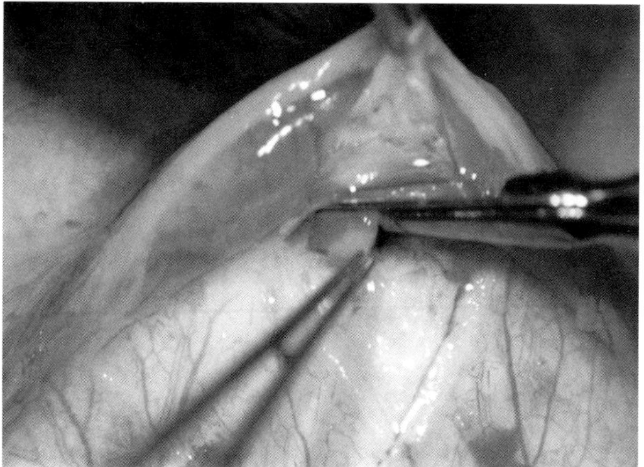

Figure 16.8 The corneo-scleral excision
After radial incisions are done with a blade, the excision is completed with Vannas scissors.

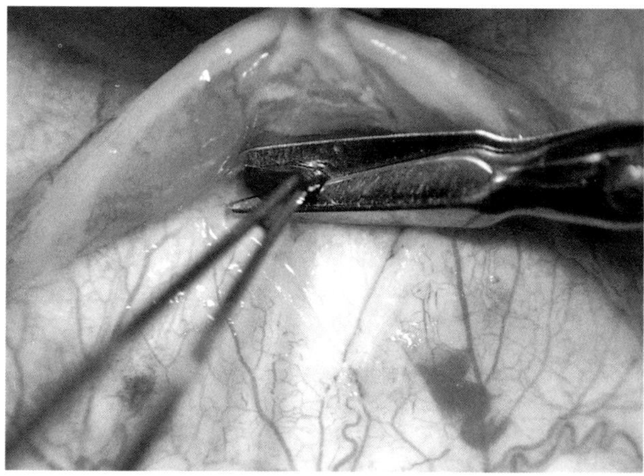

Figure 16.9 Iridectomy
An iridectomy is made with Vannas scissors.

membrane does not remain over what would otherwise appear to be a full-thickness opening. If the initial sharp-point blade incision into the anterior chamber was appropriately positioned through clear cornea, then the opening produced by the punch will be through clear cornea and perhaps trabecular meshwork, but remain anterior to scleral spur. This anterior block excision eliminates the risk of bleeding or blockage of the filtration opening by ciliary body or iris as may occur with a more posterior entry site.

The other common technique of cornea-scleral block excision is done by two parallel, radial, full-thickness incisions with the sharp-point blade. These two incisions determine the width of the block to be excised and should be positioned as described above according to the surgeon's desire to direct outflow towards one side of the flap or the other and according to the amount of aqueous egress desired. Vannas scissors are then positioned parallel to the limbus with one tip of the Vannas scissors through one of the radial incisions into the anterior chamber. Care should be taken to make certain that the tip is completely in the anterior chamber so that a full-thickness cut will be made. The scissors are then slid as far posteriorly as possible and oriented perpendicular to the plane of tissue and a full-thickness cut is made. If the radial incisions were begun in clear cornea and extended posteriorly just into the transition zone of blue limbal tissue, then the posterior Vannas incision will remain anterior to the scleral spur. The assistant must maintain anterior traction on the scleral flap while the surgeon then grasps the posterior edge of the corneo-scleral block and places it on posterior stretch. A firm stretch is required and this will deform the peripheral cornea but is necessary to make certain that the anterior extent of the block incision will be appropriately far enough anterior. The Vannas scissors are then slid as far anteriorly as possible, maintaining the orientation of the blades parallel to the limbus. Also, the lower blade should be more anterior than the upper blade so that the remaining corneal edge will be beveled posteriorly, leaving no posterior corneal ledge for iris to adhere to should the chamber shallow postoperatively (Fig. 16.8).

Iridectomy

A peripheral iridectomy is required in all cases even if there is a previous iridectomy at another site. The only instance in which an iridectomy is not required is if the filtration site is positioned directly over a previous peripheral iridectomy or sector iridectomy and there is no iris tissue visible through the internal opening. Otherwise, a peripheral iridectomy must be done after excision of the corneo-scleral tissue. The iris will often balloon into the filtration site or must be grasped with a 0.12 forceps and brought into the corneo-scleral opening. Vannas scissors should be used for the iridectomy with the blades oriented flush against the sclera and parallel to the limbus (Fig. 16.9). Care should be taken to have the assistant keep conjunctiva and Tenon's away from the blades in the case of a limbal-based conjunctival flap. The surgeon should make certain to excise enough iris tissue so that the edge of the iridectomy is free from the corneo-scleral opening. It is better to err on the side of a larger iridectomy than necessary or otherwise the iridectomy may be

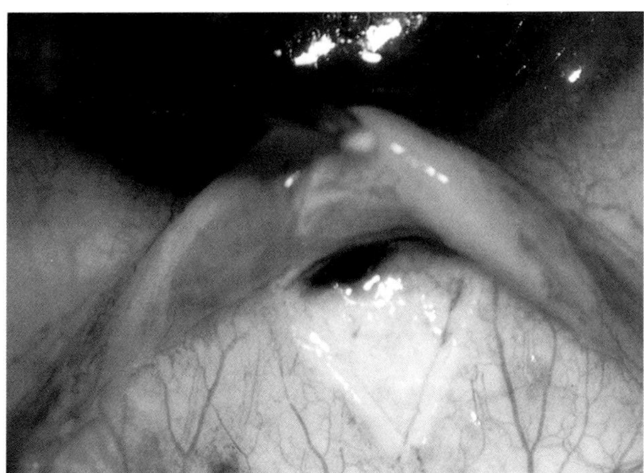

Figure 16.10 Inspecting the filtration site
Before scleral flap closure, the filtration site should be inspected for residual bleeding or blockage of the filtration opening.

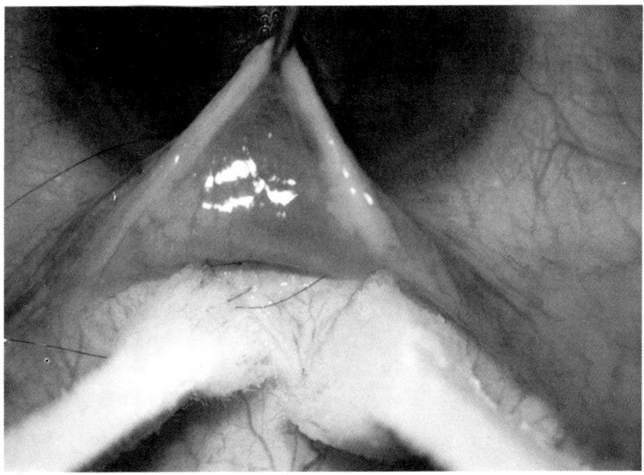

Figure 16.11 Testing for aqueous flow
Testing for aqueous flow through the trabeculectomy is done with cellulose spears at several intraocular pressure levels. When antifibrosis agents are used, there should be almost no leakage at intraocular pressures less than 10 mmHg, and only a slow ooze at levels from 10 to 15 mmHg.

only partial thickness, especially in African-American patients who have thick irides. Infrequently, there may be transient bleeding from iris vessels. In the vast majority of cases, this lasts less than a minute. The surgeon should simply continue irrigation with balanced salt solution through the filtration site to prevent residual blood remaining in the anterior chamber.

Scleral flap closure

Prior to closure of the scleral flap, the filtration site should be irrigated with balanced salt solution, and the surgeon should verify that there is no residual bleeding and that there is a clear filtration opening not blocked by Descemet's membrane, iris, ciliary body or vitreous (Fig. 16.10). The scleral flap is repositioned in its bed and closed with 10-0 nylon suture. If the flap is square or rectangular, a suture should be placed in each posterior corner of the flap. A triangular flap may be closed with one nylon suture at the apex. These sutures do not have to be particularly tight but are simply to maintain the flap in its bed. If extensive cautery was required to cauterize scleral perforating vessels, the scleral bed edges may have retracted; the flap in this case should not be pulled tight enough to result in complete apposition of the flap to its original bed edge. The sutures should be only partial thickness through the scleral flap. Otherwise, a stretch hole may result, especially if the flap is thin, and it may be very difficult to gain control over flow of aqueous through this defect. Once the flap is sutured into its bed, the anterior chamber is reformed through the previously placed clear cornea paracentesis track. The surgeon should evaluate the extent of aqueous egress around the edges of the scleral flap. The area is dried with a cellulose sponge and checked for spontaneous aqueous flow. If there is copious egress of aqueous, it may be necessary to place additional sutures to appose the anterior edge of the flap to the edge of the bed more firmly. The surgeon should remember to make these suture passes partial thickness through the flap as described above. The sutures should be trimmed at the knot so that in the case of a low or flat bleb postoperatively, the loose ends will not protrude into the conjunctiva and cause a conjunctival buttonhole leak. It is not necessary to bury the knots into the sclera. Externalized, releasable scleral flap sutures may be placed as described later in this chapter. The three steps of suture placement, anterior chamber reformation, and evaluation of aqueous outflow and level of intraocular pressure are patiently and continually repeated until the anterior chamber remains deep after reformation with a good intraocular pressure as judged by finger tension and with a continual but slow and controlled egress of aqueous from the edge of the flap (Fig. 16.11). In some cases, such as patients with a shallow anterior chamber and chronic angle closure (who are at risk for flat chamber), or young adults with significant myopia and thin sclera who are at risk for hypotony maculopathy (especially if mitomycin is used) the surgeon may wish to have minimal or no egress of aqueous visible. However, the surgeon should make certain that outflow can be induced by applying light pressure with the cellulose sponge just on the scleral-side of the edge of the flap. In cases in which the egress of aqueous is less than the surgeon

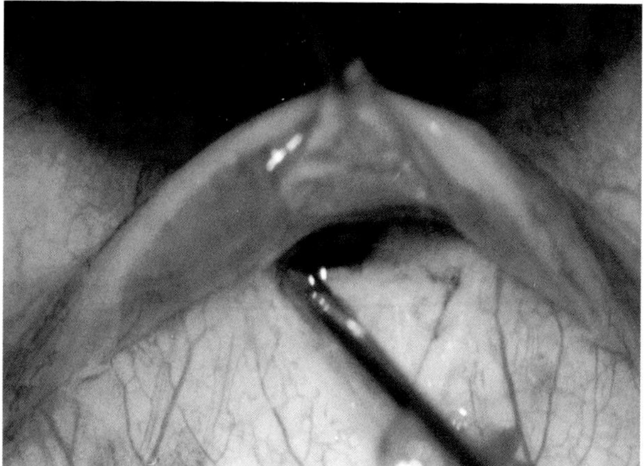

Figure 16.12 Adjusting aqueous egress
If there is insufficient flow through the filtering site, cautery can be used to shrink the scleral to lessen overlap and increase outflow.

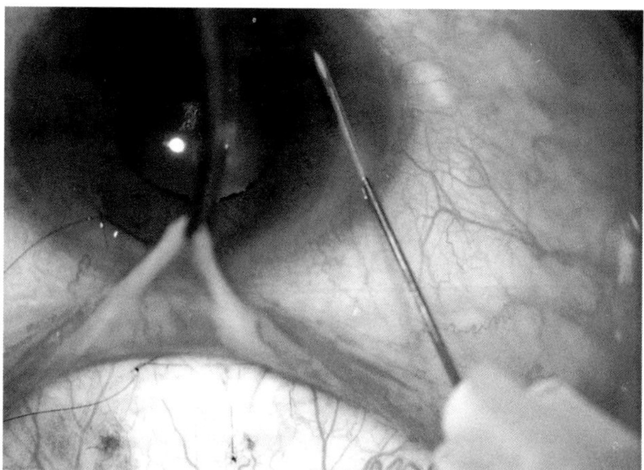

Figure 16.13 Reforming the anterior chamber
After placement of scleral flap sutures, the anterior chamber is reformed via the paracentesis track; the amount of filtration is observed and modified as judged necessary.

believes necessary, short bursts of cautery with the needle-point cautery can be applied into the cleft at the edge of the flap in order to make the edges gape and allow aqueous outflow (Fig. 16.12). Special care should be taken to apply this cautery initially in a very short burst since excessive retraction of tissue may occur, making it difficult to suture the edges close enough together to prevent overfiltration. Rather than using cautery to increase outflow, the surgeon may wish simply to remove the sutures already placed, replacing them with looser sutures. The number of sutures required to obtain the desired level of outflow may be highly variable from patient to patient depending on many factors, including the amount of flow desired (which will depend upon the type of glaucoma and the characteristics of the patient), the thickness of the scleral flap and the proximity of the corneo-scleral opening to the edge of the flap. In some cases, the posterior corner or apex sutures may be all that is required, while in other cases 6–8 sutures may be necessary for control of the amount of aqueous egress. The intraoperative evaluation and manipulation of the amount of aqueous egress is crucial for obtaining consistently good results, minimizing early postoperative complications, and avoiding unwanted surprises which may occur if the surgeon simply places a predetermined, standard number of sutures without evaluating or adjusting the flow rate intraoperatively (Fig. 16.13). The judgment of the correct amount of aqueous egress requires experience. This aspect of the surgery is a large part of the 'art' of glaucoma filtering surgery, and the glaucoma surgeon should strive to develop a 'feel' for the correct amount of outflow for each particular case.

Conjunctival flap closure

If a fornix-based conjunctival flap has been done, then the limbal incision site should be de-epithelialized by scraping with a 67 blade or by cautery. Conjunctiva should then be stretched anteriorly and either end sutured with an anterior anchoring suture of 10-0 nylon anteriorly through peripheral clear cornea. A small running or purse-string type suture will probably be required to close any gaping of conjunctiva beyond the anchoring suture. The other end of the conjunctival flap is then very tightly stretched and also sutured anteriorly with an anchoring suture. As at the other end of the wound, a small running closure may be required to prevent leakage distal to the anchoring suture, especially if a posterior relaxing incision had initially been made at that end of the conjunctival incision. The anterior chamber should then be reformed and slight pressure applied to the edge of the scleral flap if necessary to produce a filtration bleb so that the conjunctival closure can be checked for leakage. Fluorescein may need to be applied to detect any small leak. An alternative to this type of closure is a horizontal mattress-running closure as described by Liss.

As is the case for closure of the fornix-based flap, there is no uniform agreement among surgeons as to the best suturing technique. For the limbal-based conjunctival closure, especially if the conjunctival incision was appropriately high on the superior fornix, a single-layer, unlocked running closure with small, closely spaced bites incorporating Tenon's and conjunctiva is quite adequate. However, we

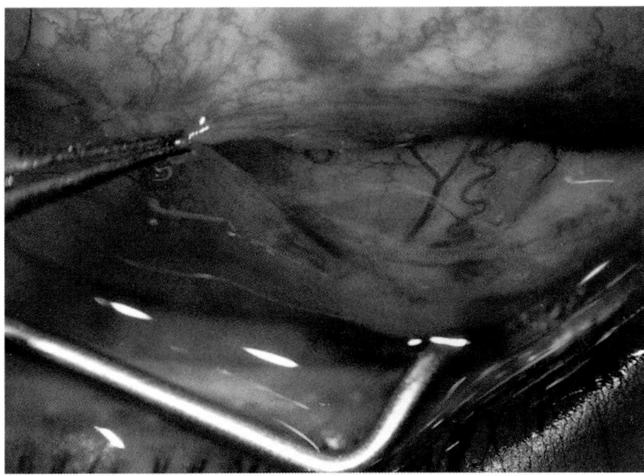

Figure 16.14 Closing the conjunctival wound
The conjunctival wound closure is facilitated by pulling up with the needle until the taut suture elevates the suture line at the point where the incision has been closed. A nontoothed forceps such as the Pierce–Hoskins is used to grasp both sides of the incision just anterior to the point where the taut suture is holding it up.

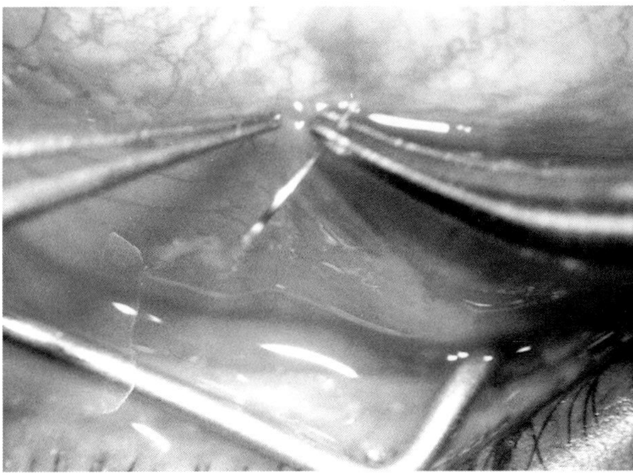

Figure 16.15 Closing the conjunctival wound
The suture tension is then relaxed and the needle passed under and just ahead of the forceps. The forceps are not released until the needle holder grabs the needle on the other side of the suture line and is ready to make the next pass.

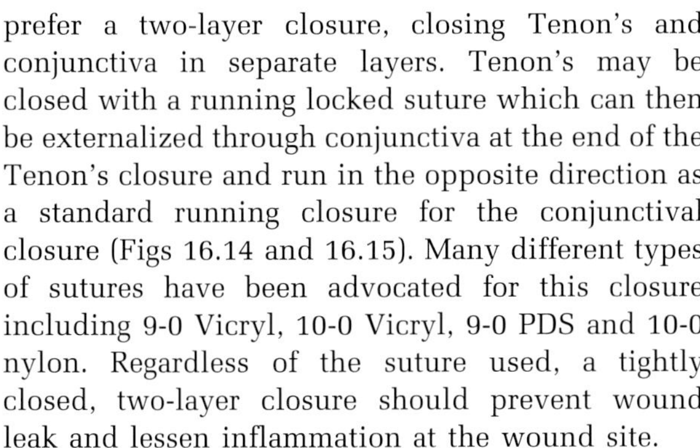

prefer a two-layer closure, closing Tenon's and conjunctiva in separate layers. Tenon's may be closed with a running locked suture which can then be externalized through conjunctiva at the end of the Tenon's closure and run in the opposite direction as a standard running closure for the conjunctival closure (Figs 16.14 and 16.15). Many different types of sutures have been advocated for this closure including 9-0 Vicryl, 10-0 Vicryl, 9-0 PDS and 10-0 nylon. Regardless of the suture used, a tightly closed, two-layer closure should prevent wound leak and lessen inflammation at the wound site.

Modifications

Releasable sutures

In cases in which the surgeon desires only minimal filtration initially, externalized releasable sutures should be considered. In these instances and perhaps when antimetabolites are used, the surgeon may plan on tightly closing the scleral flap initially with a more aggressive outflow produced later from removal of the releasable suture when it is determined that a more copious drainage is necessary and safe. This lessens the likelihood of early postoperative complications of overfiltration and flat chamber. Many surgeons also believe that removal of the externalized releasable suture is easier and safer than employing the analogous technique of postoperative laser suture lysis. The technique described below may be used with either limbus-based or fornix-based conjunctival flaps. The initial pass of the 10-0 nylon suture begins on the clear cornea side of the limbus no more than about 1 mm on to clear cornea (Fig. 16.16). The needle is passed about half thickness through cornea and sclera, exiting the sclera near the edge of the scleral flap (Fig. 16.17). The next pass is through the scleral flap into the edge of the scleral bed using the technique as described previously for routine scleral flap closure (Fig. 16.18). The final pass of the suture is done back-handed, simply reversing the initial pass of the suture, following a path roughly parallel to the initial suture pass, but far enough apart so that when the suture is eventu-

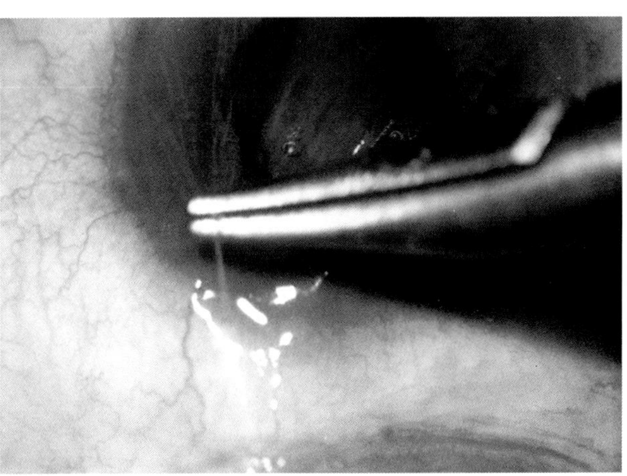

Figure 16.16 Releasable suture
This releasable suture starts in the cornea approximately 2 mm away from the trabeculectomy flap and 1 mm in front of the limbus.

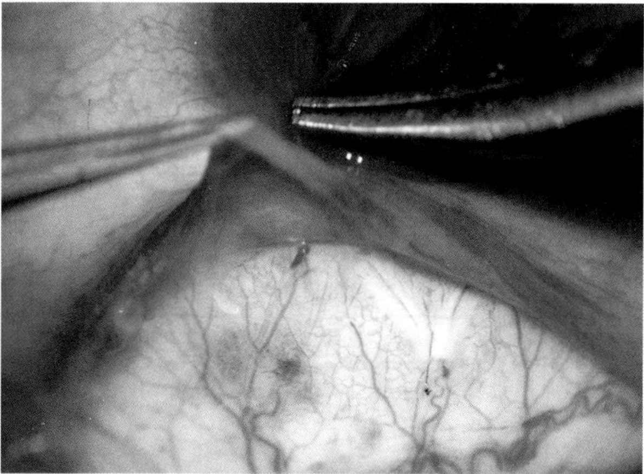

Figure 16.17 Releasable suture
The suture needle emerges on the other side of the limbus.

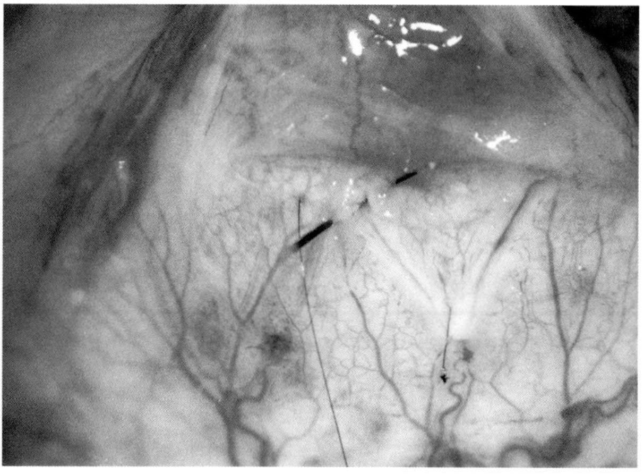

Figure 16.18 Releasable suture
A bite is taken in the trabeculectomy flap where the inner opening is closest to the edge of the flap.

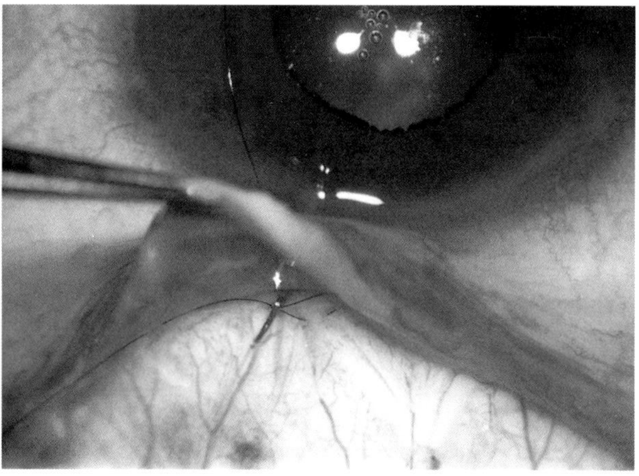

Figure 16.19 Releasable suture
The suture is then exteriorized under the limbus taking care to pass the suture away from the first suture pass to avoid touching or overlapping it. This is important so as not to restrict pulling the suture from the track when it is released.

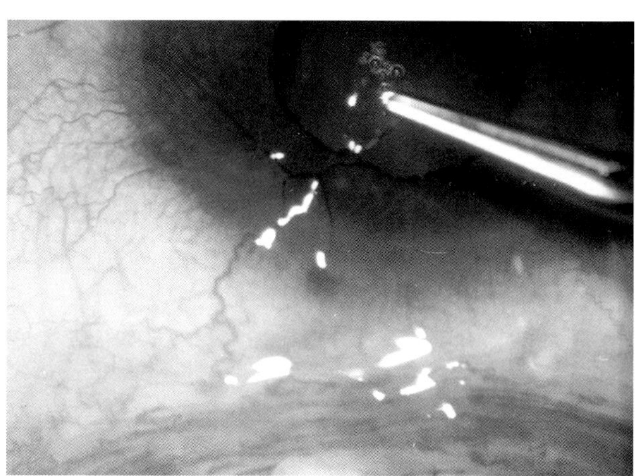

Figure 16.20 Completion of a releasable suture
The releasable suture is now tied with four throws on the first knot.

ally cut, there is enough suture exposed to be easily grasped (Fig. 16.19). The two ends of the suture which are now exposed on peripheral clear cornea are tied tightly and the ends are trimmed at the knot (Fig. 16.20). One or possibly two of this type of suture may be placed on either side of the flap. The suture may be released in the postoperative period when deemed appropriate by the surgeon. This is done at the slit lamp under topical anesthesia by simply cutting through the exposed suture with a sharp-point blade or Vannas scissors and removing it with a slow, steady pull.

Anterior chamber maintenance suture

In patients with a posterior chamber intraocular lens, the surgeon may wish to consider intraoperative placement of an anterior chamber maintenance suture in order to eliminate concern over postoperative flat chamber. This suture should be placed at the beginning of the procedure, before the eye is entered, when the eye is still firm and the anterior chamber is deep. A 9-0 nylon suture, double-armed with a straight needle, is passed from limbus to limbus to form a barrier to forward movement of the

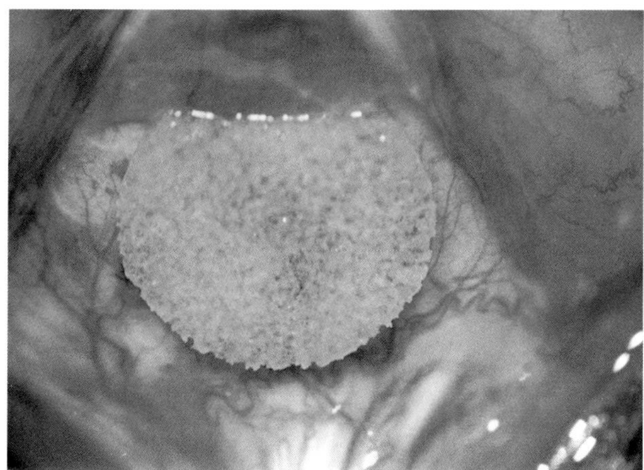

Figure 16.21 Application of mitomycin
The sponge supplied as a light shield also makes an excellent vehicle for the mitomycin soak, when it is trimmed to fit into the limbus.

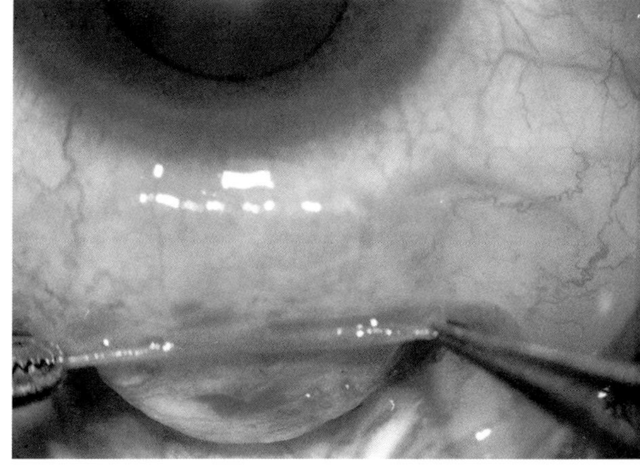

Figure 16.22 Mitomycin
The conjunctival–Tenon's flap is pulled posteriorly over the mitomycin-soaked sponge with the edge of the conjunctival incision reflected forward to eliminate any chance of contact with the sponge.

lens. The initial entry of the needle should be directed perpendicularly to the curve of the peripheral cornea just on the corneal side of the limbus. The entry point should be at the 8.30 o'clock position for a right-handed surgeon and the 3.30 o'clock position for a left-hand dominant surgeon so that the intraocular pass of the needle will be in a forehand fashion. The needle is then passed across the anterior chamber just above the iris and lens and is externalized just on the corneal side of the limbus. The other arm of the suture is passed with a similar course parallel to the initial pass with the entry site 2–3 mm superior to the initial suture pass, perhaps at about the 9.30 o'clock position for right-handed surgeons and the 2.30 o'clock position for left-handed surgeons. The two free ends are then tied tightly with four loops to prevent slippage of the knot. The suture must be cinched tight enough to deform the peripheral cornea slightly at the entry and exit sites of the suture. The suture is trimmed flush with the knot. The patient is kept on topical antibiotics postoperatively as long as this suture is in place. The suture may be removed at any time that the surgeon believes the risk of postoperative flat chamber has passed.

Antimetabolites

Certain patients have been shown to have a significantly decreased success rate with the basic trabeculectomy technique described above. The predominant risk factors for failure include neovascular glaucoma, aphakia and previous intraocular surgery with residual scar tissue remaining. Many other factors are also known to predispose patients to failure of filtration surgery. Over the last decade the antimetabolites 5-fluorouracil (5-FU) and mitomycin have been used to improve the success rate of filtering surgery in these patients. 5-FU is administered predominantly via postoperative subconjunctival injections, although it is also effective applied topically at the time of surgery. Mitomycin requires intraoperative application. There is no consensus among glaucoma surgeons as to the ideal method of intraoperative application. Differences of opinion exist as to the ideal vehicle for mitomycin application, the concentration of mitomycin to be used and the ideal application time. Regardless of the differing opinions over specific aspects of mitomycin usage, certain important principles will always apply. Whenever mitomycin is to be used, it must be applied prior to entry into the anterior chamber. If the surgeon prefers to place the mitomycin after dissection of the scleral flap, particular care must be taken not to enter the anterior chamber when extending the flap dissection anteriorly. Also, care must be taken to make certain that mitomycin does not come into contact with the edges of the conjunctival wound, especially if a fornix-based conjunctival flap has been dissected. When employing mitomycin with a fornix-based conjunctival approach, the surgeon must make certain that the limbal peritomy is broad enough and the dissection posteriorly enough to allow placement of the mitomycin sponge without contact to the wound edges. When using mitomycin the surgeon should adjust his or her basic filtration procedure in such a way as to decrease the amount of aqueous filtration obtained at the end of the case. This can be accomplished by modifications in dissection of the scleral flap, placement of the corneo-scleral filtration site and closure of the scleral flap as discussed in detail previously.

Mitomycin may be applied with a cellulose sponge which has been thinned to approximately half of its original thickness and approximately half of its original length. The sponge is saturated with mitomycin, placed over the site of the intended filtration site and conjunctiva is draped carefully over the sponge (Figs 16.21 and 16.22). We recommend a limbal-based conjunctival flap when using mitomycin, using a concentration of mitomycin of 0.4 mg/cc with an application time of 1–4 minutes. The length of application is individualized for each patient depending on the characteristics of the patient, the type of glaucoma and the health of the ocular tissues at the surgery site. The sponge is then removed from the field and the area of application is vigorously irrigated with approximately 1–15 cc of balanced saline solution. With this technique, the mitomycin is applied prior to dissection of the scleral flap to eliminate any chance of entering the anterior chamber prior to the mitomycin application and to lessen the likelihood of prolonged hypotony which may occur if mitomycin placement underneath the scleral flap results in complete ischemia with no healing at all in the bed of the flap.

Summary

In many patients, glaucoma filtration surgery can halt or at least retard what would otherwise be relentlessly progressive vision loss from glaucoma. Filtration surgery requires diligent attention to details of performance. The planned approach and intraoperative execution of the procedure must be individualized for each patient in order to maximize the likelihood of the desired result of glaucoma filtration surgery: preserved vision and preserved quality of life.

FURTHER READING

Allen RC, Bellows AR, Hutchinson TST, Murphy SD, Filtration surgery in the treatment of neovascular glaucoma, *Ophthalmology* (1982) **89**:1181–87.

Bellows AR, Johnston MA, Surgical management of chronic glaucoma in aphakia, *Ophthalmology* (1983) **90**:807–13.

Cairns JE, Trabeculectomy—preliminary report of a new method, *Am J Ophthalmol* (1968) **66**:673–79.

Chen CW, Huang HT, Barr JS, Lee CC, Trabeculectomy with simultaneous topical application of mitomycin-C in refractory glaucoma. *J Oc Pharmacol* (1990) **6**:175–82.

Heuer DK, Gressel MG, Parrish RK, Trabeculectomy in aphakic eyes, *Ophthalmology* (1984) **91**:1045–51.

Heuer DK, Parrish RK, Gressel MG, Hodapp E, Palmberg PF, 5-fluorouracil and glaucoma filtering surgery. III. Intermediate follow-up of a pilot study, *Ophthalmology* (1986) **93**:1537–46.

Heuer DK, Parrish RK, Gressel MG, Hodapp E, Palmberg PF, Anderson DR, 6-fluorouracil and glaucoma filtering surgery. II. A pilot study, *Ophthalmology* (1984) **91**:384–94.

Inaba Z, Long-term results of trabeculectomy on the Japanese: an analysis by life-table method, *Jpn J Ophthalmol* (1982) **26**:361–73.

Katz LJ, Spaeth GL, Filtration surgery. In: Ritch R, Shield MB, Krupin T, eds. *The glaucomas* (1989), 653–96.

Kimbrough RL, Stewart RM, Decker WL, Praeger TL, Trabeculectomy: square or triangular scleral flap, *Ophthalmic Surg* (1982) **13**:753.

Kronfeld P, The rise of the filter operations, *Surv Ophthalmol* (1972) **17**:168–79.

Liss RP, Scholes GN, Crandall AS, Glaucoma filtration surgery: new horizontal mattress closure of conjunctival incision, *Ophthal Surg* (1991) **22**:298–300.

Luntz M, Freedman J, Fornix-based conjunctival flap in glaucoma filtration surgery, *Ophthal Surg* (1980) **11**:516–21.

Palmer SS, Mitomycin as adjunct chemotherapy with trabeculectomy, *Ophthalmology* (1991) **98**:317–21.

Quigley HA, Slipknots for trabeculectomy flap closure, *Ophthal Surg* (1985) **16**:56–58.

Reichert R, Stewart W, Shields MB, Limbus-based vs fornix-based conjunctival flaps in trabeculectomy, *Ophthal Surg* (1987) **18**:672–76.

Schwartz AL, Anderson DR, Trabecular surgery, *Arch Ophthalmol* (1974) **92**:134–38.

Shuster JN, Krupin T, Kolker AE, et al., Limbus-based vs fornix-based conjunctival flaps in trabeculectomy, *Arch Ophthalmol* (1984) **102**:361–62.

Singh G, Effect of size of trabeculectomy on intraocular pressure, *Glaucoma* (1983) **5**:192–96.

Starita RJ, Fellman RL, Spaeth GL, Poryzees EM, Effect of varying size of scleral flap and corneal block on trabeculectomy, *Ophthal Surg* (1984) **15**:454–57.

Traverso CE, Tomey KF, Antonios S, Limbal- vs. fornix-based conjunctival trabeculectomy flaps, *Am J Ophthalmol* (1987) **104**:28–32.

Wilson RP, Moster MR, The chamber-retaining suture revisited, *Ophthal Surg* (1990) **21**:625–27.

17 Aqueous shunts

Anne L Coleman

Introduction

Aqueous shunts are drainage devices designed to lower intraocular pressure by draining aqueous humor from the interior of the eye to an encapsulated reservoir near the equator of the globe. In general, aqueous shunts have been used in eyes with poor surgical prognoses as listed in Table 17.1. The devices generally consist of a plastic plate (or plates) and a silicone or silastic tube; the tube not only serves as the means of egress of aqueous from the eye but also acts as a seton, preventing the opening into the eye from closing. Although there have been several devices used to help keep an opening in the eye patent, Anthony Molteno was the first to design an implant that helped with the formation of a posterior episcleral filtering bleb.

Most aqueous shunts have a similar design. There is a silicone or silastic tube which is placed into the eye and through which aqueous humor passes into the episcleral-subconjunctival space. In this area there is an episcleral plate that is designed to help with the formation of a filtering bleb. There are three key design features which distinguish different implants: the presence of a valve or mechanism to restrict the flow of aqueous humor from the eye, the surface area of the episcleral plate, and the material used. The reaction of the surrounding tissue to the material is a source of concern. Research is ongoing into whether these factors are important in the short- and/or long-term success of aqueous shunts.

Table 17.1 **Clinical indications for aqueous shunts**

1) Prior failed glaucoma filtering surgery
2) Aphakic/pseudophakic glaucoma
3) Neovascular glaucoma
4) Uveitic glaucoma
5) Congenital glaucoma
6) Prior penetrating keratoplasty
7) Angle-closure glaucoma
8) Epithelial downgrowth

The restriction of flow of aqueous humor from the eye is important in the prevention of immediate postoperative hypotony and its attendant complications. The implants that do not have such a mechanism (Molteno, Baerveldt and Schocket band implants) are usually inserted in a two-stage procedure or the flow of aqueous is restricted by a suture ligature around the tube or an internal stent. Several aqueous shunts, specifically the Krupin Long Valve implant, Joseph implant, White pump-shunt, Optimed Glaucoma Pressure Regulator and Ahmed Glaucoma Valve implant, have pressure-sensitive valves or internal mechanisms to restrict the flow of aqueous from the eye. These aqueous shunts prevent bidirectional flow of fluid, with the goal being to prevent ocular hypotony in the immediate postoperative period. Prata and coauthors reported that the Ahmed and Krupin implants function as flow-restricting devices at flow rates of 2–2.5 μl/min. In in vitro tests with human plasma, the Ahmed and Krupin implants had greater resistance (change in pressure/change in flow) than partially ligated Baerveldt implants.

The surface area of the episcleral plate may influence the amount of intraocular pressure reduction because of its effect on the size of the filtering bleb. In animal eyes with Molteno implants, Minckler and coauthors found that the pressure within the filtration bleb surrounding the episcleral plate is similar to the pressure in the anterior chamber. Since the main resistance to aqueous flow and pressure reduction is the capsular wall surrounding the episcleral plate, a potential advantage of a large filtration bleb is a larger surface area for diffusion. Heuer and coauthors have reported that there is a greater reduction in intraocular pressure in eyes with the double-plate Molteno implant compared to the single-plate

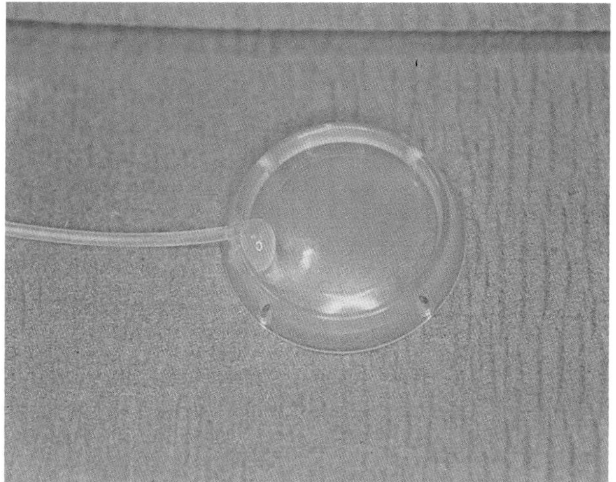

Figure 17.1 The Molteno implant
This has a surface area of 134 mm².

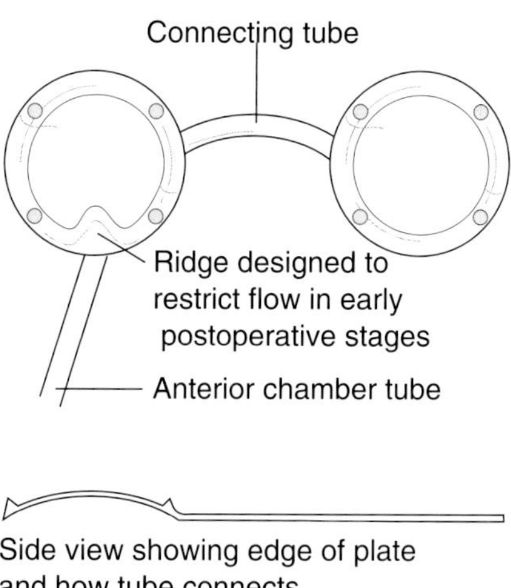

Figure 17.2 The double-plate Molteno implant
The double-plate Molteno implant has a surface area of 268 mm². The pressure ridge increases the resistance of aqueous flow from the eye during the first postoperative week.

Molteno implant, and Mills and coauthors found two-year success rates of 67% and 85% for single and double-plate Molteno implants, respectively. Although Lloyd and coauthors reported the percentage decrease in intraocular pressure to be similar for the Baerveldt 500 mm² and 350 mm² implants, eyes with the larger implant did require an average of 0.6 fewer medications postoperatively. Thus, a larger surface area may be beneficial in terms of intraocular pressure reduction. Whether better intraocular pressure reduction is associated with more postoperative complications is not clear. Heuer and coauthors reported that double-plate Molteno implants are associated with more complications than single-plate implants, while Lloyd and coauthors did not find a statistically significant difference in the number of complications between 350 mm² and 500 mm² Baerveldt implants.

Even though aqueous shunts are made of relatively nonreactive substances such as polypropylene, silicone, silastic and polymethyl methacrylate, they stimulate the formation of a collagenous and fibrovascular capsule around the episcleral plate. Histopathologically, this capsular wall has been described as a collagenous meshwork that progressively becomes more dense from inside to out. The thickness of this capsule is important in the resistance of aqueous flow from the episcleral plate to the surrounding vasculature. Currently, investigators are attempting to modify the surface of the episcleral plate to help prevent the formation of a thick capsule, but no studies have been published to date on the effects of such modifications in humans.

Types of aqueous shunts

Nonvalved aqueous shunts

Single-plate and double-plate Molteno implants

Single-plate Molteno implants (IOP Inc., Costa Mesa, CA) consist of a circular, polypropylene episcleral plate and a silicone tube (Fig. 17.1). The tube opens on to the surface of the convex, episcleral plate, and its inner diameter is 0.3 mm. The plate's diameter is 13 mm. One side of the single-plate Molteno implant has a surface area of 134 mm². Double-plate Molteno implants consist of a single-plate Molteno implant connected with a 10 mm long silicone tube to another circular episcleral plate (Fig. 17.2). The surface area of 268 mm² is twice that of the single-plate Molteno implant, and the plates are positioned on both sides of a rectus muscle. Right and left-eyed double-plate Molteno implants are available. Dual-chamber Molteno implants are single and double-plate Molteno implants that are modified with a pressure ridge. This ridge increases the resistance of aqueous flow from the eye in the immediate postoperative period by enabling swollen Tenon's tissue to create a temporary seal over the implant.

Baerveldt implant

The Baerveldt implant (Iovision, Irvine, CA) consists of a silicone tube and episcleral plate. The plate is currently available in three sizes: 250, 350 and 450 mm² (Fig. 17.3). The internal diameter of the tube is 0.3 mm. When implanted, the plate is placed

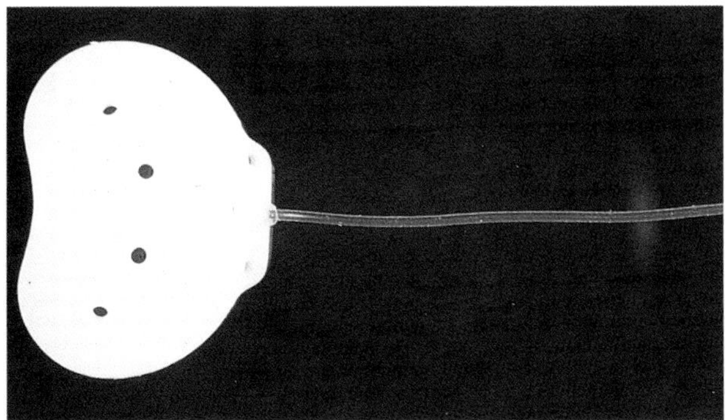

Figure 17.3 The Baerveldt implant
The Baerveldt implant has fenestrations or holes that help limit the size of the bleb and theoretically help prevent motility disturbances.

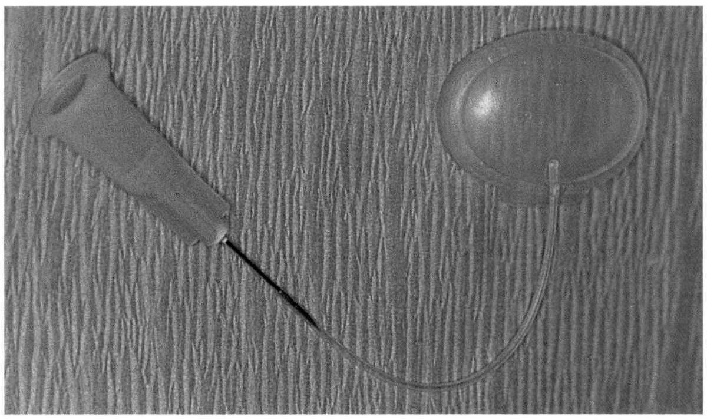

Figure 17.4 The Krupin Long Valve disc implant
The Krupin Long Valve disc implant has a surface area of 183 mm² and a slit valve.

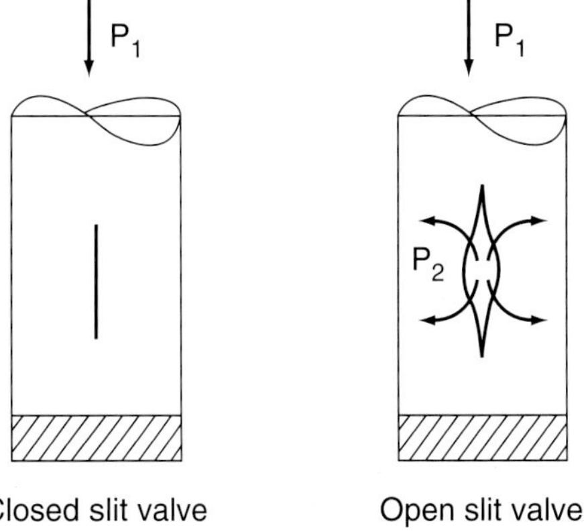

Figure 17.5 Function of a slit valve
The slit valve opens when the pressure in the eye and tube (P_1) is greater than the pressure outside the eye and tube (P_2). The Krupin Long Valve disc implant has a theoretical opening pressure between 10 and 12 mmHg and a closing pressure between 8 and 10 mmHg.

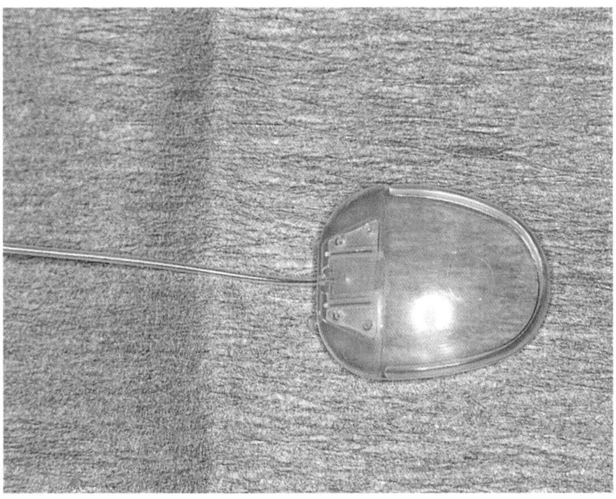

Figure 17.6 The Ahmed Glaucoma Valve
The Ahmed Glaucoma Valve implant has a surface area of 185 mm² and a unidirectional valve.

underneath two adjacent rectus muscles. Fenestration holes have been added to the plates to help limit the height of the blebs by the growth of fibrovascular tissue through these holes.

Valved implants

Krupin Long Valve disc implant

The Krupin Long Valve disc implant (Hood Laboratories, Pembroke, MA) consists of a silastic tube and disc (Fig. 17.4). The valve mechanism consists of horizontal and vertical slits in the distal end of the silastic tube. The slits are designed to open at a pressure of 11 mmHg and close at a pressure of 9 mmHg (Fig. 17.5). A silastic tube is attached to the convex, anterior surface of a silastic disc. The disc is oval, measures 13 mm posteriorly and 18 mm horizontally, and has a surface area of 183 mm².

Ahmed Glaucoma Valve implant

The Ahmed Glaucoma Valve (New World Medical Inc., Rancho Cucamonga, CA) has a silicone tube, silicone elastomer membrane and polypropylene episcleral plate (Fig. 17.6). The valve-like mechanism consists of a silicone membrane which is 8 mm long and 7 mm wide. This membrane is folded over on itself and is then stretched so that there is enough tension to restrict aqueous flow through the tube. The

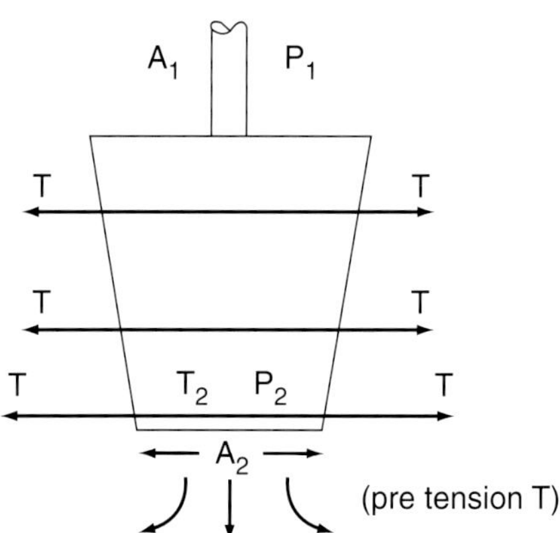

Figure 17.7 Function of the Ahmed Glaucoma Valve
The valve-like mechanism of the Ahmed Glaucoma Valve implant consists of silicone membrane folded over on itself and placed on stretch so that there is tension across the membrane (T). The tension on the membrane has been adjusted so that the opening pressure is 8–10 mmHg. The membrane is shaped so that it has a larger area at the entrance of the tube (inlet or A_1) and a smaller area where the fluid exits (outlet or A_2). Because of this venturi-shaped chamber, a smaller pressure differential than in slit valves is needed between inside (P_1) and outside (P_2) the eye for fluid to leave the eye. When P_1–P_2 is greater than T, the membranes open and aqueous flows through the valve.

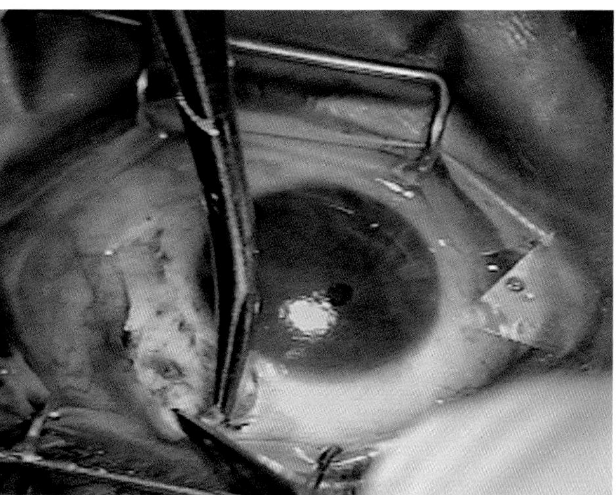

Figure 17.8 Peritomy
A fornix-based conjunctival flap is created with scissors and radialized towards the fornix at each end to permit adequate exposure posteriorly for securing the plate to the sclera.

shape of the membrane is such that the cross-section of the membrane at the entrance of the tube is wider than the cross-section of the membrane at the outlet. Bernoulli's principle suggests that this venturi-shaped chamber should help with the flow of aqueous from the eye (Fig. 17.7). The opening pressure of the Ahmed Glaucoma Valve implant is theoretically 8 mmHg. The inner diameter of the tube is 0.3 mm, and the plate has a surface area of 185 mm^2. The plate is shaped similar to a horseshoe crab and measures 16 mm posteriorly and 13 mm horizontally.

Results obtained with the various devices are summarized in Table 17.2.

Surgical techniques

One-stage surgical implantation

Conjunctival incision and scleral exposure

A limbus-based or fornix-based conjunctival incision is made (Fig. 17.8) after the placement of a traction suture through the peripheral cornea or under a rectus muscle. The length of the conjunctival incision depends on the implant to be inserted. The double-plate Molteno implant requires exposure of two quadrants while the single-plate Molteno, Baerveldt, Krupin and Ahmed implants require exposure of one quadrant. The identification of the rectus muscles in a quadrant helps with the insertion of Baerveldt and Krupin Long Valve disc implants. The sclera in the quadrant is exposed by dissection in the sub-Tenon's space so that the implant can be placed posterior to the insertions of the rectus muscles. The episcleral vessels are cauterized as needed.

Preparation of implant

The implant may be soaked in an antibiotic solution prior to implantation. The tube should then be irrigated with balanced saline solution prior to placement of the episcleral plate 8–10 mm beyond the posterior surgical limbus (Fig. 17.9a). The irrigation of the tube is important with the Molteno, Baerveldt and Krupin implants in order to check the patency of the tube. The irrigation of the tube in the Ahmed Glaucoma Valve implant not only checks patency but also helps to break the capillary attraction of the silicone membranes so that the valve-like mechanism can function (Fig. 17.9b).

Placement of implant (Fig. 17.10)

The episcleral plate should be secured 8–10 mm beyond the posterior surgical limbus with nonabsorbable sutures (5-0 to 9-0 Supramid, nylon or mersilene). The holes present on the anterior edge

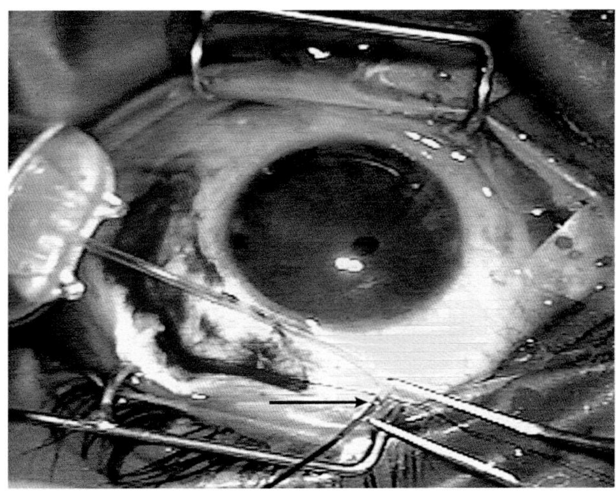

(a)

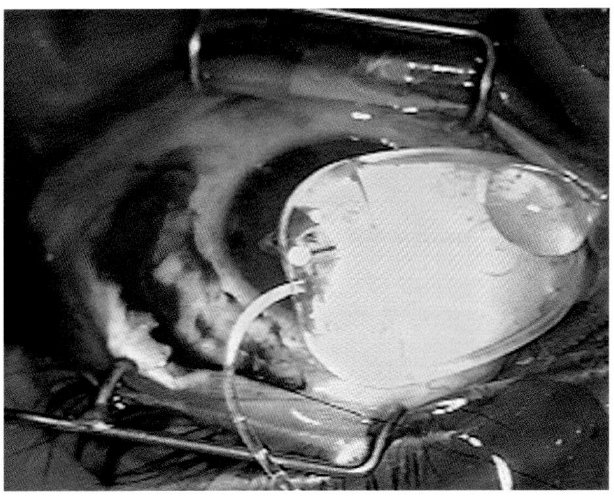

(b)

Figure 17.9 Preparation of the Ahmed Glaucoma Valve implant
It is essential to flush the device prior to implantation. This is done with a 27 gauge cannula. (a) The arrow points to the cannula in the end of the tube. (b) Irrigation of fluid through the cannula.

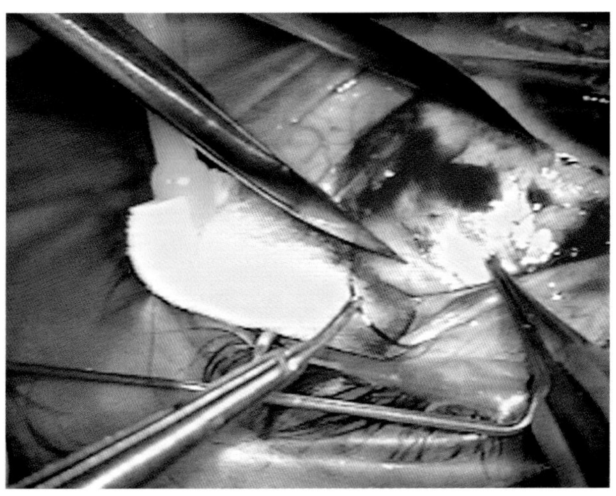

(a)

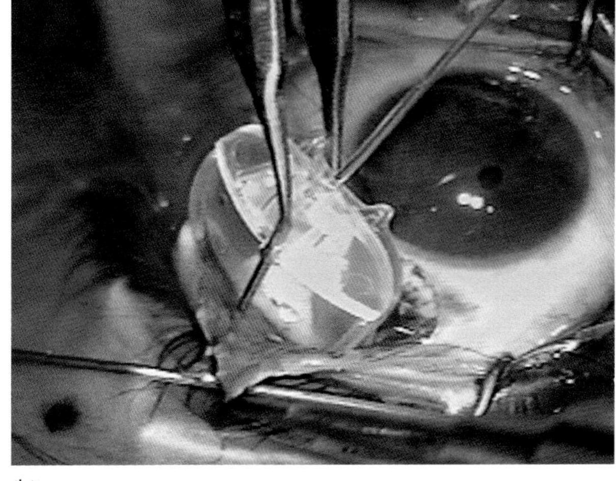

(b)

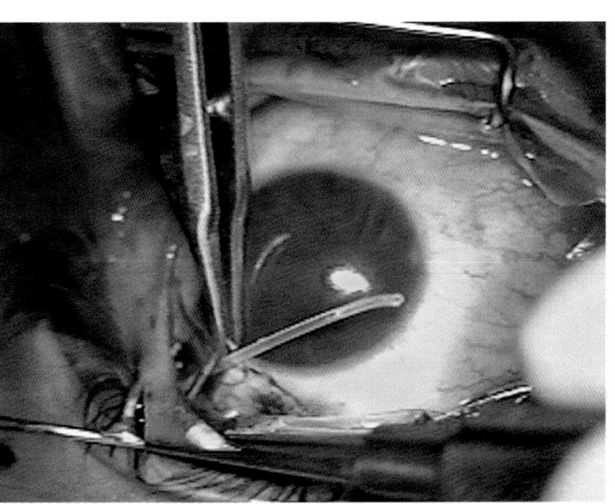

(c)

Figure 17.10 Insertion of the plate
(a) A caliper is used to measure 10 mm from the limbus. The suture used to secure the plate may be preplaced at the 10 mm mark; in this case one needle of a double-armed 9-0 nylon suture is placed through half-thickness sclera in the midportion of the quadrant. (b) The insertion is started, using a smooth forceps to grasp the device. (c) The plate easily slips into the prepared sub-Tenon's pocket.

Table 17.2 **Cumulative probability of success of different types of aqueous shunts**

Study	Type of shunt	Number of eyes (patients)	Diagnoses (no. of eyes)	Follow-up time (mean ± SD), months	Cumulative probability of success/time	Definition of success
Lloyd, Sedlak et al., 1994	Molteno single-plate	96 (96)	Aphakia/IOL (50) Failed filter (12) NVG (18) <13 yrs old (16)	47.4 ± 18.2 59.8 ± 6.6 33.8 ± 24.7 65.7 ± 8.4	74%/2 years 58%/2 years 57%/2 years 68%/2 years	1) IOP ≤ 21 and > 5 mmHg with or without meds 2) No further glaucoma surgery 3) No devastating complications 4) No loss of light perception
Mermound et al., 1993	Molteno single-plate	60 (54)	NVG (60)	24.7 ± 9.4	53%/2 years	1) IOP ≤ 21 mmHg with or without meds 2) No further glaucoma surgery 3) No development of phthisis bulbi 4) No loss of light perception
Hill et al., 1993	Molteno single-plate or double-plate in one-stage implantation	10 (10)	Uveitic glaucoma	28 ± 17	79%/2 years	1) IOP ≤ 21 and > 5 mmHg with or without meds 2) No further glaucoma surgery 3) No development of phthisis bulbi 4) No loss of light perception
Mills et al., 1996	Molteno single or double-plate	77 (71)	Aphakic/IOL (24) NVG (20) Uveitic (12) Failed filter (9) Traumatic (8) Congenital (4)	median 44 months (range 6–107)	54%/5 years	1) IOP < 22 mmHg with or without meds 2) No further glaucoma surgery 3) No devastating complications 4) No loss of light perception
Heuer et al., 1992	Molteno single-plate	37 (37)	OAG (15) ACG (21) Uveitic (5) Congenital (4) Traumatic (4) Uncertain (1)	14.9 ± 68.9	46%/2 years	1) IOP ≤ 21 and ≥ 6 mmHg with or without meds 2) No further glaucoma surgery 3) No devastating complications
Heuer et al., 1992	Molteno double-plate	38 (38)	OAG (18) ACG (17) Uveitic (8) Congenital (4) Traumatic (3) Uncertain (1)	16.4 ± 6.8	71%/2 years	1) IOP ≤ 21 and ≥ 6 mmHg with or without meds 2) No further glaucoma surgery 3) No devastating complications

Lloyd, Baerveldt, Heuer et al., 1994	Baerveldt implant (200 or 350 mm^2)	13 (13)	Aphakic/IOL (10)	16.2 ± 7.6	67%/18 months	1) IOP ≤ 21 and ≥ 6 mmHg with or without meds 2) No further glaucoma surgery 3) No devastating complications 4) No loss of light perception
Lloyd, Baerveldt, Fellenbaum et al., 1994	Baerveldt implant (350 mm^2)	37 (37)	Aphakic/IOL (33) Failed filter (4)	15.5 ± 4.8	93%/18 months	1) IOP ≤ 21 and ≥ 6 mmHg with or without meds 2) No further glaucoma surgery 3) No devastating complications 4) No loss of light perception
Lloyd, Baerveldt, Fellenbaum et al., 1994	Baerveldt implant (500 mm^2)	36 (36)	Aphakic/IOL (31) Failed filter (5)	14.1 ± 5.4	88%/18 months	1) IOP ≤ 21 and ≥ 6 mmHg with or without meds 2) No further glaucoma surgery 3) No devastating complications 4) No loss of light perception
Siegner et al., 1995	Baerveldt implant (200, 250, 350 or 500 mm^2)	103 (100)	NVG (34) Congenital (15) Uveitic (11) OAG (16) ACG (7) PKP (9) Traumatic (7) CMG (4)	13.6 ± 0.9	60.3/2 years	1) IOP ≤ 21 and ≥ 5 mmHg with or without meds 2) No further glaucoma surgery 3) No loss of light perception
Hodkin et al., 1995	Baerveldt implant (350 mm^2)	50 (50)	Aphakic/IOL (35) Failed filter (12) NVG (7) Age < 13 years (3) PKP (13) Phakic (5)	13.7 ± 19.2	70%/18 months	1) IOP ≤ 21 mmHg with or without meds 2) No further glaucoma surgery 3) No development of phthisis bulbi 4) No loss of light perception
Fellenbaum et al., 1994	Krupin eye valve with disk	25 (25)	OAG (11) ACG (7) NVG (3) CMG (2) ICE (2)	13.2, range 4–19	66%/1 year	1) IOP < 22 and > 5 mmHg with or without meds 2) No further glaucoma surgery 3) No devastating complications
Coleman et al., 1995	Ahmed Glaucoma Valve	60 (60)	OAG (18) PKP (16) NVG (14) Congenital (6) Uveitic (5) ACG (1)	median 9.3, range 3–22	78%/1 year	1) IOP < 22 and > 4 mmHg with or without meds 2) less than 20% reduction in IOP from preop value if preop IOP < 22 mmHg 3) No further glaucoma surgery 4) No devastating visual complications

Notes:
IOL = intraocular lens, NVG = neovascular glaucoma, OAG = open-angle glaucoma, ACG = angle-closure glaucoma, PKP = penetrating keratoplasty, CMG = chronic mixed glaucoma, ICE = iridocorneal endothelial syndrome.

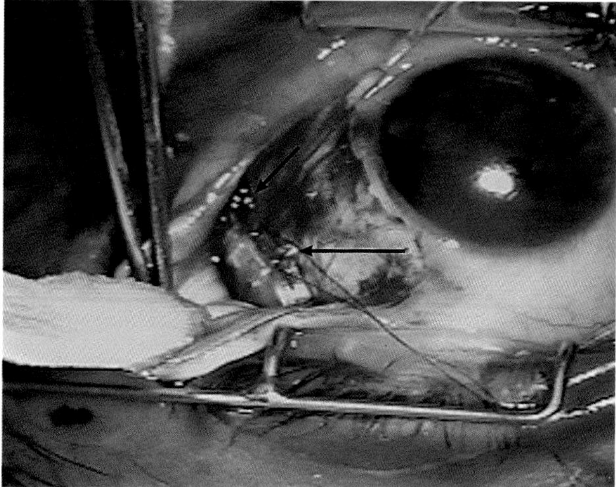

Figure 17.11 Fixating the implant to the sclera
The fixation holes (arrows) of the Ahmed Glaucoma Valve implant are used to fixate the implant to the sclera. In this case, each needle of the double-armed 9-0 nylon suture has been passed through one of the fixation holes and the two ends tied together to secure the plate. Some surgeons will place an interrupted suture through each hole.

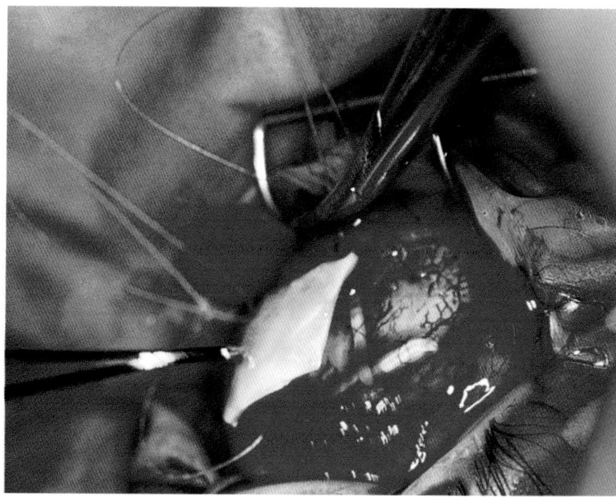

Figure 17.12 The Krupin Long Valve implant
This has a silastic ridge through which sutures may be passed (arrow).

of Molteno, Baerveldt and Ahmed implants are used to help fixate the implant (Fig. 17.11). The Krupin disc has a silastic ridge through which a needle can pass with ease (Fig. 17.12). The double-plate Molteno implant is placed so that a plate is on either side of a rectus muscle. The connecting silicone tube may be placed over or under the rectus muscle.

Methods to restrict the flow of aqueous humor through the tube in implants without an internal mechanism

Many investigators have reported on methods to restrict the flow of aqueous through the tube when Molteno or Baerveldt implants are placed in a one-stage procedure. These methods include the use of an external suture ligature, an internal stent, or both. When a vicryl, chromic, nylon or silk suture is tied around the tube posterior to the scleral flap or donor graft, it can be cut with a laser or with scissors through a conjunctival incision if it does not dissolve or is not releasable. Another method is to occlude the proximal end of the tube with a polypropylene or nylon suture. This end of the tube is then inserted into the anterior chamber and may be lysed with a laser in the immediate postoperative period (Fig. 17.13). A chromic, 5.0 nylon or 3.0 supramid suture can be threaded first through the tube and then through the episcleral plate where its distal end can be placed subconjunctivally either over the plate or 90–180 degrees away from the tube. This suture can then be removed in the immediate postoperative period as needed. Sherwood and coauthors reported on the placement of vertical slits in the tube anterior to an absorbable external suture ligature. These slits help prevent the intraocular pressure from being too high in the immediate postoperative period while the fibrotic capsule forms around the episcleral plate. Despite the restriction of flow through tubes with these methods, problems with ocular hypotony may occur.

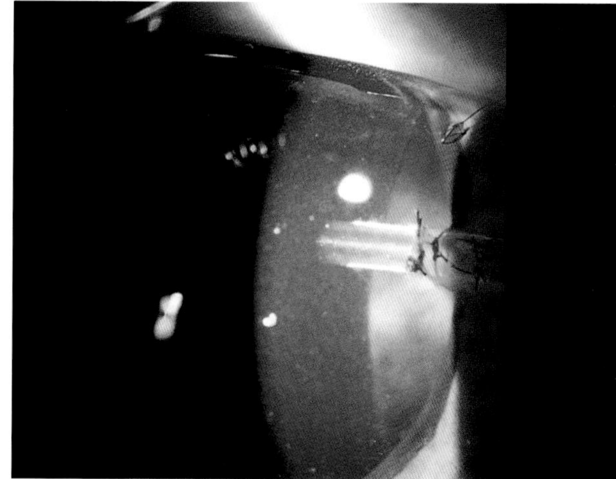

Figure 17.13 Occluding the proximal end of the tube
A suture is tied around the proximal end of a Molteno tube and is then inserted into the anterior chamber. This suture may be lysed with an argon laser during the postoperative period. (Courtesy of Jeffrey Liebmann, MD.)

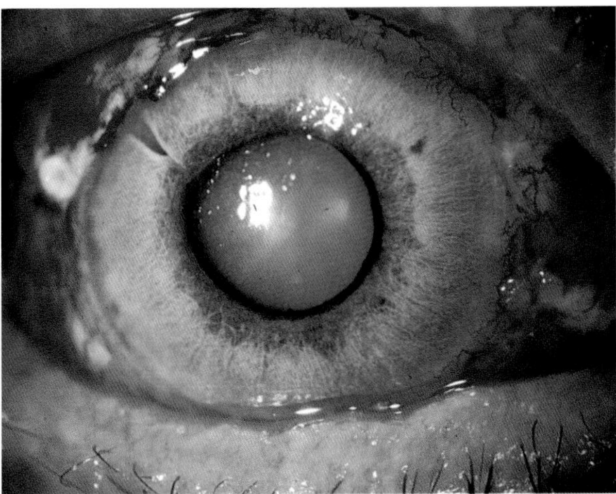

Figure 17.20 A flat anterior chamber secondary to malignant glaucoma
This patient has a flat anterior chamber secondary to malignant glaucoma. The tube is occluded by the surrounding iris.

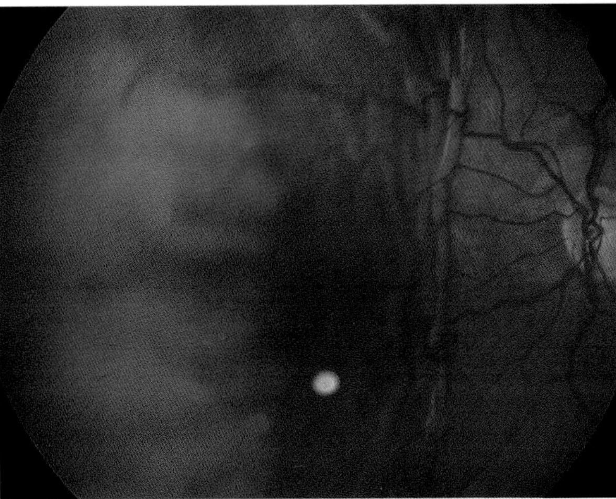

Figure 17.21 A resolving serous choroidal detachment
After the placement of a drainage device, this patient has a serous choroidal detachment that is resolving.

Complications

The complications associated with aqueous shunts can be categorized as those associated with the reduction of intraocular pressure, with the functioning and placement of the tube, with the episcleral plate and the response of surrounding tissues to it, and with intraocular surgery *per se*.

Complications associated with reduction of intraocular pressure

Flat anterior chamber

Flat anterior chamber has been reported following insertion of valved and nonvalved aqueous shunts (Fig. 17.20). When single-plate Molteno implants without modifications to restrict aqueous flow were inserted into 30 eyes in a one-stage procedure, seven (23%) of the eyes had flat anterior chambers the first postoperative week. Even when Molteno and Baerveldt implants have the placement of stents in the tube or external ligation with a suture, there are still cases of flat anterior chambers postoperatively, reported in up to 30% of cases. The incorporation of a valve into the shunt design reduces the risk of flat anterior chamber. Flat anterior chambers may require reformation of the anterior chamber with saline, viscoelastics or gas after the determination and management of their etiology, e.g. wound leak, overfiltration, pupillary block, etc.

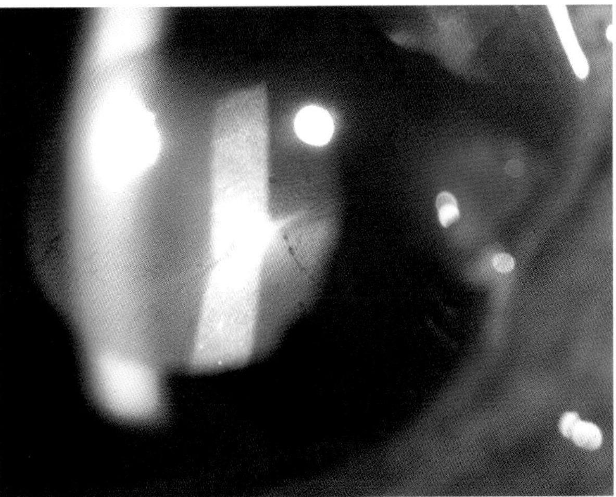

Figure 17.22 Kissing choroidal detachments
This patient with glaucoma due to the Sturge–Weber syndrome has kissing choroidal detachments that required surgical drainage. (Courtesy of Neil Choplin, MD.)

Serous choroidal effusions

Serous choroidal effusions occur in up to 32% of eyes following shunt placement (Figs 17.21 and 17.22). The presence of a valve in the device does not alter the risk of choroidal effusion, and most are probably due to ocular decompression. Drainage of the choroidal effusion may be necessary.

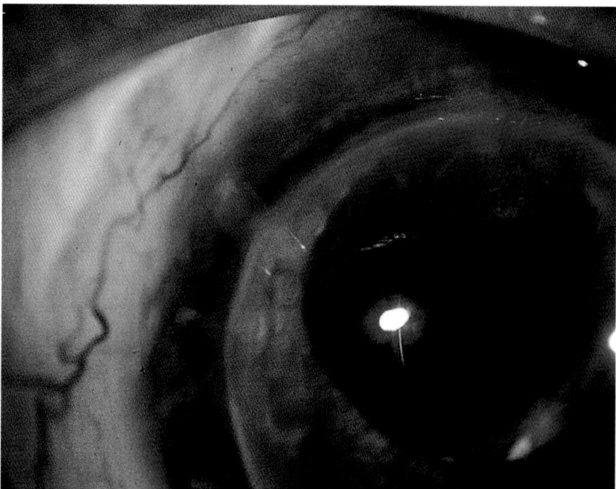

Figure 17.23 Blockage of drainage tube by vitreous
This tube was blocked by a strand of vitreous following a Nd:YAG capsulotomy (see also Fig. 15.47).

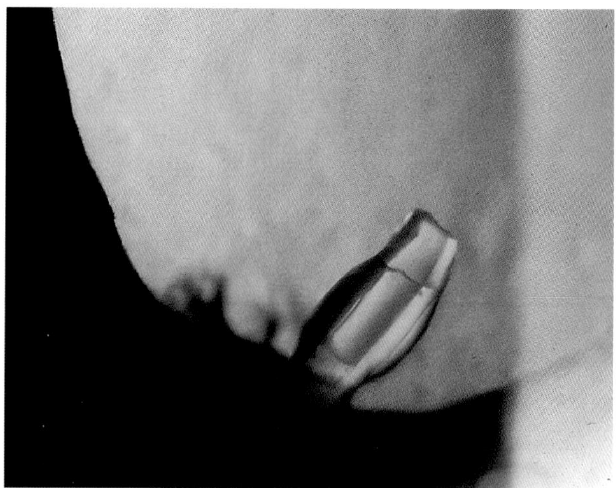

Figure 17.24 A tube blocked by silicone oil
This tube was blocked by silicone oil that entered the tube despite the placement of the tube and implant inferiorly.

Suprachoroidal hemorrhage
Suprachoroidal hemorrhage can be a devastating complication that can occur in eyes after the reduction of intraocular pressure. The presence of a device to restrict the flow of aqueous from the eye does not eliminate the risk of suprachoroidal hemorrhage in eyes that are predisposed to develop them.

Ocular hypotony
Despite restriction of aqueous flow with stents, external ligatures or internal devices, ocular hypotony may still occur following placement of Molteno, Baerveldt, Ahmed and Krupin implants. This ocular hypotony may occur because of inadequate restriction of the flow of aqueous, the leakage of aqueous around the tube or the decreased production of aqueous humor by the ciliary body.

Phthisis bulbi
The risk of phthisis bulbi ranges from 2% up to 18% following shunt placement, with neovascular glaucoma having a greater risk.

Complications associated with the functioning and placement of the tube

Tube blockage
The obstruction of tubes (Figs 17.23 and 17.24) by vitreous, fibrin, blood, inflammatory debris, silicone oil or iris has occurred in up to 20% of eyes with an aqueous shunt. The blockage of tubes seems to occur as frequently with nonvalved implants as with valved implants. The Nd:YAG laser may be used to open a tube blocked with fibrin, blood, inflammatory debris, iris or a vitreous strand. In addition, the tube may be irrigated intracamerally or may be removed from the eye prior to its being flushed.

Tube retraction or malposition
Tubes have retracted or have needed to be repositioned in up to 7% of eyes with an aqueous shunt. Tubes may retract as intraocular pressure rises following recovery from surgery, and the decompressed eye fills. Tubes which are too long (Fig. 17.25) may cause symptoms.

Tube erosion
Erosion of the tube through the conjunctiva (Figs 17.26 and 17.27) or cornea may occur in up to 5% of eyes, despite the placement of a patch graft. Treatment of tube erosion through the conjunctiva includes regrafting with a donor material while erosion through the cornea may require local corneal grafting. Foreign material such as tube shunts should not be left uncovered and exposed due to the risk of infection.

Tube–lens touch
Intermittent or persistent tube–lens touch (Fig. 17.28) may be associated with the formation of a cataract in phakic eyes. The incidence of cataract may be as high as 25% even in the absence of lens–tube touch.

Tube–corneal touch
Despite careful positioning of the tube, as many as 10% of eyes may have tube–corneal touch post-

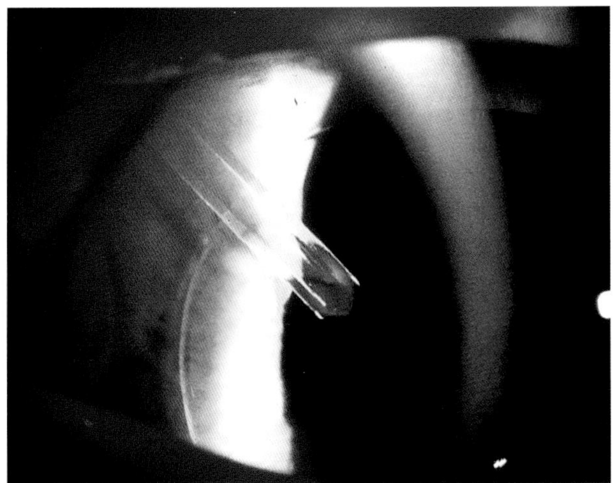

Figure 17.25 Tube too long
This tube, which is anterior to an anterior chamber intraocular lens and extends beyond the pupillary margin, is too long, since it is in the pupillary space and may cause glare or visual disturbances.

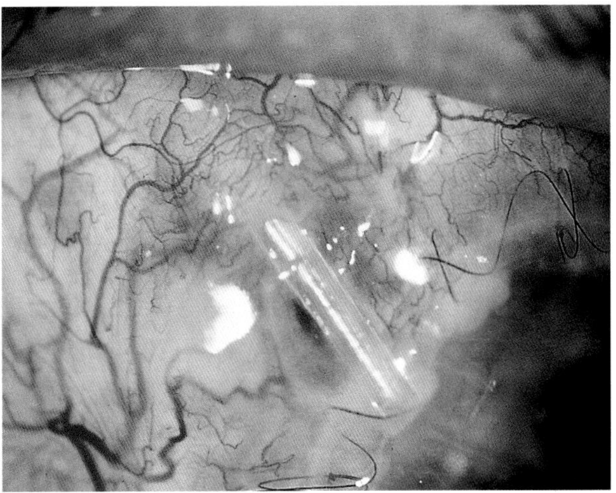

Figure 17.26 Tube erosion
This tube has eroded through the patch graft. It was repaired with a corneal patch graft.

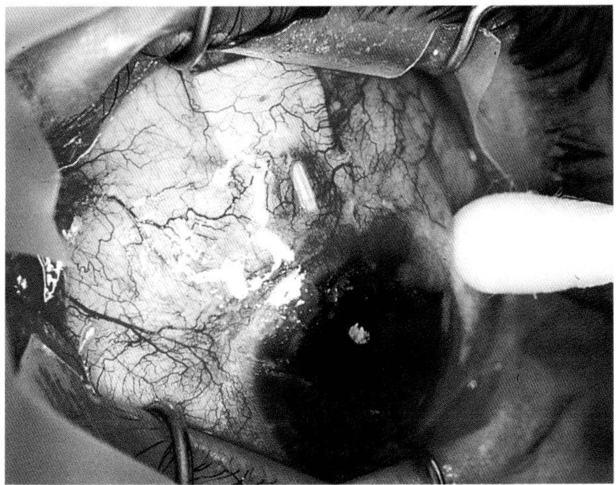

Figure 17.27 This tube has eroded through the patch graft and conjunctiva

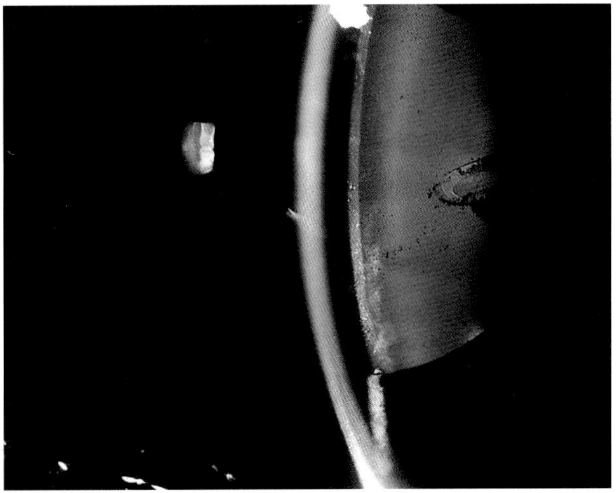

Figure 17.28 This eye has a shallow anterior chamber and tube–lens touch

operatively. This tube–corneal touch (Figs 17.29 and 17.30) may or may not result in corneal decompensation or corneal graft failure.

Corneal decompensation/edema

Corneal decompensation following placement of a tube shunt has been reported in up to 18% of eyes. Although progressive corneal endothelial cell loss after uncomplicated implantations of Molteno drainage devices has been reported, it is not believed to be clinically significant.

Corneal graft failure

In eyes with prior corneal grafts (Fig. 17.31), corneal graft failure (Fig. 17.32) has been reported in up to 45% of cases following tube-shunt implantation.

Anterior uveitis

Significant anterior uveitis may occur in up to 14% of cases, with fibrinous uveitis being reported in up to 24%.

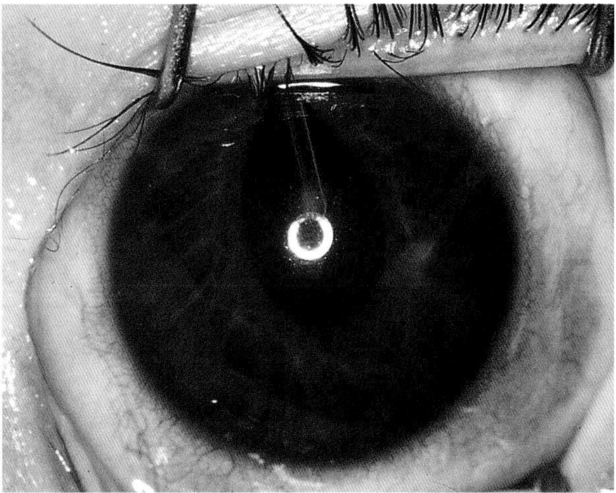

Figure 17.29 Intermittent tube–corneal touch
This eye with two Ahmed Glaucoma Valve implants has intermittent tube–corneal touch that has resulted in focal corneal edema and haze.

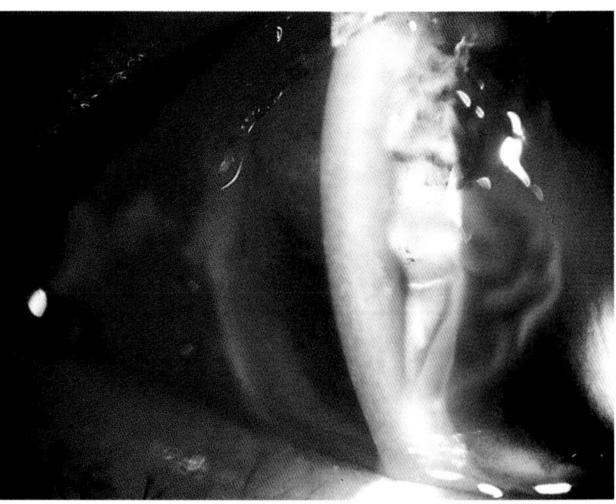

Figure 17.30 An eye with epithelial downgrowth
This eye has epithelial downgrowth and the tube was positioned posterior to the corneal endothelium and anterior to the sheet of epithelial cells.

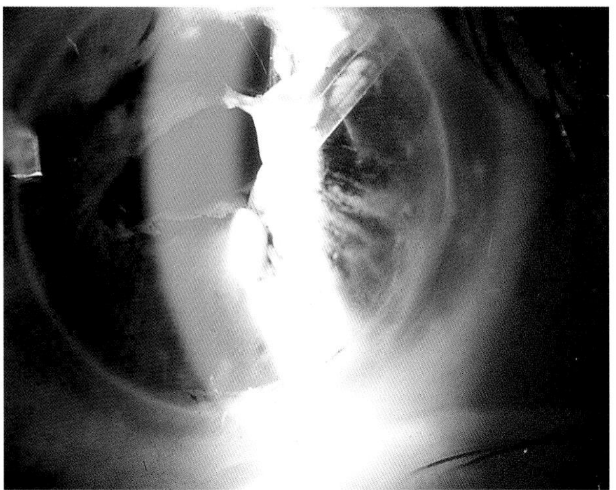

Figure 17.31 Peter's anomaly
This eye has Peter's anomaly with a clear corneal graft and Ahmed Glaucoma Valve implant.

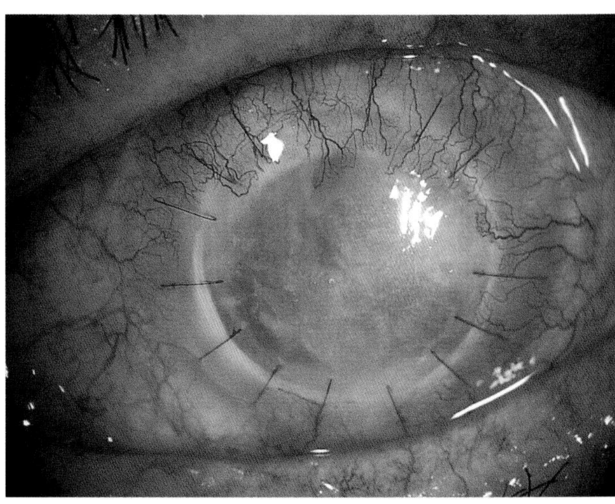

Figure 17.32 A failed corneal graft
This eye has a failed corneal graft after the placement of an Ahmed Glaucoma Valve implant.

Complications associated with the episcleral plate

Implant extrusion or erosion

Implants may erode through the conjunctiva (Fig. 17.33), with a reported incidence of about 3%. Anterior placement of the plate increases the risk, as blinking causes the conjunctiva to be rubbed over the hard plastic. Securing the plate at least 8 mm from the limbus reduces the risk of plâte erosion.

Bleb encapsulation

A rise in pressure following tube-shunt implantation commonly occurs 3–4 weeks postoperatively, and has been termed the 'hypertensive phase'. Bleb encapsulation or Tenon's cysts (Figs 17.34 and 17.35) have been reported in up to 10% of eyes with aqueous shunts. Intraocular pressure may be quite high if encapsulation occurs. They are treated similarly to the high bleb phase seen after trabeculectomies and may or may not require surgical intervention.

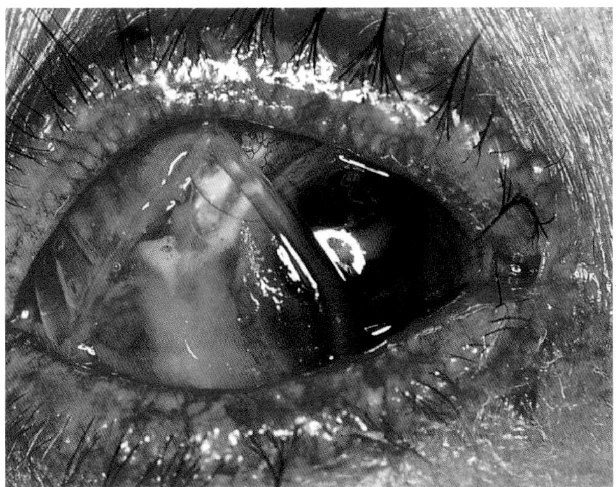

Figure 17.33 Extrusion of the plate
In this eye, the Ahmed Glaucoma Valve implant eroded through the conjunctiva. The tube remained secured to the sclera and inside the eye. Because of the risk of infection, this implant was removed.

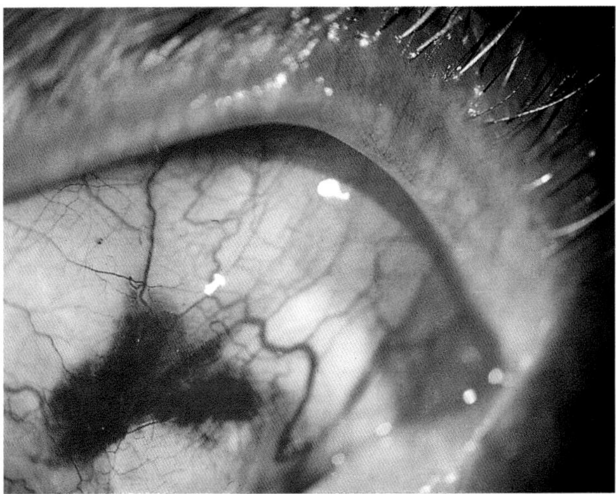

Figure 17.34 This eye has a normal-sized bleb over the Ahmed Glaucoma Valve implant

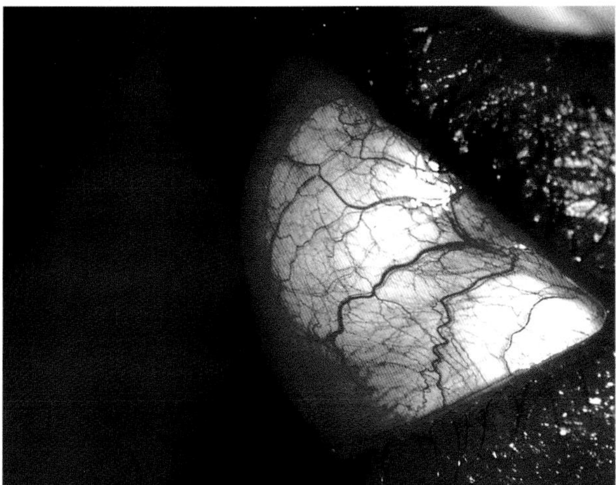

Figure 17.35 Tenon's cyst
When this patient looks straight ahead, the Tenon's cyst over the Ahmed Glaucoma Valve implant is quite prominent from the side.

Motility disturbances

Motility disturbances (Fig. 17.36) have been reported with Molteno, Baerveldt, Krupin and Ahmed implants. Acquired restrictive strabismus may occur from direct interference of muscle contraction by the plate or by involvement of the muscle sheath or tendon (superior oblique) within the bleb capsule. Placement of a shunt in the superonasal quadrant may produce an acquired Brown's syndrome with inability to look up and in. This quadrant should therefore be avoided.

Complications associated with intraocular surgery *per se*

Retinal detachment and/or vitreous hemorrhage

The incidence of retinal detachment after the placement of an aqueous shunt is up to 14%, and that of vitreous hemorrhage is as high as 11%. Vitreous hemorrhages may be secondary to underlying diseases such as proliferative diabetic retinopathy.

Endophthalmitis

The incidence of endophthalmitis after the placement of Molteno, Baerveldt, Ahmed or Krupin implants is 0–3%.

Malignant glaucoma or aqueous misdirection

Aqueous misdirection occurs in up to 4% of eyes after the placement of an aqueous shunt. The presence of a valve-like mechanism does not protect an eye from developing malignant glaucoma. Malignant glaucoma may require surgical intervention if it does not respond to cycloplegic agents and aqueous suppressants (Fig. 17.37).

Pupillary block

Pupillary block occurs in 2–3% of eyes following tube-shunt placement. The best way to treat or prevent pupillary block is with a laser iridotomy.

Epiretinal membrane and/or cystoid macular edema

Epiretinal membranes and/or cystoid macular edema have been reported in up to 14% of eyes with Molteno, Baerveldt, Krupin or Ahmed implants.

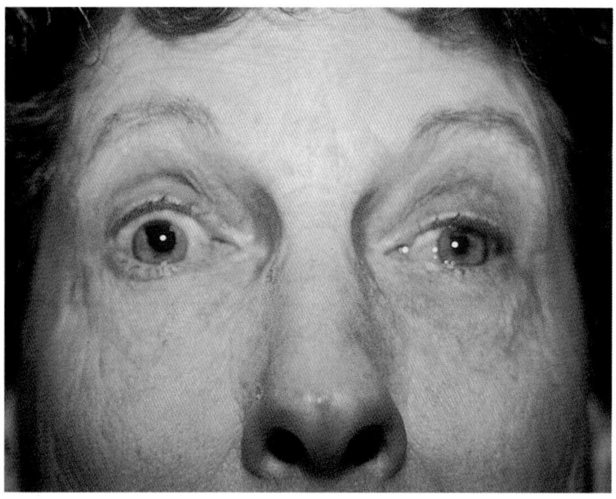

(a)

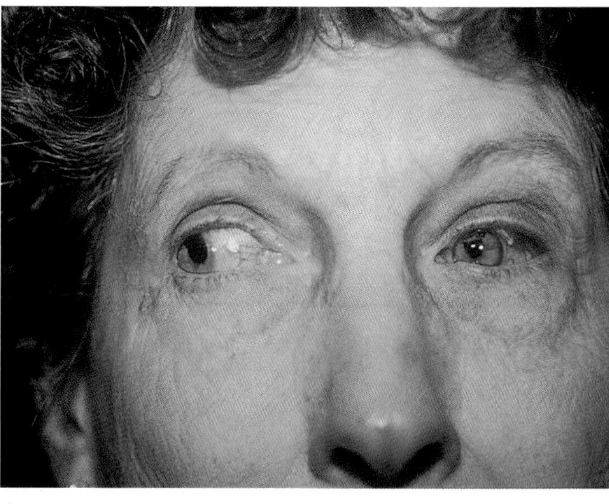

(b)

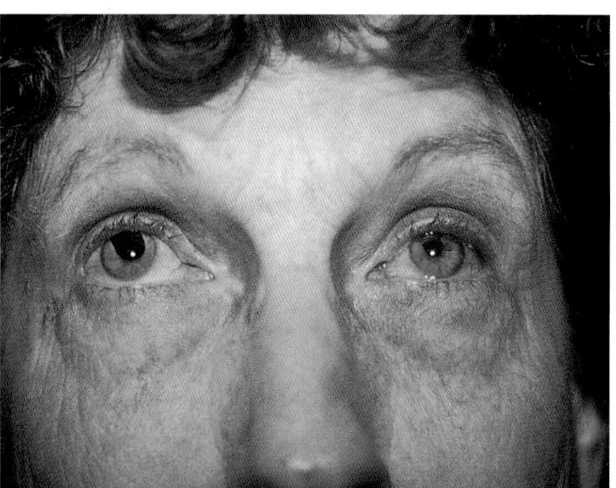

(c)

Figure 17.36 Motility disturbances
Restrictive strabismus developed following placement of an Ahmed Glaucoma Valve in the superotemporal quadrant of the left eye. (a) Primary position shows exotropia and hypertropia. (b) Adduction of the left eye is restricted on attempted right gaze. (c) Upgaze of the left eye is similarly restricted. This patient required muscle surgery to correct horizontal and vertical diplopia. At surgery, the bleb capsule was found to be adherent to the intermuscular septum of the superior and lateral rectus muscles, restricting and foreshortening the muscles. Following surgery, she has minimal diplopia in extreme positions of gaze, but is asymptomatic in most positions. (Courtesy of Neil Choplin, MD.)

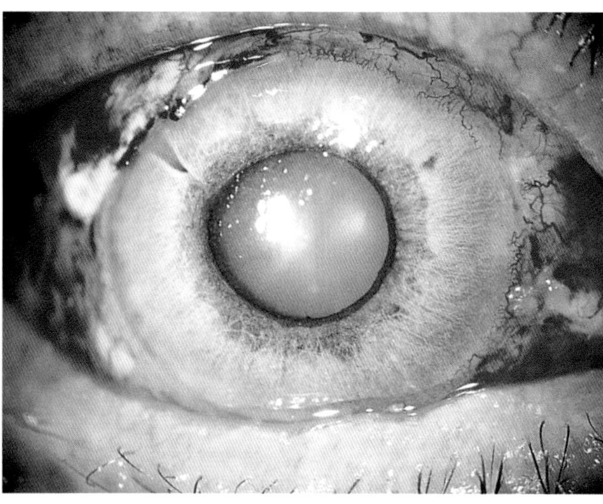

(a)

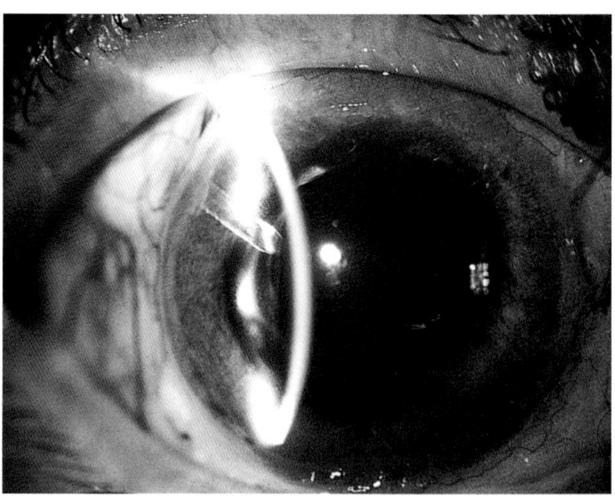

(b)

Figure 17.37 Malignant glaucoma
Malignant glaucoma developed after the placement of an Ahmed Glaucoma Valve implant which has been placed for neovascular glaucoma. (a) After this eye had a lensectomy and vitrectomy, the chamber was formed and the intraocular pressure was controlled (b).

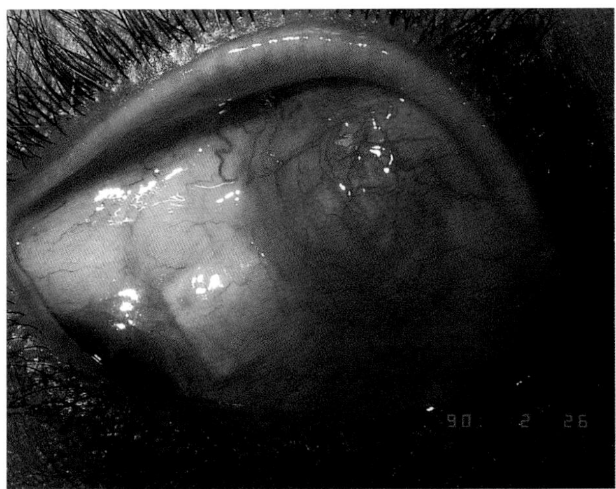

Figure 17.38 This eye has a mature, well functioning bleb after the placement of a single-plate Molteno implant

Summary

Aqueous shunts have a role in the management of eyes with glaucoma. Despite two-year success rates of approximately 50% or better in eyes with usually poor surgical prognoses, aqueous shunts are no panacea, and their use in eyes may be fraught with serious complications. Appropriate case selection and excellent surgical technique and postoperative care may help prevent some but not all of these complications (Fig. 17.38).

FURTHER READING

Brandt JD, Patch grafts of dehydrated cadaveric dura mater for tube-shunt glaucoma surgery, *Arch Ophthalmol* (1993) **111**:1436–9.

Brown RD, Cairns JE, Experience with the Molteno long tube implant, *Trans Ophthal Soc UK* (1983) **103**:297–308.

Clayton D, Hills M, *Statistical models in epidemiology* (Oxford: Oxford University Press, 1993).

Coleman AL, Hill R, Wilson MR, et al., Initial clinical experience with the Ahmed Glaucoma Valve implant, *Am J Ophthalmol* (1995) **120**:23–31.

Coleman AL, Smyth RJ, Wilson MR, Tam M, Initial clinical experience with the Ahmed Glaucoma Valve implant in pediatric patients, *Archives of Ophthalmology* (1996) **115**:186–91.

Davidovski F, Stewart RH, Kimbrough RL, Long-term results with the White Glaucoma Pump-shunt, *Ophthalmic Surg* (1990) **21**:288–93.

Egbert PR, Lieberman MF, Internal suture occlusion of the Molteno glaucoma implant for the prevention of postoperative hypotony, *Ophthalmic Surg* (1989) **20**:53–6.

Ellis BD, Varley GA, Kalenak JW, Meisler DM, Huang SS, Bacterial endophthalmitis following cataract surgery in an eye with a preexisting Molteno implant, *Ophthalmic Surg* (1993) **24**:117–18.

El-Sayad F, El-Maghraby A, Helal M, Amayem A, The use of releasable sutures in Molteno glaucoma implant procedures to reduce postoperative hypotony, *Ophthalmic Surg* (1991) **22**:82–4.

Fellenbaum PS, Almeida AR, Minckler DS, Sidoti PA, Baerveldt G, Heuer DK, Krupin disk implantation for complicated glaucomas, *Ophthalmology* (1994) **101**:1178–82.

Freedman J, Scleral patch grafts with Molteno setons, *Ophthalmic Surg* (1987) **18**:532–4.

Heuer DK, Lloyd MA, Abrams DA, et al., Which is better? One or two? A randomized clinical trial of single plate versus double-plate Molteno implantation for glaucomas in aphakia and pseudophakia, *Ophthalmology* (1992) **99**:1512–19.

Hill RA, Heuer DK, Baerveldt G, et al., Molteno implantation for glaucoma in young patients, *Ophthalmology* (1991) **98**:1042–6.

Hill RA, Nguyen QH, Baerveldt G, et al., Trabeculectomy and Molteno implantation of glaucomas associated with uveitis, *Ophthalmology* (1993) **100**:903–8.

Hitchings RA, Joseph NH, Sherwood MB, Lattimer J, Miller M, Use of one-piece valved tube and variable surface area explant for glaucoma drainage surgery, *Ophthalmology* (1987) **94**:1079–84.

Hoarne Nairne JEA, Sherwood D, Jacob JSH, Rich WJCC, Single stage insertion of the Molteno tube for glaucoma and modifications to reduce postoperative hypotony, *Br J Ophthalmol* (1988) **72**:846–51.

Hodkin MJ, Goldblatt WS, Burgoyne CF, Ball SF, Insler MS, Early clinical experience with the Baerveldt implant in complicated glaucomas, *Am J Ophthalmol* (1995) **120**:32–40.

Honrubia FM, Grijalbo MP, Gomez ML, Lopez A, Surgical treatment of neovascular glaucoma, *Trans Ophthalmol Soc UK* (1979) **99**:89–91.

The Krupin Eye Valve Filtering Surgery Study Group, Krupin eye valve with disk for filtration surgery, *Ophthalmology* (1994) **101**:651–8.

Krupin T, Podos SM, Becker B, Newkirk JB, Valve implants in filtering surgery, *Am J Ophthalmol* (1976) **81**:232–5.

Latina MA, Single stage Molteno implant with combination internal occlusion and external ligature, *Ophthalmic Surg* (1990) **21**:444–6.

Liebmann JM, Ritch R, Intraocular suture ligature to reduce hypotony following Molteno seton implantation, *Ophthalmic Surg* (1992) **23**:51–2.

Lloyd MA, Baerveldt F, Fellenbaum PS, et al., Intermediate-term results of a randomized clinical trial of the 350-versus the 500-square mm Baerveldt implant, *Ophthalmology* (1994) **101**:1456–64.

Lloyd MAE, Baerveldt F, Heuer DK, Minckler DS, Martone JF, Initial clinical experience with the Baerveldt implant in complicated glaucomas, *Ophthalmology* (1994) **101**:640–50.

Lloyd MA, Sedlak T, Heuer DK, et al., Clinical experience with the single-plate Molteno implant in complicated glaucomas: update of a pilot study, *Ophthalmology* (1992) **99**:679–87.

Mascati NT, A new surgical approach for the control of a class of glaucomas, *Int Surg* (1967) **47**:10–15.

McDermott ML, Swendris RP, Shin DH, Juzych MS, Cowden JW, Corneal endothelial cells counts after Molteno implantation, *Am J Ophthalmol* (1993) **115**:93–6.

Mermoud A, Salmon JF, Alexander P, Straker C, Murray ADN, Molteno tube implantation for neovascular glaucoma: long-term results and factors influencing the outcome, *Ophthalmology* (1993) **100**:897–902.

Mills RP, Reynolds A, Emond MJ, Barlow WE, Leen MM, Long-term survival of Molteno glaucoma drainage devices, *Ophthalmology* (1996) **103**:299–305.

Minckler DS, Heuer DK, Hasty B, Baerveldt G, Cutting RC, Barlow WE, Clinical experience with the single-plate Molteno implant in complicated glaucomas, *Ophthalmology* (1988) **95**:1181–8.

Minckler DS, Shammas A, Wilcox M, Ogden TE, Experimental studies of aqueous filtration using the Molteno implant, *Tr Am Ophth Soc* (1987) **84**:368–92.

Molteno ACB, New implant for drainage in glaucoma: clinical trial, *Br J Ophthalmol* (1969) **53**:606–15.

Molteno ACB, The dual chamber single plate implant—its use in neovascular glaucoma, *Aust NZ J Ophthalmol* (1990) **18**:431–6.

Molteno ACB, Polkinghorne PJ, Bowbyes JA, The vicryl tie technique for inserting a draining implant in the treatment of secondary glaucoma, *Aust NZ J Ophthalmol* (1986) **14**:343–54.

Noureddin BN, Wilson-Holt N, Lavin M, Jeffrey M, Hitchings RA, Advanced uncontrolled glaucoma: Nd:YAG cyclophotocoagulation or tube surgery, *Ophthalmology* (1992) **99**:430–7.

Perkins TW, Endophthalmitis after placement of a Molteno implant, *Ophthalmic Surg* (1990) **21**:733–4.

Prata JA, Mermoud A, LaBree L, Minckler DS, In vitro and in vivo flow characteristics of glaucoma drainage implants, *Ophthalmology* (1995) **102**:894–904.

Rajah-Sivayoham ISS, Camero-venous shunt for secondary glaucoma following orbital venous obstruction, *Br J Ophthalmol* (1968) **52**:843–5.

Rollett M, Moreau M, Traitement de le hypopyon par le drainage capillaire de la chambre antérieure, *Rev Gen Ophthalmol* (1906) **25**:481–9.

Rubin B, Chan CC, Burnier M, Munion L, Freedman J, Histopathologic study of the Molteno glaucoma implant in three patients, *Am J Ophthalmol* (1990) **110**:371–9.

Schocket SS, Lakhanpal V, Richards RD, Anterior chamber tube shunt to an encircling band in the treatment of neovascular glaucoma, *Ophthalmology* (1982) **89**:1188–94.

Schocket SS, Nirankari VS, Lakhanpal V, Richards RD, Lerner BC, Anterior chamber tube shunt to an encircling band in the treatment of neovascular glaucoma and other refractory glaucomas: a long-term study, *Ophthalmology* (1985) **92**:553–62.

Scott DR, Quigley HA, Medical management of a high bleb phase after trabeculectomies, *Ophthalmology* (1988) **95**:1169–73.

Sherwood MB, Smith MF, Prevention of early hypotony associated with Molteno implants by a new occluding stent technique, *Ophthalmology* (1993) **100**:85–90.

Siegner SW, Netland PA, Urban RC, Clinical experience with the Baerveldt glaucoma drainage implant, *Ophthalmology* (1995) **102**:1298–307.

Smith MF, Sherwood MB, McGorray SP, Comparison of the double-plate Molteno drainage implant with the Schocket procedure, *Arch Ophthalmol* (1992) **110**:1246–50.

Smith SL, Starita RJ, Fellman RL, Lynn JR, Early clinical experience with the Baerveldt 350-square mm glaucoma implant and associated extraocular muscle imbalance, *Ophthalmology* (1993) **100**:914–18.

Spiegel D, Shrader RR, Wilson RP, Anterior chamber tube shunt to an encircling band (Schocket procedure) in the treatment of refractory glaucoma, *Ophthalmic Surg* (1992) **23**:804–7.

White TC, Clinical results of glaucoma surgery using the White Glaucoma Pump Shunt, *Ann Ophthalmol* (1992) **24**:365–73.

Wilson RP, Cantor L, Katz LJ, Schmidt CM, Steinmann WC, Allee S, Aqueous shunts: Molteno versus Schocket, *Ophthalmology* (1992) **99**:672–8.

18 Combined cataract and glaucoma surgery

Mary Fran Smith, James William Doyle, Maher M Fanous and Mark B Sherwood

Introduction

In the 1980s, the surgical management of patients with visually significant cataract and glaucoma generally revolved around three different approaches: 1) extracapsular cataract extraction (ECCE) alone; 2) glaucoma filtering surgery alone with cataract extraction later; and 3) combined cataract and glaucoma surgery (with either one incision or two separate incisions). The indications for, and limitations of, each approach were well recognized. For example, cataract extraction alone was associated with the risk of uncontrollable intraocular pressures (IOPs) in the postoperative period. Glaucoma filtering surgery first was once thought to guarantee immediate IOP control following cataract surgery, but this has not been shown necessarily to be so. This approach also carried the risk of losing the bleb in the postoperative period following the cataract extraction, with failure rates of up to 50%. Combined surgery had the advantage of addressing both cataract and glaucoma problems simultaneously, while reducing the risk of an early IOP spike. However, long-term pressure control was not usually as good as with trabeculectomy surgery alone, and the surgery itself was technically more difficult and more prone to complications. Because of these limitations with combined extracapsular cataract extraction and trabeculectomy, many surgeons opted for a two-stage approach.

Phacoemulsification

Technological advances in cataract removal technique, e.g. the advent of phacoemulsification and small incision (foldable) intraocular lenses, have changed the way surgeons approach coexisting cataract and glaucoma. Figure 18.1 illustrates one approach to the decision making when choosing which procedure is most appropriate for a glaucoma patient with a cataract. Phacoemulsification-style cataract removal does not appear to have as high an incidence of postoperative IOP spikes as did extracapsular surgery. Additionally, there is an increased tendency for IOP to drop following phacoemulsification surgery. Therefore, many patients with cataracts and mild to even moderate glaucoma may do well with phacoemulsification cataract surgery alone.

Preoperative evaluation

During the preoperative evaluation of a patient with cataract and glaucoma, the question of whether to do phacoemulsification alone or a combined phacotrabeculectomy is considered. One approach is to make this decision based on the number of medications the patient requires preoperatively to control the glaucoma—modified by optic nerve and field appearance—as well as by the patient's life expectancy. For example, a patient requiring few medications to control the glaucoma might do well with phacoemulsification alone, but if the patient is young and already has advanced nerve and field changes, a combined procedure might be the better choice.

Another consideration is that glaucoma associated with narrow angles or angle-closure glaucoma is likely to have improved IOP control following phacoemulsification alone. A final point worth mentioning is that certain glaucoma patients, e.g. those with iridocorneal endothelial syndrome or Fuch's dystrophy, deserve special attention to the

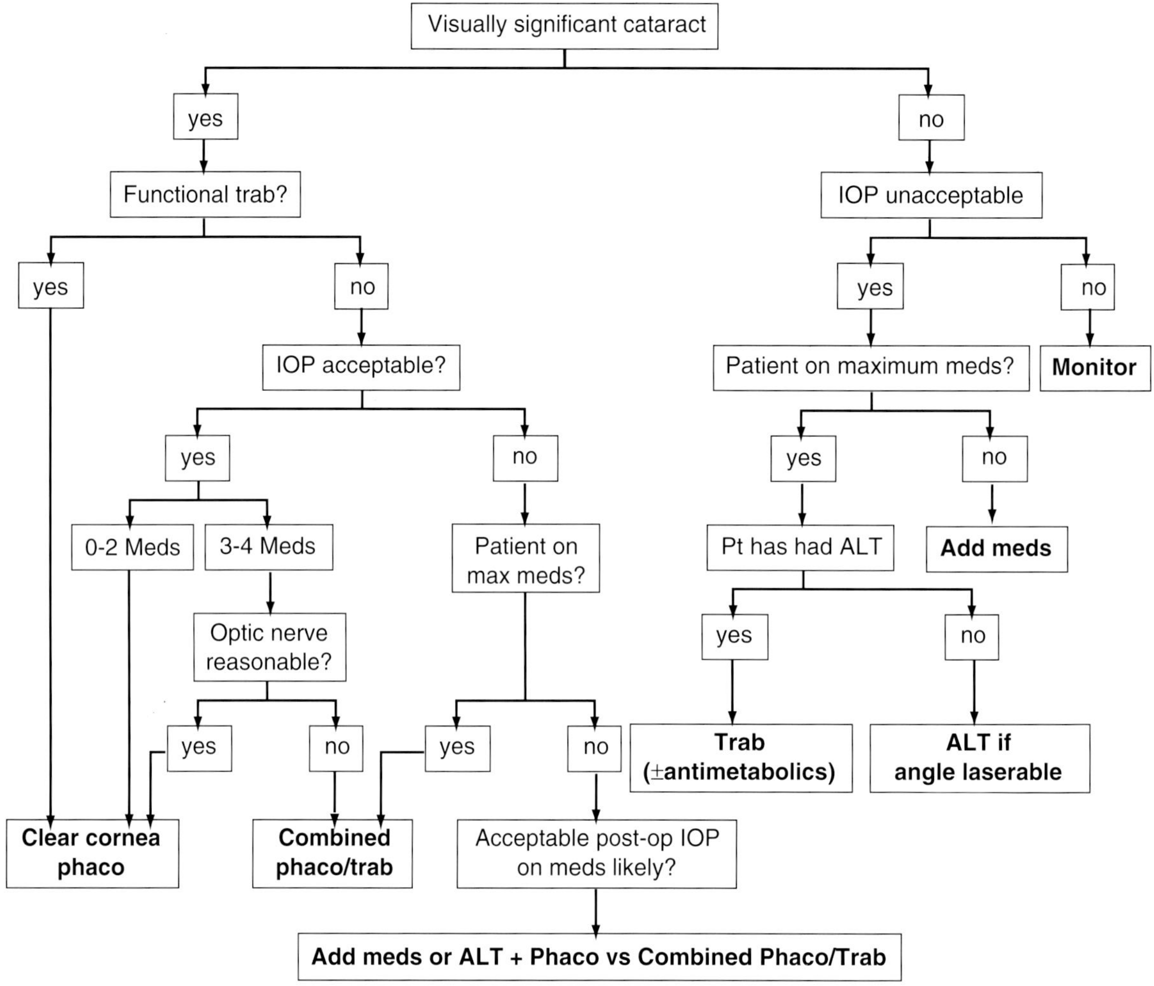

Figure 18.1 Choosing the appropriate surgical procedure

Flow chart illustrating the decision-making involved in choosing the appropriate surgical procedure for the glaucoma patient with a cataract.

status of their corneas prior to proceeding with routine phacoemulsification surgery. Consideration should be given to the use of an enhanced irrigating solution, such as BSS Plus™ (Alcon, Fort Worth, Texas), to protect the corneal endothelium.

Phacoemulsification alone

The options for phacoemulsification alone are a temporal clear corneal approach or a superior scleral tunnel approach. A temporal approach through a scleral tunnel may also be considered. The clear corneal approach may be preferable because it leaves the conjunctiva undisturbed. This may enhance the success of trabeculectomy should it ever be needed in the future. Temporal clear corneal phacoemulsification should also be considered in patients with pre-existing filtering blebs to decrease conjunctival manipulation and decrease the risk of scarring within the bleb. Figures 18.2–18.4 illustrate one approach to creating a clear corneal incision.

Management of the pupil

Glaucoma patients frequently have pupils that dilate poorly, either because of sphincter fibrosis from years of miotic therapy, posterior synechiae, or from primary conditions such as exfoliation syndrome. The surgeon therefore may need to enlarge the pupil in order safely to perform phacoemulsification, unless he or she is very experienced with the procedure and is comfortable working through a suboptimal pupil. Figure 18.5–18.11 show management options for the pupil.

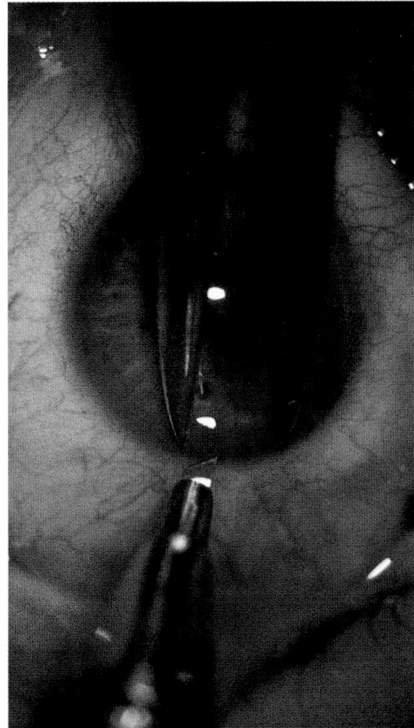

Figure 18.2 Creating a clear corneal incision
One approach to temporal clear corneal phacoemulsification begins with outlining a 3 mm incision, in this case with a diamond blade.

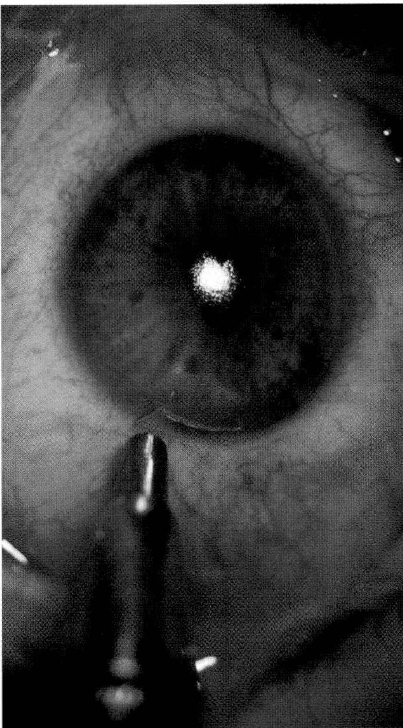

Figure 18.3 Clear corneal incision
A partial thickness groove is completed with the diamond blade for the width of the incision.

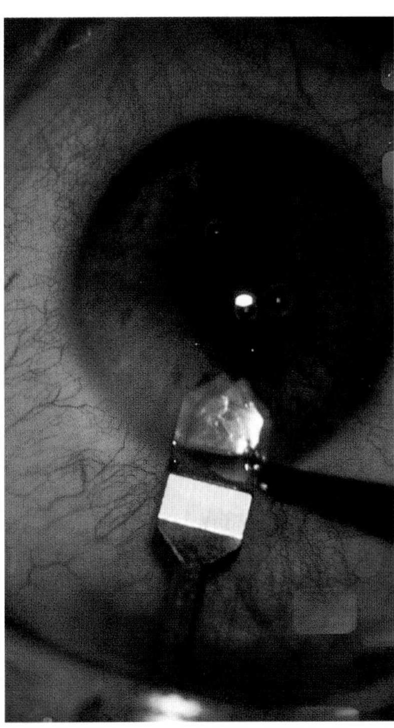

Figure 18.4 Clear corneal incision
A diamond keratome is used to complete the stepped incision through clear cornea.

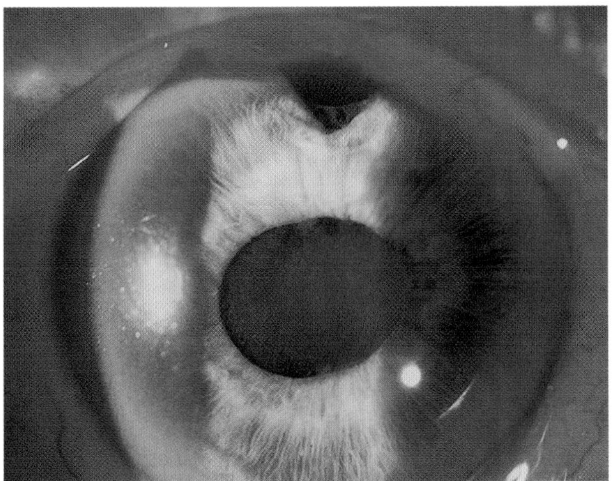

Figure 18.5 Pseudoexfoliation glaucoma
This 80-year-old female with pseudoexfoliation glaucoma was status post successful trabeculectomy surgery performed two years previously. A bleb is present superiorly. She complained of glare and reading difficulties attributable to a cataract. Note poor pupillary dilatation.

Zonules

Glaucoma patients are often at risk of weak zonules due to such factors as advanced age or the exfoliation syndrome. Extra care must thus be taken in these patients to avoid complications due to weak zonules, such as vitreous loss or loss of lens material posteriorly into the vitreous cavity. To avoid stress on what may be weak zonules, thorough hydrodissection and hydrodelineation must be performed to free the nucleus from all its cortical attachments, allowing free rotation within the bag, and care must be taken to avoid pushing the nucleus with the tip of the phacoemulsification handpiece during sculpting, which could cause the zonules to be disrupted. Figures 18.12–18.14 illustrate some of these points.

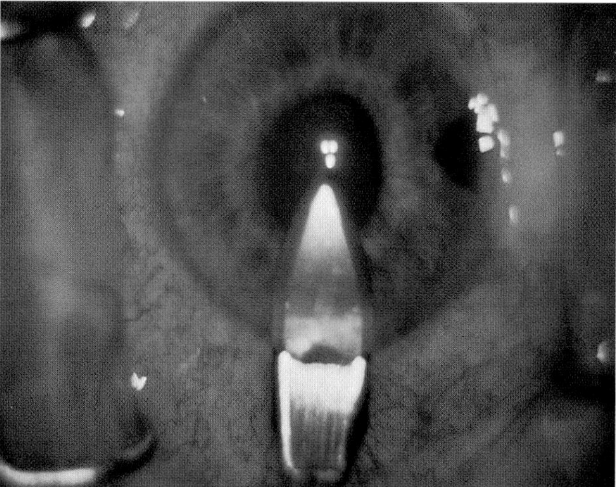

Figure 18.6 3 mm temporal incision
A standard 3 mm temporal incision was made temporally with a keratome. The bleb is to the surgeon's right.

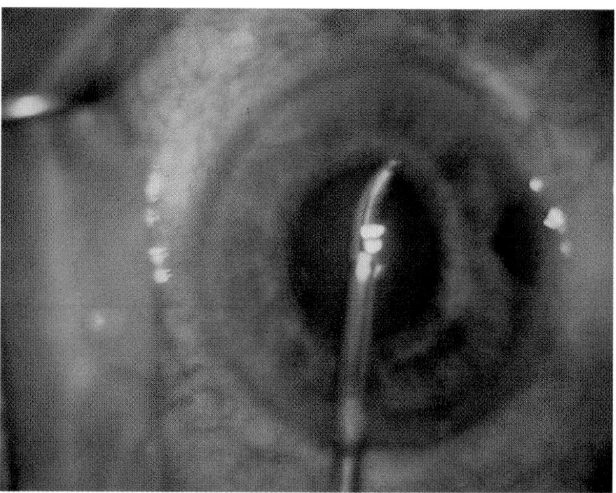

Figure 18.7 Multiple small sphincterotomies
Either Rapazzo scissors or intraocular retinal scissors may be used for this procedure. Following 8–12 small cuts in the sphincter, viscoelastic can be used to open the pupil.

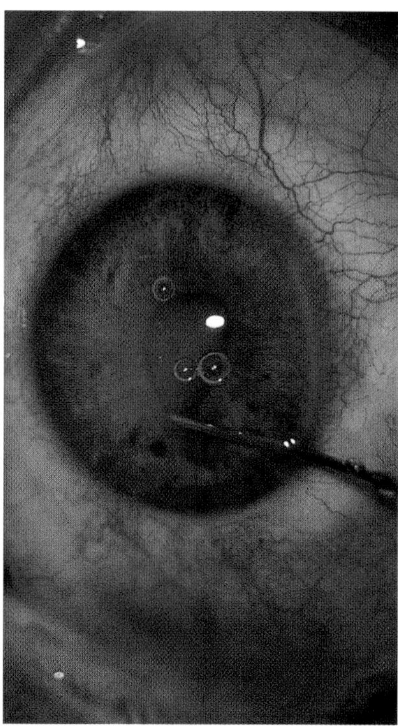

Figure 18.8 Posterior synechiae
If posterior synechiae are present they may be broken by injecting viscoelastic and sweeping with the cannula.

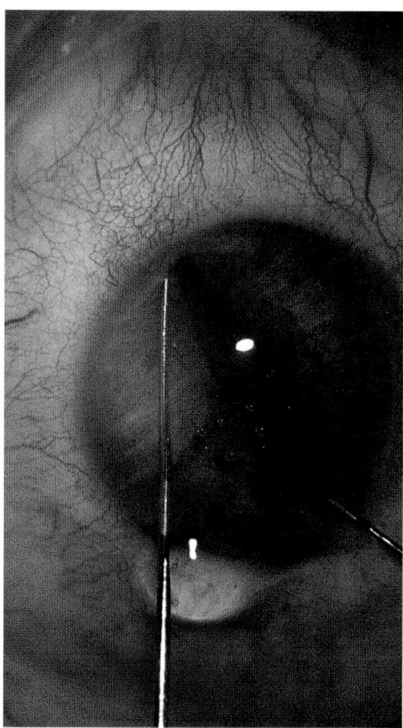

Figure 18.9 Enlarging the pupil
Another useful way to enlarge the pupil is by stretching using two hooks, first in the six to twelve o'clock direction and then three to nine.

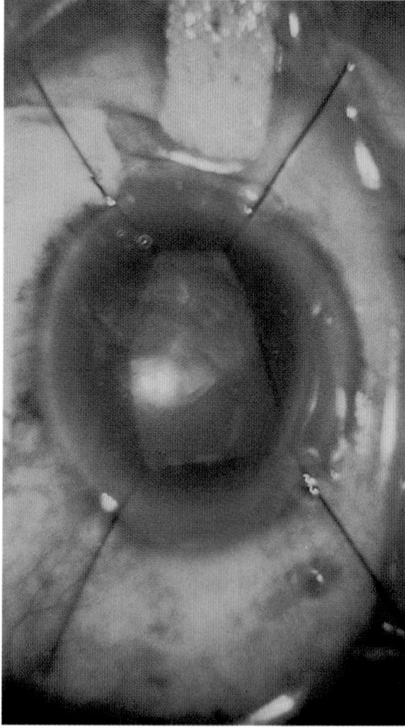

Figure 18.10 Dilating the pupil with disposable hooks
The pupil may also be dilated with disposable iris hooks, such as those available from Grieshaber, Switzerland. The hooks are inserted through limbal stab incisions approximately 90 degrees apart. An adjustable silicone sleeve holds the hook (and the pupil) in place.

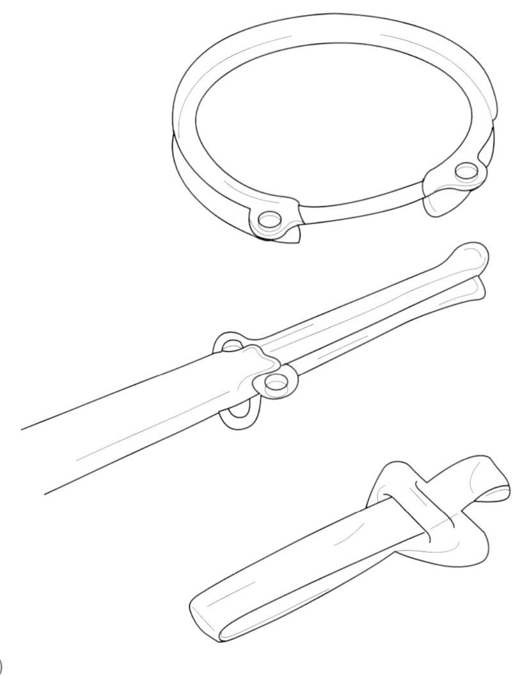

(a)

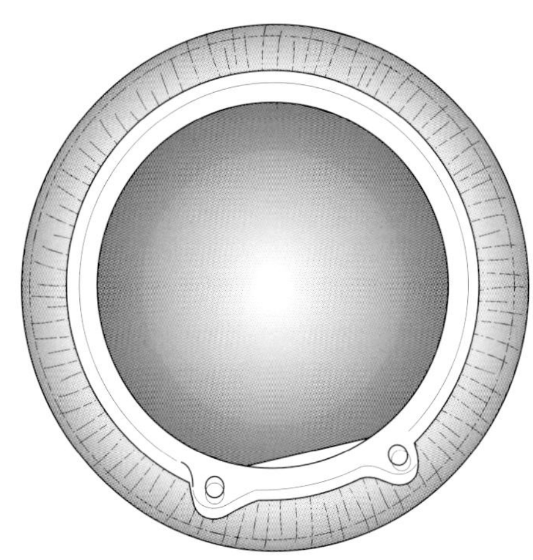

(b)

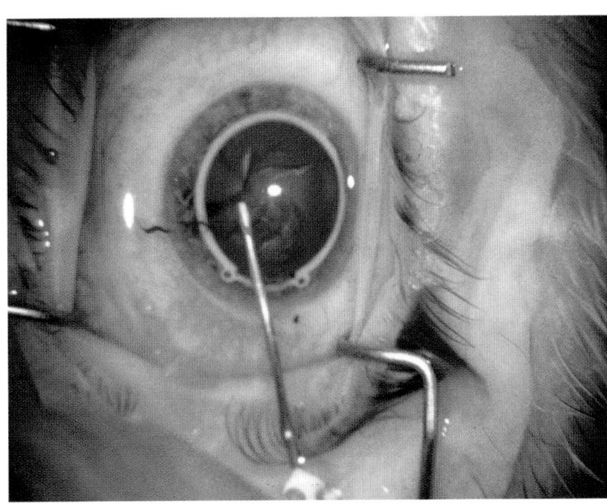

(c)

Figure 18.11 The Graether Pupil Expander
The Graether Pupil Expander offers another alternative for enlarging a small pupil. (a) The device inserter. (b) Drawing of the device in place. (c) Clinical photograph.

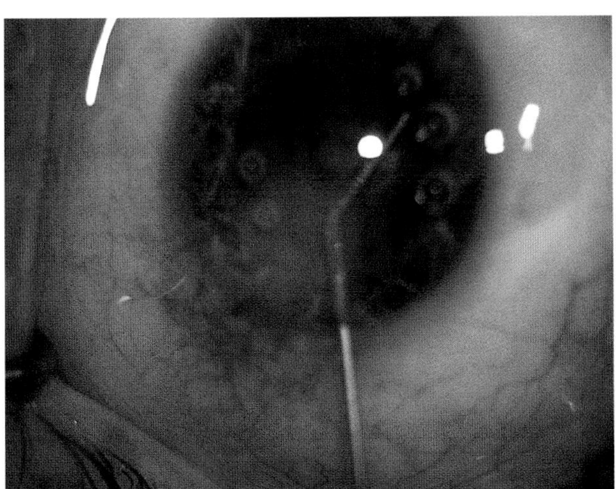

Figure 18.12 Hydrodissection and hydrodelineation
Hydrodissection and hydrodelineation is performed with balanced salt solution using a 27 or 30-gauge blunt cannula.

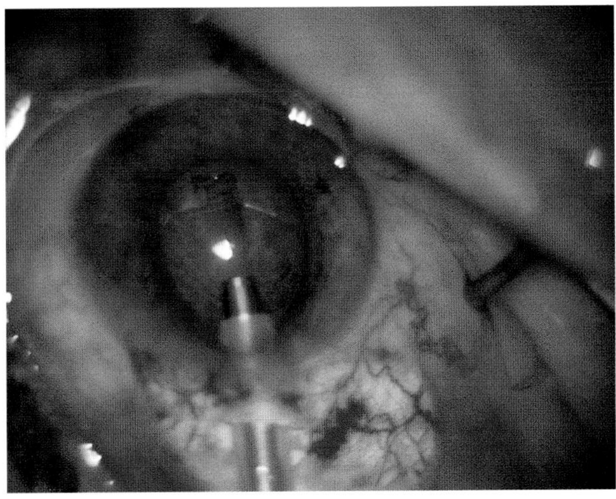

Figure 18.13 Initial nuclear grooving
During the 'divide and conquer' stage of phacoemulsification in glaucomatous eyes, suboptimal pupil dilatation (even after manual pupillary enlargement) may limit groove extension into the peripheral nucleus.

Completion of surgery

After quadrant removal and cortical clean-up, a polymethyl methacrylate (PMMA) or foldable intraocular lens (Fig. 18.15) may be inserted into the bag. If there has been a disruption in the capsular bag or torn zonules, the lens may be placed in the ciliary sulcus provided the surgeon is able to determine that there is sufficient capsular support. Foldable-style lenses include plate haptic silicone lenses, prolene or PMMA loop haptic silicone lenses, and acrylic lenses. All PMMA and some foldable lenses may require wound enlargement prior to insertion.

If a bleb is overfunctioning at the time of phacoemulsification, viscoelastic may be left in the eye postoperatively to slow aqueous flow through the bleb, and allow some bleb healing. If no bleb is present or bleb function is appropriate, extra care should be taken to remove all viscoelastic from these eyes to prevent a postoperative pressure rise. If advanced nerve damage is noted preoperatively, it may be prudent to check intraocular pressure 3–6 hours after surgery, and treat medically if there is a significant spike.

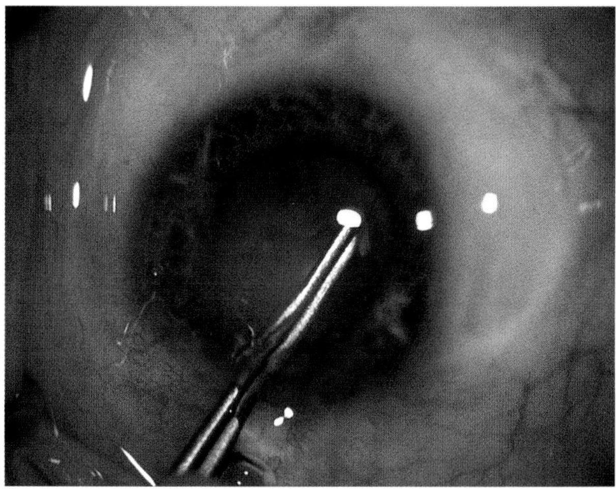

Figure 18.14 A nucleus splitter
One option for splitting the nucleus into pieces is the use of a nucleus splitter, provided the grooves are made sufficiently deep. This figure illustrates the use of a Salz-style nucleus-cracking instrument.

Combined phacotrabeculectomy

Small incision size and the potential for less postoperative inflammation than that seen with ECCE are two advantages of phacoemulsification which make it the theoretical procedure of choice for combination with filtering surgery in the comanagement of cataract and glaucoma. As compared with combined extracapsular cataract extraction and trabeculectomy surgery, combined phacoemulsification/trabeculectomy surgery is associated with earlier visual rehabilitation, less postoperative astigmatism, higher blebs, and improved long-term IOP control. Equally important, antimetabolite use to modulate wound healing following filtering surgery has made combined phacotrabeculectomy a better option for many patients.

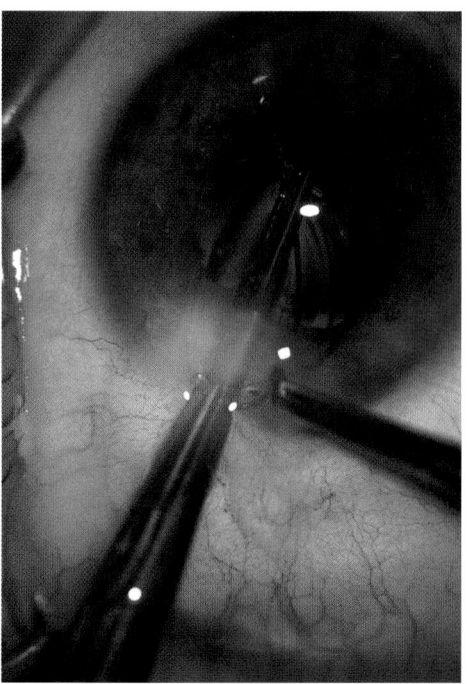

Figure 18.15 A foldable intraocular lens
Insertion of a foldable intraocular lens, using a Fine folding forceps.

One or two-site approach

Combined surgery may be performed either with two separate incisions (one temporally for cataract extraction, and a superior trabeculectomy flap) or through one incision superiorly through which phacoemulsification is performed, with subsequent conversion to a trabeculectomy flap. The advantages of two separate incisions include theoretical decreased inflammation at the trabeculectomy site, and the ability easily to make a limbus-based conjunctival flap for enhanced antimetabolite application over the planned sclerostomy site. In two-incision surgery, phacoemulsification is performed temporally first, followed by routine trabeculectomy superiorly.

The advantages of a single incision include greater ease of surgery and decreased operating time. One

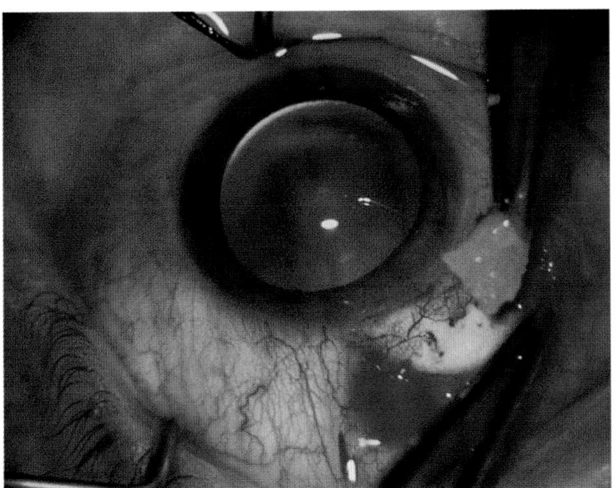

Figure 18.16 Application of mitomycin-C
Intraoperative low-dose mitomycin-C (200 μg/cc × 5 minutes) on a cellulose sponge is applied following development of a fornix-based conjunctival flap.

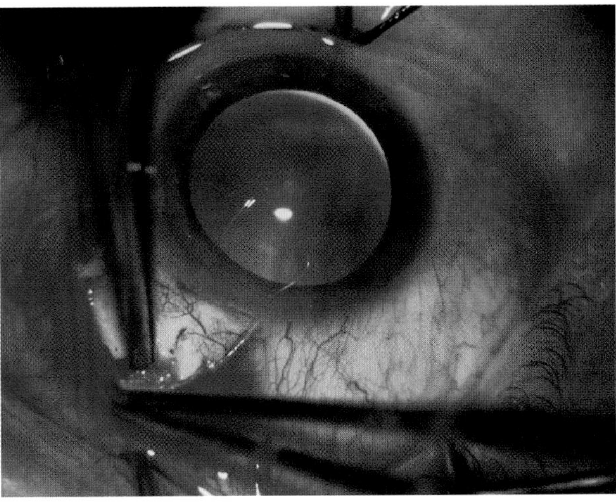

Figure 18.17 Application of mitomycin-C
The sponge is inserted underneath the conjunctival flap

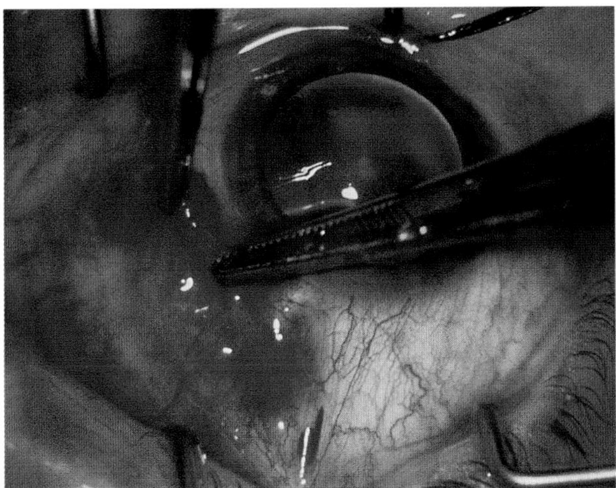

Figure 18.18 Application of mitomycin-C
The conjunctiva is draped over the sponge, taking care to avoid contact between the sponge and the conjunctival wound edge. After the 5-minute application, the site should be thoroughly irrigated with balanced salt solution.

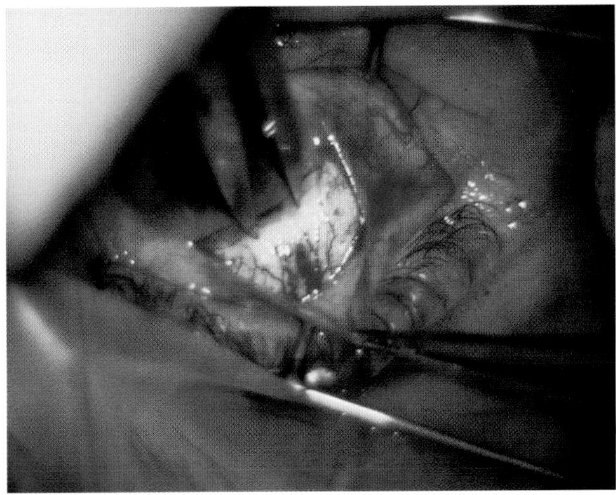

Figure 18.19 Creation of scleral tunnel
Phacoemulsification may be performed through a 2 mm long by 3 mm wide tunnel. The width of the incision is determined by the width of the tip being used and that of the keratome used to create the opening into the anterior chamber.

incision phacotrabeculectomy begins with a conjunctival incision superiorly. A fornix-based conjunctival flap allows for better visualization during surgery and, in one prospective study, was associated with equally successful final outcomes compared to eyes having a limbus-based conjunctival flap (although this study did not use adjunctive antimetabolites).

Many surgeons have the impression that intraoperative antimetabolite application augments postoperative filter function in combined surgeries. A prospective study looking at 5-fluorouracil (5-FU) augmentation noted no difference between patients receiving and not receiving 5-FU. Another prospective study noted that adjunctive mitomycin-C (MMC) improved the filtration success rate of combined

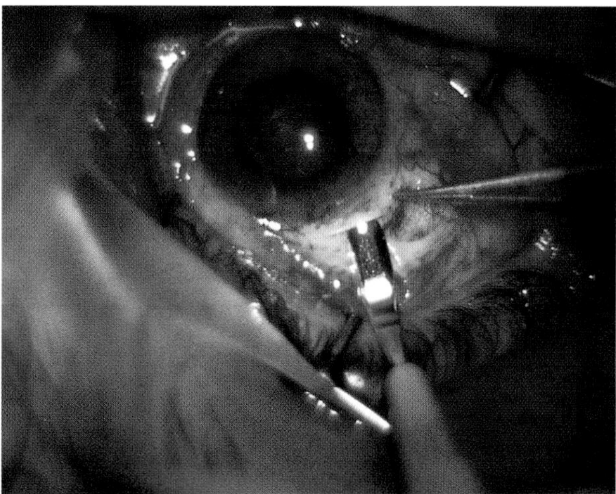

Figure 18.20 Creation of scleral tunnel
A crescent-type blade is used to create the scleral tunnel

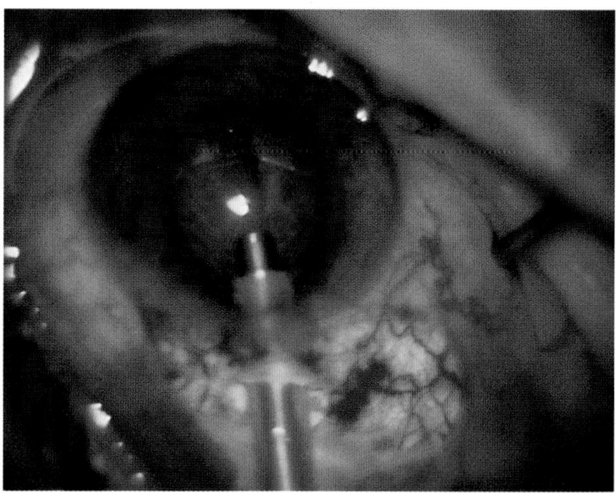

Figure 18.21 Phacoemulsification
The lens is removed by the appropriate phacoemulsification technique.

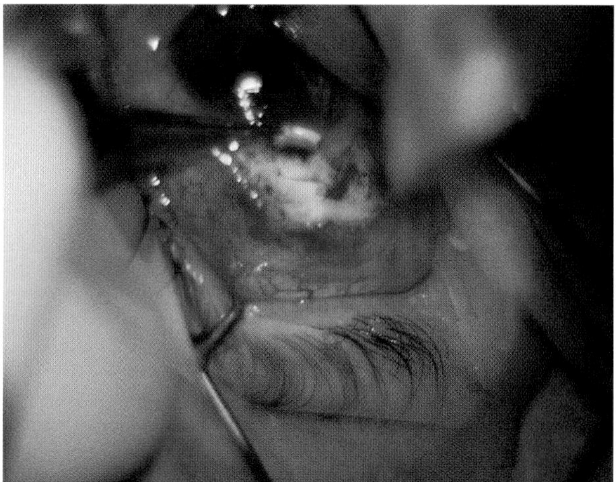

Figure 18.22 Insertion of intraocular lens
Lens insertion may be simplified by first converting the scleral tunnel to a flap with Vannas scissors. If the surgeon prefers, the lens may be inserted and the tunnel converted afterwards. Some surgeons perform the filtering portion of the procedure without radializing the flap, using a punch under the roof of the tunnel to remove a piece of the inner wall, thus creating a 'no-stitch phacotrabeculectomy' which requires no flap sutures.

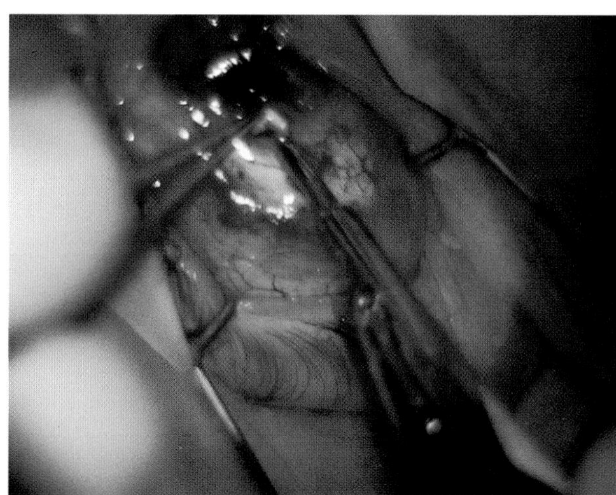

Figure 18.23 Removing a block of inner tissue
A block of inner tissue beneath the converted trabeculectomy flap is removed with a punch. Some surgeons prefer to remove the block of tissue by free-hand dissection.

procedures in selected patients with glaucoma and one or more risk factors for failure. Other retrospective studies have reported excellent IOP success rates with MMC or 5-FU use. Figures 18.16–18.18 illustrate the application of low dose Mitomycin C to the surgery site. Figures 18.19–18.30 illustrate the remaining steps in performing a phacotrabeculectomy.

Following phacotrabeculectomy with mitomycin-C, success rates as high as 90% for IOP control and visual acuity better than 20/40 in 80% of patients have been reported. Possible complications, often secondary to either bleb leak or simple overfiltration, may include shallow anterior chambers, fibrin formation (associated with chronic use of miotics,

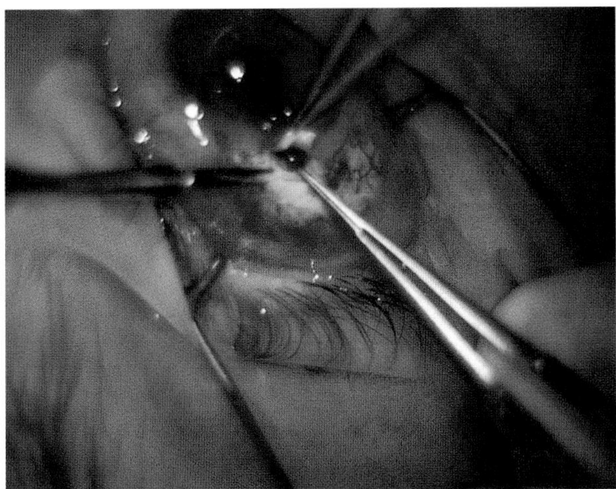

Figure 18.24 A peripheral iridectomy is performed

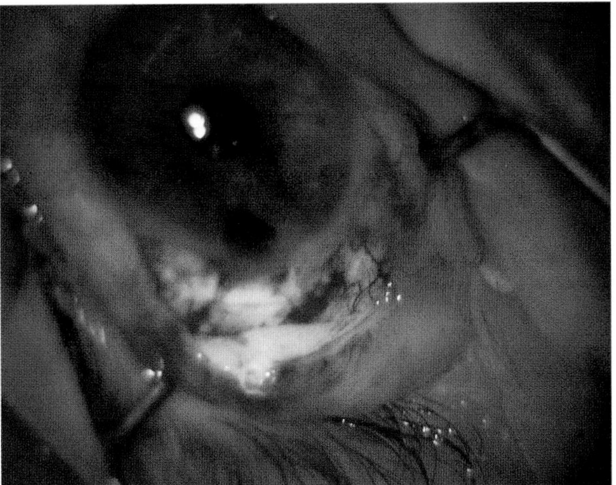

Figure 18.25 Appearance following peripheral iridectomy
In this case, viscoelastic has been left in the eye for stabilization purposes.

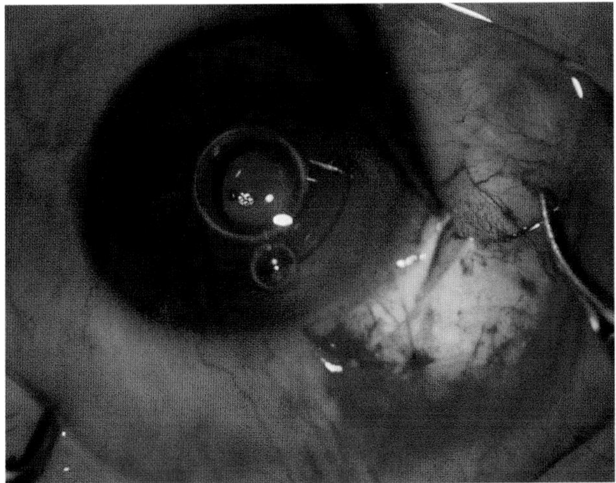

Figure 18.26 Closing the flap
The flap is securely closed with a combination of releasable and 'permanent' 10–0 nylon sutures.

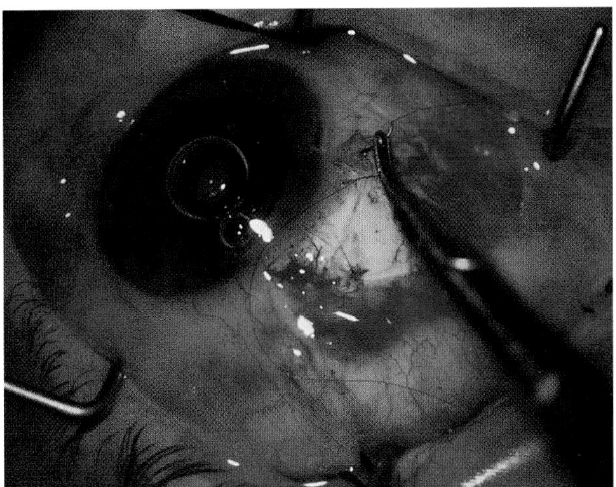

Figure 18.27 The releasable suture technique
The releasable suture technique involves a three-throw slip knot formation, with externalization of the suture beyond the anticipated conjunctival 'hood'. Releasable sutures are useful in these cases because laser suture lysis may cause conjunctival wound disruption when a fornix-based conjunctival flap has been used.

exfoliation syndrome, iris manipulation such as stretching), hyphema, choroidal effusions, and hypotony maculopathy.

With the incision size for phacotrabeculectomy similar to that of trabeculectomy alone, the combined procedure appears to be a reasonable approach to the patient requiring cataract surgery who has concomitant glaucoma. Separating the treatment into two operations guarantees that the patient will have two operations, whereas the combined procedure offers the opportunity for the surgeon to control both problems with a single operation. In the small percentage of patients whose

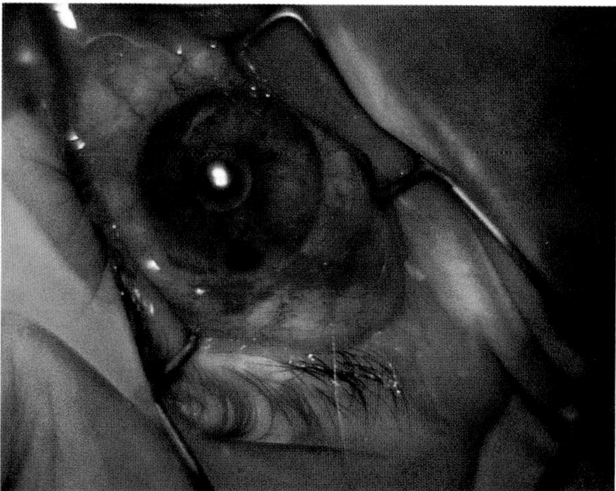

Figure 18.28 Conjunctival closure
The conjunctiva is brought forward to the limbus. Peripheral superior corneal epithelium is removed with cautery to help establish a conjunctival/corneal anterior bond.

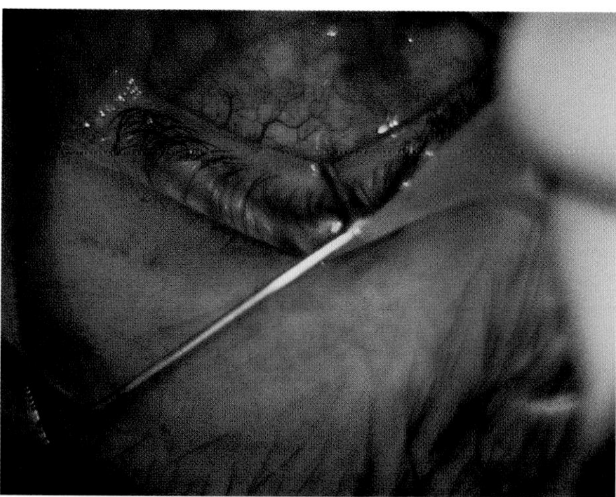

Figure 18.29 Stretching the conjunctiva across the superior peripheral cornea
Conjunctiva is stretched tightly across the superior peripheral cornea, forming a 'hood' and the conjunctiva is anchored on either side with 10–0 nylon suture bites through episclera.

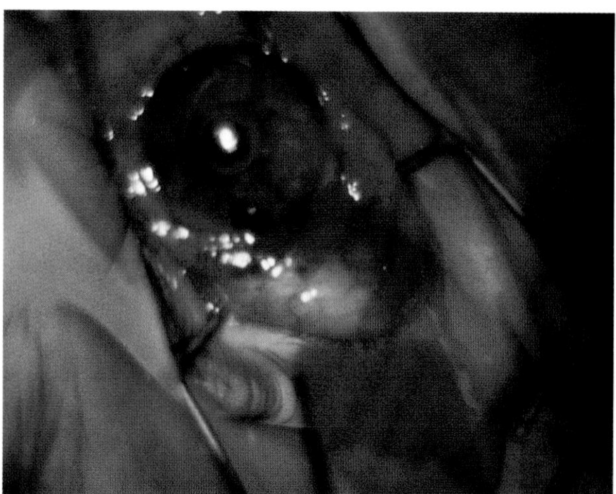

Figure 18.30 Closing the conjunctival relaxing incision
The conjunctival relaxing incision is closed with a running 8-0 polyglactin suture on a vascular needle.

glaucoma remains uncontrolled, the small incision of the phacotrabeculectomy leaves plenty of untouched conjunctiva on either side of the incision for additional glaucoma surgery, should it ever be necessary.

FURTHER READING

Allan BD, Barrett GD, Combined small incision phacoemulsification and trabeculectomy, *J Cataract Refract Surg* (1993) **19**:97–102.

Arnold PN, No-stitch phacotrabeculectomy, *J Cataract Refract Surg* (1996) **22**:253–60.

Colin J, Exfoliative syndrome and phacoemulsification, *J Fr Ophthalmol* (1994) **17**:465–9.

Costa VP, Moster MR, Wilson RP, Schmidt CM, Grandham S, Smith M, Effects of topical mitomycin-C on primary trabeculectomies and combined procedures, *Br J Ophthalmol* (1993) **77**:693–7.

Day SE, Fanous MM, Smith MF, Doyle JW, Phacotrabeculectomy: which is better? Single or separate incisions? *Invest Ophthalmol Vis Sci* (1996) **37**:252.

Gimbel HV, Meyer D, Small incision trabeculectomy combined with phacoemulsification and intraocular lens implantation, *J Cataract Refract Surg* (1993) **19**:92–6.

Hughes BA, Song MS, Shin DH, et al., Primary glaucoma triple procedure with or without adjunctive subconjunctival mitomycin and risk factors for failure, *Invest Ophthalmol Vis Sci* (1995) **36**:876.

Hurvitz LM, 5-FU-supplemented phacoemulsification, posterior chamber intraocular lens implantation, and trabeculectomy, *Ophthalmic Surg* (1993) **24**:674–80.

Kim DD, Doyle JW, Smith MF, Intraocular pressure reduction following phacoemulsification cataract extraction with posterior chamber intraocular lens implantation in glaucoma. *Invest-Ophthalmol Vis Sci* (1994) **38**:4940.

Lederer CM, Combined cataract extraction with intraocular lens implant and mitomycin-C augmented trabeculectomy, *Ophthalmology* (1996) **103**:1025–34.

Lyle WA, Jin JC, Comparison of a 3 and 6-mm incision in combined phacoemulsification and trabeculectomy, *Am J Ophthalmol* (1991) **111**:189–6.

Munden PM, Alward WL, Combined phacoemulsification, posterior chamber intraocular lens implantation, and trabeculectomy with mitomycin-C, *Am J Ophthalmol* (1995) **119**:20–9.

O'Grady JM, Juzych MS, Shin DH, Lemon LC, Swendris RP, Trabeculectomy, phacoemulsification, and posterior chamber lens implantation with and without 5-fluorouracil, *Am J Ophthalmol* (1993) **116**:594–9.

Shields MB, *Textbook of glaucoma* (Williams & Wilkins: Baltimore, Md, 1992).

Stewart WC, Crinkley CM, Carlson AN, Results of trabeculectomy combined with phacoemulsification versus trabeculectomy combined with extracapsular cataract extraction in patients with advanced glaucoma, *Ophthalmic Surg* (1994) **25**:621–7.

Stewart WC, Crinkley CM, Carlson AN, Fornix- vs limbus-based flaps in combined phacoemulsification and trabeculectomy, *Doc Ophthalmol* (1994) **88**:141–51.

Wedrich A, Menapace R, Radax U, Papapanos P, Amon M, Combined small incision cataract surgery and trabeculectomy—technique and results, *Int Ophthalmol* (1992) **16**:409–14.

Wishart PK, Austin MW, Combined cataract extraction and trabeculectomy: phacoemulsification compared with extracapsular technique, *Ophthalmic Surg* (1993) **24**:814–21.

19 Treatment of developmental glaucoma

Carlo E Traverso

Medical management before surgery

Medical treatment of developmental glaucoma is used mostly as a temporizing measure pending surgical treatment, as it has little chance to obtain and maintain the target IOP in most cases. Topical beta blockers and other aqueous suppressants, such as acetazolamide and other carbonic anhydrase inhibitors, are commonly used in preparation for surgery with the hope of improving corneal transparency, thus facilitating gonioscopy and fundoscopy. Caution must be exercised with infants and small children when using medical therapy, as the relatively small blood volume may lead to high systemic levels of many medications if used in adult dosages, leading to significant side-effects.

Surgical management

The purpose of surgery is to preserve vision. Since visual disability in developmental glaucoma seems to be related to pressure-induced optic nerve atrophy and to surgical complications, a balance must be struck between surgical risks and the maintenance of the target intraocular pressure. A team approach may be necessary in many cases to treat anisometropia, amblyopia, strabismus, corneal opacity, and cataract. Prompt lowering of the intraocular pressure can be helpful to clear cornea edema, which can rapidly cause irreversible amblyopia.

Surgical treatment can be divided into the following categories: angle surgery, filtration surgery, cyclodestructive procedures, and aqueous shunts.

Angle surgery

Since angle surgery is rarely performed on adults, most surgeons have little experience with these types of procedures. However, success rates can be very high. Poor prognostic factors include larger corneal diameters, longer intervals from diagnosis to treatment, and newborn developmental glaucoma. Various methods have been described and each surgeon develops his or her own modifications. The techniques described below are illustrative.

Goniotomy

This technique, nowadays facilitated by the availability of viscoelastics, is recommended when the cornea is sufficiently clear to allow good intraoperative visualization of the angle. In some cases the removal of edematous epithelium may be necessary.

Goniotomy technique

After positioning the operating microscope with a 40-degree tilt, the globe, is exposed with a speculum and rotated with a bridle suture. A goniolens with an irrigating handle is then positioned over the cornea. After obtaining a clear view of the angle sectors to be incised, the goniolens is removed. A small paracentesis tract is performed in the opposite quadrant (i.e. on the surgeon's side), and a viscoelastic is introduced into the anterior chamber. The tip of the goniotomy knife is then introduced and brought forward (Fig. 19.1). As soon as the knife is pushed safely across the anterior chamber beyond the pupil, the goniolens is again positioned. The tip of the knife is then pushed to incise the trabecular tissue right above the scleral spur or the apparent iris insertion, whichever is the most anterior. The knife is then swept from side to side. During the cut it is often possible to see the iris tissue fall posteri-

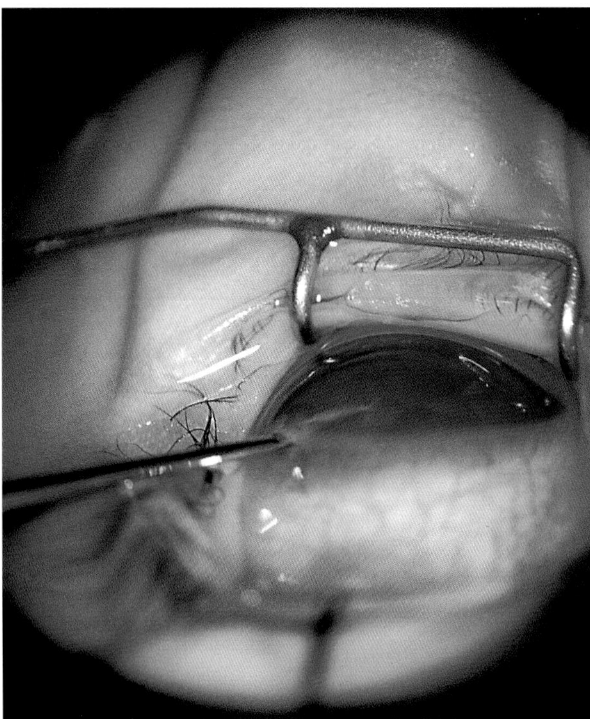

Figure 19.1 Goniotomy technique
The goniotomy knife is introduced into the anterior chamber.

orly. The site of the incision will appear strikingly white in contrast to the grayish surrounding tissue (Fig. 19.2). In order to reach around 150 degrees of the angle, some rotation of the globe and goniolens is usually necessary. The knife is then withdrawn, the anterior chamber is irrigated, and the viscoelastic aspirated. A single 10-0 nylon suture is placed at the entry site to prevent leakage and iris incarceration; the knot should be carefully buried. Blood 'ex-vacuo' and from direct damage to the angle vessels is commonly observed at the end of the procedure (Fig. 19.3).

Trabeculotomy

The principle of trabeculotomy is to open Schlemm's canal to the anterior chamber by cutting in towards the dysgenetic trabecular tissue after probing Schlemm's canal from an external approach. Since the procedure is based on the ab externo recognition of the Schlemm's canal area, it can be difficult in buphthalmic eyes with abnormal and distorted limbal anatomy. The main advantage of trabeculotomy is its applicability in cases with corneal edema that prevents a gonioscopic view of the anterior chamber, thus precluding goniotomy.

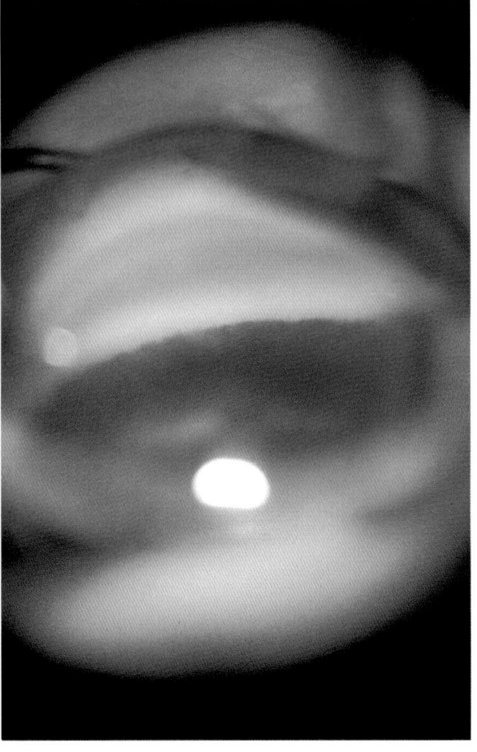

(a)

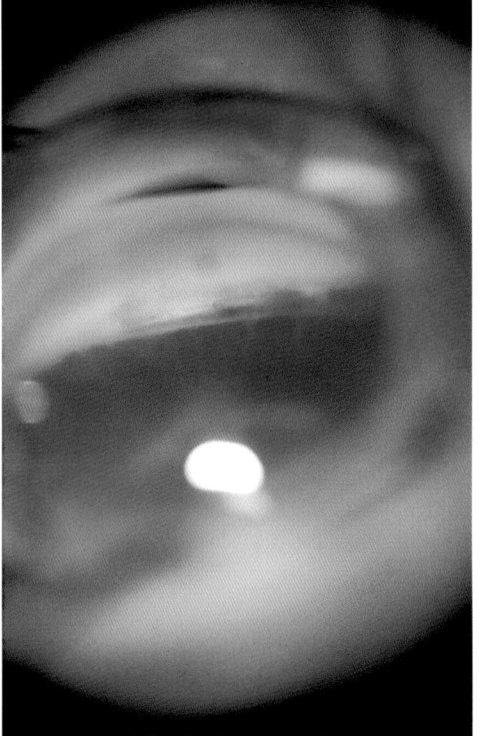

(b)

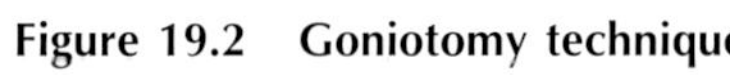

Figure 19.2 Goniotomy technique
Intraoperative gonioscopic view before (a) and immediately after (b) goniotomy. The incised site appears strikingly white in contrast to the surrounding tissue. Some blood is also seen.

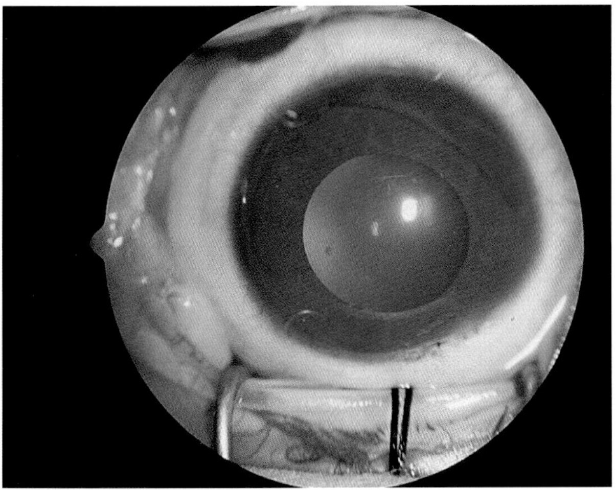

Figure 19.3 Goniotomy technique
At the conclusion of the procedure, a moderate amount of blood is frequently seen in the anterior chamber.

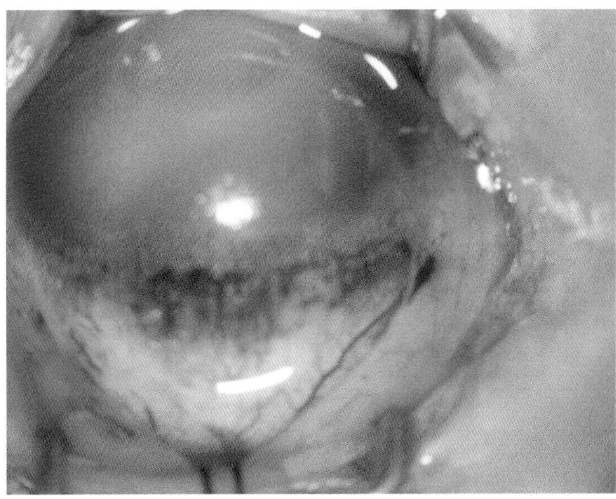

Figure 19.4 Trabeculotomy technique
A fornix-based conjunctival flap is prepared.

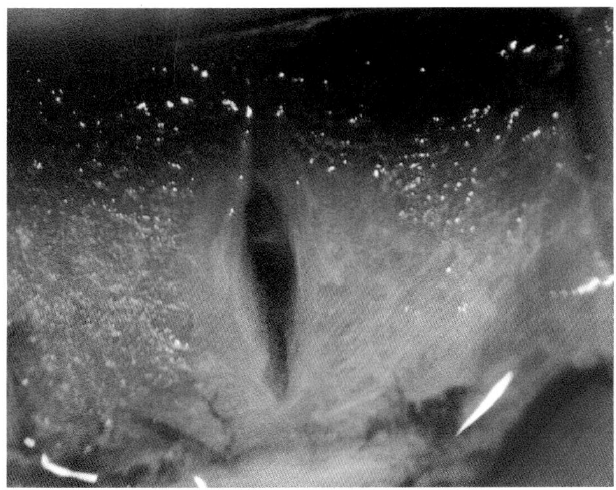

Figure 19.5 Trabeculotomy technique
Underneath a scleral flap, a radial incision is made until a change in the pattern of the connective fibers is seen, indicating the location of Schlemm's canal.

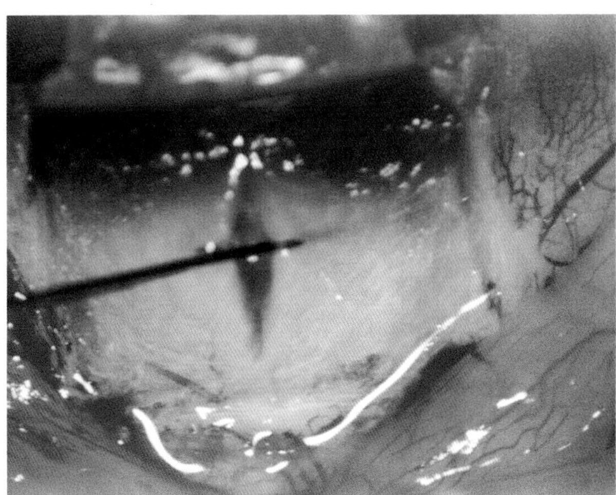

Figure 19.6 Trabeculotomy technique
Schlemm's canal is probed with a 6-0 nylon suture.

Trabeculotomy technique

After positioning the microscope with a 20-degree tilt, the eye is exposed with a speculum and a fornix-based conjunctival flap is dissected (Fig. 19.4). A bridle suture is then passed under the superior rectus muscle. The globe is rotated downwards and a limbus-based, two-thirds thickness scleral flap dissected. A small paracentesis is made 120 degrees away. At maximum microscope magnification, radial, layer-by-layer incisions are made centered on the corneoscleral transition zone at the limbus, in the bottom of the scleral bed. As the cutting proceeds very slowly, the assistant continuously dries the incision site with sponges. As soon as minimal amounts of aqueous begin to percolate from the bottom the incision is halted. With the help of sponges the exact origin of the aqueous ooze is identified. A change in the pattern of the connective fibers is typical (Fig. 19.5). A few very delicate radial cuts are then sufficient to open the outer wall of Schlemm's canal. Aqueous leakage will be evident. Care must be taken not to enter the

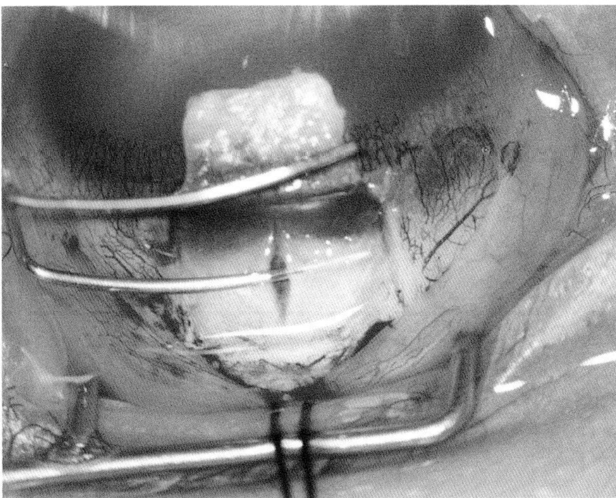

Figure 19.7 Trabeculotomy technique
The lower arm of a Harms' trabeculotome is introduced into Schlemm's canal.

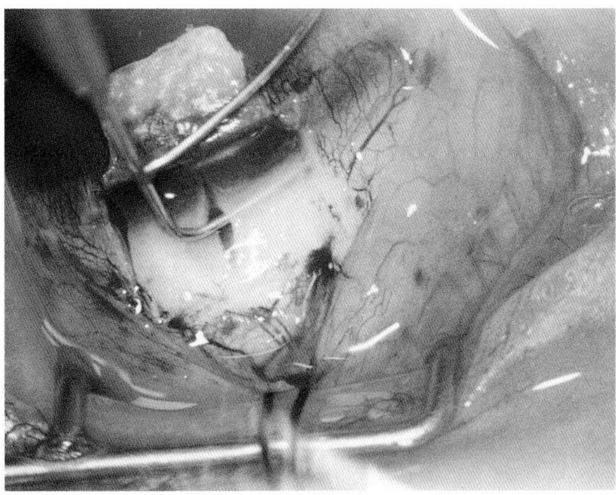

Figure 19.8 Trabeculotomy technique
The handle of the trabeculotome is rotated and the lower arm is pushed forward through the trabecular tissue into the anterior chamber.

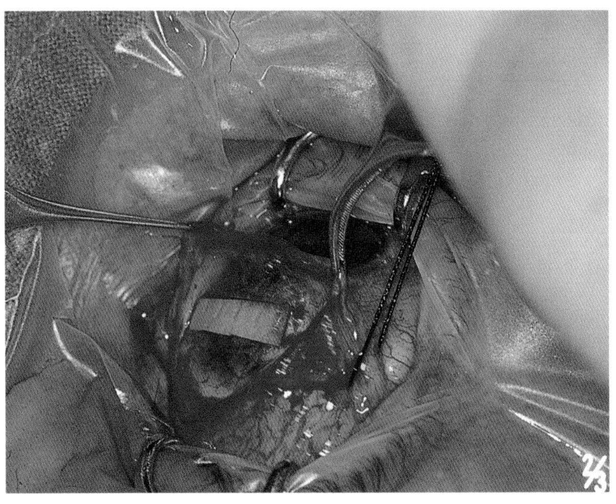

(a)

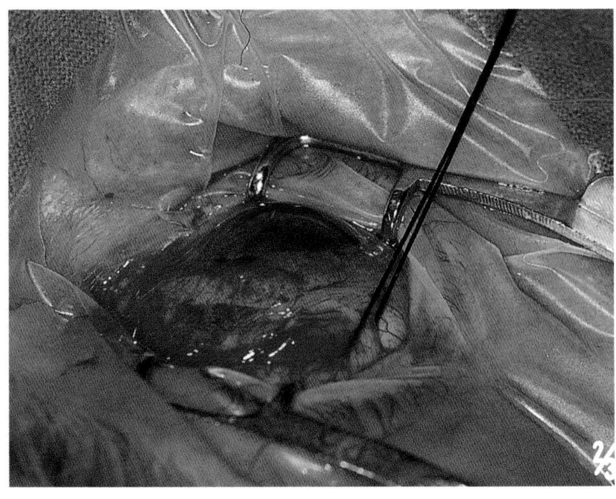

(b)

Figure 19.9 Trabeculectomy for developmental glaucoma
Mitomycin is applied with a filter paper (a). The conjunctival flap can be easily draped over the paper, keeping the incision margins away from the antimetabolite (b).

anterior chamber. Schlemm's canal is then probed with a piece of 6-0 nylon suture, the cut end of which has been blunted with mild cautery to facilitate a smooth movement, decreasing the chances of creating false routes. Using two tying forceps, the nylon probe is held parallel to the limbus and introduced into Schlemm's canal with a gentle push (Fig. 19.6). It should advance for at least one centimeter on each side, meeting some resistance. If the tip appears in the anterior chamber, a conversion to trabeculectomy should be considered. The introduction of the probe can be facilitated by snipping the walls of the radial incision with a 15-degree blade, right over the Schlemm's canal area. A double-armed Harms' trabeculotome is then introduced on one side (Fig. 19.7). Its lower arm is pushed forward, parallel to the limbus, keeping a mild constant outward pressure to maintain it against the sclera; if the anterior chamber is inadvertently entered, conversion to trabeculectomy

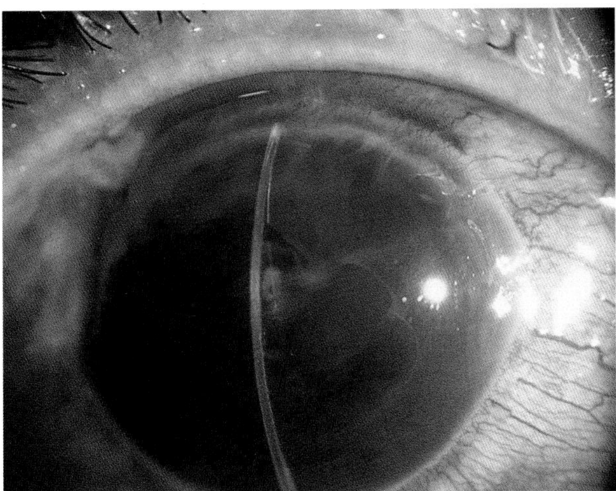

Figure 19.10 Trabeculectomy for developmental glaucoma
Massive postoperative suprachoroidal hemorrhage. This hemorrhage occurred two days after uneventful trabeculectomy. The eye had undergone multiple previous procedures, was buphthalmic, and aphakic. Blood and retinal membranes can be seen in the anterior chamber.

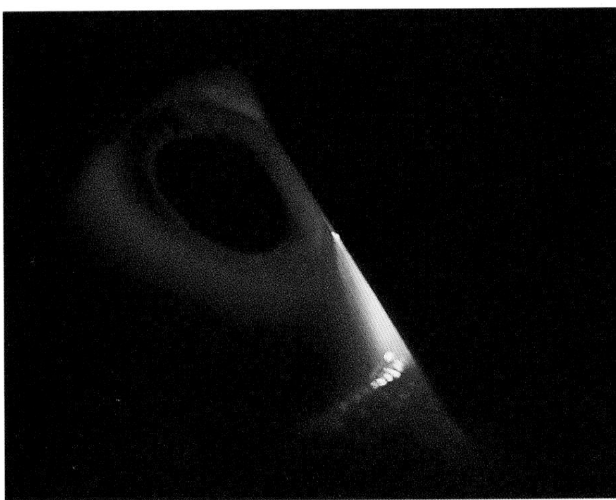

Figure 19.11 Ciliodestructive procedures
Application of a cryoprobe for cyclocryotherapy. Exposure time should be reduced from standard adult settings (e,g, one minute freeze at –60°C) in cases with thin sclera.

should be considered. When the arm is introduced fully, the handle is very gently rotated in both directions for 10 degrees; slight alternate bulging and depression of the sclera over the tip of the trabeculotome should be observed, confirming its correct positioning. If during the maneuver the anterior chamber is entered without resistance, once again conversion to trabeculectomy should be considered. Trabeculotomy is performed by rotating the handle of the instrument so as to move the distal part of its arm towards the pupil (Fig. 19.8); the sweep should be aimed between the iris plane and the corneal endothelium, to avoid damage to the lens (Fig. 19.9). The trabeculotome is then quickly withdrawn and the procedure repeated on the other side. If the anterior chamber is shallow or flat after the first sweep, it must be deepened with viscoelastic injected through the paracentesis. The second sweep is not to be attempted with a shallow anterior chamber. The scleral flap and conjunctiva are then closed. Although trabeculotomy can be performed without first preparing a scleral flap, there are advantages in using one. From a deeper scleral bed the radial, layer-by-layer incisions are less difficult to make and the approach for the nylon probe is less angled. In addition, a scleral flap allows a prompt conversion to trabeculectomy should it be necessary. As an alternative technique, Schlemm's canal can be probed for 360 degrees with a polypropylene suture which is then pulled to rip open the trabecular tissue.

Filtration surgery

Trabeculectomy is the filtration procedure of choice, and is detailed in Chapter 16. Variable success rates have been reported in developmental glaucomas, and many factors must be considered when evaluating these patients. Since these eyes are at high risk for failure due to episcleral fibrosis, antimetabolites are often necessary. Considering the difficulty of administering 5-fluorouracil injections in this age group without general anesthesia, intraoperative mitomycin is the most practical choice in the pediatric age. A combination of trabeculotomy and trabeculotomy has also been used.

For the application of mitomycin it is convenient to use filter paper rather than sponges. Filter paper is easily cut to a shape fitting the contour of the limbus; it does not swell after being soaked with the solution, and the solution is not easily squeezed out of the paper. The conjunctiva can be easily draped over a thin piece of filter paper, keeping the edges of the incision away from the antimetabolite (Fig. 19.9). Consideration of the long-term risk/benefit ratio of the use of antimetabolites in the pediatric age group must realistically weigh the chances of infection and bleb rupture in such patients. All complications described for filtration surgery in Chapter 16 can occur in developmental glaucoma, including delayed massive suprachoroidal hemorrhage (Fig. 19.10).

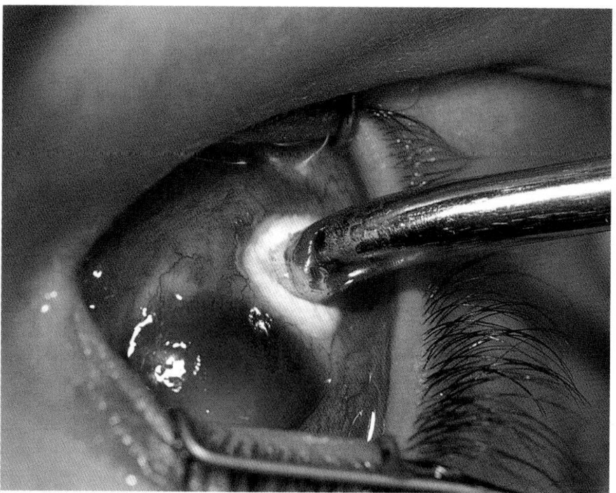

Figure 19.12 Cyclodestructive procedures
Transpupillary retroillumination to localize the ciliary body.

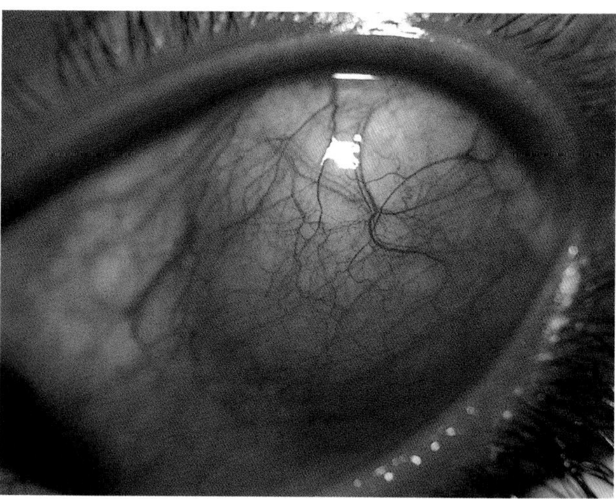

Figure 19.13 Drainage devices
A large posterior bleb may interfere with extraocular muscle contraction, leading to strabismus. Amblyopia is of concern in this age group.

Cyclodestruction

In developmental glaucomas, cyclodestructive procedures such as cyclocryotherapy and transscleral laser cyclophotocoagulation can be performed with the same modalities used for adults (Fig. 19.11) (see Chapter 15). Special attention should be paid to the localization of the ciliary body, since the anterior segment anatomy can be distorted. In most cases, transpupillary retroillumination with a penlight will be sufficient (Fig. 19.12). Postoperative pain following cyclocryotherapy can be excruciating; therefore when the procedure is performed under general anesthesia a retrobulbar block with a long-acting anesthetic such as bupivacaine is advisable to blunt the pain when the patient awakens. Postoperative chemosis can be severe in children; a peritomy can avoid the freezing of conjunctiva, and aspirin pretreatment can decrease the swelling.

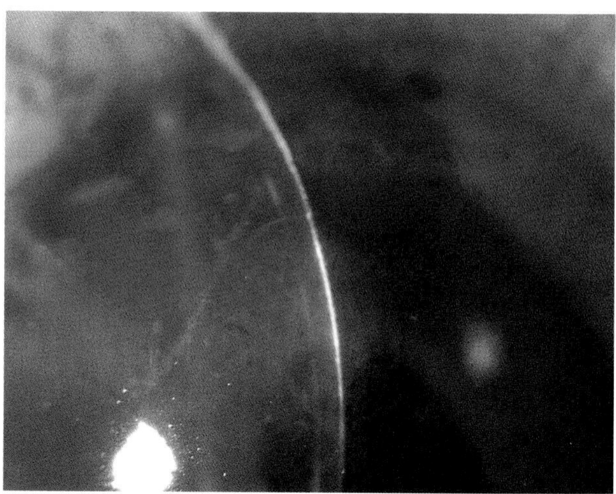

Figure 19.14 Drainage devices
Localized corneal decompensation over an anterior chamber tube. The tube is positioned too anteriorly and is touching the cornea.

Drainage devices (aqueous shunts)

Drainage implants are detailed in Chapter 17. All types of implants have been tried in children with varying degrees of success and some frustration. In the long term, failures due to occlusion, fibrosis, and dislocation of the tube and/or plate are of concern. Oversized blebs can cause muscle imbalance (Fig. 19.13). Even minor additional procedures, in this age group, like the removal of releasable sutures, might need general anesthesia. In order to prevent corneal decompensation, iris atrophy, and cataract formation, the tube should be appropriately positioned in the anterior chamber (Fig. 19.14).

FURTHER READING

Akimoto M, Tanihara H, Negi A, Nagata M, Surgical results of trabeculotomy ab externo for developmental glaucoma, *Arch Ophthalmol* (1994) **112**:1540–4.

Beck AD, Lynch MG, 360° trabeculotomy for primary congenital glaucoma, *Arch Ophthalmol* (1995) **113**:1200–2.

Costa VP, Katz LJ, Spaeth GL, Primary trabeculectomy in young adults, *Ophthalmology* (1993) **100**:1071–6.

Elder MJ, Combined trabeculotomy–trabeculectomy compared with primary trabeculotomy for congenital glaucoma, *Br J Ophthalmol* (1994) **78**:745–8.

Munoz M, Tomey KF, Traverso CE, Day SH, Senft SH, Clinical experience with the Molteno implant in advanced infantile glaucoma, *J Pediatric Ophthalmol Strabismus* (1991) **28**:68–72.

Quigley H, Childhood glaucoma: results with trabeculotomy and study of reversible cupping, *Ophthalmology* (1982) **89**:219–23.

Susanna R Jr, Oltregge EW, Carani JCE, Mitomycin as an adjunct chemotherapy with trabeculectomy in congenital and developmental glaucomas, *J Glaucoma* (1995) **4**:151–7.

Traverso CE, Tomey KF, Al-Kaff A, The long-tube single plate Molteno implant for the treatment of recalcitrant glaucoma, *Int Ophthalmol* (1989) **13**:159–62.

Traverso CE, Tomey KF, Day SF, Senft SH, Jaafar M, Surgical treatment of primary congenital glaucoma. Analysis of prognostic factors on 519 cases, *Boll Oculist* (1990) **69 (suppl 2)**:255–62.

Index

Page numbers in *italics* refer to figures, where they occur on pages without accompanying text. The alphabetical order of the index is letter-by-letter.